CW00631909

Paul J

Monoclonal antibodies have an important and wide-ranging role in many areas of biomedical research and this volume is among the first to combine technical and clinical aspects of the subject. Monoclonal antibodies provide highly specific reagents with which to identify, analyse, quantitate and manipulate molecules, both in solution and in solid phase, such as at a cell surface. The aim of this book is to provide a unique combination of information concerning the production (by both cellular and molecular biology techniques), and structural and functional characteristics of monoclonal antibodies, together with detailed discussions of the various analytic, diagnostic and therapeutic applications of these antibodies in many areas of clinical medicine, including histopathology, oncology, transplantation, infectious diseases, rheumatology, haematology and dermatology.

Monoclonal antibodies

POSTGRADUATE MEDICAL SCIENCE

This important new series is based on the successful and internationally well-regarded specialist training programme at the Royal Postgraduate Medical School in London. Each volume provides an integrated and self-contained account of a key area of medical science, developed in conjunction with the course organisers and including contributions from specially invited authorities.

The aim of the series is to provide biomedical and clinical scientists with a reliable introduction to the theory and to the technical and clinical applications of each topic.

The volumes will be a valuable resource and guide for trainees in the medical and biomedical sciences and for laboratory-based scientists.

In the series:

Radiation protection of patients by R. Wootton

Image analysis in histology: conventional and confocal microscopy by D. Springall, R. Wootton and J. Polak

POSTGRADUATE MEDICAL SCIENCE

Monoclonal antibodies

Production, engineering and clinical application

EDITED BY

MARY A. RITTER and
HEATHER M. LADYMAN

Department of Immunology
Royal Postgraduate Medical School

Published in association with the Royal Postgraduate Medical School
University of London by

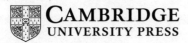 CAMBRIDGE
UNIVERSITY PRESS

Published by the Press Syndicate of the University of Cambridge
The Pitt Building, Trumpington Street, Cambridge CB2 1RP
40 West 20th Street, New York, NY 10011-4211, USA
10 Stamford Road, Oakleigh, Melbourne 3166, Australia

© Cambridge University Press 1995

First published 1995

Printed in Great Britain at the University Press, Cambridge

A catalogue record for this book is available from the British Library

Library of Congress cataloguing in publication data available

ISBN 0 521 47354 3 hardback
ISBN 0 521 42503 4 paperback

KT

Contents

11A.10   References   255

11B   Monoclonal antibodies in infectious disease: prophylaxis and therapy   260
           J. Cohen

           11B.1   Introduction   260
           11B.2   Bacterial infections   261
           11B.3   Viral and chlamydial infections   266
           11B.4   Additional applications of monoclonal antibodies 268
           11B.5   Conclusions   268
           11B.6   References   269

12A   Monoclonal antibodies in transplantation: immunohistology   274
           M. L. Rose

           12A.1   Introduction   274
           12A.2   Nature of the infiltrate   274
           12A.3   Major histocompatibility complex antigens   276
           12A.4   Adhesion molecules   285
           12A.5   Cytokines   287
           12A.6   References   288

12B   Experimental studies on *in-vivo* immunosuppression   292
           N. M. Parish and A. Cooke

           12B.1   Introduction   292
           12B.2   Monoclonal antibody treatments directed towards T cell   294
                    surface markers
           12B.3   Monoclonal antibody therapies targeted at   304
                    antigen-presenting cells
           12B.4   Monoclonal antibody therapies targeting cytokines 305
           12B.5   Monoclonal antibody therapies targeting adhesion molecules   308
           12B.6   Monoclonal antibodies directed towards miscellaneous cell   309
                    markers
           12B.7   References   310

12C   Monoclonal antibodies in transplantation: prophylaxis and treatment of
           graft-versus-host disease after bone marrow transplantation   317
           L. Boström and O. Ringden

           12C.1   Introduction   317
           12C.2   Prevention of GVHD with *in-vitro* use of monoclonal   319
                    antibodies
           12C.3   Randomized clinical studies comparing pharmacological   324
                    GVHD prophylaxis with T cell depletion
           12C.4   Monoclonal antibodies *in vivo* for prevention of GVHD   325
           12C.5   Treatment of GVHD with monoclonal antibodies   326
           12C.6   Monoclonal antibodies in the diagnosis of GVHD   328
           12C.7   Outlook   329
           12C.8   References   329

Contributors

Dr R. Baatard
Service de Néphrologie, Immunologie Clinique et Unité de Recherche,
INSERM U. 211, CHU Nantes, France

Dr A. Bamias
Imperial Cancer Research Fund Laboratories, Hammersmith Hospital, Du
Cane Road, London W12 0NN, UK

Dr L. Boström
Department of Clinical Immunology, The Karolinska Institute, Huddinge
Hospital, Stockholm, Sweden

Dr D. Cantarovich
Service de Néphrologie, Immunologie Clinique et Unité de Recherche,
INSERM U. 211, CHU Nantes, France

Dr A. C. Chu
Unit of Dermatology, Hammersmith Hospital, Du Cane Road, London W12
0NN, UK

Dr J. Cohen
Department of Bacteriology, Royal Postgraduate Medical School, Du Cane
Road, London W12 0NN, UK

Dr A. Colfor
Department of Histopathology, Royal Marsden Hospital, Fulham Road,
London SW3 6JJ, UK

Dr D. B. Cook
Department of Clinical Biochemistry, The Medical School, Framlingham
Place, Newcastle-upon-Tyne, NE2 4HH, UK

Dr A. Cooke
Immunology Division, Department of Pathology, Cambridge University,
Tennis Court Road, Cambridge CB2 1QP, UK

Dr N. S. Courtenay-Luck
Antisoma plc, Samaritan Hospital for Women, 153–173 Marylebone Road,
London NW1 5QH, UK

Dr J. Dantal
Service de Néphrologie, Immunologie Clinique et Unité de Recherche,
INSERM U. 211, CHU Nantes, France

Dr A. A. Epenetos
Imperial Cancer Research Fund Laboratories, MRC Building, Hammersmith
Hospital, Du Cane Road, London W12 0HS, UK

Dr A. J. T. George
Department of Immunology, Royal Postgraduate Medical School, Du Cane
Road, London W12 0NN, UK

Dr M. Giral
Service de Néphrologie, Immunologie Clinique et Unité de Recherche,
INSERM U. 211, CHU Nantes, France

Dr J. J. Gray
Clinical Microbiology and Public Health Laboratory, Level 6, Addenbrookes
Hospital, Hills Road, Cambridge CB2 2QW, UK

Prof. P. A. Hall
Pathology Department, Ninewells Hospital and Medical School, University of
Dundee, Dundee DD1 9SY, UK

Dr E. Hillhouse
Department of Clinical Biochemistry and Metabolic Medicine, The Medical
School, Framlingham Place, Newcastle-upon-Tyne NE2 4HH, UK

Dr M. Hourmant
Service de Néphrologie, Immunologie Clinique et Unité de Recherche,
INSERM U. 211, CHU Nantes, France

Dr J. D. Isaacs
Division of Immunology, Department of Pathology, Cambridge University,
Tennis Court Road, Cambridge CB2 1QP, UK

Dr Y. Jacques
Service de Néphrologie, Immunologie Clinique et Unité de Recherche,
INSERM U. 211, CHU Nantes, France

Prof. P. J. Lachmann
Molecular Immunopathology Unit, Medical Research Council Centre and
University of Cambridge Clinical School, Cambridge CB2 2QH, UK

Ms H. M. Ladyman
Department of Immunology, Royal Postgraduate Medical School, Du Cane
Road, London W12 0NN, UK

Dr B. Le Mauff
Service de Néphrologie, Immunologie Clinique et Unité de Recherche,
INSERM U. 211, CHU Nantes, France

Dr R. J. Morris
Laboratory of Neurobiology, National Institute for Medical Research, The
Ridgeway, Mill Hill, London NW7 1AA, UK

Dr N. M. Parish
Division of Immunology, Department of Pathology, University of Cambridge,
Tennis Court Road, Cambridge CB2 1QP, UK

Mr K. M. Price
Zeneca, Cambridge Research Biochemicals Ltd, Gadbrook Park, Northwich,
Cheshire CW9 7RA, UK

Prof. O. Ringden
Department of Clinical Immunology, The Karolinska Institute, Huddinge
Hospital, Stockholm, Sweden

Prof. M. A. Ritter
Department of Immunology, Royal Postgraduate Medical School, Du Cane
Road, London W12 0NN, UK

Dr M. L. Rose
Immunology Department, Harefield Hospital, Harefield, Uxbridge UB9 6JH,
UK

Dr A. Sa'adu
Division of Immunological Medicine, Clinical Research Centre, Northwick
Park Hospital, Watford Road, Harrow HA1 3UJ, UK

Prof. C. H. Self
Department of Clinical Biochemistry and Metabolic Medicine, The Medical
School, Framlingham Place, Newcastle-upon-Tyne, NE2 4HH, UK

Dr S. Songsivilai
Department of Immunology, Faculty of Medicine, Siriraj Hospital, Mahidol
University, Bangkok 10700, Thailand

Dr J. P. Soulillou
Service de Néphrologie, Immunologie Clinique et Unité de Recherche,
INSERM U. 211, CHU Nantes, France

Dr E. Tsele
Department of Dermatology, Royal Postgraduate Medical School, Du Cane
Road, London W12 0NN, UK

Dr T. G. Wreghitt
Clinical Microbiology and Public Health Laboratory, Level 6,
Addenbrookes Hospital, Hills Road, Cambridge CB2 2QW, UK

Dr A. Zumla
School of Medicine, University Teaching Hospital, PO Box 50110, Lusaka,
Zambia

1

Introduction

M. A. RITTER

1.1 Introduction

The production of antibodies (also referred to as immunoglobulins, Ig) forms
an integral part of an individual's immune response to an invading pathogen.
The structure of these molecules is designed such that they are bifunctional:
they carry specificity for their antigen and they activate a variety of effector
functions that lead ultimately to the destruction of the specific target pathogen.
These two properties mean that antibodies are critical to the successful defence
of the host; they have also led to the use of antibodies as indispensible tools in
experimental research, clinical investigation and diagnosis and, more recently,
clinical therapy. However, there is a major difference between the role of
antibodies in host defence and in the laboratory or clinic. Invading pathogens
are complex organisms, carrying on their surface a multitude of different
antigenic determinants (epitopes). It is therefore advantageous for the host to
produce as wide a range as possible of antibody molecules to ensure that the
pathogen is effectively targeted and destroyed. In contrast, laboratory and
clinical reagents are usually required to recognize a single molecule and
frequently a single epitope on that single molecule. It is with the production
and use of such reagents that this book is concerned.

1.2 Generation of an immune response

Immune responses are generated as a consequence of the recognition of foreign
material by antigen-specific lymphocytes. Activation of B lymphocytes leads to
the production of antibody whereas activation of T lymphocytes leads to
destruction of infected host cells by different mechanisms. A brief account of B
cell activation will be given here as a knowledge of this will provide the
framework within which the techniques of monoclonal antibody production can
be placed.

Lymphocytes recognize antigen by means of specific cell surface receptors;
for B cells these receptors consist of membrane-bound antibody molecules.
Each cell carries approximately 50 000 receptor molecules on its surface, each

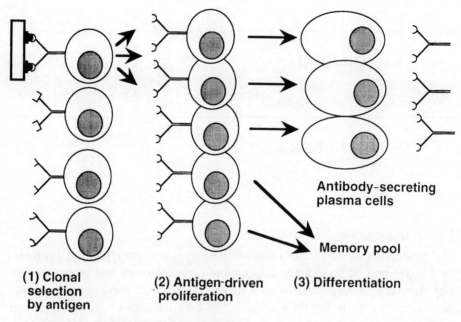

Figure 1.1. Clonal selection of B cells.

with an identical specificity. Hence, each B cell has a single specificity although at any one time an individual will possess many millions of different B cells as part of their immune repertoire. When an antigen enters the body it will bind to and activate any B cell whose receptor can recognize an epitope on that antigen. Activation leads to two main events (Figure 1.1). First, the B cell undergoes several mitotic divisions, thus giving rise to a 'clone' of identical cells. Second, these daughter cells differentiate to form either plasma cells or 'memory' B cells. The function of plasma cells is to secrete large amounts of soluble antibody of the same specificity as that which formed the cell surface receptor on the original, activated B cell. The function of memory cells is to mount an enhanced immune response on subsequent re-exposure to the same antigen. Moreover, the antibodies produced during this 'secondary' immune response are of higher affinity as development of memory B cells involves a process of hypermutation in the receptor gene loci followed by stringent antigen selection ('affinity maturation'). An individual, therefore, contains a repertoire of potential immune responses but it is the invading pathogen that directs and enhances the actual response against itself.

1.3   Antibody structure

Antibody molecules are glycoproteins whose basic unit comprises two identical 'heavy' and two identical 'light' polypeptide chains (Figure 1.2). Each chain is composed of domains: heavy chains contain four or five, according to their

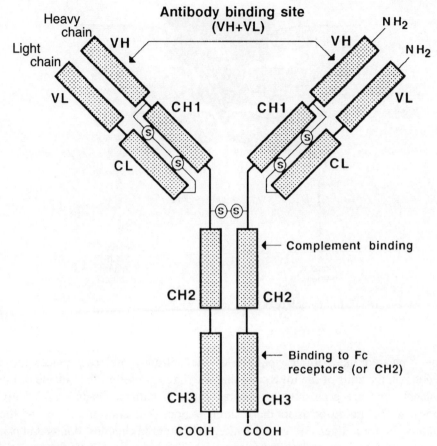

Figure 1.2. Basic structure of an antibody molecule.

class (4, IgG, IgA, IgD; 5, IgM, IgE) and light chains contain two. The ability to bind to antigen is controlled by the N-terminal domains, one binding site for antigen being created by the combination of one domain from the heavy and one from the light chain. The remaining domains control the effector functions of the antibody molecule (for example by activating the complement cascade or by activating phagocytosis via binding to Fc receptors on the surface of macrophages). This bifunctionality is controlled by differences in the primary structure of the various domains. Those at the N-terminus vary considerably between antibodies of differing specificities (and are therefore termed 'variable' or 'V' domains) whereas all other domains are relatively 'constant' ('C' domains). In a single antibody molecule, the two heavy chains are identical to each other as also are the two light chains, thus the antibody contains two identical binding sites for antigen.

How is the specificity of antibody determined? Variability in the V domains is not spread throughout the domain but is focused in three main areas that are termed the 'hypervariable' (or complementarity determining, CDR) regions.

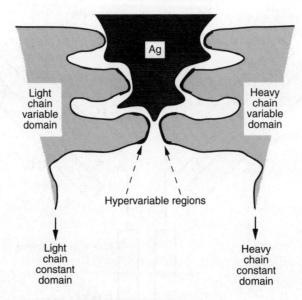

Figure 1.3. Interaction between antibody and antigen.

The β-pleated sheet folding pattern of the antibody molecule places these regions on the ends of the folds such that they are exposed to the outside of the molecule and are accessible for interaction with antigen (Figure 1.3). Variations in the amino acids in these three regions will alter the shape of the binding site for antigen and will also alter the potential chemical bonds that can form to hold antigen and antibody together. The alteration of the amino acid sequence in the hypervariable regions will control both antibody specificity and affinity (point mutations that occur in the genes encoding the V domains during B memory development can generate antibodies of enhanced affinity).

1.4   Generation of the B cell repertoire

How is the bifunctional antibody protein encoded in the genome? In the past, theories have ranged from the proposal that there is a single gene which encodes a single protein whose specificity is instructed by the antigen around which it moulds itself, to the idea that there is a separate gene for each antibody specificity. The first theory was discounted once the relationship between primary and secondary structure of proteins was understood; the impossibility of the second theory was appreciated once it had been calculated that, if true, antibody-encoding genes would occupy almost the entire mammalian genome. The truth, as often is the case, lies somewhere between these two extremes.

Each antibody polypeptide chain is encoded within a separate genetic locus (heavy chain locus, IgH; kappa light chain locus, κ; lambda light chain locus, λ). Within each locus there are exons that encode the constant domains of the appropriate chain (these determine the isotype, i.e. κ and λ for the light chains, α, δ, ε, γ and μ for the heavy chains). In addition, each locus has clusters (families) of exons that the B cell uses to create its own unique V region encoding gene. Three rearranging gene families are present in the IgH locus (variable, V; diversity, D; joining, J), while the κ and λ have only two (variable, V; joining, J). During B cell development each B cell randomly 'selects' one V and one J exon within a light chain locus (from a choice of approximately 200 V and 4 J) and one V, one D and one J within the IgH locus (from a choice of approximately 100 V, 50 D and 4 J) to create its own unique variable region genes for its light and heavy chains (Figures 1.4 and 1.5). In this way each B cell creates its own unique specificity from a potential repertoire (total rearrangements and recombinations possible) of approximately 10^{10}. It is likely that around 10^{8} specificities are present in an individual at any given time. The B cell receptor repertoire is created randomly; it is for antigen to select out those B cells of the appropriate specificity.

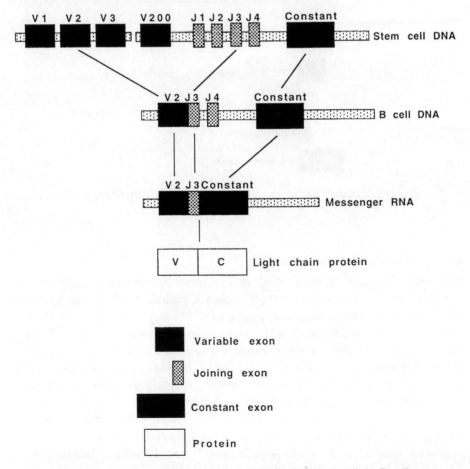

Figure 1.4. Gene rearrangements in the light chain locus of the B cell receptor.

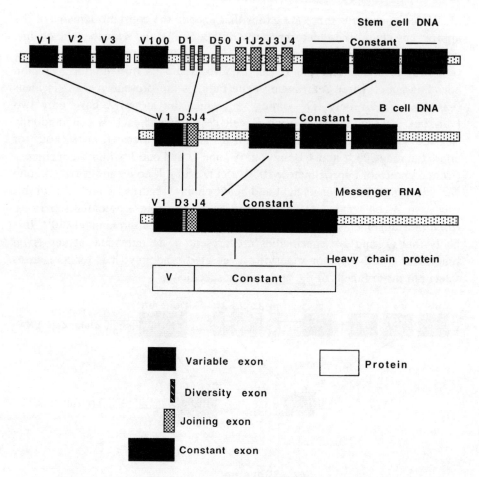

Figure 1.5. Gene rearrangements in the heavy chain locus of the B cell receptor.

1.5   What is a monoclonal antibody?

When antigen enters the body, there may be many B cells whose receptors can recognize some aspect of the foreign molecule/pathogen. These are likely to differ from each other both in the epitope to which they bind and in the affinity of their binding. This diversity will then be reflected in the secreted antibodies that are produced after clonal expansion and differentiation of the antigen-activated B cells. Many B cells will have undergone clonal expansion and so the antibodies will be the product of many clones: they are therefore 'polyclonal'. A polyclonal response, as discussed above, is highly advantageous in combating an invading pathogen, both in terms of the quantity of antigen–antibody binding and in the range of effector functions that can be activated. However, polyclonal antibodies do not in general provide clearly defined and reproducible reagents for use in the laboratory. (Although in fairness it should be pointed out that polyclonality can be an advantage in certain experimental situations, such as anti-Ig antibodies for use as secondary reagents in immuno-staining, where binding of several anti-Ig molecules to the first layer reagent will provide useful amplification of the signal.)

In the majority of situations, however, it is highly beneficial to have an homogeneous reagent that is of a single specificity and affinity and which is, therefore, predictable: the product of a single B cell clone, i.e. monoclonal antibody (mab). To obtain such an antibody it is necessary to isolate and propagate single antibody-secreting B cell clones, something that is not directly possible but which is made possible by the combination of methods of *in vitro* cell fusion, selection and cloning. This technique of monoclonal antibody production was developed by Georges Köhler and Cesar Milstein as part of their research into mechanisms underlying the diversity of antibodies (Köhler & Milstein, 1975). It is an excellent example of how basic academic research can lead to the more applied aspects of science, industry and clinical medicine. In recognition of the significance of their findings, Köhler and Milstein were awarded the Nobel prize for medicine in 1984 (Milstein, 1985).

In essence the technique involves the fusion of a B lymphocyte that has the property of specific antibody production, but which cannot live for more than a few days in culture, with a myeloma cell that has lost the ability to produce antibody but which has the property of immortality. The product of this union is a 'hybridoma' cell which can live forever (via mitotic cell division to give an ever expanding clone of identical cells) and which can secrete antibody of the desired specificity. The actual technique is obviously more complex than this as in reality the source of immune B cells (usually rodent spleen or lymph node) is a mixture of many different cell lineages. It is therefore necessary to put the hybridoma cells through a series of stringent selection procedures to eliminate hybrids that are either producing no antibody or, importantly, antibody that is of either the wrong specificity or of too low an affinity to be useful. The separation of individual clones to ensure monoclonality of the hybridoma cells and of the antibody that they secrete is also of crucial importance (Chapter 2).

More recently, molecular strategies have been devised so that, by manipulating the genes that encode the heavy and light chains, 'designer' mab can be produced with properties suited to their final use (Chapters 7 and 8). For example, antibodies can be 'humanized' by genetically grafting their hyper-variable regions (CDRs) into a human antibody; these reagents can be then used *in vivo* without inducing an anti-mouse Ig response in the patient. 'Phage techniques can be used to create very small monovalent antibodies (single chain antibodies) with the property of excellent tissue penetration, while 'phage display libraries may make it possible to generate a vast array of unique antibody specificities without the need for active immunization. This is of considerable importance for the generation of novel reagents particularly in the human system where it has been difficult to apply conventional monoclonal techniques (Chapter 5).

1.6   The aim of this book

We have designed this book to provide our readers with a full perspective of
mab in both the laboratory and clinical setting because there is an important
interplay between the experimental development of new reagents and their
subsequent application. The initial chapters deal with the use of cellular and
molecular techniques for the production (Chapters 2, 5 and 7) and modification
(Chapters 6 and 9) of monoclonal reagents, the mapping of the epitopes
recognized by antibodies (Chapter 4) and the use of these reagents in novel and
enhanced assay systems (Chapter 9). To complete this aspect of the book,
Chapter 3 provides an important and 'user-friendly' consideration of the nature
of antibody affinity and its practical implications for those who wish to use
monoclonal antibodies in the laboratory and clinical setting. The second part of
this book contains a series of chapters covering the many clinical areas in which
mab are currently used, both in routine application as well as in experimental
investigations.

We hope that after reading these chapters you will not only successfully raise
your own monoclonal reagents but that you will have a good appreciation of
the many and varied applications of these reagents to clinical medicine. Even if
you do not go on to produce your own antibodies, we hope that a knowledge of
how they are made will enhance your appreciation of these unique reagents.

1.7   References

Köhler, G. & Milstein, C. (1975). Continuous cultures of cells secreting antibody of
    defined specificity. *Nature*, **256**, 495–497.
Milstein, C. (1985). From the structure of antibodies to the diversification of the
    immune response. *EMBO Journal*, **4**, 1083–1092.

2

Production of monoclonal antibodies

H. M. LADYMAN and M. A. RITTER

2.1 Introduction

In this chapter we discuss the various techniques currently used during the production of monoclonal antibodies (mab), their application and their relative merits. The actual protocols are detailed in Chapter 16 (Technical appendix). As you will discover, although all are based on the original method of Kohler and Milstein (Kohler & Milstein, 1975; Galfre & Milstein, 1981) there are many variations in the methods used by different laboratories. The final design of such techniques is determined in part by logical consideration and in part by empiricism. When establishing the monoclonal system in your own laboratory it is important to try to dissociate these two aspects, so that you can 'filter' the often conflicting advice of others in the field (we all have our idiosyncracies). We hope that this chapter will help you to do this.

2.2 Antigens and immunization

2.2.1 Antigen

When planning the production of a mab you must first consider the antigen that you wish it to recognize. The method of antigen preparation, the immunization procedure and the choice of animal to immunize will differ according to the species of origin, chemical structure, size and source (e.g. whole cells, crude tissue extract, purified protein or peptide). You may wish to use mab techniques to discover novel molecules or you may be interested in producing reagents to a known molecule whose structure and function you wish to investigate further. Obviously the choice of antigen is a personal one, determined by your own particular interests, but certain general points are worth considering.

An antigen is a molecule that can be recognized by an antibody (or T cell receptor). The immunogenicity of a molecule is determined by its ability to activate the immune system. Not all antigens are immunogenic, although by definition they can be recognized by an antibody, because they may be too small on their own to generate an immune response *de novo*. To initiate an immune response the molecule must obviously bind to and activate specific B lymphocytes such that clones of specific antibody-producing cells and memory B cells can be generated. On their own, B lymphocytes will only generate a primary immune response that is characterized by relatively limited clonal expansion, IgM antibody and no memory. To induce B cell memory and the consequent Ig class switching (switch from IgM to IgG, A or E), enhanced affinity and increased level of antibody production that characterize the secondary immune response to re-exposure to the same antigen, it is necessary to also activate T lymphocytes. This dependence on T cells is because they provide growth and maturation signals via cell–cell contact and secreted soluble molecules (cytokines). In contrast to B lymphocytes which can recognize whole macromolecules in their native configuration, T lymphocytes can only respond to enzymatically processed protein antigen that is presented to them on the surface of an 'antigen presenting cell' (the processing cell, e.g. dendritic cell, macrophage, B lymphocyte). This processed antigen is in the form of a small peptide (approximately 15 amino acids, for the T cells that help B cells) sitting in a specialized groove in class II major histocompatibility complex (MHC) molecules on the surface of the antigen-presenting cell. The two populations of lymphocytes, B and T, therefore have very different ways of looking at antigen and these will influence the outcome of immunization.

The major parameters that you should consider when selecting your immunogen are size, heterogeneity, chemical nature, quantity and conformation.

2.2.1.1 Size and quantity

Molecules whose molecular weight is less than 1000 are unlikely to be large enough to be able to stimulate both T and B cells and are therefore likely to generate only an IgM 'primary' type immune response. This is important to remember when trying to raise antibodies to peptide antigens (Chapter 4). The problem can be circumvented by coupling the peptide to a larger 'carrier' macromolecule such as bovine serum albumin (BSA) or keyhole limpet haemocyanin (KLH), both old favourites of immunologists owing to their very effective immunogenicity (Dadi *et al.*, 1984). Conjugation to a carrier can also be useful for larger molecules which, although structurally immunogenic, may be available in only very small quantities.

2.2.1.2 Heterogeneity

Experiments with synthetic polymers have shown that molecular heterogeneity is an important component of immunogenicity. Homopolymers were shown to be non-immunogenic, copolymers were sometimes immunogenic while heteropolymers were regularly effective in generating an immune response. Heterogeneity will not be a problem with macromolecules or more complex cellular and tissue antigens but may be important in the selection of peptides for immunization.

2.2.1.3 Conformation

B lymphocytes bind and respond to whole macromolecules, thus the antigenic determinants (epitopes) that a B cell recognizes may be dependent on the conformation of the molecule. It is therefore important to consider the state of the antigen to which you want your mab to bind; will it be in its native configuration or will it be denatured? Your immunogen preparation and method of screening should obviously take account of this. T cells respond only to processed peptide antigen, therefore conformation is not a problem.

2.2.1.4 Chemical structure

Different types of molecule differ considerably in their immunogenicity. Proteins and glycoproteins provide the best immunogens, generating good, enhanced memory responses with IgG antibodies. In the absence of protein, carbohydrates tend to generate a 'T independent' response with little or no memory and Ig class switching. This reflects the fact that T cells, required for memory generation and Ig class switching, can only be activated by peptides derived from processed protein antigens. Lipids are very poorly immunogenic. The optical configuration of a molecule will also affect its immunogenicity. Mammalian L-forms will generate good immune responses whereas bacterial D-forms are poor immunogens, presumably because they cannot be effectively 'processed' by enzymes and so cannot be presented to T cells in the immunized mammalian host.

2.2.2 Immunodominant molecules

Some molecules are, because of their structure, more immunogenic than others and can dominate an immune response if present in a crude antigen preparation. This should not normally cause a problem in the generation of mab as an appropriate antigen-specific screening system will simply ignore B cells that have responded to the dominant antigen. However, if the antigen-specific B cell yield is very low, partial purification of the antigen preparation, either by enrichment for the specific antigen or depletion of the immunodominant component, may help. In addition, if your antigen is present quantitatively as only a small component of your immunogenic preparation, some form of enrichment, if feasible, may improve the efficiency of antibody generation. It is sometimes found, however, that in purified antigen preparations it is the smallest contaminant that gives the best antibody response.

2.2.3   Production of antigens

Having selected your antigen the next step is to identify an appropriate source
and to prepare your antigen in a form that can be used for immunization. The
preparation does not have to be pure, as the screening method is the most
effective stage at which to select for cells that are producing antibody of the
appropriate specificity. Moreover, the preparation can be physically quite
crude, e.g. tissue homogenate or whole cells in suspension, because the host
animal's own enzymes will rapidly further breakdown the antigen such that, for
proteins, both B and T cells can respond. The most appropriate preparations
for immunization are soluble molecules in solution, small molecular aggregates
in suspension, whole cells in single cell suspension and tissue homogenates.

2.2.4   Adjuvants

The immunogenicity of an antigen can be enhanced by the addition of an
adjuvant to the preparation used for immunization, providing that the route of
immunization is not intravascular (see 2.2.9). Most adjuvants are of two main
types: colloidal, such as aluminium hydroxide, or oils that can be used to form
an emulsion with an aqueous antigen preparation (e.g. Freund's complete and
incomplete adjuvants). These are mixed thoroughly with the immunogen prior
to immunization and, after injection, provide long-lasting local depots of
antigen from which small amounts can be released over a long period of time,
providing continuous *in vivo* boosting of the immune response. This is important as it has been calculated that in the absence of adjuvant approximately only
0.1% of antigen administered as a single dose actually reaches the immune
system. Some adjuvants contain additional components that enhance immune
responsiveness, for example complete Freund's adjuvant contains killed mycobacteria in addition to oil and an emulsifying agent; these stimulate granuloma
formation (localized accumulation of immune cells) and cause polyclonal
activation of lymphocytes. Complete Freund's adjuvant should be used for the
first immunization but should be replaced by incomplete Freund's adjuvant (oil
and emulsifying agent only) for all subsequent immunizations to avoid excessive inflammation. There are also several new more clearly defined and highly
effective adjuvants on the market such as Optivant (Universal Biologicals Ltd,
U.K.).

   Nitrocellulose membranes have also been shown to have adjuvant activity.
Antigens that can be identified by Western blotting can be cut out on strips of
membrane and used as immunogen by dissolving the nitrocellulose and bound
antigen in minimal organic solvent; then, on adding an aqueous bicarbonate
buffer, the nitrocellulose forms a fine precipitate. These fine particles can then
be injected with or without emulsification in traditional adjuvant (Abou-Zeid
et al., 1987; Larsson & Nilsson, 1988).

2.2.5 Choice of host to be immunized

This will be determined by the source of the antigen, the myeloma line that is to be used for the fusion and the use to which you wish to put the monoclonal antibodies that you raise.

Unless the antigen is an alloantigen, the antigen and host to be immunized must belong to different species; moreover, the greater the genetic disparity between the two species the greater the degree of structural difference there is likely to be between your immunogenic molecule and the equivalent molecule in the host and hence the greater the potential range of antibody specificities that can be raised. Where the target antigen is of human origin, both mouse and rat monoclonal antibodies have been successful, however, where mouse or rat antigens are used, rodent monoclonal antibodies have not always been easily generated. Interestingly, mice appear to generate good immune responses to rat antigens, as evidenced by the large number of very successful reagents that have been produced. The reverse situation has been less productive and, although some very good rat anti-mouse antibodies have been generated, for some mouse antigens (e.g. CD4) the best reagents have been produced in Armenian hamsters. Unfortunately these have not been readily available in the UK and the Syrian hamster, which is available, is not a good substitute because the spleen gives rise to a population of very aggressive fibroblasts that quickly overgrow the hybridoma cells in culture.

Another point to consider, if you have chosen mouse or rat as recipient, is whether to use an inbred strain (Balb/c mouse or Lou rat, to match the available myeloma lines) or whether to use an F_1 hybrid (to include Balb/c or Lou as one of the two parental strains). The advantage of a hybrid is that different strains may vary in their responses to an antigen according to their MHC haplotype, as it is the MHC molecules that control the ability of their antigen-presenting cells to present antigen peptides to T cells. By using an F_1 hybrid derived from strains that differ in their MHC haplotypes you will increase the chance of obtaining a good response to your antigen.

Your choice of myeloma cells also to some extent dictates the species of animal to be immunized because intraspecies hybrids are more stable than interspecies hybrids. For mouse and rat reagents this is not a problem as myeloma lines exist for both species and the genetic similarities between the two render rat–mouse hybrids relatively stable. It does, however, lead to problems for the human and other systems where there are no good myeloma lines (Chapter 5). The solution in these cases may be to either clone the Ig-encoding genes as soon as possible after antigen-specific hybridomas have been selected and cloned, or to generate the reagents *de novo* by molecular biology techniques (Chapters 7 and 8).

The final use to which you wish to put your antibodies will also affect your choice of host for immunization. First, if the mab is required for *in vivo* use it is optimal if the mab and the recipient are of the same species so as to avoid the generation of a host anti-mab response (Chapter 10B). Antibody engineering techniques can now circumvent this problem (Chapters 7, 8 and 10B). Second, if large quantities of mabs are to be produced using the ascites method, the hybridoma cells should be genetically compatible with the host in which the ascites is to be produced; if they are not, then an immunocompromized host must be used.

Finally, the immunization schedule should be started with fairly young animals as the number of fibroblasts in the spleen will increase with age. Excessive fibroblasts in the primary fusion plate can lead to hybridoma cells being outgrown by this cellular competition. Moreover, as a general rule, females give a better immune response than do males. Therefore, female mice of about 6–8 weeks or female rats of about 8–10 weeks should be used.

2.2.6   *Route of immunization*

The route of immunization will depend on the nature of the antigen. Intraperitoneal (i.p.), intramuscular (i.m.), intradermal (i.d.) or subcutaneous (s.c.) routes can be used for any antigen preparation with or without adjuvant. These routes will predominantly give an immune response in the local regional lymph nodes. Intravenous (i.v.) immunization will ensure that the predominant response occurs in the spleen; however, only soluble antigen or cells in single-cell (i.e. no aggregates) suspension, without adjuvant can be administered intravenously. The spleen is the most accessible source of B lymphocytes for the fusion so it is advantageous to make the final boost prior to the fusion without adjuvant, via the tail vein. Nevertheless, it is frequently impossible to do this and in practice, after several boosts, i.p., i.m., i.d. or s.c., in mice the spleen will also contain many specific B lymphocytes and very successful fusions can be achieved using splenic lymphocytes without a final i.v. immunization. Unfortunately, in rats the spleen is not a good source of immune B cells unless the animal has been immunized i.v. In this case, it is possible to use the regional lymph nodes as the source of activated B lymphocytes.

For the production of IgM mab or if the antigen is in very short supply or has a very short half-life it is possible to perform intrasplenic immunization (Gearing *et al.*, 1985). This requires some delicate surgery and can only be performed once.

Another method that may be useful if you have very little antigen or if you wish to raise human mab where it is not feasible to immunize *in vivo*, is that of *in-vitro* immunization (Reading, 1983). In this system, splenic or peripheral blood leucocytes (i.e. B lymphocytes, T lymphocytes and antigen-presenting cells) are cultured together with the antigen; following this *in-vitro* priming, cells are subsequently fused with myeloma cells in the conventional way (see 2.3). The culture conditions are critical and require much patience to optimize (Vaux *et al.*, 1990). Commercial kits are also now available for *in-vitro* immunization. These supply all the necessary reagents, apart from your cells and immunogen, and may help to optimize your chances of success.

2.2.7 Frequency and timing of immunization

The number of times you immunize the animal prior to the fusion will determine to some extent the class of antibody that you are likely to produce. If you need IgM mab you should immunize once, or at the most twice, as you only require to provoke a primary immune response, with no class switching. If you want IgG mab then you need to provoke a secondary response and three or more immunizations are recommended. Such multiple immunizations will not only induce class switching but will also enhance the magnitude of the immune response and the affinity of the antibodies produced. For antigens that cannot activate T cells, a primary IgM-type response will always be generated.

The length of time between immunizations can also influence the affinity of antibodies that you produce. The physiological purpose of antibody production is to clear the antigen from the body. After immunization and subsequent initial antibody production, antigen levels will become progressively reduced. When a low concentration is reached, only high affinity B cells will be activated and clonally expanded (see Chapter 3). The longer the interval between immunizations the lower the level of residual antigen and the greater the preferential selection for high-affinity B cells. In practice, 3–4 weeks is the most usual interval used, although intervals of up to 3 months have certainly been used with success in rabbits. In shorter-lived rodents you will have to balance the number of immunizations and the length of interval between them with the risk of fibroblasts in the older animals. The final boost should always be 3–4 days before the fusion because this will ensure the presence of many B immunoblasts (antigen activated B cells that are in division), which are the most successful fusion partners for myeloma cells.

2.3 Cell fusion (Figure 2.1)

2.3.1 Choice of myeloma cells

There is a range of mouse and rat myeloma lines available (for the human system, see Chapter 5). These lines were originally derived from tumours of antibody-secreting plasma cells; it is therefore important that you choose a line that has been selected so that it can no longer produce either light or heavy chains of its own. This is important, because if both myeloma cell and B cell partners in a hybridoma cells can produce immunoglobulin, the two different heavy and light chains can randomly associate to give several different hybrid antibody molecules in addition to the specific antibody for which you selected.

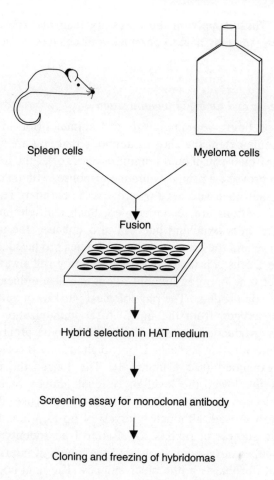

Spleen cells   Myeloma cells

Fusion

Hybrid selection in HAT medium

Screening assay for monoclonal antibody

Cloning and freezing of hybridomas

Figure 2.1. Hybridoma technology: fusion and screening.

These hybrid molecules reduce the efficiency of your system and can lead to problems of non-specificity (this mixing can be an advantage if you specifically want bispecific antibodies (Chapter 6)).

The second consideration is that, if possible, the myeloma cells should be genetically compatible with your source of B cells (2.2.8).

The myeloma cells are usually stored in liquid nitrogen and should be thawed out and grown up for at least 1 week prior to the fusion. About 2 days after thawing the cells will begin to divide. They should be expanded into larger flasks as necessary, as they become confluent. The day before the fusion the myeloma cells should be divided into fresh medium at approximately 3×10^5 cells/ml so that they will be in the exponential growth phase ready for the fusion.

2.3.2 Choice of fusogen

Variables that are involved during a fusion are the fusogen, cell ratio, medium, conditions for achieving contact, time, temperature and processing after the fusion.

The fusion of cell membranes occurs at very low frequencies when cells are brought into close contact with each other but this fusion rate can be increased by the use of substances called fusogens.

The original fusogen used was Sendai virus but this has now been superseded by polyethylene glycol (PEG) which is much safer to use and does not require culturing of virus. Different batches of PEG have different fusogenic efficiencies; however, this does not seem to relate to the molecular weight of the PEG. It is therefore advisable to test new batches of PEG prior to carrying out an important fusion. Despite reports to the contrary, the speed at which the PEG is added to the pellet of spleen and myeloma cells does not appear to be too critical, providing you are not too rough (i.e. 30 s is as successful as 4 min). The ratio of spleen:myeloma cells should be approximately 10:1; however, this is not absolutely critical and ratios as low as 2:1 have certainly generated successful hybrids. In contrast, temperature is important and for a successful fusion you should ensure that all reagents are at 37 °C.

Electrofusion is an alternative method which may give a higher ratio of hybrids but fewer cells can be manipulated at a time and it requires some practice to set up the correct operating conditions. Basically, it involves the application of an alignment current (alternating current field, approximately 4.5 V) to the mixed spleen and myeloma cells such that small strings of cells form. One or more fusion pulses (direct current field, approximately 55 V) are then applied; this electric current interferes with the cell membrane breaking its continuity so that after the current ceases and the membranes repair themselves, if two cells are touching their cell membranes will join to make one large cell. An alternating current electric field is continued after the fusion pulse to hold the cells together during recovery. The voltage and timing of these pulses is critical to cause fusion without complete disruption of the cells (Lo *et al.*, 1984).

The cheapest, simplest, most reliable and therefore the most popular method is with PEG. Initially, whichever fusion method is used, only the plasma membranes of the cells fuse and two separate nuclei can be seen within the cell. Nuclear fusion occurs during mitosis and results in a cell that contains a complete diploid set of chromosomes from each parent cell. In subsequent mitotic divisions there is a tendency for the hybrid cells to lose some chromosomes, a tendency that is greater if the two cells are of different genetic origin (interspecies hybrids). Although some chromosome loss may be inconsequential, loss of the chromosomes carrying either the B cell's immunoglobulin genes or the myeloma cell's genes that are responsible for immortality in culture would be disasterous.

2.3.3   Medium

The choice of medium for the fusion should be that in which the myeloma cells have been growing successfully but without serum; this is usually RPMI-1640, with sodium pyruvate and penicillin and streptomycin (to inhibit possible bacterial growth). After the fusion the cells should be plated in the same medium but with the addition of 10% FCS. During the fusion the medium should be buffered with Hepes but for plating out and subsequent growth of cells the medium should be bicarbonate buffered and the cultures kept at 37 °C in an atmosphere of 5% CO_2 in air. Cells prefer long-term culture in the latter but for ease of operation while working in the hood outside the CO_2 environment, Hepes buffer is used to keep the pH correct.

It should be noted that other media (e.g. DMEM (Dulbecco's modified Eagle's medium), Iscove's) and other sera (newborn calf, horse, human cord blood) are also successful. Serum substitutes and serum-free media are not good at the fusion stage but can be invaluable at later stages, especially for bulk production and subsequent purification (2.6.2 and 2.7.2) where it is an advantage to reduce the number of contaminating proteins to a minimum.

2.4   Growth and selection of hybrids

2.4.1   Feeder cells

Feeder cells are used because they secrete cytokines and other factors into the medium which help the hybridoma cells to survive and proliferate. Also, if phagocytic cells are used they will ingest the cell debris and thus eliminate some of the toxic substances released into the medium by the dying cells. For this reason, peritoneal macrophages are frequently used as feeder cells. These are normally taken from an animal of the same species, although this is not an absolute requirement, for example mouse macrophages very successfully support the growth of rat hybridoma cells. Nevertheless, other non-phagocytic cells are also good feeders, for example rat thymocytes and 3T3 fibroblasts. The latter have the advantage that, being a cell line, they are readily grown in large numbers but it is important to inactivate them by irradiation before use to prevent them from rapidly expanding throughout the cultures which is at the expense of the hybridoma cells. It is possible to make monoclonal antibodies without using feeder cells, although success rates are likely to be lower. Commercially available 'hybridoma growth factors' can be very useful in replacing feeders. Finally, although it is common practice to use feeders at the fusion stage of mab production, this is probably unnecessary as the spleen contains many phagocytic cells which will therefore be present in the suspension that is used for fusion with myeloma cells. It is likely, however, that if feeder cells are plated out in advance, then the supernatant will contain cytokines from day 0 and the fusion will get off to a good start.

2.4.2 HAT selection

Immediately after the fusion, the first problem that you must deal with is the presence of unwanted cells in your cultures. Not all cells will have formed hybrids during the fusion. Unfused spleen cells will not cause any problems because they will die in culture within a few days. The major problem will be the unfused myeloma cells as these are immortal (hence their use in the immortalization of your antibody-producing B cells) and will rapidly grow throughout the culture, to the detriment of the hybrids which will be growing more slowly at this stage. These unwanted unfused myeloma cells can be removed using selective HAT medium (Figure 2.2).

The myeloma cells used as fusion partners have been selected so that they lack the enzyme hypoxanthinephosphoribosyltransferase (HPRT) and are therefore unable to utilize the salvage pathway for RNA synthesis. By adding aminopterin (A) to the culture medium thus blocking the main pathways of DNA and RNA synthesis, the unfused myeloma cells are unable to grow. Hybrids made from the fusion of a myeloma cell and a spleen cell will have the HPRT enzyme, inherited from the spleen cell parent, and will be able to utilize the salvage pathway if they are provided with exogenous hypoxanthine (H) and thymidine (T). Although some methods recommend delaying the addition of HAT medium for 24 h after fusion, it can be added immediately without harming the newly-formed hybrids. Cultures are kept in HAT medium for approximately 2 weeks. After this time, only hybrids will be surviving in the cultures and the cells can be weaned gently off the salvage pathway by using HT in the medium for a further week before reverting to normal tissue culture medium. This is important as the aminopterin has a longer half-life in culture than either H or T.

As soon as the HAT is removed, the growth rate of the hybrids will increase and small clones will become visible in the cultures (if you have used NS0

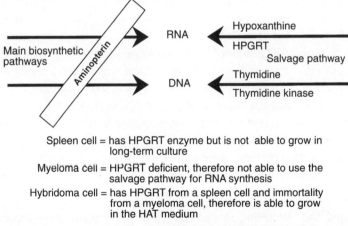

Figure 2.2. Mechanism of hybrid cell selection in HAT medium.

myeloma cells, hybrid clones will appear even in the presence of HAT). The second major problem now arises: that of unwanted hybrids. Not every spleen cell that formed a hybrid with a myeloma cell will have been a B cell (spleen contains T cells, macrophages, neutrophils, etc.). Moreover, even if a B cell were involved in hybrid formation, it may not be producing antibody of the specificity that you require.

2.4.3   Screening method

As soon as clones of cells are visible and the medium has started to turn slightly acidic (yellow), a small aliquot of supernatant medium should be removed for testing. If the screening assay proves positive the cells from that well should be cloned as soon as possible, preferably within 24 h. Negative wells should be rescreened a few days later or when the wells have become nearly confluent with cells.

Your screening assay is a critical stage in the production of monoclonal antibodies because the reagents that you generate will only be as good as the selection system that you use in their production. The immune response will generate a wide range of specificities and affinities; it is for you to select those that perform optimally for the purpose to which you wish to put them. It is therefore critical that you include appropriate controls and that you choose a screening method that is the same or very close to the method in which you will ultimately be using the antibodies. This is particularly important as different antibodies will be best suited to different assay systems (Chapter 3). The screening method should also be rapid, reliable and feasible to carry out with large numbers of small samples; you could have 200 samples, each of only 100 μl (approximately 1 μg of antibody) in volume, to screen in a day.

When the medium turns yellow it indicates that the cells are growing rapidly and fresh medium should be added to maintain the cells.

Obviously the purpose of screening is to detect, at the earliest possible stage, which wells of the fusion plate contain clones of hybridoma cells secreting antibody of the desired specificity. However, you can also design your screening system to detect only mab of a particular class or subclass. For instance, you may want your mab to bind complement for use in cytotoxicity assays or for the prevention of graft-versus-host disease after bone marrow transplantation (Chapter 12C) and therefore require a subclass that will fix complement, or you may want to use your mab for immunoprecipitation when it would be useful if it bound protein A.

The exact type of screening assay that you choose is therefore dependent on the nature of the antigen and the final use for which you want the antibody.

The basic rules for a primary screening assay are:

1 Rapid (non-secreting clones can quickly overgrow your specific mab-producing clone in the well of a 24-well plate).

2 Possible on a large scale (you may have supernatants from 100 to 200 wells to screen on a single day).

3 Possible with a small quantity of antibody (approximately 1 μg)

4 Include a positive and a negative control each time, otherwise you may lose valuable time and valuable hybrids due to false positives or false negatives.

5 Well established. It is essential to have your screening assay working well before your clones are ready for screening as they will not wait for you to perfect it.

After screening, cells that are producing antibody of interest (give a good positive reaction in your screening assay) must be cloned (see 2.5). Wells that are negative or borderline may contain several clones and the slowest growing clone could be the one producing specific antibody, therefore, even from a well with a large number of cells growing you may get a negative or borderline result. It is often worthwhile to rescreen these wells after a few days.

2.4.3.1 *Screening assays for mab against soluble antigens*

The most suitable screening assays for soluble antigens are the ELISA (enzyme-linked immunosorbant assay) and Dot blot assays. Briefly, soluble antigen is bound to either the plastic of the wells of a 96-well plate or to nitrocellulose or nylon membrane. Mab supernatants are incubated with this bound antigen and those mabs which are antigen specific will bind. An enzyme-linked secondary antibody with specificity for the monoclonal immunoglobulin (e.g. anti-mouse Ig if you are making mouse monoclonals) is used to detect wells/dots where the primary mab have bound. This binding is then visualized by the addition of an appropriate enzyme substrate that after reaction with the enzyme yields a coloured product. Where the enzyme peroxidase is used the substrate chromogens *ortho*-phenyl diamine (OPD), 2,2'azino-di-3-ethylbenzthiazoline-6-sulphonic acid (ABTS) or 3,3',5,5'-tetramethylbenzidine (TMB) are used for ELISA (reaction product is soluble) and 3,3'-diamino-benzidine tetrahydrochloride (DAB), 4-chloro-1-napthol or enhanced chemiluminescence (ECL) for Dot blots (reaction product is insoluble). Alternatively, alkaline phosphatase-linked secondary antibodies can be used with *p*-nitrophenol phosphate (soluble product) or napthol-AS-MX phosphate (free acid) with fast red TR or fast blue BB salt (insoluble product) as substrates.

Western blotting provides a higher resolution screening assay that is particularly useful when the molecular weight of the antigen is known but where pure antigen is not available for screening. A cell/tissue lysate containing the antigen of interest is first separated into its different molecular weight components by SDS-PAGE (polyacrylamide gel electrophoresis in the presence of sodium dodecyl sulphate). These proteins are then electrophoretically transferred onto a nitrocellulose/nylon membrane and strips of this are tested for mab binding in the same way as for Dot blots. Equipment is available (see Appendix, Chapter 16) to enable you to screen 56 supernatants simultaneously by Western blotting.

2.4.3.2 Screening methods for monoclonal antibodies against cellular and insoluble antigens

There are several techniques that can be used for screening mab against cellular and insoluble antigens, the major one being immunohistochemistry. This is the method of choice for characterizing tissue or cellular antigens and it can be carried out on frozen tissue sections, fixed paraffin wax embedded tissue sections or on cell smears or cytospins. The principle of immunohistochemistry is the same as that of ELISA and Dot blotting. The mab is incubated with the antigen (tissue section or cell preparation); after washing, a secondary labelled antibody is applied that can have either a fluorochrome, an enzyme or biotin conjugated to it. The fluorochrome can be visualized directly by UV light microscopy whereas the enzyme-linked antibody requires a substrate to produce a coloured product which is detectable by light microscopy. Biotin-linked antibodies require subsequent incubation with avidin or streptavidin (both of which have a high affinity for biotin); either of these can be conjugated to a fluorochrome or an enzyme in order to detect your mab staining. This technique has the advantage of being able to distinguish qualitatively different monoclonals at the first screening stage. This is easily done as they will have different staining patterns on the tissues, so that you can select clones that are going to be different at a very early stage. By screening on various tissues you can detect cross-reactivity on other tissues.

Mab to cell surface and intracellular molecules can also be screened by immunofluorescence analysis of cells in suspension (live or fixed cells for surface or internal molecules, respectively). The principle of the labelling technique is the same as for immunohistochemistry. Immunolabelling can be analysed by flow cytometry. This permits quantitative analysis of fluorescence intensity, together with other cell parameters such as size, granularity and, for more sophisticated screening, simultaneous labelling of other cell markers, using up to three additional fluorochromes of different emission wavelengths. Finally, the ELISA technique can be modified to study mab that bind to either whole cells or a particulate antigen, such as cell membranes, platelets or aggregated molecules. The conditions for coating these antigens onto the ELISA plate will be different for each antigen; therefore, you will have to spend some time finding the optimal conditions for your antigen (type of plate, coating buffer, coating temperature, coating time).

2.5   Cloning techniques

The next problem that must be addressed is that of clonality. When the fused cells are first plated out, many different cells will be present in a single well;

hence, after growth in culture, there may be many clones in each well. Your specific antibody-secreting clone is therefore likely to be mixed with clones that are either non-secreting or which are producing antibody of an undesired specificity. It is therefore essential to separate your specific cells from these contaminants to ensure that you have a single clone of cells and therefore that the antibody produced is genuinely monoclonal. This is critical for the production of the monoclonal reagent. It is also critical in a more practical way; non-secreting clones will often proliferate more rapidly than those that secrete antibody and can completely overgrow a culture, leading to loss of the valuable hybridoma.

The aim of every cloning technique is to grow a clone of cells from an isolated single cell. There are various methods that can be used. The easiest method is by limiting dilution. In this you dilute the cells to a set concentration calculated so that each well of a 96-well plate will have either one cell or no cell at all (in fact you will always get more variation than this because it follows a Poisson distribution). A dilution that gives, on average, 0.3 cells per well is that most frequently used. The major problem with this technique is that of cell viability: the hybridoma cells dislike sudden changes in concentration. This can be overcome in two ways. First, the use of feeder cells greatly enhances the survival of hybridomas during cloning. Second, a preliminary cloning under less stringent conditions (e.g. six cells per well) will help the hybrids to acclimatize to low density. This should then be followed by two sequential clonings at 0.3 cells per well to ensure monoclonality. Obviously, between each cloning you must screen the supernatant medium from each well to follow the location of the hybrids that are specific for your antigen.

An alternative approach is to titrate the cells by doubling dilution across the plate so that each row of wells contains half the number of the previous row until the final row has theoretically 0.25 or fewer cells per well. This method has the advantage of having cells at a high density (e.g. 16 cells per well) at the left side of the plate which provides an 'insurance policy' against cell loss, whereas the right hand side of the plate is at very low density for cloning. Clones should be chosen from wells furthest to the right as they will have the greatest chance of being a true clone, but this choice should be augmented by visual clues, i.e. checking by inverted light microscopy for discrete clones of cells. This is particularly useful if the fusion partner used is NS0 as they usually form tight, discrete and clearly discernible clones of cells (Figure 2.3).

The most accurate method of cloning is by single cell manipulation. This is done best by using a cell sorter machine with a laser detection system that detects droplets containing a single cell; by giving each droplet a small electric charge they are deflected into separate wells of a 96-well plate. All major flow cytometry machines that are designed for fluorescence-activated cell sorting can be used in this way. Cloning by this method is very accurate but is also very time consuming. It is therefore usually advisable to carry out the initial cloning steps by limiting dilution and to employ cell sorting for a final high stringency step.

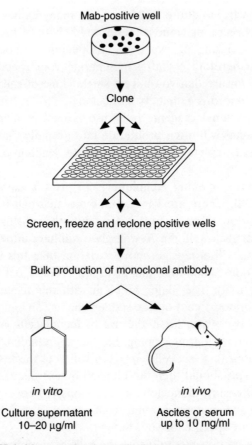

Figure 2.3. Hybridoma technology: cloning and bulk production.

2.6   Cell maintenance and bulk production of antibody

2.6.1   Cell preservation

Once you have cloned out your hybridoma cells you will need to freeze some down in liquid nitrogen so that you have a permanent supply. This is a critical step in mab production and you are advised to freeze stocks at regular intervals during production. Even in the best laboratories contamination of cultures or failures in incubators can occur. It is also wise to store your cells in more than one place because liquid nitrogen tanks are vulnerable to drying out.

To freeze cells they must be cryoprotected; if you were to freeze them in ordinary medium they would be destroyed by ice crystals that form inside the cells during the freezing procedure, rupturing the cell membrane. A mixture of 10% dimethylsulphoxide (DMSO), 90% fetal calf serum (FCS) should be prepared and kept cold (4 °C) as the freezing medium. When frozen this mixture does not increase in volume, so the cells remain intact (although some cells are more sensitive than others and may require the amount of DMSO to be reduced to 5%). The cells should be suspended in this medium at between 10^5 to 10^6 cells per ml and cooled very slowly, at a rate of about 1–2 °C per min. This can be achieved by a variety of methods and does not require an expensive freezing machine (Chapter 16). Once they have reached −70 °C they can be transferred to the liquid nitrogen storage vessel.

To thaw cells after liquid nitrogen storage, they should be treated as for myeloma cells, i.e. thawed quickly and the DMSO diluted out immediately. They should then be incubated at 37 °C, with 5% carbon dioxide (CO_2) in air, and after 2–3 days the cells will have recovered and will start to grow and divide.

2.6.2 Bulk production of monoclonal antibodies

When you have successfully cloned your hybridoma cells, you will probably possess approximately 10^6 cells in 200 μl in one well of a cloning plate. Your next task is to grow up the cells to ensure a good stock of both hybridoma cells and of the antibody that they secrete.

Large amounts of mab can be produced by either bulk tissue culture or by production of ascites. For bulk culture, the hybridoma cells should be progressively transferred into larger and larger containers until a suitable size is reached (the cells do not like abrupt changes in density and volume of the container). For many uses, sufficient antibody can be produced by static cultures in large flasks. Alternatively, larger amounts can be produced using roller cultures, or by utilizing one of the many specialized containers that are commercially available (e.g. hollow fibre systems, multilayered culture containers). These methods, however, are quite expensive and are not successful with all hybridomas. A simple alternative for large scale production is to set up a continuous culture of hybridoma cells in dialysis tubing (Sjogren-Jansson & Jeansson, 1985). Supernatant from standard flask cultures will contain between approximately 10 and 50 μg/ml of mab, although this will vary according to the individual hybridoma and the degree of confluence of the cultures at the time of harvesting.

Alternatively, the mab can be produced in much larger amounts as an ascitic fluid. Hybridomas will grow in the peritoneal cavity of animals of the same strain as the tumour cell line and spleen cell donor (i.e. donor and recipient must be genetically compatible) and secrete mab into the ascitic fluid formed within the abdominal cavity. The animal should be primed with either pristane (2,6,10,14-tetramethylpentadecane) (Hoogenraad *et al.*, 1983) or incomplete Freund's adjuvant; this will activate the peritoneal macrophages causing them to produce cytokines which assist the growth of the hybridoma cells. Some hybridoma cells are reluctant to grow *in vivo*; injection of a larger number of cells in the inoculate may overcome this problem. Once the cells are acclimatized to growing *in vivo* they can be passaged from one animal to another and it is worthwhile cryopreserving some of these cells for future ascites production.

With this technique, the fluid collected can contain up to 10 mg/ml of monoclonal antibody.

2.7 Characterization and purification of antibody

2.7.1 Monoclonal antibody isotype determination

It is useful to know the isotype of your mab so that you know in which assays it will be most useful or what method to use to purify it. For example IgM mab are useful for cytotoxicity assays but they do not bind protein A. Alternatively, if you want to use two-colour immunostaining you can use isotype-specific secondary antibodies, provided that you have mabs of different isotypes.

There are several methods available for determining the mab isotype; all involve the use of isotype-specific secondary anti-Ig antibodies combined with a visual detection system. The quickest and simplest method is a commercially available 'dipstick' assay. This system uses the Dot blot technique and comprises a strip of specially-prepared membrane with separate dots, each one containing a different specific anti-isotype antibody. You simply dip this strip into first your mab (which will bind to the appropriate anti-isotype dot) then, after washing, into a species specific anti-mouse Ig antibody (to locate the dot to which your mab has bound) and finally into the substrate solution (to visualize the binding). You obtain a coloured product at the spot to which your mab has bound. An alternative commercial kit utilizes a haemagglutination system. This provides you with red blood cells (RBC) coated with isotype-specific antibodies. An aliquot of each RBC preparation is placed into separate wells of a 96-well plate together with an aliquot of your mab and incubated for 30 min. Whichever RBC preparation your mab haemagglutinates is the isotype of your mab. Another kit available is an ELISA, again using isotype-specific antibodies to detect the mab isotype. Alternatively, you could make cytospin preparations of your hybridoma cells and use isotype-specific labelled (enzyme or fluorochrome) antibody to detect the mab isotype as expressed in/on the hybridoma cells. It is also possible to use the Ouchterlony technique but this is dependent on having equivalent antibody concentrations and is therefore less reliable. These and several other kits are available commercially.

2.7.2 Antibody purification

Once you have prepared a large quantity of your mab, either by bulk culture or as ascitic fluid, you may wish to purify it. The major contaminants will differ according to which method of bulk production you have used. For tissue culture supernatant the main contaminants come from the FCS (bovine albumin, transferin, maternal IgG). This can be reduced/eliminated by using a low serum/serum-free medium in which to grow the cells in bulk. For ascites, the major contaminants will be mouse Ig and lipoproteins from the host peritoneal fluid.

2.7.2.1 *Partial purification of immunoglobulins by salt fractionation*

This technique relies on the fact that proteins behave differently depending on their relative solubility at different salt concentrations. The salt ions interfere with the hydrophilic bonds formed between the protein and water molecules; as the salt–water reaction is more stable than the protein–water reaction, the protein will precipitate out of solution. Larger protein molecules precipitate at lower salt concentrations than smaller ones. Immunoglobulins being fairly large molecules compared with other serum proteins can thus be precipitated from either serum samples or culture supernatant leaving the other major serum proteins (e.g. albumin) in solution. This also serves to concentrate the antibody as the precipitate is then redissolved in a minimal volume. The salts that are most useful for precipitating immunoglobulin are sodium sulphate and ammonium sulphate. The solubility of ammonium sulphate is less sensitive to temperature change and only varies by about 3% between 0 °C and 25 °C whereas the solubility of sodium sulphate is fivefold greater at 25 °C than at 0 °C. If your mab is stable at room temperature it is convenient to use sodium, sulphate but if your mab is labile at room temperature you should use ammonium sulphate at 4 °C. Ammonium sulphate, however, can interfere with some labelling techniques (e.g. FITC (fluorescein isothiocyanate) and biotin). Sodium sulphate should be used if these procedures are to be followed.

2.7.2.2 *Chromatography*

Proteins can be separated according to their size and shape, overall molecular charge or their biological activity. The properties of the protein to be isolated should be carefully considered when choosing an isolation method (Table 2.1).

Size exclusion chromatography

Size exclusion chromatography separates proteins according to their molecular size and shape. It utilizes a column packed with beads made of polymerized agarose (e.g. Sepharose, Pharmacia, U.K. or Biogel-A, Bio-rad, U.K.), cross-linked Dextran (Sephadex, Pharmacia), polyacrylamide (Biogel-B, Bio-rad) or a dextran covalently linked with methyl bisacrylamide (Sephacryl, Pharmacia). The beads (matrix) are porous and are available with different pore sizes.

Table 2.1. *Choice of chromatographic technique according to molecular property*

Molecular property	Chromatographic technique
Size and shape	Size exclusion
Charge	Ion exchange
Biological activity	Affinity

Separation takes place because large molecules can be excluded from the pores, and so pass through the spaces between the beads, whereas smaller molecules enter the pores and are thus retarded within the matrix. The smaller the molecule the more able it is to permeate the gel matrix and so the longer it will take to elute from the column. Molecules that are larger than the exclusion limit of the gel matrix are eluted in the void volume (volume of the column not occupied by the beads – space between the beads). Molecules smaller than the exclusion limit will elute in decreasing order of size. Very small molecules that can freely permeate the pores will elute at the volume equal to the total internal volume of the column.

This method is very useful for purifying IgM mabs as they have a much greater molecular mass (970 kDa) than any other serum protein. If a gel with an exclusion limit of 200 kDa is used, all proteins except IgM will be retarded within the matrix and the IgM will be eluted with the void volume.

Ion exchange chromatography

Ion exchange chromatography relies on the fact that the charge of a protein varies according to the pH of the ambient solution. In this technique, the beads used for the matrix of the column carry either a positive or negative charge and therefore have an affinity for molecules with the opposite charge. Diethyl-aminoethyl (DEAE) cellulose beads are positively charged and at pH 8, when Ig will be negatively charged, the Ig molecules will bind to the beads. Ig can then be eluted from the matrix by changing the pH or ionic strength of the elution buffer, thus changing either the charge of the Ig or competing the Ig from the beads with excess ions. It is less harmful to the Ig to change the ionic strength. In either case it is better to change the buffer as an increasing gradient. This is called an anion exchanger. A cation exchanger works on the same principle except that the beads, carboxymethyl (CM) cellulose, are negatively charged. Therefore, they will bind molecules that have an overall positive charge and these can be competed from the beads by an increasing concentration of cations in the same way as with the anion exchanger, using either a pH or increasing ionic strength buffer gradient.

Affinity chromatography

In affinity chromatography the specific protein binding molecules are co-valently bound to agarose beads and used to isolate your specific mab. The nature of the protein-binding molecule will define the specificity of the affinity column. Protein A, protein G, isotype-specific antibody or specific antigen can be used according to the mab you wish to isolate. Protein A and protein G are both Fc-binding proteins isolated from bacteria, their Fc specificity varies, as does their specific binding pH (Akerstrom & Bjorck, 1986). The known Ig binding for mouse and rat monoclonal antibody isotypes is given in Table 2.2. Protein G binds Ig at a lower pH than protein A and can therefore be eluted at a high pH, which is less damaging to the Ig than the very low pH buffer

Table 2.2. *Binding properties of protein A and protein G*

Species/isotype		Protein A	Protein G
Mouse	IgG1	±	+
	IgG2a	+	+
	IgG2b	+	+
	IgG3	+	+
Rat	IgG1	±	+
	IgG2a	±	+
	IgG2b	−	+
	IgG2c	±	+

required for Ig elution from protein A. Most Ig will bind to protein G at pH 5–7 and can be eluted between pH 9 and pH 10. In contrast, most binding of Ig to protein A occurs between pH 8 and pH 9 and is eluted at pH 2–4. The semi-purified mab solution is added to the affinity column, the mab will bind to the ligand on the beads and the contaminant components will flow through the column. The mab can then be removed from the column by changing either the pH or the eluting buffer.

2.7.3 *Determination of protein concentration*

Once you have purified your mab you will need to estimate the concentration of Ig in the preparation. The easiest way to do this is by spectrophotometry, by measuring its optical density (OD) at 280 nm. This technique takes advantage of the fact that light waves passing through a solution are impeded by molecules in the solution, depending on their concentration. Every molecule will deflect the light to a greater or lesser extent, according to its unique folding conformation. This is expressed as its extinction coefficient (ε). Once you have measured the OD of your mab solution, you can substitute it into the equation $OD = \varepsilon c l$ (where OD = optical density, ε = extinction coefficient, c = concentration and l = length (in cm) of the light path through the solution) and thereby calculate the concentration of antibody.

2.7.4 *Polyacrylamide gel electrophoresis in the presence of sodium dodecyl sulphate (SDS-PAGE)*

Once you have estimated your mab concentration, you can check the purity of your preparation by SDS-PAGE. In electrophoresis proteins migrate through the matrix according to their charge, size and shape. Boiling protein in the detergent SDS denatures the protein molecules and binds the SDS to the protein at the rate of 1.4 g SDS/g protein. Thus all the protein molecules have the same charge to weight ratio and they migrate according to their relative molecular mass. There are some exceptions to this rule, for example glyco-sylated proteins will bind less SDS than non-glycosylated proteins of the same molecular mass and molecules with disulphide bonds will not bind the optimum amount of SDS unless they are reduced.

On polymerization the polyacrylamide forms a porous gel, the pore size being determined by the concentration of acrylamide (low concentration, larger pores, high concentration, smaller pores). A modified version of the Laemmli method is usually used; this method uses a discontinuous buffer system (the gel buffer is of a higher molarity than the electrode buffer) and a stacking gel to increase the resolution (Laemmli, 1970). The protein–SDS complexes are all negatively charged at pH 8.3 (electrode buffer) so they migrate quickly into the stacking gel; once in the stacking gel, pH 6.8, their electrophoretic mobility decreases and they concentrate to form a narrow band. They enter the separating gel, pH 8.8, as a neat band and then migrate according to their relative molecular mass. Thus a crude cell/tissue lysate preparation, of diverse protein composition, can be separated into individual protein components. Molecular weight standards, treated in the same way as the sample, must always be included in any SDS-PAGE experiment as each gel will run slightly differently according to the temperature, acrylamide concentration, electric current and length of time it is run.

This technique is useful to test the purity of your mab preparation. You should find only one band under non-reducing conditions (IgG, 150 kDa; IgM, 970 kDa) and two under reducing conditions (IgG, 50 and 25 kDa; IgM, 65 and 25 kDa). Alternatively, it can be used in combination with Western blotting to identify the molecular weight and characteristics of the antigen to which your mab binds.

2.8   Storage

Antibodies are fairly robust molecules but should nevertheless be treated with care. It should also be noted that different antibodies differ considerably in their stability during storage (e.g. some may survive well at $+4\,°C$ for many months whereas others may maintain activity at this temperature for a week or less).

Antibodies should be stored at between $-20\,°C$ and $-70\,°C$, preferably the latter. Repeated freezing and thawing will destroy antibody activity. They should therefore be stored in aliquots of a size appropriate to the use to which they will be used. If your antibody is to be kept at $+4\,°C$, and is stable at that temperature, it should be kept sterile or should contain an antibacterial agent. Tissue culture supernatants store well. Purified antibody should be stored in neutral isotonic buffer (Tris buffered saline, phosphate buffered saline). Low protein concentrations should be avoided. If your antibody is present at a low concentration, a carrier protein (e.g. bovine serum albumin (BSA)) should be added (e.g. 0.1% BSA).

2.9 Analysis of the structure of the antigen to which your monoclonal binds

This is a very large area and depends on the nature of your target antigen. Only an overview will be given here (for further details see Johnson & Thorpe, 1992).

Once you have an antibody, you can use it to analyse the structure of the target antigen. The three main primary techniques by which this can be achieved are immunoprecipitation, Western blotting and affinity purification. Many additional techniques, which are beyond the scope of this volume, are obviously also involved.

2.9.1 Western blotting

If your mab recognizes a cellular/tissue antigen you can define the molecular weight and characteristics of its antigen by SDS-PAGE and Western blotting. First, you will have to prepare an antigen lysate from the particular cells or tissue that express the specific antigen and separate them by SDS-PAGE. These are then transferred onto nitrocellulose or nylon membrane with the aid of an electric current. The membrane can then be either inserted into a slot blotter equipment or cut into strips and incubated with your mab, in the same way as described (2.4.3).

The protein band recognized by your mab is visualized by incubating with a secondary enzyme-labelled antibody and a coloured product developed with the specific substrate. By comparing the position of the identified band with those of the molecular weight markers, the relative molecular mass of your mab antigen can be determined.

2.9.2 Immunoprecipitation

If your mab recognizes a cell surface protein this can be further characterized by immunoprecipitation. First, the cell surface proteins are radiolabelled with ^{125}Iodine (^{125}I) in the presence of lactoperoxidase and hydrogen peroxide, then the cells are lysed so that the membrane is fragmented and only proteins that are closely associated within the membrane will be included in individual micelles. These micelles are sedimented and dialysed to remove the free ^{125}I, pre-cleared to remove any proteins that bind non-specifically to protein A or immunoglobulin. Your mab can then be added to the lysate and incubated to allow specific recognition of antigen. This antibody/antigen (Ab/Ag) complex can then be precipitated with protein A Sepharose beads. The Ab/Ag/protein A bead complex is then washed to remove all non-complexed proteins. The complex is boiled in SDS-PAGE sample buffer to dissociate the molecules prior to separation on SDS-PAGE, together with radiolabelled molecular weight markers. The position of the mab-precipitated protein bands are visualized by exposing the gel onto X-ray sensitive film which is subsequently developed. The relative molecular mass of the mab-precipitated protein is estimated by comparison with the molecular weight standards. If more bands are precipitated in this technique than in SDS-PAGE and Western blotting then the extra bands must be proteins that are closely associated with the specific protein within the cell membrane (Cone, 1987).

2.9.3   *Metabolic labelling*

If your mab antigen is not expressed as a cell surface molecule, or cannot be iodinated due to the lack of tyrosine residues then it is possible to radiolabel it metabolically. This uses a radiolabelled amino acid (e.g. ^{35}S-methionine) which is incorporated into the protein as it is synthesized. A cell line is required which expresses your antigen in culture. The technique can also be used to study the rate of antigen synthesis and turnover. It involves washing the cells with methionine-free medium to remove unlabelled methionine, adding ^{35}S-methionine and incubating for a predetermined time, then washing with complete medium to remove the labelled methionine. The length of time necessary for the incorporation of the radiolabelled amino acid is dependent on the rate of synthesis of your protein antigen. An initial experiment using several time points is required to determine the optimum incubation time. The cells can then be lysed and processed by SDS-PAGE and Western blotting or immuno-precipitation. Either the gel or the Western blot can be exposed to X-ray sensitive film and developed, as for immunoprecipitation, to visualize the radioactive bands (Newman, 1987).

2.10   Summary

Mab production is difficult but can be very rewarding. You could be very lucky and produce the reagent that you want within 3–6 months; however, it could take longer. No matter how thoughtful and careful you are, there is an unpredictable element involved. Good luck!

2.11   References

Abou-Zeid, C., Filley, E., Steele, J. & Rook, G. A. W. (1987). A simple new method for using antigens separated by polyacrylamide gel electrophoresis to stimulate lymphocytes *in vitro* after converting bands cut from Western blots into antigen-bearing particles. *Journal of Immunological Methods*, **98**, 5–10.

Akerstrom, B. & Bjorck, L. (1986). A physicochemical study of protein G, a molecule with unique immunoglobulin G-binding properties. *Journal of Biological Chemistry*, **26**, 10240–10247.

Cone, R. E. (1987). Strategies for the isolation of cell surface receptors of lymphoid cells. *Methods in Enzymology*, **150**, 388–399.

Dadi, H. K., Morris, R. J., Hulme, E. C. & Birdsell, N. J. M. (1984). Antibodies to a covalent agonist used to isolate the muscarinic cholinergic receptor from rat brain. In *Investigation of Membrane Located Receptors*, ed. E. Reid, G. M. W. Cook & D. J. Morre, pp. 425–428. New York, Plenum Press.

Gearing, A. J. H., Thorpe, R., Spitz, L. & Spitz, M. (1985). Use of 'single shot' intrasplenic immunisation for production of monoclonal antibodies specific for human IgM. *Journal of Immunological Methods*, **76**, 337–343.

Galfre, G. & Milstein, C. (1981). Preparation of monoclonal antibodies: strategies and procedures. *Methods in Enzymology*, **73B**, 3–46.

Hoogenraad, N., Helman, T. & Hoogenraad, J. (1983). The effect of pre-injection of mice with pristane on ascites tumour formation and monoclonal antibody production. *Journal of Immunological Methods*, **61**, 317–320.

Johnstone, A. P. & Thorpe, R. (1992). *Immunochemistry in Practice*. Oxford, Blackwell Scientific Press.

Kohler, G. & Milstein, C. (1975). Continous cultures of fused cells producing antibodies of predefined specificity. *Nature*, **256**, 495–497.

Laemmli, U. K. (1970). Cleavage of structural proteins during assembly of the head of bacteriophage T4. *Nature*, **227**, 680–685.

Larsson, A. & Nilsson, B. O. (1988). Immunisation with nanogram quantities of nitrocellulose-bound antigen, electroblotted from sodium dodecyl sulphate-polyacrylamide gels. *Scandinavian Journal of Immunology*, **27**, 305–309.

Lo, M. M. S., Tsong, T. Y., Conrad, M. K., Strittmatter, S. M., Hester, L. D. & Synder, S. H. (1984). Monoclonal antibody production by receptor-mediated electrically induced cell fusion. *Nature*, **310**, 792–794.

Newman, R. A. (1987). Lymphoid receptors for transferin. *Methods in Enzymology*, **150**, 723–746.

Reading, C. (1983). Theory and method for immunisation in culture and monoclonal antibody production. *Journal of Immunological Methods*, **53**, 261–291.

Sjogren-Jansson, E. & Jeansson, S. (1985). Large scale production of monoclonal antibodies in dialysis tubing. *Journal of Immunological Methods*, **84**, 359–364.

Vaux, D., Tooze, J. & Fuller, S. (1990). Identification by anti-idiotype antibodies of an intracellular membrane protein that recognises a mammalian endoplasmic reticulum retention signal. *Nature*, **345**, 495–502.

3

Antigen–antibody interactions: how affinity and kinetics affect assay design and selection procedures

R. J. MORRIS

3.1 Introduction

Antibodies are used to detect antigens under a wide range of conditions. To ensure efficient interaction under the particular circumstances of any given assay, it is necessary to know something about the main parameters influencing the binding of antibody and antigen. For those undertaking the production of new mab such knowledge is even more important as the astute choice of screening methods will ensure the selection of hybridomas with the properties required by the investigator.

This chapter explains in simple terms those features of antibody binding which will affect how you use them. I cannot avoid making some use of equations and numbers but the points being made are intuitively obvious and should pose no problems, whatever your level of mathematical literacy.

3.2 What is affinity?

3.2.1 Association constant, K_a

Antibodies do not react irreversibly (covalently) with their antigen, rather, the antibody–antigen complex formed is able to dissociate. When antibody is added to antigen, two related reactions occur. The first (Figure 3.1a) is the association of Antigen (A) with antiBody (B) to form the Antigen–antiBody complex (AB). This reaction proceeds fastest at the very beginning when the concentration of A and B is at its highest and slows down until a stage is reached where AB dissociates as fast as it is formed. This point, where the reaction appears not to proceed at all (at the molecular level, association and dissociation is proceeding as before but the concentration of all the reactants is steady) is called equilibrium. The second reaction, already alluded to, is the dissociation of AB, which starts off slowly and builds to a maximum as AB accumulates (Figure 3.1b).

We are interested in how much complex, AB, is formed. The convention to

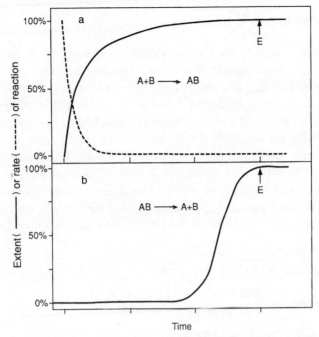

Figure 3.1. The association (a) and dissociation (b) of antigen and antibody as equilibrium (E with arrow) is approached for a reaction starting with equimolar antigen (A) and antibody (B). (—) Progress of the reaction (i.e. extent of formation of AB in (a) or its dissociation in (b)). (---) (a) shows the rate of the association reaction, equal to $k_{+1}[A][B]$. Thus when [A] and [B] are reduced 50%, the rate is 25% its initial value and when the reactants are 90% complexed, the rate is 1% its initial value. The rate at which equilibrium is approached is extremely slow when equimolar concentrations of reactants are used. The rate of the dissociation reaction is equal to $k_{-1}[AB]$ and so when plotted as a percentage is identical to the extent of the reaction.

denote concentration of AB is [AB]. The two reactions can be summarized as:

$$A + B \rightleftharpoons AB$$

The concentration of product formed [AB] must depend on [A] and [B] (because if you were to increase either or both of [A] and [B], more product would form). Thus:

$$[AB] = ?[A][B]$$

On what other factors does [AB] depend? There are a variety of other parameters: temperature, pH and ionic composition being the most important. We discuss their contribution below, but for the moment, let us take these as standard (e.g. deal with the reaction at 20 °C in isotonic salt at pH 7.4). Then the only other factor influencing [AB] is the intrinsic affinity of the antibody and antigen. This is a constant property of these reactants (at any given temperature, etc.) and is called K. Then:

$$[AB] = K[A][B]$$

$$\text{And so } K = \frac{[AB]}{[A][B]}$$

K, the affinity constant for the association of the antibody and antigen, is called the association constant. It is given a bewildering variety of names in the literature (e.g. K_a, K_0, K_1) and is best identified because its units are always the reciprocal of concentration (M^{-1} or 1 mole^{-1}). Note that [A], [B] and [AB] are the concentrations of these reactants at equilibrium, *not* the concentration initially added to the solution.

To appreciate what the association constant means, let us take an example. Suppose 10^{-8} M antigen (1 μg/ml for a MW 100 000 protein) is mixed with 10^{-8} M antibody (1.5 μg/ml for an IgG, the concentration present in about a 1:3 dilution of tissue culture supernatant) and at equilibrium the concentration of free antigen is 10^{-10} M. What is the affinity constant of the reaction?

Since $[A] = 10^{-10}$ M,

then $[AB] = [A]_{total} - [A]$

$$= (100 \times 10^{-10}) - (1 \times 10^{-10}) \text{ M}$$

$$= 99 \times 10^{-10} \text{ M}$$

and $[B] = [B]_{total} - [AB] = 10^{-10}$ M

$$K_a = \frac{99 \times 10^{-10}}{10^{-10} \times 10^{-10}} = 99 \times 10^{10} = 10^{12} \text{ M}^{-1}$$

Antibodies are regarded as having a high affinity if their K_a lies within the region 10^7 to 10^{12}; low affinity antibodies have K_as of 10^5 to 10^7 M^{-1}. To stress the obvious but easily forgotten, in surveying a list of K_as, the higher the number the higher the affinity.

3.2.2   Dissociation constant, K_d

The association constant is used less frequently than the dissociation constant, K_d, for a reason of simple convenience. The K_d is the affinity constant for the dissociation of AB (in other words, the association constant for the reverse reaction).

$$K_d = \frac{[A][B]}{[AB]} \left(= \frac{1}{K_a} \right)$$

Its units are M.

Its popularity as a measure of affinity stems from the practice of determining the 50% endpoint of a reaction. As equilibrium is approached asymptotically, determining the level of [A], [B] or [AB] at equilibrium is tedious and requires great accuracy. On the other hand, determining the concentration of antibody which complexes with half the antigen is much faster and can be done very accurately.

At 50% completion, $[A] = [AB]$ by definition,

therefore, $K_d = [B]$.

Thus, the dissociation constant is equal to the concentration of antibody required to keep the reaction at 50% completion. A high affinity antibody is one which requires a very low concentration (typically 10^{-7} to 10^{-12} M) of *free* antibody to keep the antibody–antigen complex associated; a low affinity antibody is one which requires a much higher concentration of *free* antibody to do this. In surveying a list of K_ds, the lower the number the higher the affinity.

Tissue culture supernatants should have 1–10 μg antibody/ml (1×10^{-8} to 7×10^{-8} M), ascitic fluid should have 1000-fold higher levels of antibody (1–10 mg/ml). (For comparison, the concentration of antibody in a really good polyclonal antiserum is usually about 1 mg/ml, although many are in the range of 0.1–1 mg/ml). The antibody concentration in different culture supernatant or ascitic fluid preparations varies over relatively narrow ranges, considering the great diversity of antibody affinities, and to a first approximation you can assume similarly produced supernatants or ascitic fluid have the same concentration of antibody. Thus, simply titrating different antibodies to the same antigen (or to different antigens present at the same concentration in the assay; 3.5.4) gives a reasonable approximation of their relative affinities, provided you have allowed the reactions to reach equilibrium. For more accurate determinations of affinity, see van Heyningen *et al.* (1983) and Roulston (1983).

3.3   Kinetics of association and dissociation

3.3.1   On rates, off rates and affinity

The foregoing has dealt with events at equilibrium, a state of affairs for which few scientists have the patience to wait. While 90% of a reaction can proceed in minutes or hours, it will take several times longer for the reaction to proceed from 90% to 99% completion and much longer still to advance to 99.9% completion as $[A]$ and $[B]$ diminish to extremely low levels. We almost always deal with short-term events, where the reaction is still some distance from equilibrium, and we should therefore consider the kinetics of antibody–antigen interactions.

The rate of formation of AB (provided temperature, etc. are kept constant) depends on $[A]$, $[B]$ and an intrinsic property of each antibody–antigen reaction, called the rate constant, denoted with a small k.

Rate of forward reaction (on rate) $= k_{+1}[A][B]$ M^{-1}s^{-1}

Rate of reverse reaction (off rate) $= k_{-1}[AB]$ s^{-1}

Here, $[A]$, $[B]$ and $[AB]$ (and so the forward and reverse rates) are constantly changing until equilibrium is reached (Figure 3.1). Then, by definition:

on rate = off rate

$$k_{+1}[A][B] = k_{-1}[AB]$$

$$\frac{k_{+1}}{k_{-1}} = \frac{[AB]}{[A][B]} = K_a$$

So the association constant is simply the ratio of the forward to reverse rate constants. It should immediately be apparent that reactions can have identical K_as but quite different rate constants. Thus:

1. $k_{+1} = 5 \times 10^7 \, M^{-1} s^{-1}$
   $k_{-1} = 1 \, s^{-1}, \qquad K_a = 5 \times 10^7 \, M^{-1}$
2. $k_{+1} = 5 \times 10^5 \, M^{-1} s^{-1}$
   $k_{-1} = 10^{-2} \, s^{-1}, \qquad K_a = 5 \times 10^7 \, M^{-1}$

The first reaction will proceed 100 times faster than the second, yet has the same affinity. More importantly for most applications, the product of the second reaction is much more stable than that of the first and so will better survive washing procedures, addition of secondary antibody, etc. When people say they want 'a high affinity antibody', they often mean they want one with a slow dissociation time, so the complex formed is stable; but if, for instance, they are doing immunoaffinity purification a fast on time (allowing fast column flow rates) may be more important.

Forward rate constants vary over the range 10^5 to 10^8, with most falling within the range of 10^6 to $10^7 \, M^{-1} s^{-1}$. This relatively restricted range reflects the fact that antibody–antigen interactions are very fast but cannot exceed the limit imposed by the need for molecules to diffuse to each other (approximately $10^{-8} \, M^{-1} s^{-1}$) (Pecht, 1982). In stressing the relative homogeneity of association rates, it should be remembered that even tenfold differences are highly significant in terms of laboratory time and experienced workers have been misled by not allowing sufficient time for certain antibodies to react (Mason & Williams, 1980). It has been known for many years that the affinity of antibodies increases during the course of immunization; it would appear that increase in the rate of association (as responding B cell clones compete for the immunogen) is a major component of this increase (Foote & Milstein, 1991). Prolonged immunization should favour fast associating antibodies.

Dissociation rate constants range from 6000 to $10^{-5} \, s^{-1}$ (see Table 1 in Pecht, 1982 or Table 2 in Karush, 1978) and it is their variation which predominantly produces the range in antibody affinity (Froese, 1968). As the dissociation rate depends on the concentration of only one reactant, the complex AB, there is a very simple relationship between k_{-1} and the time taken for the complex to 50% dissociate.

$$t_{\frac{1}{2}} \text{ dissociation} = 0.693/k_{-1} \, s$$

where 0.693 is $(-\ln 0.5)$ (50% dissociation, expressed as a ln as this linearly transforms the exponential curve of the rate).

3.3.2 Effect of increasing the antibody concentration

For any given antibody–antigen interaction, you can do comparatively little (3.5.2) about its affinity but its rate is very easily changed simply by changing the concentration of one of the reactants. Thus, if you mix 10^{-8} M antigen with 10^{-8} M antibody (here we assume an infinite affinity; the figures apply well for K_a of 10^{-10} M^{-1} or better) or with ten times more antibody, the rate of the reactions, and consequently the time taken to reach equilibrium, will be very different (Figure 3.2.). Given that most investigators use relatively short incubation times, their choice of optimum titre for any antibody almost certainly reflects its k_{+1} rather than K_a.

3.3.3 Effect of decreasing the antigen concentration

Suppose you have a reaction working well but for some reason the amount of antigen available is going to be reduced, say tenfold. If you increase the antibody concentration tenfold the reaction will proceed initially at the same rate and you can retain the same time of incubation. However, this is not always the best way to proceed. You cannot avoid having a tenfold lower signal. Whether you can detect this or not will depend on the sensitivity of your

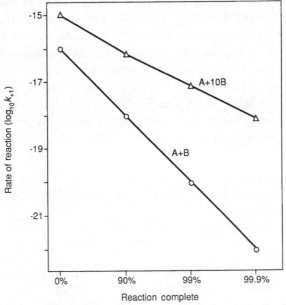

Figure 3.2. Increasing the antibody concentration tenfold maintains a much faster rate of reaction as it approaches equilibrium. In the lower curve (○), 10 nM antigen and 10 nM antibody have been mixed; in the upper curve (△) the initial antibody concentration has been increased to 100 nM. The K_d of the reaction is 10^{-10} M. Note both axes are to the log$_{10}$, the rate with higher antibody is nearly 1000-fold higher at 99.9% completion than the rate with equimolar antigen/antibody.

detection system, and your background. It is possible, using appropriate detection systems, to increase sensitivity enormously (see below), and the factor limiting detection most commonly is the level of background binding. It is impossible to generalize about background because what contributes to it will differ in different situations. However, in raising the antibody concentration tenfold you risk increasing the background substantially. You must remember that in the normal situation, most of your added antibody will be quickly bound by antigen and not available to contribute to the background; with ten times lower antigen and ten times higher antibody, the effective antibody concentration available for background binding will be about 1000-fold higher (Table 3.1).

Conversely, lowering the antibody concentration will almost always lower the background, giving you a cleaner detection system, with excellent signal to noise. You must, however, allow much longer for the reaction to proceed. Often an overnight or over-weekend incubation can be very effective. Note that this approach is only possible if the antigen is stable. A common source of instability is loss of antigen from the assay matrix, particularly when using paper (immunoblots, Dot blots). In such situations, shorter incubations are unavoidable.

These considerations about background and kinetics of reactions apply not only to monoclonals but also to the secondary (and any additional) antibodies where these are used. Indeed, they apply more so in most cases. Secondary antibodies are normally polyclonal and in the immune serum they are 10% or less of the total immunoglobulin. Where the secondary antibodies have been affinity-purified (i.e. adsorbed to and eluted from a column containing the relevant Ig), all the immunoglobulin is active antibody. A good preparation should give as clean a reaction as the primary mab. In most cases, however, the antibodies have not been affinity-purified before labelling and carry with them a major component of antibodies to the diverse pathogens encountered by the rabbit or sheep. These invariably contribute to the background.

Table 3.1. *When the concentration of antigen falls, maintaining the rate of the reaction by proportionately increasing the concentration of antibody produces a marked increase in concentration of free antibody*

	Equimolar antigen:antibody		Lower antigen/higher antibody	
	Concentration reactants		Concentration reactants	
	Added	At equilibrium	Added	At equilibrium
[AB]	0 nM	9.9 nM	0 nM	0.999 nM
[A]	10 nM	0.1 nM	1 nM	0.001 nM
[B]	10 nM	0.1 nM	100 nM	99.9 nM

Calculated for a reaction with $K_a = 10^{-10}$ M^{-1}.

3.4 Sensitivity, and its relationship to affinity

3.4.1 Inherent sensitivity of different detection systems

Each detection system used has an inherent sensitivity level. An assay such as immunodiffusion, which requires the investigator to see antigen–antibody complexes, is inherently less sensitive than one using radioactivity or enzymatic detection systems. At the moment, enzyme-based methods are the most sensitive (see Figure 3.3). Of these, alkaline phosphatase is more sensitive that horseradish peroxidase, partly because the latter enzyme generates highly reactive intermediates which decrease the enzymatic activity (and all antigenicity in its immediate microenvironment) within 10–20 min whereas alkaline phosphatase can be left reacting for 24–48 h. In certain immunohistochemical applications, however, the greater resolution obtainable with peroxidase substrates, and the clarity of a brown signal standing out from blue nuclear counterstains, makes peroxidase the label of choice. Immunofluorescence techniques can be as sensitive as peroxidase and have the advantage (in immunocytochemical applications) of giving a readily-photographed signal and being simpler than the enzymatic methods. ^{125}I-labelled antibodies, whose

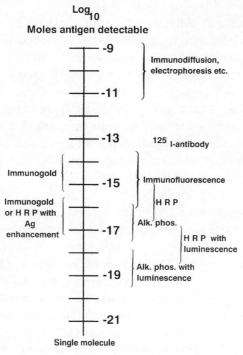

Figure 3.3. Approximate sensitivity of common detection systems. Calculated for a protein of MW 100 000 from the data in Ouchterlony & Nilsson (1986) for immunodiffusion. Provided by BioCell Research Laboratories (Cardiff) for immunogold and Amersham International for ^{125}I, horseradish peroxidase (HRP) and alkaline phosphatase (Alk. phos.)-labelled antibodies or from experience in my own laboratory.

binding can be quantified, and immunogold procedures also lie in this general area of sensitivity.

Any such list of relative sensitivity is complicated by the fact that techniques are constantly improving. The chemiluminescent techniques introduced within the past year, for instance, have greatly extended the peroxidase and alkaline phosphatase methods. Optical enhancement methods can enormously augment any of these detection systems in immunohistochemistry. Immunogold labelling, seen in the electron microscope, detects individual molecules of antigen; low energy emission cameras and computer signal-to-noise enhancement procedures can increase the sensitivity of fluorescence methods to the point where single molecules can be detected; and even techniques as old as dark-field illumination can extend the sensitivity of peroxidase in immunohistochemistry by about tenfold.

3.4.2 *The antibody component, and the biotin–avidin alternative*

The quality of the antibodies, and the skill with which they have been conjugated, stored and used, are also important determinants of sensitivity. Novices may benefit from a detailed account that I have given elsewhere (Morris, 1991).

The IgG molecule is dimeric and it should always be possible to get two molecules of any label onto it. In some cases, it is possible to get four to eight fluorescent or enzyme molecules onto a single antibody molecule without affecting its antigen binding or its background labelling. The most common 'label' applied to any primary antibody is the secondary antibody and again between two and eight molecules of anti-Ig antibody will bind for each primary antibody. The secondary antibody is, in its turn, labelled with some detection system and so the degree of augmentation of signal that can be achieved may vary from fourfold (two molecules of secondary antibody, each labelled with two detection molecules) to about 40-fold.

The ratio of secondary antibody which will bind to a primary antibody, and the level of labelling of the secondary antibody with the detection molecule, are variables which are not cited by commercial firms selling the antibodies nor by the vast majority of investigators who have tried to relate sensitivity to a particular detection system. This failure undermines a vast literature on the relative merits of direct and indirect conjugation systems and alternatives such as biotin–avidin systems. You are best advised to ask experienced investigators for advice because some relatively cheap and unpurified secondary antibodies out-perform the more expensive products of other firms.

Some commercially available biotin–avidin systems do perform superbly when properly used and merit specific comment. Avidin is a tetrameric (and so tetravalent) protein of MW 67 000 which binds the small, essential vitamin biotin with a high affinity ($K_d < 10^{-15}$ M, i.e. its binding is diffusion limited and virtually irreversible under physiological conditions) (Green, 1975). It functions in egg white as a bacteriostatic and can be used to form complexes with biotin-labelled antibodies and enzymes which rapidly build up a large collection of enzyme molecules around the primary antibody. Avidin (particularly when complexed to biotin) is extremely stable to heat and enzymatic digestion (although not to oxidizing agents, including strong light) and so is a robust laboratory reagent. Its disadvantage is that it is very basic (pI of 10) and tends to have high non-specific binding to tissues in immunohistochemistry. This can be avoided by using the bacterial homologue, streptavidin, which has an acid pI (although it does not appear to be as stable). The non-specific binding may also be avoided by using the minimum amount of avidin–biotinylated enzyme complex necessary, often much less (10–100-fold, if the antigen is in low abundance) than the manufacturer's recommendation, and allowing a longer incubation time (3.3.3; note that it is essential to maintain the ratio of the two components in forming the avidin–biotinylated enzyme complex, to ensure free biotin-binding sites are left for the biotinylated second antibody (Figure 3.4a). The amount of complex used, however, is at the discretion of the

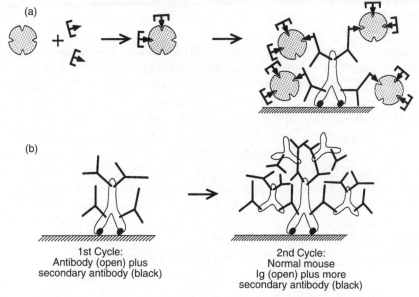

1st Cycle:
Antibody (open) plus
secondary antibody (black)

2nd Cycle:
Normal mouse
Ig (open) plus more
secondary antibody (black)

Figure 3.4. Use of multivalency to form complexes in detecting bound antibody. (a) Complex formation with avidin and biotinylated enzyme and antibody. The secondary antibody is shown as binding to two different epitopes, each present twice on the dimeric primary antibody, and itself having only one biotin group attached. In practice, the secondary antibody is likely to carry 2–8 biotin groups. (b) Cycles of addition of mouse immunoglobulin (Ig) (the first addition is the monoclonal; thereafter, normal mouse immunoglobulin suffices and can be added as a 0.1% solution of normal mouse serum) and anti-mouse immunoglobulin increase the number of molecules of detecting enzyme by a factor of n per cycle, where n = number of epitopes on the mouse immunoglobulin recognized by the secondary antibody. Each molecule of secondary antibody can be labelled with 2–8 molecules of enzyme, fluorochrome etc.

investigator). It is also worth noting that avidin complexes seem to have very little background binding to paper and are ideal for sensitive immunoblot or dot blot assays.

Finally, the multivalency of antibodies, or of avidin, can be used to build up large molecular complexes by repeated cycles of antibody addition. Provided the background binding is kept minimal, the antigen is stable and the process is not hurried, considerable augmentation can readily be achieved (Figure 3.4b).

3.4.3 Relation of sensitivity to affinity

Strictly speaking, these properties are unrelated. However, affinity is an important determinant of the background binding of an antibody. The lower the affinity, the higher the concentration of free antibody needed and it is this which binds non-specifically to the tissue, plastic, paper matrix, etc. If the assay system is one in which the antibody is labelled (immunohistochemistry, ELISA, immunoblot, etc.), this non-specific labelling will produce the background above which you need to detect specific signal. Thus the benefits of a very sensitive assay will not be realized unless the antibody is of high affinity. Where the labelled species is the antigen (e.g. radioimmunoassay), these considerations do not apply.

Suppose you have an assay which will detect (at 50% completion) 10^{-15} moles of antigen in an assay volume of 0.100 ml (10^{-4} l). If the antibody has a K_d of 10^{-12} M, you will need $10^{-12} \times 10^{-4} = 10^{-16}$ moles of free antibody to keep the reaction at 50% completion, plus a further 10^{-15} moles bound to the antigen. Thus, of 11×10^{-16} moles of antibody added, less than 10% is available to contribute to background binding. Without any washes or other measures to improve the signal-to-noise ratio, you already have quite a useful assay. Suppose, however, the antibody affinity is 10^{-9} M. Then you will require 10^{-13} moles of free antibody, and again 10^{-15} moles bound, and so 101×10^{-15} moles in total of which 99% is free and contributing to the background. Good washing procedures are now essential to reduce the noise, and if these are not effective, you have no alternative but to increase the signal (i.e. the amount of antigen) and so sacrifice sensitivity.

3.5   Other parameters affecting affinity

3.5.1 Multivalency

3.5.1.1 Solid-phase antigen binding to a single antibody

IgG antibodies are bivalent, IgM pentavalent. When binding to soluble, monovalent antigen, binding at each site is independent of binding at the other(s) (Figure 3.5a). However, when the antigen is on a solid matrix, binding

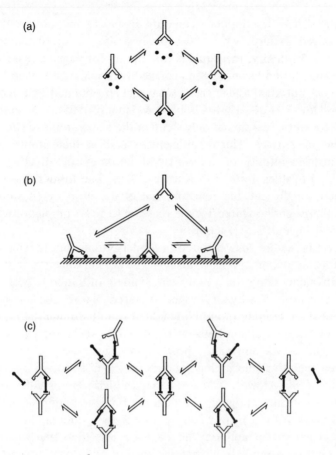

Figure 3.5. Situations in which multivalent binding increases affinity. (a) With soluble antigen and one antibody, binding of antigen to each site on an IgG antibody is independent of binding at the other site and there is no increase in affinity. (b) Immobilized, repeated antigen, on binding antibody at both sites on the IgG, will not allow it to dissociate until both sites release the antigen simultaneously, with a consequent increase in affinity. (c) The equilibria involved in partial dissociation (to release half the antigen) from a complex formed between an antigen with two epitopes, bound by the corresponding two antibodies. In this scheme, two more dissociation steps are required before the antigen is fully dissociated.

at each additional site dramatically increases the affinity of the reaction, to an extent that could readily change the specificity.

Suppose we have an epitope which is repeated, e.g. in a polymer such as the cytoskeletal proteins, or on paper or plastic in a Dot blot or ELISA assay. An IgG antibody, on binding at one site to such an epitope, is immediately immobilized near the adjacent epitopes so that the diffusion-limited element of its association reaction is vastly reduced. However, the real augmentation of affinity comes into effect once the antibody has bound at both its antigen-binding sites. Then, the antibody can only dissociate and move away from the epitope-covered surface, when *both* binding sites dissociate *simultaneously* (Figure 3.5b). In theory, this squares the affinity for each increase in valency; this full augmentation has not been achieved (as some monovalent binding will always occur) but 1000-fold increases have been obtained (see Karush, 1978 pp. 104 ff; Dower *et al.*, 1984*a*; Babbitt & Huang, 1985). IgM antibodies are restricted, for steric reasons, to only three of their potential five sites binding to epitopes on one surface. This is sufficient to increase their affinity 10^6-fold, so that an intrinsic affinity of $K_d = 10^{-4}$ M becomes an effective affinity of $K_d = 10^{-10}$ M (Tables 4 and 5 in Karush, 1978). The former K_d is so low we would not normally call the reaction that of an antibody (it would require 45 mg/ml of *free* antibody to drive the reaction to 50% completion), the second is a genuinely high affinity reaction.

This effect is readily demonstrated in model systems but to what extent is it likely to affect real immunological assays? The answer depends on the extent to which multivalent, rather than univalent, binding of antibody occurs. There is obviously a certain density of antigen required before bivalent binding can occur but also the amount of antibody added will determine the ratio of multi-to univalent binding. If antibody were added in sufficient excess, its initial binding would all be univalent; how rapidly this re-equilibrates to give a dominance of multivalent binding depends on the dissociation kinetics (Mason & Williams, 1980; Dower *et al.*, 1984*b*). In these two studies of antibody binding to cell surface antigens, the degree of augmentation of the affinity of binding of bivalent $F(ab')_2$ over Fab' was three to tenfold in most cases (Table 3.2). If the amount of antibody added were less than that of antigen, the binding would be essentially all multivalent (an additional advantage of long incubation times with low concentrations of antibody).

This enhancement of affinity with multivalency of binding could obviously lead to loss of specificity as unwanted cross-reactions occur. In the first wave of production of monoclonals, there were a number of reports of 'unexpected cross-reactivity' of antibodies, in each case with a polymer such as actin or tubulin, and IgM antibodies (e.g. Dulbecco *et al.*, 1981; Dales *et al.*, 1983). A similar effect has been reported with affinity-purified polyclonal IgG antibodies (Nigg *et al.*, 1982). Such a change in specificity is particularly possible in immunohistochemistry, where the natural density of an epitope in a tissue could vary greatly. For example, the hypothalamic neuropeptides, oxytocin and vasopressin, differ in two of nine amino acids. Antibodies to either are considered highly specific if their affinity for one peptide is 1000-fold higher than for the other (Berzofsky & Schechter, 1981), a property usually deter-mined by radioimmunoassay (i.e. with monovalent antigen in liquid phase). These peptides are packed at very high density into secretory vesicles *in vivo*, to which divalent antibody binding could readily occur on tissue sections. The consequent augmentation of affinity could, in principle, be sufficient to allow an anti-oxytocin antibody to bind to vasopressin and *vice versa*. The normal control, of pre-incubating the antibody with soluble peptides to show selective blocking of the reaction, would be misleading as this is a monovalent reaction. Specificity, however, would be restored simply by diluting the antibody further so that the concentration of *free* antibody was also reduced 10–1000-fold. Alternatively, monovalent Fab antibodies completely avoid this specificity trap.

This property is also important in the biochemical characterization and purification of immobilized (e.g. membrane-bound or cytoskeletal) antigens. An IgM antibody, of low intrinsic affinity, can be excellent for detecting such antigens on cells or sections; however, when the antigen is solubilized, and rendered monovalent, reactivity can disappear. This happens even with an IgG antibody (e.g. Williams *et al.*, 1977). It is frequently, and incorrectly, attributed to the antibodies concerned detecting 'conformationally determined epitopes', which are supposedly denatured by the detergents used. Such antibodies cannot be used for immunoprecipitation or immunoaffinity purification of their antigens. (Although the antibody is immobilized in immunoaffinity purification, the state of the antigen (here solubilized and monomeric) is the only determinant of affinity enhancement produced by multivalent binding.) As proteins are concentrated in discontinuous electrophoresis systems (Laemmli, 1970), reactivity with a fast dissociating (low affinity) antibody could well be recovered on an immunoblot where multivalent interactions with immobilized antigen are restored.

In producing mab, it is therefore important to match your screening assay to your eventual purpose. If you require them for solid phase assays, use a solid phase assay for screening. If you intend to use them for a liquid phase assay, screen with RIA or immunoprecipitation.

3.5.1.2 Two antibodies binding to different epitopes on a single antigen

The basic principle of affinity enhancement can also be brought to bear on soluble, monomeric antigens, if you have two antibodies directed to different epitopes on the molecule. Again, the antigen can only dissociate from the complex when both antibodies simultaneously dissociate (Figure 3.4c). Hence two low affinity antibodies combine to give a high-affinity reaction, a property which can be made use of in designing radioimmunoassays or immunoaffinity purification (Ehrlich *et al.*, 1982, 1983; Ehrlich & Moyle, 1983; Holmes & Parham, 1983). This property can also cause loss of immunoreactivity during hybridoma cloning, as a promising high affinity 'clone' is split into two of lesser affinity (Hughes-Jones *et al.*, 1984).

This situation, where multiple antibodies bind to different epitopes on the same molecule, is that found with any conventional antiserum to protein antigens (even to quite small proteins such as lysozyme and myoglobin (Atassi & Lee, 1978; Harper *et al.*, 1987)). The high affinity (and therefore specificity) of many polyclonal antibodies is achieved by the complex interaction of individual antibodies of lower intrinsic affinity (Sperling *et al.*, 1983).

3.5.2   Temperature and chemical crosslinking

In the few cases where it has been studied, raising the temperature of the antibody–antigen interaction from 4 °C to 24 °C causes a twofold increase in the rate of association and tenfold or more increase in the rate of dissociation, resulting in an overall drop in affinity of five to tenfold (Mason & Williams, 1980). The reason for this lies in the balance of hydrophilic (temperature sensitive) to hydrophobic (temperature insensitive) interactions involved in antibody binding (Berzofsky & Berkower, 1984) and is likely to be fairly general. In theory it is better to carry out your incubations at 4 °C. In practice, the loss in affinity with temperature is often insignificant (e.g. a change from a K_d of 10^{-12} to 10^{-11} M will be largely academic). The shorter incubations needed at room temperature or 37 °C often are more convenient than, and as sensitive as, longer incubations in the cold. The beneficial effect of higher temperature is on the association reaction and so it often pays to set up and leave the incubation at room temperature for some hours, transfer it to 4 °C overnight and carry out subsequent washes and incubations for longer times at the lower temperature (this has been a strategy in immunochemistry for many years).

Temperature is a natural way to influence both association and dissociation rates. There is another way to influence dissociation rates in assays like immunoblotting, dot blots, ELISAs and immunohistochemistry and that is to cheat by fixing the primary antibody to the antigen (1% paraformaldehyde for 5 min at room temperature, followed by 2% defatted milk powder in PBS to block the reaction). In fact the conditions for cross-linking the components of soluble multimolecular complexes in solution using low concentrations of glutaraldehyde (without incorporating the monomeric species) have been determined with great accuracy (see Craig, 1988) and could be applied to fast-dissociating antibody–antigen complexes in solution.

3.5.3   pH and ionic strength

pH has a marked effect on antibody–antigen interactions. I have seen a strong polyclonal antibody completely dissociate at pH 5.0, as does a monoclonal (to a different antigen) which I commonly use. It is worth noting that the pH optimum for horseradish peroxidase is 5.2, although this can be extended to pH 7 by including immidazole at 10–25 mM in the buffer. Alkaline (pH 11) buffers can be effectively used to dissociate antigen from an immunoaffinity column.

The antibody–antigen interaction, on the other hand, is relatively insensitive to ionic strength although background binding is likely to be affected by it.

Thus hydrophobic interactions (e.g. with plastic) will be greater at high ionic strength whereas ionic interactions will dominate at low ionic strength.

3.5.4 Amount of antigen

This will not in any way affect the affinity of the reaction but it is often the main determinant of the concentration of antibody used. Affinity determines the concentration of *free* antibody needed to drive the reaction whereas most of the added antibody is bound to antigen. I illustrate this, in Table 3.2, for three antibodies to rat thymocyte surface glycoproteins (Mason & Williams, 1980) and two antibodies to class I histocompatibility antigens on mouse spleen cells (Dower *et al.*, 1984*b*). Of the former, values for both the Fab' (i.e. monovalent) and F(ab')$_2$ (i.e. divalent, equivalent to IgG) fragments of the OX7 anti-Thy-1.1 antibody are shown, along with the F(ab')$_2$ fragments of W3/13 and W3/25 antibodies to CD43 and CD4, respectively. (F(ab')$_2$ fragments or their Fab' monovalent derivatives are used for such exact work to avoid additional antibody binding through the Fc receptor (Jensenius & Williams, 1974)). For the anti-histocompatibility antibodies, data for both the Fab' and F(ab')$_2$ are available. I have assumed a reaction volume of 0.1 ml, containing 10^6 thymocytes or splenocytes, and calculated for each the concentration of antibody which needs to be added to drive the reaction to 50% completion. Despite the more than 10^4-fold range in antibody affinities

Table 3.2. *It is the amount of antigen (A), not the affinity of the antibody (B), that most commonly determines the concentration of antibody used: data calculated for monoclonal antibodies to lymphocyte surface antigens*

					at 50% reaction		
Antigen	Antibody	$K_d{}^a$	No. per cell[b]	$[A]_{total}{}^a$	$[AB]^a$ +	$[B]^a$	= $[B]_{total}{}^a$
Thy-1	OX7 Fab'	3.7	105	169	85 +	3.7	= 89
	OX7 F(ab')$_2$	0.01	105	169	85 +	0.01	= 85
CD43	W3/13	4.4	3.75	6	3 +	4.4	= 7
CD4	W3/25	0.16	1.5	2.4	1.2 +	0.16	= 1
H-2K	36-7 Fab'	110	5	8	4	+ 110	= 114
	36-7 F(ab')$_2$	37.5	5	8	4	+ 37.5	= 42
H-2D	27-11 Fab'	140	11	18	9	+ 140	− 149
	27-11 F(ab')$_2$	27	11	18	9	+ 27	= 36

$^a 10^{-10}$ M

[b] $\times\ 10^4$ = the number of antigenic sites per cell

represented, the concentration of antibody required (far right column) is determined by the amount of antigen, which varies over a 70-fold range. Thy-1 is an unusually abundant glycoprotein on the surface of thymocytes but many viral antigens, cytoskeletal and secretory products can be present at higher levels within cells.

It is a common, but erroneous, oversimplification to assume that an antibody that must be used at a high concentration must therefore be of low affinity; it may simply be that its antigen is abundant. You need to know the concentration of *free*, not total, antibody to determine affinity.

3.6   The nature of a protein epitope and its influence on antibody binding

3.6.1   *What defines an epitope?*

Approximately five to eight amino acids are usually critically involved in determining an epitope although a further ten amino acids interact with the antigen-binding site of the antibody (Crumpton, 1974; Amit *et al.*, 1986; van Regenmortel *et al.*, 1988). If antibodies had equal access to all chemical moieties on a protein, the dominant antigenic determinants would probably be hydrophobic, as experience with small haptens shows the hydrophobic ones generally elicit higher affinity antibodies (Karush, 1978). The hydrophobic groups on a protein cluster internally to minimize exposure to water and hence to an antibody trying to gain access to them. The surfaces of proteins are covered with hydrophilic groups and it is from among these that the major epitopes are formed (Crumpton, 1974; Berzofsky, 1985; Novotny *et al.*, 1987; Getzoff *et al.*, 1988). The inherent predilection for hydrophobic groups remains, however, and single 'buried' hydrophobic residues (particularly proline, phenylalanine and leucine), within an otherwise exposed hydrophilic sequence, are often involved in strong epitopes (Getzoff *et al.*, 1988).

All antigenic determinants are conformationally dependent (Crumpton, 1974). Any part of the polypeptide chain exposed on the surface of a protein flips rapidly through a number of different conformational variants (the higher the temperature, the faster the flipping). One of these forms will be recognized by the antibody, which will bind and 'freeze' that preferred conformation. This was beautifully shown by Crumpton (1966) who made an antibody to myoglobin from which the haem group had been removed. Under physiological conditions, the association of haem with the myoglobin is reversible, so that a minute proportion of the protein exists in the haem-free condition. When the antibody to haem-free myoglobin was added to a solution of normal, haem-containing myoglobin, a white haem-free protein precipitate quickly formed, leaving the brown haem in the supernatant. It should be noted that the association rates of antibodies to proteins are distinctly lower than those for small haptens (Karush, 1978; Mason & Williams, 1986), which in general have much simpler conformational choices, presumably reflecting the complex contribution of protein conformation in binding to the former. (This description of antibody–antigen binding is somewhat oversimplified; should you read the primary literature you will find binding occurs in multiple stages as both antibody and antigen adjust to each other's presence, rather like a hand (the primary determinant of conformation, and so the antibody) going into a silk glove.)

Some parts of proteins are conformationally constrained and can adopt only a few, or perhaps a unique, conformation. Thus regions around disulphide bonds, or beta-pleated sheets, are relatively rigid. Antibodies have a proportionately lower chance of recognizing one of these limited conformational forms and these regions are less likely to function as immunological epitopes (Tainer *et al.*, 1985). If, however, you are lucky enough to have an antibody that does recognize a constrained conformation, it will almost certainly have a fast on-time as the epitope spends most or all of its time in the required conformation (e.g. small haptens or the small rigid snake toxins (Novotny *et al.*, 1987); you can put your hand into a stiff leather glove, of the right size, faster than you can slip on a silk glove).

Most epitopes are a sequential run of amino acids along the polypeptide chain (Crumpton, 1974; Atassi & Lee, 1978; van Regenmortel *et al.*, 1988). When a protein is denatured, and the denaturing solvent then removed (e.g. in immunoblotting), the protein is most unlikely to fully regain its original conformation. Every part of the polypeptide chain, however, will resume flopping in and out of a multitude of conformations, among which ones identical to that defining the epitope on the native molecule are likely to recur. This is why immunoblotting works. If you have an antibody which recognizes the native protein, you would be well advised not to reduce it before electrophoresis. Intact disulphide bonds will preserve gross structure and so increase the probability that when the denaturant is removed the required conformation will be regained. Denaturation, especially if combined with reduction, can expose new epitopes not previously accessible to antibodies (Crumpton, 1974). This is useful if you find anti-peptide antibodies will not react with the native protein. Antibodies characterized as 'specific' for one protein, however, have been found to react with an epitope exposed by reduction on a different protein (Crumpton, 1974; Walter & Werchau, 1982).

There are some epitopes which are composed of amino acids drawn from different parts of the polypeptide chain that are brought together by the conformational folds of the protein. The classical case is the three epitopes of lysozyme, one of which, for instance, consists of residues Lys33, Phe34, Arg114, Asn113 and Lys116. Atassi & Lee (1978) proved that these were the residues involved by synthesizing the peptide Lys-Phe-Gly-Arg-Asn-Lys, where the Gly residue gave approximately the correct spacing (deduced from the crystallographic structure) between the active residues. This peptide inhibited antibody from binding to the epitope. Such epitopes are unlikely to be recovered after full denaturation of the protein.

3.6.2   Protein recognition by anti-peptide antibodies

The generation and use of anti-peptide antibodies, often to identify a protein whose sequence has been determined by molecular biological methods, is one of the more common endeavours of recent biomolecular research. Such antibodies will potentially include some which recognize the native protein, although others recognize conformations which are not accessible, or not present, in the native protein. There is therefore a general preference for producing polyclonal (rabbit) antibodies to peptides as these are more likely to include reactive clones. I include here some general notes, applicable to both monoclonal and polyclonal antibodies, to guide further reading. The short book of van Regenmortel *et al.* (1988) on this subject can be highly recommended.

To raise the antibodies, you need to choose a peptide and couple it to a protein carrier. If structural data are available, choose a peptide which is exposed on the surface (preferably a convex 'corner') with hydrophilic sequences, although a single hydrophobic residue (especially Pro, Phe and Leu) will help (see Getzoff *et al.*, 1988). Couple the peptide to the carrier by a single, defined linkage, preferably at the amino or carboxy terminals. Two exceptions come to mind. If the peptide has a Cys residue involved in disulphide bonding, then couple it thus to the carrier. If you intend to use the antibody to detect antigen in aldehyde-fixed tissue, then use aldehydes to couple the peptide to the carrier (3.6.3). In reacting protein with anti-peptide antibodies you will promote conformational flexibility by using higher temperatures and partial denaturation (e.g. reduction of disulphide bonds).

3.6.3   Antibodies to small molecules (neurotransmitters, amines, etc.)

Again, antibodies can only be made to such small molecules by first coupling them to a protein carrier. In many cases (e.g. serotonin; Milstein *et al.*, 1983; Flurkey *et al.*, 1985) such molecules are so small that the antibodies elicited will react not with the free, native molecule but with the conjugated version (and in some cases, with the conjugating linkage and not with serotonin at all). This can be put to good use if the antibodies are wanted for immunohistochemistry, where the antigen itself will have to be fixed to proteins in the tissue. Provided the method of conjugation used to produce the immunogen is the same as that used in fixing the tissue, high affinity, specific reagents can be produced (Milstein *et al.*, 1983; Burgeon *et al.*, 1991; Meyer *et al.*, 1991). If what is required is an antibody which recognizes the unconjugated molecule (e.g. in RIA), the coupling procedure, and stability of the coupled molecule, have to be examined very carefully (Flurkey *et al.*, 1985; Hayes, 1990).

3.6.4   Recognizing fixed antigens

Fixation is the process of immobilizing an antigen at its biological location in a tissue so that subsequent addition of a labelled antibody can be used to identify the location of the molecule. There are two ways of fixing molecules. One is precipitation, using organic solvents (e.g. dry acetone, acetic alcohol) or acids (trichloroacetic or picric acids); the other is chemical crosslinkage, almost invariably carried out with aldehydes.

The precipitating methods have the advantage that they do not change the antigen and so reactivity with the antibodies remains maximal. To react with the antibody, however, the section must be restored to physiological, non-precipitating conditions and many antigens redissolve during this step and float away (with their antibody attached). This approach is therefore best for antigens which have an inherent tendency to be insoluble (cytoskeletal or extracellular matrix components, membrane-bound molecules, etc.) and at its worst with soluble antigens (cytoplasmic proteins, small molecules normally found in cellular or extracellular fluids, etc.). This approach also does not preserve cytoarchitecture very well and cannot be used for electron microscopic observation.

The commonly used aldehydes are glutaraldehyde and paraformaldehyde. Curiously, the chemistry of their interaction with proteins under the conditions used for tissue fixation remains a puzzle (Johnson, 1987; Quicho, 1976) although the main group on the protein which reacts is the -NH_2 group on the lysine side chain (see Quicho, 1976; Morris & Barber, 1983; Johnson, 1987; Cheung *et al.*, 1990). This is also true for the periodate-lysine-paraformaldehyde fixative (Hixson *et al.*, 1981) despite the hopes of its designers that it would crosslink carbohydrates (McClean & Nakane, 1974). Thus chemical fixation puts epitopes containing Lys residues directly at risk and there is a stabilization of conformation which will further restrict immunoreactivity more generally. The best way around this problem is to screen antibodies using fixed antigen. Where the antigen is a small molecule, using aldehyde fixation to couple it to a carrier during the initial immunization is advantageous (3.6.3) and immunohistochemistry of such small molecules on well-fixed tissue has been relatively simple. If you are dealing with a protein, fixation prior to immunization may not be the answer, as it can impede proteolytic processing by antigen-presenting cells, leaving the fixed protein poorly immunogenic. There is little you can do to improve the immunoreactivity of the tissue once it is fixed, although higher temperatures of incubation, and limited proteolysis (e.g. 0.1% trypsin for several minutes at room temperature) to 'nick' the proteins and re-introduce a degree of conformational flexibility, are worth trying.

3.7 So what is antibody specificity?

Antibodies, as molecular reagents, have unparalleled specificity. In Table 3.3 some examples from the classic book by Pressman & Grossberg (1968) are reproduced, which summarizes many years of study on the specificity of reactions with haptens. No other research tool could so simply distinguish such similar chemical forms in complex mixtures like tissue or biological fluid. The sensitivity of antibodies to protein conformation, in addition to sequence (see examples in Crumpton, 1974), further underlines their exquisite specificity. Undoubtedly this could be improved on even further if antibody–antigen complexes were (by analogy to gene probes) washed under increasingly more stringent conditions during the assay (e.g. at higher temperatures or lower pH).

No antibody has absolute specificity, in the sense that it will react with only one epitope, whatever the conditions; an antibody can always react to some extent with chemically similar epitopes. Its affinity for its proper epitope, however, is usually around 10^3 times greater than its affinity for closely related epitopes (Table 3.3). This means that in practice the choice of an appropriate dilution of antibody will ensure complete specificity in most assays. We can illustrate this by returning to the example given in 3.4.3. There we considered the case of an antibody with a K_d of 10^{-12} M detecting 2×10^{-15} moles of antigen, in a reaction mixture of 10^{-4} l. For 50% completion, 1×10^{-15} moles plus 0.1×10^{-15} moles of antibody need to be added to bind 50% of the antigen and maintain a concentration of 10^{-12} M free antibody, respectively. Now suppose that the antibody also detects a second epitope, present in equal quantities, but detected with 10^3-fold lower affinity, i.e. with a K_d of 10^{-9} M. Let us call this second epitope A' and the epitope recognized with high affinity, A. In order to recognize 50% of A', you need to add 1×10^{-15} moles plus 10^{-13} moles of antibody, totalling 101×10^{-15} moles of antibody. Thus if you

Table 3.3. *Antibody specificity shown in two anti-hapten systems*

A. Relative affinity of anti-maleanilate antibodies for various related haptens

1.00

0.00

0.016

0.004

B. Relative affinity of anti-3-nitro-5-carboxybenzene antibodies for various related haptens

1.00

0.0013

0.0005

0.0001

0.013

0.0001

add 100 times more antibody than you need to detect A, you will detect 50% of A'. Do you need to dilute the antibody 100-fold for it to become specific for A? Consider what happens with a tenfold dilution, i.e. 10×10^{-15} moles of antibody are added. This is a 100-fold excess over that needed to bind 50% of A, and so this epitope is saturated with antibody, removing 2×10^{-15} moles of the added antibody. The remaining 8×10^{-15} moles are sufficient to saturate only a few percent of A'; unless you are using an exceptional assay which detects such low levels of binding above the high levels of binding to A, you will miss this altogether. Thus in practice, you do not have to dilute your antibody very much to make it specific.

It is unwise to assume that specificity demonstrated in one situation applies to all others. Where possible, use complementary methods (e.g. HPLC (high performance liquid chromatography) or electrophoretic mobility) to demonstrate that the specificity you require actually exists in your system.

3.8   Summary

In optimizing an antibody–antigen interaction, it is frequently necessary to balance opposing requirements. If these have been considered and incorporated into the choice and design of the screening assays, the antibodies selected will be better suited to your requirements. The main variables you can alter, and the conditions under which you might opt for them, are as follows.

> *Higher temperatures* (20–45 °C): to maximize conformational flexibility of the antigen (e.g. with anti-peptide antibodies, or when using chemically-fixed tissue); whenever short incubation times are desirable (e.g. antigen unstable or washes free of assay matrix); in immuno-affinity chromatography (provided the dissociation rate is slow enough, and antigen stable), to maximise both the association and dissociation rates.
>
> *Lower temperatures* (4 °C): to maximize stability of the antibody–antigen complex for quick-dissociating antibodies.
>
> *Longer incubation times*: to enable lower antibody concentrations to be used, usually giving a better signal-to-noise (e.g. for very sensitive assays or where a clean background is desirable, as in immunohisto-chemistry).
>
> *Solid matrix* (antigen immobilized on paper, plastic, cell surface or tissue sections): usually adopted for ease of assay, if the antigen density is high enough to enable multivalent binding it will also augment affinity.
>
> *Liquid phase assay*: use for screening when you want an antibody to bind antigen in liquid phase (RIA (radioimmunoassay), immunoprecipitation, immunoaffinity purification).
>
> *Multiple antibodies to different epitopes*: give greatly enhanced affinity for soluble antigen.

Dilution of antibody: titrate your antibody in your assay; do not use it in excess. Remember the dilution you *add* to an assay will usually reflect the amount of antigen present, only the dilution *free* after the reaction has proceeded (e.g. to 50%) reflects the affinity; higher antibody concentrations will increase the rate of reaction but also the background and the opportunity for unwanted, low-affinity cross-reactions.

3.9   References

Amit, A. G., Mariuzza, R. A., Phillips, S. E. V. & Poljak, R. J. (1986). Three-dimensional structure of an antigen–antibody complex at 2.8 A resolution. *Science*, **233**, 747–753.

Atassi, M. Z. & Lee, C. L. (1978). The precise and entire antigenic structure of native lysozyme. *Biochemical Journal*, **171**, 429–434.

Babbitt, B. P. & Huang, L. (1985). Effects of valency on thermodynamic parameters of specific membrane interactions. *Biochemistry*, **24**, 2186–2194.

Berzofsky, J. A. (1985). Intrinsic and extrinsic factors in protein antigenic structure. *Science*, **229**, 932–940.

Berzofsky, J. A. & Berkower, I. J. (1984). Antibody–antigen interaction. In *Fundamental Immunology*, ed. W. E. Paul, pp. 595–644. New York, Raven Press.

Berzofsky, J. A. & Schechter, A. N. (1981). The concepts of crossreactivity and specificity in immunology. *Molecular Immunology*, **18**, 751–763.

Burgeon, E., Chapleur, M., Schoenen, J., Remicheus, D., Legros, J. J., Greenan, V. & Robert, R. (1991) Monoclonal antibodies to oxytocin: production and characterization. *Neuroimmunology*, **31**, 235–244.

Cheung, D. T., Tong, D., Perelman, N., Ertl, D. & Nimni, M. E. (1990). Mechanism of crosslinking of proteins by glutaraldehyde. IV. *In vitro* and *in vivo* stability of a crosslinked collagen matrix. *Connective Tissue Research* **25**, 27–34.

Craig, W. S. (1988). Determination of quaternary structure of an active enzyme using chemical cross-linking with glutaraldehyde. *Methods in Enzymology*, **156**, 333–345.

Crumpton, M. J. (1966). Conformational changes in sperm whale metmyoglobin due to combination with antibodies to apomyoglobin. *Biochemical Journal*, **100**, 223–232.

Crumpton, M. J. (1974). Protein antigens: the molecular basis of antigenicity and immunogenicity. In *The Antigens*, Vol. II, ed. M. Sela, pp. 1–79. New York, Academic Press.

Dales, S., Fujinami, R. S. & Oldstone, M. B. A. (1983). Serological relatedness between Thy-1.2 and actin revealed by monoclonal antibody. *Journal of Immunology*, **131**, 1332–1338.

Dower, S. K., Ozato, K. & Segal, D. M. (1984*a*). The interaction of monoclonal antibodies with MHC class I antigens on mouse spleen cells. I. Analysis of the mechanism of binding. *Journal of Immunology*, **132**, 751–759.

Dower, S. K., Titus, J. A. & Segal, D. M. (1984*b*). The binding of multivalent ligands to cell surface receptors. In *Cell Surface Dynamics*, ed. A. Perelson, pp. 277–328. New York, Marcel Dekker.

Dulbecco, R., Unger, M., Bologna, M., Battifor, H., Syka, P. & Okada, S. (1981). Cross-reactivity between Thy-1 and a component of intermediate filaments demonstrated using a monoclonal antibody. *Nature*, **292**, 772–774.

Ehrlich, P. H. & Moyle, W. R. (1983). Cooperative immunoassays: ultrasensitive assays with mixed monoclonal antibodies. *Science*, **221**, 279–281.

Ehrlich, P. H., Moyle, W. R. & Moustafa, Z. A. (1983). Further characterisation of cooperative interactions of monoclonal antibodies. *Journal of Immunology*, **131**, 1906–1912.

Ehrlich, P. H., Moyle, W. R., Moustafa, Z. A. & Canfield, R. E. (1982). Mixing two monoclonal antibodies yields enhanced affinity for antigen. *Journal of Immunology*, **128**, 2709–2713.

Flurkey, K., Bolger, M. B. & Linthicum, D. S. (1985). Preparation and characterisation of antisera and monoclonal antibodies to serotonergic and dopaminergic ligands. *Journal of Neuroimmunology*, **8**, 115–127.

Foote, J. & Milstein, C. (1991). Kinetic maturation of an immune response. *Nature*, **352**, 530–532.

Froese, A. (1968). Kinetic and equilibrium studies on 2,4 dinitrophenyl hapten-antibody systems. *Immunochemistry*, **5**, 253–264.

Getzoff, E. D., Tainer, J. A., Lerner, R. A. & Geysen, H. M. (1988). The chemistry and mechanism of antibody binding to protein antigens. *Advances in Immunology*, **43**, 1–98.

Green, N. M. (1975). Avidin. *Advances in Protein Chemistry*, **29**, 85–133.

Harper, M., Lema, F., Boulot, G. & Poljak, R. J. (1987). Antigen specificity and cross-reactivity of monoclonal anti-lysozyme antibodies. *Molecular Immunology*, **24**, 97–108.

Hayes, E. C. (1990). Preparation of antibodies directed against leukotrienes. *Methods in Enzymology*, **187**, 116–124.

Hixson, D. C., Yep, J. N., Glenney, J. K., Hayes, T. & Walborg, E. F. (1981). Evaluation of periodate/lysine/paraformaldehyde fixation as a method for cross-linking plasma membrane glycoproteins. *Journal of Histochemistry and Cytochemistry*, **29**, 561–566.

Holmes, N. J. & Parham, P. (1983). Enhancement of monoclonal antibodies against HLA-A2 is due to antibody bivalency. *Journal of Biological Chemistry*, **258**, 1580–1586.

Hughes-Jones, N. C., Gorick, B. D., Miller, N. G. A. & Howard, J. C. (1984). IgG pair formation on one antigenic molecule is the main mechanism of synergy between antibodies in complement-mediated lysis. *European Journal of Immunology*, **14**, 974–978.

Jensenius, J. C. & Williams, A. F. (1974). The binding of anti-immunoglobulin antibodies to rat thymocytes and thoracic duct lymphocytes. *European Journal of Immunology*, **4**, 91–97.

Johnson, T. J. (1987). Glutaraldehyde fixation chemistry: oxygen-consuming reactions. *European Journal of Cell Biology*, **45**, 160–169.

Karush, F. (1978). The affinity of antibody: range, variability and the role of multivalence. In *Comprehensive Immunology. Immunoglobulins*, vol. 5, ed. G. W. Litman & R. A. Good, pp. 85–116. New York, Plenum Medical Book Company.

Laemmli, U. K. (1970). Cleavage of structural proteins during the assembly of bacteriophage T4. *Nature*, **227**, 680–681.

McClean, I. W. & Nakane, P. W. (1974). Periodate-lysine-paraformaldehyde fixative, a new fixative for immunoelectron microscopy. *Journal of Histochemistry and Cytochemistry*, **22**, 1077–1083.

Mason, D. W. & Williams, A. F. (1980). The kinetics of antibody binding to membrane antigens in solution and at the cell surface. *Biochemical Journal*, **187**, 1–20.

Mason, D. W. & Williams, A. F. (1986). Kinetics of antibody reactions and the analysis of cell surface antigens. In *Handbook of Experimental Immunology*, 4th edn, vol. 1, ed. D. M. Wier, L. A. Herzenberg, C. Blackwell & L. A. Herzenberg, Chap. 38. Oxford, Blackwell Scientific Publications.

Meyer, K. H., Behringer, D. M. & Veh, R. W. (1991). Antibodies against neuroactive amino acids and neuropeptides. I. A new two-step procedure for their conjugation to carrier proteins and the production of an anti-Met-enkephalin antibody with glutaraldehyde-fixed tissues. *Journal of Histochemistry and Cytochemistry*, **39**, 749–760.

Milstein, C., Wright, B. & Cuello, A. C. (1983). The discrepancy between the cross-reactivity of a monoclonal antibody to serotonin and its immunohistochemical specificity. *Molecular Immunology*, **20**, 113–123.

Morris, R. J. (1991). Immunoperoxidase staining of gene products in cultured cells using monoclonal antibodies. In *Methods in Molecular Biology. Gene Transfer and Expression Protocols*, vol. 7, ed. E. J. Murray, pp. 339–359. Clifton, N. J., Humana Press Inc.

Morris, R. J. & Barber, P. C. (1983). Fixation of Thy-1 in nervous tissue for immuno-histochemistry: a quantitative assessment of the effect of different fixation conditions upon retention of antigenicity and the cross-linking of Thy-1. *Journal of Histochemistry and Cytochemistry*, **27**, 263–274.

Nigg, E. A., Walter, G. & Singer, S. J. (1982). On the nature of crossreactions observed with antibodies directed to defined epitopes. *Proceedings of the National Academy of Sciences USA*, **79**, 5939–5943.

Novotny, J., Handschumacher, M. & Bruccoleri, R. E. (1987). Protein antigenicity: a static surface property. *Immunology Today*, **8**, 26–31.

Ouchterlony, O. & Nilsson, L. A. (1986). Immunodiffusion and immunoelectro-phoresis. In *Handbook of Experimental Immunology*, 4th edn, vol. 1, ed. D. M. Wier, L. A. Herzenberg, C. Blackwell & L. A. Herzenberg, Chap. 32. Oxford, Blackwell Scientific Publications.

Pecht, I. (1982). Dynamic aspects of antibody function. In *The Antigens*, vol. IV, ed. M. Sela, pp. 1–69. New York, Academic Press.

Pressman, D. & Grossberg, A. L. (1968). *The Structural Basis of Antibody Specificity*. New York, W. A. Benjamin Inc.

Quicho, F. A. (1976). Immobilised proteins in single crystals. *Methods in Enzymology*, **44**, 546–558.

Roulston, J. E. (1983). Estimation of the equilibrium constant for an antibody using data derived from an antiserum dilution curve. *Journal of Immunological Methods*, **63**, 133–138.

Sperling, R., Francus, T. and Siskind, G. W. (1983). Degeneracy of antibody specificity. *Journal of Immunology*, **131**, 882–885.

Tainer, J. A., Getzoff, E. D., Paterson, Y., Olson, A. J. & Lerner, R. A. (1985). The atomic mobility component of protein antigenicity. *Annual Review of Immunology*, **3**, 501–535.

Van Heyningen, V., Brock, D. J. H. & van Heyningen, S. (1983). A simple method for ranking the affinities of monoclonal antibodies. *Journal of Immunological Methods* **62**, 147–153.

Van Regenmortel, M. H. V., Briand, J. P., Muller, S. & Plaue, S. (1988). *Synthetic Polypeptides as Antigens*. Amsterdam, Elsevier.

Walter, G. & Werchau, H. (1982). Cross-reactivity of antibodies against synthetic peptides. *Journal of Cellular Biochemistry*, **19**, 119–125.

Williams, A. F., Barclay, A. N., Letarte-Muirhead, M. & Morris, R. J. (1977). Rat Thy-1 antigens from thymus and brain: their tissue distribution, purification and chemical composition. *Cold Spring Harbor Symposia on Quantitative Biology*, **41**, 51–61.

4

Production and characterization of synthetic peptide-derived antibodies

K. M. PRICE

4.1 Introduction

Synthetic peptides are used extensively in life science research for a great variety of purposes. This review will attempt to cover just two applications: monoclonal antibody production and the subsequent analysis of their epitopes.

The use of synthetic peptides as immunogens has proved to be an important route for the production of antibodies to previously uncharacterized proteins. Once the nucleotide sequence of a gene has been determined the amino acid sequence for any protein encoded by that gene may be predicted. Peptides selected from such a sequence may then be used to raise antibodies that may prove cross-reactive with the native protein. Many antibodies have been raised for the first time using this approach (Lerner, 1982; Sutcliffe *et al.*, 1983; Shinnick *et al.*, 1983; Walter & Dolittle, 1983).

The synthetic peptide approach to antibody production has several advantages over other methods. For example, the antibodies may be raised to

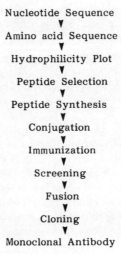

Figure 4.1. Summary of the peptide approach to antibody production.

specific areas of a protein in order to probe biochemical function or to block normal biological activity. It is also possible to raise antibodies to peptides which have sequences that are conserved between members of a family of closely-related proteins so as to produce pan-reactive reagents. Conversely, antibodies specific to individual members of protein families may be generated by careful selection of unique amino acid sequences. A summary of the approach is shown in Figure 4.1.

Peptides, as fragments of antigens, can also be used to precisely define or map the epitope recognized by an antibody. This process is usually applied to antibodies raised to large antigens. Two methods employing peptides will be described which enable the epitope within a large protein to be determined.

However, the use of peptides as immunogens presents some problems. The main one being how to select from a protein a peptide that will be antigenic, and also induce antibodies that are able to recognise their epitope when contained in the whole native protein.

4.2   Prediction and selection of antigen determinants

The literature on the structure of antigens and their interaction with antibody is enormous and beyond the scope of this chapter. Interested readers are referred to Getzoff *et al.* (1988) who provides an authoritative review of the subject.

Proteins are complex molecules which adopt a particular conformation or shape depending on the conditions under which they are analysed. For example, a protein that has been processed for microtome sectioning will have been crosslinked using formaldehyde as well as subjected to temperatures of 60 °C during wax embedding; these procedures will alter the shape of the molecule from its natural form. If antibodies are to be used to detect these antigens they must have access to their epitope. Proteins, being three-dimensional structures, will have regions completely inaccessible to antibody (e.g. within the protein structure). An antibody is a large molecule and may be unable to penetrate the matrix. Peptides should be selected from an accessible region of the protein if the resulting antibody is to be of use. The most accessible areas will be those parts of the molecule that are exposed or on the outside of the structure. As these regions are in contact with an aqueous environment they are usually hydrophilic (Getzoff *et al.*, 1988). The peptide should also adopt a conformation that mimics its shape when contained within the native protein. Finally, the peptide must be immunogenic or be coupled to a carrier molecule.

Using the hydrophilicity plot as a starting point the following sections deal with the various factors that can be used to identify an optimally conformed, immunogenic peptide. There are predictive algorithms available that can aid in the detection of hydrophilic areas (Kyte & Dolittle, 1982; Hopp & Woods, 1983). These computer programs assign a 'hydrophilic index' to each amino acid in the protein and then plot out a profile. The regions of hydrophilicity can then be seen.

There have also been attempts to produce algorithms to predict flexibility (Weshof *et al.*, 1984) and secondary structure (Chou & Fasman, 1978), parameters that may be important in antigenicity; however, a hydrophilicity plot is a good starting point and is easily performed. A hydrophilicity program is contained within most protein database management systems (e.g. PCGENE, Intelligenetics Inc.) or can be obtained from the literature (Hopp & Woods, 1983).

Using this as the starting point, the protein can be checked for the following characteristics.

There are data available that suggest that longer peptides have a greater conformational similarity to the native protein and therefore are more likely to induce antibodies that recognize the natural protein (van Regenmortel, 1987). There are also data to suggest that a single antigenic determinant (i.e. the smallest immunogenic peptide) is between five and eight amino acids (Geysen *et al.*, 1987). Consequently, a peptide length of 15–20 amino acids is preferable as it should contain at least one epitope and adopt a limited amount of native conformation.

Studies have also been made on the occurrence of particular amino acids within actual epitopes (Geysen *et al.*, 1991). This work on 82 different sera showed that particular amino acids differed in the frequency with which they occurred in epitopes. For example, glutamic acid was the most likely whereas arginine was the least likely. An appreciation of this finding may help in the selection of one sequence over another.

Clearly, any peptide selected must be synthesizable and also be readily soluble in an aqueous buffer for conjugation and use in biological assays. If a hydrophilic region has been selected then solubility should not be a problem. Even these regions, however, may contain hydrophobic residues (e.g. tryptophan, valine, leucine, isoleucine and phenylalanine) and if there is a choice, a peptide with as few hydrophobic residues as possible should be selected.

Glutamine may also cause insolubility as it can form hydrogen bonds between peptide chains, so multiple glutamines are to be avoided. A cysteine in the selected sequence is useful for conjugation; however, if there are two cysteines present, inter- and intra-peptide disulphide bonds may form leading to insolubility and structural alteration. Conjugation to a carrier molecule is necessary to render the peptide immunogenic (4.3). The cysteine should be positioned at the N- or C-terminus for optimal conjugation.

Two useful amino acids to look for during the selection process are proline and tyrosine. Proline has an angular backbone (due to a *cis* bond) which means that it can give the peptide a shape that may mimic more closely the shape of the peptide in the protein (Atherton & Sheppard, 1989). Normally, peptide chains tend to be rather linear; the introduction of a proline puts an angle into it and so enhances its potential. Tyrosine serves two purposes: first, it is a large amino acid and so confers shape to the peptide and second, it can be used to couple the peptide to a carrier using *bis*-diazotized tolidine.

It should also be appreciated that peptides which span sites within a protein may be modified in nature (e.g. glycosylation sites) and may induce antibodies that do not recognize the modified (native) version of the protein. Equally, transmembrane regions of membrane-bound proteins may not be accessible in nature and will not, therefore, induce useful antibodies.

The selection process will finally narrow down the candidates to two or three peptides. If possible at least two and preferably three should be selected and synthesized. This greatly increases the chance of at least one peptide being successful. The actual synthesis of peptides is an area covered extensively elsewhere (Atherton & Sheppard, 1989) and readers are referred to it.

The purity of the peptide used for antibody production will greatly influence the quality of the antibody response. Material less that 80% pure should not be used and it is preferable to have greater than 90% purity. It is essential to establish the integrity of the peptide and its purity, amino acid composition and molecular weight prior to use.

4.3 Conjugation

Normally, an immunogenic antigen is a large, complex molecule with a molecular weight greater than 10 000 and, as such, is able to promote a good immune response and induce high levels of specific antibody. Peptides, however, are very small molecules, typically 1000–2000 Daltons, which even when emulsified in adjuvant are able to elicit only a very poor immune response.

A normal immune response which results in a good level of antibody production usually requires the stimulation of T cell help to induce the B cells to recognize the antigen. Clearly a hapten or peptide is unable to do this. The probable explanation is that at least two different 'epitopes' are required within the antigen: one to stimulate the T cells, the other the B cells. A small peptide may not be large enough to contain two clear epitopes (Francis *et al.*, 1987). The solution to this problem is to couple the peptide to a larger carrier molecule (e.g. bovine serum albumin) which is inherently immunogenic. The T and B cells now have a whole range of 'epitopes' to react to and a vigorous response results in which antibody is made to the carrier as well as to the peptide. The immune system responds to the hapten–carrier conjugate as if it were a single molecule and in so doing makes antibody to the peptide as well.

The proportion of antibody made to the peptide is small compared with the overall response but is far higher than with peptide alone. The penalty for this is that there will be high levels of anti-carrier antibody produced which may have to be removed to make the reagent useable. Such problems do not occur with monoclonal antibody production because careful screening will remove those clones responding to carrier. Carrier proteins are, by nature, immunogenic and include bovine serum albumin, ovalbumin and keyhole limpet haemocyanin. Another system has been developed using a purified protein derivative from *Mycobacteria tuberculae*. This carrier is reported (Lachmann,

1985) to simulate T cell help but not induce antibody to itself. This means the whole response can be directed towards the peptide.

The choice of carrier is wide but, as a general all purpose protein, bovine serum albumin fulfils most purposes; it is cheap, soluble and easily available (for review see Sela, 1987).

The next step, after carrier selection, is to chemically bind the peptide to the protein. This is not a random process and can be finely manipulated to ensure that the peptide is bound in a known orientation. The reagents used to link the peptide to the carrier are termed heterobifunctional as they have a reactive group at each end of the molecule that can crosslink proteins.

These reagents can be used to link the peptide in a particular way to achieve an antibody that reacts with a particular part of the peptide. For example, CCK and gastrin have the same five C-terminal residues. If an antibody specific for CCK is required, then clearly antibodies to the common sequence must be avoided. Consequently, if the C-terminus of the peptide is coupled to the carrier, the likelihood of cross-reactivity to this region is reduced, simply because it is now 'hidden' by the conjugating agent.

There are numerous reagents for crosslinking proteins; however, there are four that are in common use.

4.3.1   Glutaraldehyde

Glutaraldehyde crosslinks primary amino groups on the peptide to those on the carrier. The primary amino groups are at the N-terminus of the peptide and/or the epsilon amino group of lysine. So conjugation using glutaraldehyde will usually result in an N-terminally coupled peptide. The linkage formed by glutaraldehyde is such that there is a degree of flexibility between peptide and carrier. This will reduce the possibility of steric hindrance, which might interfere with access of the immune system to the peptide, and so result in a better response.

4.3.2   m-maleimidobenzoic acid N-hydroxysuccinimide ester (MBS)

MBS will link peptides via the -SH group on cysteine to $-NH_2$ groups. This is a widely used reagent because it unequivocally links the peptide through a specific residue. A cysteine can be added to the peptide, either N- or C-terminally, to facilitate conjugation. Again, conjugation through one of the termini will usually produce antibody to the other.

4.3.3   bis-diazotized tolidine (Bdt)

Bdt will link peptides via the aromatic side chain of tyrosine and, to a lesser extent, histidine to the same residues on the carrier proteins. This linker is a large molecule that provides a 'spacer' between peptide and carrier that usually results in an enhanced anti-peptide antibody response, due to the increased accessibility of the peptide.

4.3.4 Carbodiimides (CDI)

Carbodiimides condense any free carboxyl and primary amino groups, whether C- or N-terminal or on side chains (i.e. lysine, aspartic acid or glutamic acid) to form CO—NH bonds. These are peptide bonds and so are extremely rigid. This can cause considerable steric hindrance as the peptide is tightly bound and is unable to rotate. The agent, however, is rather non-specific and so can couple at various places in the peptide giving rise to several alternative conjugates which give rise to a variety of antibody responses. This can be advantageous as it presents multiple alternatives to the immune system.

The methods for all of these conjugation techiques are given in Appendix 4.7. For a more detailed account, the reader is referred to the excellent review of Szelke (1983). The ratio of peptide to carrier has been the subject of much debate (Erlanger, 1980). Peptide carrier ratios of around 5:1 appear to give the best antibody response; this corresponds to about 5–25 molecules of peptide per 50 000 Daltons of carrier protein. However, the ratios used in Appendix 4.7 have given reproducibly good titres. If feasible, a variety of carrier and/or coupling agents should be used so that the peptide is presented in a variety of ways to the immune system. This will increase the chances of generating an antibody with the desired characteristics.

In addition to this classic approach to antibody production using peptide conjugates, there are several novel systems currently being evaluated that do not require a carrier to be used. For example, Tam *et al*. (1981) has developed a novel way of building up large immunogenic peptides. This is done using an unusual property of lysine. Lysine has two amino groups, one at the N-terminus and one on a side chain. Normally peptide synthesis occurs by coupling through the N-terminal amino group but by using the side chain group as well a branching poly-lysine molecule can be built up.

In brief, a single lysine is attached to the resin support. This has two sites for attachment. Lysine is now added and binds at these sites. As each lysine has two sites, there are now four sites available to couple fresh lysine molecules. Subsequent steps give eight and finally 16 available coupling sites. The peptide is then synthesized on the end of each lysine branch. This therefore, when it is cleaved from the resin, results in a molecule containing 16 copies of the peptide. As its molecular weight may now be 20 000–30 000, it is immunogenic in its own right and does not require conjugation to a carrier molecule. Such an approach results in a higher proportion of anti-peptide response as there is no contaminating anti-carrier response.

Success has also been achieved using *in-vitro* immunization procedures using free peptides (Borrebaeck, 1988).

4.4   Immunization

Standard immunization schedules are used to produce the antibodies. Typically a primary immunization in complete Freund's adjuvant followed at 14 day intervals with boosters in incomplete Freund's adjuvant give good results in mice, rabbits and sheep.

For mouse mab production the primary injection is given subcutaneously (s.c.) with the boosters given intraperitoneally (i.p.). Each injection contains 5–10 μg of antigen. The actual amount is calculated from the peptide content of the conjugate only, the carrier is ignored. It is assumed that all peptide used in the conjugation is present in the immunogen. For larger animals, such as rabbit or sheep, immunization doses of up to 50 μg of antigen per injection are appropriate.

The development of the antibody response is monitored by taking test bleeds from the animals. This is done during the week between injections. It is important to monitor the response for mab (as well as polyclonal) so that the spleen may be removed at an optimal moment.

4.5   Screening

The design of the assay system is crucial to the overall outcome. As mentioned previously, the peptide used to immunize the animal may not represent the bioactive conformation of the peptide. Consequently, an assay must include a test to detect activity towards the native protein. It is therefore inadvisable to rely on a single assay against the peptide, such as an ELISA (enzyme-linked immunosorbent assay), which may give positive results with antibodies that recognize the peptide but are unable to react with the whole bioactive protein. A two-stage screening strategy is therefore recommended. This strategy must be applied to the test bleeds as well as to the supernatants. The very nature of mab production generates enormous numbers of samples for screening, so the chosen systems must be rapid.

An ELISA system is the usual choice to screen for anti-peptide activity. However, problems may occur in the adsorption of some peptides to the plastic surface of the wells. If the peptide binds to the plastic by the amino acids that are contained in the epitope recognized by the antibody, then the antibody may not be able to bind the peptide, owing to steric hindrance, and will give a false negative result. Although this only occurs with some peptide antibody combinations it is impossible to predict. Consequently, it is better to use a peptide conjugate to coat the plastic wells. If a carrier molecule has been used in the immunogen, then a different carrier molecule must be used for coating the ELISA plate as the polyclonal antibody response will give a mixture of antibodies, many of which will be directed against the carrier molecule. The same coupling chemistry must be used so that the peptide is in the same orientation. This screening conjugate can be made at the same time as the one for immunization.

When peptides are synthesized there will always be a proportion that are not full length. It is therefore important to ensure that the antibodies are reacting only with the full length sequence and so it is critical that highly-purified peptide is used in the screening assay. Lower quality peptide may result in false positives which will increase the workload at the second screen.

The ELISA procedure is described elsewhere and the reader is referred to Engvall & Perlmann (1971) for a review. The ELISA system is rapid and provides a result in 4 h or less. This will identify which clones recognize the peptide. A second assay should now be performed with these positive clones to determine which are also reactive with the bioactive protein.

The choice of second assay may be dictated by the final use for which the antibody is intended. Consequently, if it is to be used for immunocytochemistry then this is how it should now be screened. Alternatively, Western blotting may be an appropriate technique, as this can give added information on the molecular weight of the target protein to aid the detection of positives. These and other techniques are described elewhere (Harlow & Lane, 1988).

An advantage of the peptide route is in the confirmation of a specific anti-protein response. If the antibody is pre-incubated with excess free peptide (50 μg of peptide per ml of supernatant) it can be blocked and so is unable to detect the protein or indeed the peptide in an ELISA. Thus if confirmation of the specificity of a particular band or staining pattern is required a second test is done using the blocked antibody. On this sample the band or staining will be absent, thus confirming the specificity of the response.

The use of peptides as immunogens, especially in mab production, is quite labour intensive; however, because a completely synthetic antigen is used antibodies can be made to proteins that cannot be purified or obtained in large enough quantities.

As we have seen earlier, if the nucleotide sequence is known, an antibody can be made to the protein encoded by that gene and the antibody can then be used as a probe to map the distribution of that protein. Such an approach has been used in the study of oncoproteins by ourselves and others (Evan *et al.*, 1985; Kris *et al.*, 1985; Price *et al.*, 1990; Muller *et al.*, 1989).

To illustrate the entire process, consider the following example. It was decided to make a mab that would recognize all members of the *myc* proto-oncogene family of which there are several members, each of which varies by a small number of amino acids. I do not intend to review the area of oncoproteins and the interested reader is referred to the many texts available (Bradshaw & Prentis, 1987).

The sequence chosen had to be common to all the *myc* family members as well as to be antigenic.

A hydrophilicity profile of the human c-*myc* sequence was run and the result is shown in Figure 4.2. The point of maximal hydrophilicity was around residue 260 (shown by small arrow). However, there were no areas of homology between the various types in this area. Fortunately, an area of similarity was

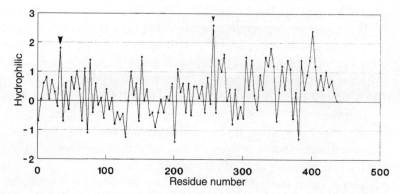

Figure 4.2. Hydrophilicity plot of the human c-*myc* oncoprotein using a Hopp & Wood (1983) format.

myc Type	Species*	Amino acid sequence
c–	H,M,R,A	[QPP]APSEDIWKKFEL[LPT]
L–	H,M	[ST] APSEDIWKKFEL[VPS]
B–	R	[QPP]APSEDIWKKFEL[LPT]
v–		[QPP]APSEDIWKKFEL[LPT]
N–	H,M	[ST] PPGEDIWKKFEL[LPT]

Figure 4.3. Comparative alignment of *myc* monoclonal antibody peptide. H, human; M, mouse; R, rat; A, avian.

found that coincided with a hydrophilicity peak around residue 40 (shown by arrow head) and this was chosen as the immunizing peptide. Figure 4.3 shows the alignment of this peptide with the various *myc* types and species.

The sequence APSEDIWKKFEL was synthesized and a C-terminal cysteine was added so that it could be conjugated using MBS. Keyhole limpet haemocyanin was used as the carrier protein. Balb/c × CBA F_1 female mice were immunized with 50 µg of immunogen (dose based on peptide content only) emulsified in complete Freund's adjuvant given s.c., followed every 2 weeks by a similar dose in incomplete Freund's adjuvant, given i.p.

Test bleeds were taken during the intervening weeks and assayed for peptide reactivity by ELISA and protein reactivity using Western blots. The antigen preparation used in the Western blots was derived from cell lines which possess elevated levels of the appropriate type of *myc* antigen (Price *et al.*, 1990).

When an adequate polyclonal response was obtained the animals were given a 50 µg intravenous (i.v.) boost of immunogen (no adjuvant) and the spleen removed 4 days later. Fusions were performed using polyethylene glycol as described elsewhere (Campbell, 1987). The resulting clones were screened first by ELISA for anti-peptide activity and the positives from this rescreened for their ability to detect proteins in Western blots from cell lines expressing various *myc* forms. Clones that were positive in both screening assays were recloned until stable using a limiting dilution process.

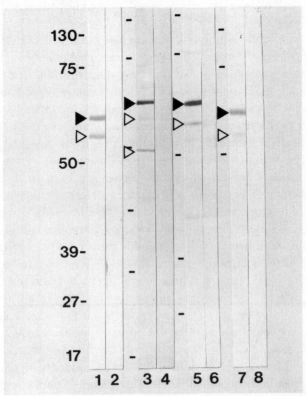

Figure 4.4. Strip 1: N417 (c-*myc* expressing) cell lysate. Strip 3: HL-60 (c-*myc* expressing) stimulated with phorbol ester (TPA) cell lysate. Strip 5: IMR-32 (N-*myc* expressing) cell lysate. Strip 7: L88 (L-*myc* expressing) cell lysate. Strips 2, 4, 6 and 8 are peptide-blocked controls. Arrowheads indicate the major bands at 62/64 kDa and at 56/58 kDa (*myc* proteolytic fragment) on strips 1, 3, 5 and 7. A 50 kDa *myc*-related protein is detected in the TPA-stimulated HL-60 blotted lysate (strip 3).

The results obtained with this antibody are shown in Figure 4.4. The antibody can detect various *myc* forms (e.g. C-N-L) at a molecular weight consistent with those found by other workers (Evan *et al.*, 1985).

It would have been impossible to produce these antibodies other than by the recombinant technique which is both complex and time consuming. Thus peptides can be a powerful tool by providing antibody probes to hitherto unavailable antigen.

4.6   Epitope detection and analysis

As we have seen, peptides can be used as synthetic antigens to make antibodies. Once made, the epitope recognized by these antibodies is fairly precisely delineated, i.e. within the peptide used as immunogen. In cases where the antibody is raised to a large antigen, perhaps containing several hundred amino acids, the precise epitope recognized by the antibody could be anywhere within the protein.

There are numerous methods that have been developed to determine the epitopes recognized within proteins, such as chemical modification, proteolytic digestion, phage expression and competitive fingerprinting (Berzofsky *et al.*, 1982; East *et al.*, 1982; Smith-Gill *et al.*, 1982; Jemmerson & Paterson, 1986*a*, *b*). These techniques are time consuming, laborious and inflexible.

Two recent developments involving peptides greatly simplify the approach, improve its flexibility and are in a format specifically designed for use with antibodies. The techniques allow the precise delineation of the sequence of amino acids which make up an epitope recognized by a particular antibody. Further characterization can be performed to determine the relative importance of each of its constituent residues to the overall binding of the antibody.

The strategy for detecting epitopes within a protein involves breaking the protein up into small peptides. Each peptide must be large enough to bind an antibody and, as mentioned previously, this has been shown to be between five and eight amino acid residues. Consequently, peptides between eight and ten residues will suffice. The protein sequence is then broken up into a series of peptides which differ by only one amino acid from the next. This is shown in Figure 4.5. This technique is referred to as Epitope Scanning or Pepscan (Geysen *et al.*, 1984).

Such a system by its nature requires that many hundreds of peptides may be needed to scan a relatively small protein of 250–300 amino acids. There are currently two systems available that enable such large numbers of peptides to be made rapidly and simply. In addition, both systems have been developed to scan antibodies and to rapidly determine their epitopes.

The Multipin system developed by Geysen *et al.* (1987) uses a polyethylene pin inserted into a holder in the familiar 8×12 microtiter plate format. A single peptide can then be synthesized on each pin totalling 96 per holder. Several holders may be used simultaneously, thus fulfilling the requirement for several hundred peptides. Once complete, the pin-bound peptides are incubated in antibody and after washing, the bound antibody is detected using an enzyme-conjugated secondary antibody and a chromogenic indicator. The pins may be regenerated and the pin-peptides reprobed with the same or another antibody.

The SPOTs system developed by Frank & Döring (1988) utilizes a specially

```
myc protein    A-P-S-E-D-I-W-K-K-F-E-L....etc.
peptide 1      A-P-S-E-D-I-W-K
peptide 2        P-S-E-D-I-W-K-K
peptide 3          S-E-D-I-W-K-K-F
peptide n                        ....etc.
```

Figure 4.5. Illustration of the epitope scanning strategy.

derivatized cellulose membrane on which are 96 SPOTs which will support the synthesis of a peptide. Each spot is 4 mm in diameter and the 96 are in the spacing of a microtiter plate. Once synthesized, the membrane is probed just like a dot blot. The SPOTs that have bound antibody change colour. The membrane may be regenerated for re-use.

4.6.1 Multipin system

The methods involved in the preparation of the pins are described in depth elsewhere (Geysen *et al.*, 1984, 1987). However, a brief summary of the chemistry is given here.

The polyethylene pins are radiation-grafted with acrylic acid. This provides a reactive functionality predominantly on the surface of the otherwise inert polyethylene, on which synthesis of peptides may be initiated. A linker is then coupled to the polyacrylic acid matrix (mono-t-butyloxycarbonyl-1, 6-diamino-hexane) (HMD), which has a backbone consisting of six carbon atoms. This has the dual purpose of acting both as a spacer as well as a coupling molecule. The spacer is added so that once synthesized the peptide is accessible from all sides by the antibody, thus reducing the possibility of steric hindrance.

Finally, an Fmoc (fluorenylmethoxycarbonyl) β-alanine is coupled to the linker; β-alanine is an unnatural amino acid, it does not occur in nature. Consequently, it will not interfere with any antibody interaction. The Fmoc β-alanine acts as a further spacing molecule but also, as it is an amino acid, is the point at which peptide synthesis can occur. The derivatization procedure is summarized in Figure 4.6. Pins derivatized ready for use are commercially

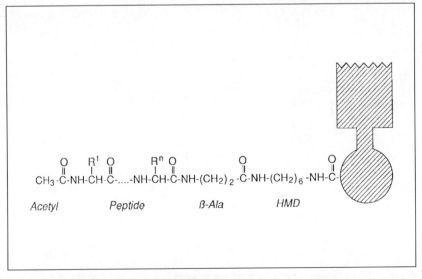

Figure 4.6. Pin-peptide schematic.

available (Cambridge Research Biochemicals, Northwich, Cheshire, CW9 7RA UK).

The Fmoc mode of peptide synthesis employing active esters is used to build up the peptides on the pins. A full description is given elsewhere (Atherton & Sheppard, 1989) but briefly the synthesis proceeds as follows.

An Fmoc-protected amino acid is represented in Figure 4.7. They have a carbon backbone, an N- and C-terminus and side chains some of which contain amino groups (e.g. lysine). Amino acids link to each other by a condensation reaction between the C-terminal -COOH group of one with the N-terminal -NH$_2$ group of the other.

To ensure that this reaction only occurs when and where you want it, other groups are added to the amino acids to block other reactivities. An Fmoc group is added to the N-terminus. This prevents the amino acid coupling to itself during synthesis and causing polymer formation. It is linked to the -NH$_2$ group by a base labile bond. The side chains of some amino acids contain groups that can also bind to amino acids (e.g. -NH$_2$ in the side chain of lysine). Consequently, various protecting groups (e.g. t-butoxycarbonyl (BOC) on lysine) are added to these side chains to block the reactivity. These molecules are linked to the side chain by acid-labile bonds.

Finally, the amino acids are activated at their C-terminus to give Opfp active esters (pentafluorophenyl esters) which are stable as solids but are extremely reactive in solution and give rapid, high-efficiency couplings. In addition, they are easy to use and ideally suited for use in this system by non-chemists.

The synthesis proceeds as follows:

The Fmoc group of β-alanine on the pin is removed by dipping the pin in a tray of 20% piperidine in dimethylformamide (DMF). This solution is basic and so removes the Fmoc group (base labile) but leaves any side chain (acid labile)-protecting groups on the β-alanine intact.

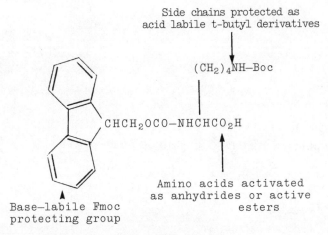

Figure 4.7. Diagram of an Fmoc amino acid.

The first amino acid is weighed out and dissolved in DMF. As soon as it is dissolved the active ester (Opfp) is activated. The pin is now placed in the amino acid solution and the amino acid binds rapidly to the free -NH$_2$ on the β-alanine. This reaction is allowed to run to completion overnight.

The following day the pin is washed in DMF. The amino acid that has just coupled has an Fmoc group at its C-terminus and this is now removed using piperidine/DMF and the whole coupling cycle is repeated. Each addition takes 24 h.

Once assembled, the peptide must now be made 'natural', i.e. all the non-natural groups are removed.

The Fmoc group on the last amino acid is removed and the -NH$_2$ group is acetylated by dipping the pin in a solution of acetic anhydride. This is done to reduce any charge difference in the peptide and renders the N-terminus unreactive.

Finally, the side chain-protecting groups (acid labile) are removed by dipping the pin in trifluoroacetic acid. After a final wash the pin-peptide is ready for use.

While the above description confines itself to one pin, obviously many hundreds of pins could be done simultaneously and a software program has been developed which records each amino acid addition. This is important if several hundred different peptides are being made as at each cycle each pin could have any one of 20 possible amino acids.

The set of peptides represents a complete overlapping 'walk' through the protein. The antibody assay is a slightly modified ELISA-type procedure.

The pins are first incubated in a protein-rich blocking buffer containing bovine serum albumin (BSA) and ovalbumin in phosphate buffered saline (PBS). This serves to block any non-specific binding to either the pins or the peptides. All the incubation steps are carried out in microtiter plates.

After washing in phosphate buffered saline containing Tween 20, the pins are placed into microtiter plates that have the test antibody optimally diluted in each well. Typically, monoclonal supernatant is used neat or ascites is diluted to 1:2000. This incubation should take place overnight to ensure detection of both high and low-affinity interactions.

After washing again, the pins are placed in microtiter plates of horseradish peroxidase-conjugated secondary antibody (typical dilution 1:2000). After 1 h at room temperature, the pins are washed again and placed in a microtiter plate containing a chromogen/substrate solution. The chromogen is ABTS (azinobisthiosulphonic acid) in a citrate-phosphate buffer pH 4.0 with hydrogen peroxide as the substrate. The positive wells will turn green after 30 min; this will indicate which pins have peptides that represent epitopes that are recognized by the antibody.

The results may be read using a plate reader and the data acquired by the software to provide a graphical print out.

If we continue to use the example of the monoclonal antibody raised to a

Table 4.1. *Hexapeptide synthesis for epitope scanning analysis of the pan-*myc *monoclonal antibody*

Pin no.	S E L Q P P A P S E D I W K K F E L L P	Assay results (mean O.D.)
1	S E L Q P P	0.36
2	E L Q P P A	0.37
3	L Q P P A P	0.35
4	Q P P A P S	0.79
5	P P A P S E	0.81
6	P A P S E D	0.82
7	A P S E D I	3.21
8	P S E D I W	2.20
9	S E D I W K	0.52
10	E D I W K K	0.28
11	D I W K K F	0.31
12	I W K K F E	0.58
13	W K K F E L	0.77
14	K K F E L L	0.35
15	K F E L L P	0.67

peptide from *myc* and study its interaction we can illustrate the specificity of the response.

A series of pins were made which scanned into and then out of the *myc* peptide APSEDIWKKFELL. The peptides were hexapeptides and overlapped by one residue. The results of the assay are shown in Table 4.1.

The specificity is extremely precise with only two pins with the sequences APSEDI and PSEDIW giving a good reaction with a small shoulder region on either side. In this case the epitope is a hexapeptide residing at the N-terminus of the peptide. This is not surprising as the peptide was conjugated through its C-terminus leaving the N-terminus the most accessible.

At this point it is worth mentioning that any system using linear sequences to represent epitopes will only ever detect linear or continuous epitopes. Those epitopes that are discontinuous, or assembled, cannot be detected using this system. Clearly, immunization with this peptide has resulted in the production of an antibody which recognizes a linear epitope.

Once the epitope has been defined the relative importance for antibody binding of each amino acid within the epitope can be investigated, i.e. which are essential for binding and which are not. This is done by making every analogue of the epitope. Replacing the residue at position 1, alanine in the example, with each of the other 19 L amino acids will result in 20 peptides including the 'parent' sequence. The same is now done at position 2 and so on through the sequence. For a hexapeptide this will give 120 peptides.

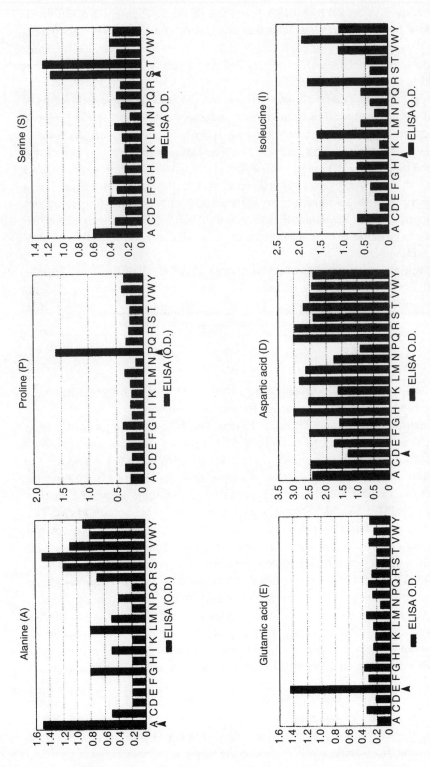

Figure 4.8. Analogue analysis of the hexapeptide, APSEDI, epitope. Each graph of 20 ELISA values represents the results of the pan-*myc* antibody binding to peptides containing the single amino acid substitution identified by the single letter code beneath each bar. The APSEDI sequence result (positive control) is identified by an arrow.

If these are now tested by ELISA the result shown in Figure 4.8 is obtained. The arrow head in each set indicates the result obtained with the parent (APSEDI) as this occurs in each set. It acts as an internal control. The other lines represent the ELISA OD (optical density) given by the peptide with that substitution in the particular position.

The results show that if proline (P), serine (S) and glutamic acid (E) are replaced with any other amino acid (with the exception of serine (S) replaced by threonine (T)) then antibody binding is lost. As mentioned previously, proline is a 'structural' amino acid and has a crucial role in the formation of this epitope. The alanine (A) and isoleucine (I) can be replaced with variable numbers of amino acids but aspartic acid (D) is the most interesting, as a replacement here with several amino acids actually enhances binding, i.e. there are analogues of this sequence that give higher binding than the parent. Such analyses can provide extremely important data concerning antibody and antigen interactions.

The Multipin system is a robust, reusable method. The antibody can be removed from the pins by sonication in a bath containing sodium dodecyl sulphate and β-mercaptoethanol. This allows the pins to be probed with another antibody thus whole panels of antibodies to be screened.

4.6.2   SPOTs system

This system was originally invented by Frank & Döring (1988) and has now been developed into a kit (Cambridge Research Biochemicals).

The cellulose membranes (8 cm × 12 cm) are first covered with a single amino acid which esterifies to the free hydroxyl groups found on the cellulose. With the entire membrane coated with an amino acid, a second amino acid is spotted onto the membrane such that 96 equidistant SPOTs in an 8 × 12 format are fitted on a single membrane. The entire sheet is then acetylated so that only functionalities on which synthesis may occur are on the small SPOTs. The chemistry used to build up peptides on the SPOTs is the same as that for the multipin system and a software package enables sequences to be typed in, manipulated and a pipetting schedule produced.

The SPOTs system has been specially developed so that it is quick, cheap and easy to use by non-chemists. The membranes are supplied, Fmoc-deprotected and ready to use. A blue indicator is incorporated into the SPOTs which is used to monitor each coupling as it proceeds. The indicator is bromophenol blue which binds to free amino groups. As the membrane is already Fmoc deprotected, the SPOTs have many free amino groups and so are blue.

The synthesis cycle pathway is very similar to that used in the multipin system with rounds of coupling, washing and deprotection, followed, when complete, by acetylation and side chain deprotection. There are, however, a few improvements which greatly speed up the whole process.

The schedule produced by the software assigns a number to each of the SPOTs. The appropriate number of SPOTs are then taken and each is numbered using a pencil. Each SPOT corresponds to one peptide and so epitope scans or analogue studies can be performed.

A cycle of coupling is as follows. If it is not the first addition then the whole membrane is Fmoc deprotected by incubating for 30 min in 20% piperidine in dimethylformamide. The membrane is then incubated in bromophenol blue indicator which binds to the free amino groups on the SPOTs and stains them blue.

A 1 μl drop of the appropriate Fmoc acid active ester is then added to the SPOT. After 15–30 min the SPOT turns yellow. As the amino acid binds to the free amino groups on the SPOT it causes the dye to change colour. This provides a simple indication that coupling has proceeded efficiently. The membrane is now washed, deprotected and dyed ready for the next addition. The method is very rapid taking only 90 min for one entire cycle of amino acid addition. This compares with 24 h for the multipin system.

The process of addition continues until the peptides have been assembled. The membranes are then incubated in acetic anhydride to acetylate the peptides and then side chain deprotected using trifluoroacetic acid. The SPOTs membranes are now ready for the antibody assay which is similar to a Dot blot. First of all the membranes are incubated overnight in a buffered, high-protein solution consisting of BSA and horse serum. After rinsing, the primary antibody is added and incubated for 3–4 h. The membrane is then washed again. A β-galactosidase-conjugated secondary antibody is then added and incubated for 2 h. The membrane is washed again. A chromogenic substrate containing BCIG (5-bromo-4-chloro-3-indoyl-β-D-galactopyranoside) is then added and after 20 min some of the SPOTs will have turned blue indicating a positive reaction.

If a synthesis is performed using the *myc* sequence (APSEDIWKKFEL), as for the multipin system, the result shown in Figure 4.9. is obtained. The positive SPOTs correspond to sequences (APSEDI and PSEDIW) which were those also obtained using the multipin system. The two systems thus give identical results.

The SPOTs membrane can be regenerated using a urea-sodium dodecyl sulphate buffer which removes the antibody and allows the peptides to be reprobed again. The membrane is fragile and reusability is limited to 6–10 uses.

Both these systems offer a unique perspective on antibody–antigen inter-actions and have been specifically developed for use by immunologists.

Peptides play a very important role within life science research and recent developments, such as those described above, further demonstrate their utility. These particular applications are in no way exhaustive but illustrate how peptides may be used to aid the solving of immunological problems that cannot be readily achieved by more conventional means.

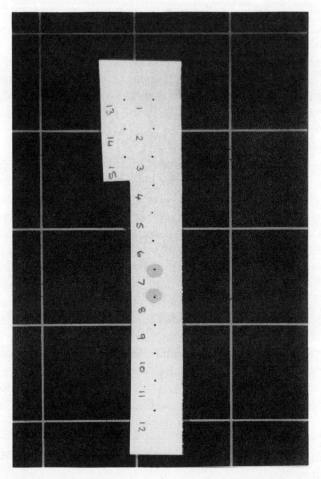

Figure 4.9. 15 SPOTs corresponding to pins 1–15 in Table 4.1. SPOTs 7 and 8 represent
sequences APSEDI and PSEDIW, respectively.

4.7   Appendix

4.7.1   Conjugation of peptide antigens to keyhole limpet haemocyanin (KLH) using glutaraldehyde

Freshly distilled or commercial high-grade (Sigma Chemical Co.) or specially
purified grade 1 glutaraldehyde stored at −20 °C or below should be used for
conjugation. Glutaraldehyde will crosslink via free amino groups, i.e. the
amino terminal of the peptide and/or the epsilon amino group of lysine. KLH
is also available from Sigma.

1. To 8 mg of KLH add 500 µl of 0.1 M sodium hydrogen carbonate
   buffer (pH 8.4; see 4.7.5) and mix by suction and expulsion from a
   pipette tip and then by rolling or gentle agitation. The KLH is

generally readily soluble under these conditions but allow to mix for 1 h prior to use. The KLH solution may remain slightly turbid but this is quite normal.

2. Dissolve 10 mg peptide in 1 ml sodium hydrogen carbonate buffer, pH 8.4.
3. Add to a cleaned glass vial the KLH solution plus (in the following order): 2.5 ml 0.1 M sodium hydrogen carbonate buffer, pH 8.4, 1.0 ml peptide solution, 10 μl glutaraldehyde. Seal the vial and stir or agitate on a roller for 3–4 h at room temperature or overnight at 4 °C.
4. The conjugate should be dialysed in about 30 cm of dialysis tubing (Sigma) against 0.9% sodium chloride solution for 24–48 h at 4 °C (e.g. 2 × 4 l) with stirring.

Note: The 30 cm sections of dialysis tubing should be washed extensively in running tap and deionised or distilled water to remove all traces of preservative. Tie a double knot in the tubing about 5 cm from one end and pour 5–10 ml distilled water into the sac formed (this may be easily achieved using a funnel). Check for leaks. Pour away distilled water and replace with conjugate. A 30 cm section of tubing will easily hold the 4 ml of conjugate. Depress tubing to eliminate as much air as possible and tie a second knot about 5 cm from the other end of the sac, so sealing the conjugate inside.

After dialysis, empty the conjugate into a vial and store at −20 °C until required for immunization.

4.7.2 Conjugation of peptide antigens to keyhole limpet haemocyanin (KLH) using m-maleimidobenzoic acid N-hydroxysuccinimide ester (MBS)

m-maleimidobenzoic acid N-hydroxysuccinimide ester (MBS) will link peptides via -SH groups on cysteine to -NH$_2$ groups on carrier proteins. Cysteine may be added to synthetic peptides at one terminus to facilitate MBS coupling.

1. The KLH must be activated with MBS before linkage to the peptide is possible. Activated KLH will need to be desalted and this is easily achieved using gel filtration (e.g. Pharmacia Sephadex G25 (medium or coarse) or Bio-Rad P-30). The column (e.g. 18 cm × 1 cm) shold be equilibrated and eluted with 50 mM sodium phosphate buffer pH 6.0 (see 4.7.5).
2. Add 1 ml 10 mM sodium phosphate buffer (pH 7.2; see 4.7.5) to 8 mg of KLH. Mix by suction and expulsion from a pipette tip and then by gentle rolling.

   Allow to mix for 1 h prior to use. The KLH solution may remain slightly turbid but this is quite normal.
3. Weigh 2 mg MBS (Sigma) and dissolve this in 300 μl dimethylformamide (DMF). The DMF should be as fresh as possible and should be stored over a molecular sieve.

4. Add 160 μl of the dissolved MBS reagent to the vial containing the KLH, reseal the vial and mix by rolling or gentle swirling for 30 min at room temperature.

5. Centrifuge the activated KLH (1000 g × 10 min) and load on to the desalting column and pool the peak fractions. The passage of the activated KLH down the column should be monitored using a flow-through spectrophotometer set at 280 nm. Alternatively, collect 250–500 μl fractions and determine protein content in each be absorbance at 280 nm. The activated KLH should elute in a peak volume of about 1.0–1.5 ml. Collect the two shoulders of the peak and, if required, use these to make up the peak volume to 1.5 ml. This procedure minimizes the loss of KLH on the column.

6. To a sealable cleaned glass vial, add in the following order 1.5 ml activated KLH (approximately 6 mg; assume 4 mg/ml recovered), 2–10 mg peptide (dissolved in 500 μl 50 mM sodium phosphate buffer, pH 6.0), 700 μl distilled water, 300 μl 1 M sodium phosphate buffer pH 7.4 (see 4.7.5)

7. Dialyse the conjugate against 0.9% sodium chloride overnight at 4 °C before use.

8. Conjugate should be stored at or below −20 °C until required for use.

4.7.3   Conjugation of peptide antigens to keyhole limpet haemocyanin (KLH) using bis-diazotized tolidine

bis-diazotized tolidine will crosslink the aromatic side chain of tyrosine and to a lesser extent histidine residues on both peptides and carrier protein.

4.7.3.1 Diazotization of o-tolidine

1. Pipette 1 ml 0.2 M HCl into a vial containing 25 mg of o-tolidine (Sigma) and allow to dissolve. Transfer the solution to a larger glass vial and add a further 3.5 ml 0.2 M HCl.

2. Pipette 0.5 ml distilled water into a vial containing 17.5 mg sodium nitrite (Sigma) and add this solution to the vial containing the o-tolidine-HCl mixture. An orange colour should develop immediately. Stir for 1 h at 4 °C.

3. Pipette 1 ml 0.16 M sodium borate-buffered saline (pH 9.0) (see 4.7.5) into a vial containing 8 mg KLH. Mix by suction and expulsion from a pipette tip and then by rolling or gentle agitation for 1 h prior to use. The KLH solution may remain slightly turbid but this is quite normal.

4. Prepare a 10 mg/ml peptide solution in phosphate buffer pH 6.0 (50 mM buffer concentration).

5. Chill a cleaned, sealable, glass vial (5–10 ml volume) in an ice-bath and add in the following order: 1 ml KLH solution, 1 ml peptide

solution, 500 μl *bis*-diazotized tolidine solution. Adjust final volume to 4 ml with distilled water and pH to about 7.4 with sodium hydroxide or boric acid as necessary. There should be a colour change from orange to red which may be immediate or may develop with increasing time. Leave mixture on ice for 2 h in the dark. Swirl occasionally.

6. Dialyse conjugate against 0.9% sodium chloride solution overnight at 4 °C before use. The conjugate may be stored at −20 °C until required for use.

4.7.4 Conjugation of peptide antigens to keyhole limpet haemocyanin (KLH) using carbodiimide

Carbodiimide condenses any free carboxyl and primary amino groups, whether C- or N-terminal or side chain (e.g. lysine) to form CO—NH bonds. A water-soluble carbodiimide 1-ethyl-3-(dimethylaminopropyl)-carbodiimide (EDC) is the most commonly used.

1. Dissolve 100 mg of KLH in 1 ml of distilled water.
2. Dissolve 10 mg of peptide in 1 ml of distilled water.
3. Adjust the pH of 100 ml of distilled water to pH 8.5 with 0.1 M sodium hydroxide.
4. Dissolve 40 mg of EDC (Sigma) in 1 ml of distilled water pH 8.5.
5. Add, to a clean glass vial, in the following order: 1 ml KLH, 1 ml of peptide, 1 ml of EDC, 7 ml of distilled water pH 8.5.
6. Mix at 4 °C for 3 h.
7. Dialyse the conjugate against 0.9% sodium chloride overnight at 4 °C.
8. The conjugate may be stored at −20 °C until required.

4.7.5 Reagents

Note: The pH of the distilled water used in the solutions described below was between 5.5 and 6.0. The pH of each solution prepared should be carefully checked. It is recommended that buffer solutions are made immediately before use, i.e. stock solutions should not be used. Sodium azide or any other preservative MUST NOT be added to any of the solutions.

1. Sodium hydrogen carbonate buffer (0.1 M, pH 8.4). Sodium hydrogen carbonate 0.8 g dissolved in 100 ml distilled water. pH adjust to 8.4 with sodium hydroxide.
2. Sodium phosphate buffers. Make up a 1 M stock solution of sodium dihydrogen orthophosphate (NaH_2PO_4 anhydrous) and a 1 M stock solution of di-sodium hydrogen orthophosphate (Na_2HPO_4 anhydrous).

   The stock solutions should be kept for no more than 1 week at room temperature.

(a) Sodium phosphate buffer (1 M, pH 7.5)
Mix the two stock solutions until the pH is 7.5.
The solution is then ready for use.

(b) Sodium phosphate buffer (10 mM, pH 7.2)
Mix the two stock solutions until the pH is 7.2.
Dilute this solution 1 part + 99 parts of distilled water, then check the pH.
The buffer is now 10 mM and ready for use.

(c) Sodium phosphate buffer (50 mM, 6.0)
Mix the two stock solutions until the pH is 6.0.
Dilute this solution 1 part + 19 parts of distilled water, then check the pH.
The buffer is now 50 mM and is ready for use.

3. Sodium borate-buffered saline (0.16 M, pH 9.0)

Dissolve 6.09 g di-sodium tetraborate decahydrate and 0.99 g boric acid in 200 ml distilled water. Check pH and adjust to 9.0 if necessary. Add 1.8 g sodium chloride.

4.8   References

Atherton, E. & Sheppard, R. C. (1989). *Solid-phase peptide synthesis*. IRL Press, Oxford University.

Berzofsky, J. A., Buckenmeyer, G. K., Hicks, G., Gurd, F. R. N., Feldman, R. J. & Minna, J. (1982). Topographic antigenic determinants recognised by monoclonal to sperm whale myoglobin. *Journal of Biological Chemistry*, **257**, 3189.

Borrebaeck C. A. (1988). A critical appraisal of the *in vitro* immunisation technology for the production of mouse and human monoclonal antibodies. *Advances in Drug Delivery Reviews*, **2**, 15.

Bradshaw, R. A & Prentis, S. (1987). *Oncogenes and Growth Factors*. Amsterdam, Elsevier Science Publishers.

Campbell, A. M. (1987). *Monoclonal antibody technology: laboratory techniques in biochemistry and molecular biology*. Amsterdam, Elsevier Science Publishers.

Chou, P. & Fasman, G. (1978). Prediction of protein secondary structure. *Advances in Enzymology*, **47**, 251–276.

East, I. J., Hurrell, J. G. R., Todd, P. E. E. & Leach, S. J. (1982). Antigenic specificity of monoclonal antibodies to human myoglobin. *Journal of Biological Chemistry*, **257**, 3199–3202.

Engvall, E. & Perlmann, P. (1971). Enzyme-linked immunosorbent assay (ELISA). Quantitative assay of immunoglobulin G. *Immunochemistry*, **8**, 874–879.

Erlanger, B. F. (1980). The preparation of antigenic hapten–carrier conjugates: a survey. *Methods in Enzymology*, **7**, 85–104.

Evan, G. I., Lewis, G. K., Ramsay, G. & Bishop, J. M. (1985). Isolation of monoclonal antibodies specific for human c-*myc* proto-oncogene product. *Molecular and Cellular Biology*, **5**, 3610–3616.

Francis, M. J., Hastings, G. Z., Syred, A. D., McGinn, B., Brown, F. & Rowlands, D. J. (1987). Non-responsiveness to a foot and mouth disease virus peptide overcome by addition of foreign helper T-cell determinants. *Nature*, **330**, 168–170.

Frank R. & Döring R. (1988). Simultaneous multiple peptide synthesis under continuous flow conditions on cellulose paper discs as segmental solid synthesis. *Tetrahedron*, **44**, 6031–6040.

Getzoff, E. D., Tainer, J. A., Lerner, R. A. & Geysen, H. M. (1988). The chemistry and mechanism of antibody binding to protein antigens. *Advances in Immunology*, **43**, 1–98.

Geysen, H. M., Mason, T. J. & Rodda, S. J. (1991). Peptides as specific recognition devices. In *Rapid Methods and Automation in Microbiology and Immunology*, ed. A. Vaheri, R. C. Tilton & A. Balows. Berlin, Springer.

Geysen, H. M., Meloen, R. H. & Barteling, S. J. (1984). Peptide synthesis used to probe viral antigens for epitopes to a resolution of a single amino acid. *Proceedings of the National Academy of Sciences U.S.A.*, **81**, 3998–4002.

Geysen, H. M., Rodda, S. J., Mason, T. J., Tribbick, G. & Schoofs, P. G. (1987). Strategies for epitope analysis using peptide synthesis. *Journal of Immunological Methods*, **102**, 259–274.

Harlow, E. & Lane, D. (1988). *Antibodies – a Laboratory Manual*. C. S. H, New York Cold Spring Harbor Laboratory.

Hopp, T. & Woods, K. (1983). A computer program for predicting protein antigenic determinants. *Molecular Immunology*, **20**, 483–489.

Jemmerson, R. & Paterson, Y. (1986*a*). Mapping epitopes on a protein antigen by the proteolysis of antigen-antibody complexes. *Science*, **232**, 1001–1004.

Jemmerson, R. & Paterson, Y. (1986*b*). Mapping antigenic sites on proteins: implications for the design of synthetic vaccines. *Biotechniques*, **4**, 18–31.

Kris, R. M., Lax, I., Gullick, W., Waterfield, M. D., Ullrich, A., Fridkin, M. & Schlessinger (1985). Antibodies against a synthetic peptide as a probe for the kinase activity of the avian EGF receptor and V-erB protein. *Cell*, **40**, 619–625.

Kyte, J. & Dolittle, R. F. (1982). A simple method for displaying the hydropathic character of a protein. *Journal of Molecular Biology*, **157**, 105–132.

Lachman, P. J. (1985). Synthetic peptides as antigens. In *Ciba Foundation Symposium*, ed. R. Porter & J. Whelan, pp. 25–57. Chichester, John Wiley.

Lerner, R. (1982). Mapping the immunologic repertoire to produce antibodies of predetermined specificity. *Nature*, **199**, 592–596.

Muller, C. P., Buhring, H. J., Becker, G., Jung, C. C., Jung, G., Troger, W., Saalmuller, A., Wiesmuller, K. H. & Bessler, W. G. (1989). Specific antibody response towards predicted epitopes of the epidermal growth factor receptor induced by a thermostable synthetic peptide adjuvant conjugate. *Clinical and Experimental Immunology*, **78**, 499–504.

Price, K. M., Cuthbertson, A. S., Varndell, I. M. & Sheppard, P. W. (1990). The production and characterisation of monoclonal antibodies to *myc*, c-*erbB*-2 and EGF-receptor using synthetic peptide approach. *Development of Biological Standards*, **71**, 23–31.

Sela, M., (1987). The choice of carrier. In *Synthetic Vaccines*, vol. 1, ed. R. Arnon, pp. 83–92. Boca Raton, Florida, CRC Press.

Shinnick, T., Sutcliffe, J., Green, N. & Lerner, R., (1983). Synthetic peptide immunogens as vaccines. *Annual Reviews of Microbiology*, **37**, 425–446.

Smith-Gill, S. J., Wilson, A. C., Potter, M., Pager, E. M., Feldmann, R. J. & Mainhart, C. R. (1982). Mapping the antigenic epitope for a monoclonal antibody against lysozyme. *Journal of Immunology*, **128**, 314–322.

Sutcliffe, J., Shinnick, T., Green, N. & Lerner, R. (1983). Antibodies that react with predetermined sites on proteins. *Science*, **219**, 660–666.

Szelke, M. (1983). Raising antibodies to small peptides. In *Immunocytochemistry: Practical Applications in Pathology and Biology*, ed. J. M. Polak & S. Van Noorden. pp. 53–68. Bristol, Wright.

Tam, J. P., Riemen, M. W. & Merrifield, R. B. (1981). Mechanisms of aspartimide formation: the effects of protecting groups, acid, base, temperature and time. *Peptide Research*, **1**, 6–18.

Van Regenmortel, M. H. V. (1987). Antigenic cross-reactivity between protein and peptides: new insights and applications. *Trends in Biochemical Science*, **12**, 237–240.

Walter, G. & Dolittle, R. (1983). Antibodies against synthetic peptides. *Genetic Engineering*, **5**, 61–69.

Westoff, E., Altschuh, D., Moras, D., Bloomer, A. C., Mondragon, A., Klug, A., & van Regenmortel, M. H. V. (1984). Correlation between segmental mobility and the location of antigenic determinants in proteins. *Nature*, **316**, 656–657.

5

Human monoclonal antibodies: production, use, problems

A. SA'ADU and A. ZUMLA

5.1 Production of human monoclonal antibodies

Human monoclonal antibodies (Humab) are generated by immortalizing human B lymphocytes. Immortalization can be achieved by fusion with neoplastic cells (fusion partners) or by transformation with Epstein–Barr virus (EBV). To augment these conventional techniques, transfection of normal B lymphocytes with tumour cell-derived DNA (Jonak *et al.*, 1984), the transfection of permanent cell lines with DNA from antibody-secreting lines (Strelkauskas *et al.*, 1987) or the introduction of natural or recombinant antibody genes into suitable cell lines, is still in its infancy but shows a lot of promise. This genetic engineering approach has been reviewed by Neuberger (1985) and by Oi & Morrison (1986) and will not be discussed further here (see also Chapters 7 and 8).

5.1.1 *Immortalization procedures*

Polyethylene glycol (PEG) has emerged as the most widely used fusion agent after the initial use of Sendai virus (Brahe & Serra, 1981). The molecular weight, source, pH and duration of exposure of cells to PEG, all influence the rate and relative success of fusions (Davidson & Gerrard, 1976; Lane *et al.*, 1984). The actual fusion protocol used varies from group to group.

It has been suggested that resting B cells do not fuse well and that cell activation is necessary for the efficient generation of hybridomas (Burnett *et al.*, 1985). Indeed peripheral blood lymphocytes fuse more readily when transformed with pokeweed mitogen (PWM).

5.1.2 *Human–human fusion*

The human myeloma fusion partners currently available have been derived from the U-266 cell line (Table 5.1). Although several different clones have been generated from this parental cell line, development of other myeloma cell

Table 5.1. *Commonly used human fusion partners*

Parent cell line	Reference	Cell type	Fusion partner	Reference
U-266	Nilsson *et al*. (1970)	Myeloma	SKO-007	Olsson & Kaplan (1980)
GM 1500	Croce *et al*. (1980*a*)	LCL	GM 4672	Osband *et al*. (1981)
W1-L2	Levy *et al*. (1968)	LCL	UC 729-6	Glassy *et al*. (1983)
ARH 77	Burk *et al*. (1978)	LCL	LICR-LON-Hmy^2	Edwards *et al*. (1982)

Table 5.2. *Examples of human monoclonal antibodies produced using human–human fusion*

Antigen	References
Measles virus	Croce *et al*. (1980*a*)
Dinitrochlorobenzene	Olsson & Kaplan (1980)
Single-stranded DNA	Shoenfeld *et al*. (1982)
Tetanus toxoid	Larrick *et al*. (1983)
Strep. pneumoniae	Schwaber *et al*. (1984)
Sheep erythrocytes	Strike *et al*. (1984)
Carcinoma cells	Glassy *et al*. (1985)
Colorectal tumour antigens	Borup-Christensen *et al*. (1986)
Malaria	Schmidt-Ullrich *et al*. (1986)
Mycobacterium leprae (*M. leprae*)	Locniskar *et al*. (1988)
Haemophilus influenzae (*H. influenzae*) type B capsular polysaccharide	Hunter *et al*. (1982)

lines has been limited because of the difficulty involved in growing these cells in culture.

The majority of human fusion partners are lymphoblastoid cell lines (LCL), derived by EBV transformation of lymphocytes (Table 5.1). They are positive for the Epstein–Barr virus nuclear antigen (EBNA). Clones derived from these parental cell lines are the most widely used human fusion partners. However, Kozbor & Croce (1985) have stressed that LCL are not in as appropriate a state of differentiation for high antibody secretion as myeloma cells, which have abundant polyribosomes and extensive Golgi apparatus.

A number of Humab have been produced by the human–human hybridoma technique (Table 5.2). The GM 4672 fusion partner appears to form hybridomas predominantly secreting IgM autoantibodies which react with polyspecific epitopes on a wide variety of antigens (Shoenfeld *et al*., 1982, 1983; Locniskar *et al*., 1988).

Table 5.3. *Examples of human monoclonal antibodies produced using human–mouse fusion*

Antigen	References
Bombesin	Ho *et al*. (1985)
Herpes simplex	Masuho *et al*. (1986)
Cytomegalovirus (CMV)	Matsumoto *et al*. (1986)
Tetanus toxoid	Burnett *et al*. (1985)
H. influenzae type B	Gigliotti *et al*. (1984)
Pseudomonas aeruginosa	Sawada *et al*. (1985)
Hepatitis B surface antigen	Tiebout *et al*. (1985)

5.1.3 Human–mouse fusion

Mouse myelomas, which have high fusion frequencies and do not secrete immunoglobulin (Ig), have been used because of the difficulties involved in the development of the human LCL and myelomas. The human–mouse hetero-hybridomas generated thrive in culture, clone easily and produce high levels of Humab. They can also be adapted to grow as ascitic tumours in nude mice (Tiebout *et al*., 1985). The human–mouse hybridoma technique has produced several Humab (Table 5.3).

5.1.4 Human–heterohybridoma fusion

Several groups have generated heterohybridoma fusion partners in the hope that they will have the growth and fusion characteristics of mouse myelomas while retaining sufficient human chromosomes so that stable Humab-secreting heterohybridomas will result after fusion with immune B cells. These hetero-hybridomas (Kozbor *et al*., 1984; Foung *et al*., 1985*a*; Teng *et al*., 1985*b*) have the added advantage that many are non-secretors of Ig themselves and are EBNA-negative (Boyd & James, 1989).

Fusing immune human lymphocytes to heterohybridoma fusion partners has resulted in the production of useful Humab (Table 5.4). Despite these succes-ses, however, no single heterohybridoma fusion partner has been consistently shown to be superior to any human or mouse fusion partners in terms of fusion frequency, stability of hybridomas developed or levels of Ig secretion. Indeed few comparative studies have been performed.

5.1.5 EBV transformation

EBV infects human B cells and inserts into the genome, transforming and immortalizing a small proportion (1%) of infected cells. It binds specifically to CD 21, a 140 kDa glycoprotein which is the receptor for the C3d complement component (Jondai *et al*., 1976; Frade *et al*., 1985). Aman et al. (1985) have

Table 5.4. *Examples of human monoclonal antibodies produced using human–heterohybridoma fusion*

Antigen	References
Tetanus toxoid	Ichimori *et al.* (1985)
Rhesus D antigen	Bron *et al.* (1984)
E. coli	Teng *et al.* (1983)
Varicella-zoster virus (VZV)	Foung *et al.* (1985*b*)
Epstein–Barr virus (EBV)	Foung *et al.* (1985*b*)
Prostatic acid phosphatase	Yamaura *et al.* (1985)
H. influenzae	Brodeur *et al.* (1987)

Table 5.5. *Examples of human monoclonal antibodies produced using Epstein–Barr virus (EBV) transformation*

Antigen	References
Rhesus D antigen	Crawford & Callard (1983)
X31 influenza virus nucleoprotein	Crawford & Callard (1983)
Genus-specific chlamydial antigen	Rosen *et al.* (1983)
Tetanus toxoid	Boyd *et al.* (1984*b*)
Cytomegalovirus (CMV)	Redmond *et al.* (1986)
Epstein–Barr virus (EBV)	Koizumi *et al.* (1986)
Plasmodium falciparum	Udomsangpetch *et al.* (1986)
Sperm	Winger *et al.* (1983)
Thyroid antigens	Garzelli *et al.* (1984)

suggested that a small, high density resting population of B cells are immortalized; however, Chan *et al.* (1986) have claimed that it is an activated large, low density cell population.

EBV is a polyclonal activator of Ig secretion by B cells (Rosen *et al.*, 1977). Transformation is usually achieved by incubating lymphocytes with culture supernatant derived from the EBV-shedding B95-8 marmoset cell line (Miller & Lipman, 1973), a method now termed 'viral-driven' transformation (Crawford, 1985). It may occur, however, if lymphocytes are co-cultured with EBNA-positive LCL, a process known as 'cell-driven' transformation (Siadak & Lostrom, 1985). 'Cell-driven' transformation appears to lead to more stable LCL which secrete higher levels of Humab (Boyd *et al.*, 1984*a*; Stricker *et al.*, 1985).

At around 1 in 10^4 cells compared with 1 in 10^5 to 10^8 cells, EBV immortalization is more efficient than most fusion protocols. It has been widely used and has resulted in production of many Humab (Table 5.5).

Table 5.6. *Examples of human monoclonal antibodies produced using combined Epstein–Barr virus (EBV)/fusion technique*

Antigen	References
Tetanus toxoid	Kozbor *et al.* (1982)
Carcinoma cells	Kozbor *et al.* (1984)
M. leprae	Atlaw *et al.* (1985)
Cytomegalovirus (CMV)	Emanuel *et al.* (1984)
Human lymphocyte antigen (HLA)	Hulette *et al.* (1985)
Endotoxin	Teng *et al.* (1985*a*)
Lung carcinoma	Cote *et al.* (1984)
Breast carcinoma	Campbell *et al.* (1987)
Rhesus D antigen	Thompson *et al.* (1986)
Ps. aeruginosa	Siadak & Lostrom (1985)
Exotoxin	Larrick *et al.* (1983)

5.1.6 Combined EBV/fusion technique

To circumvent the instability of Humab secretion by EBV-transformed LCL, a combination of transformation followed by fusion has been pioneered by Kozbor *et al.* (1982). B cells transformed with EBV fuse with greater efficiency than those transformed with PWM. The resultant hybridomas (Table 5.6) clone more readily than LCL and Humab scretion may be increased five to tenfold (Kozbor & Roder, 1983, 1984; Foung *et al.*, 1985*a*; Ichimori *et al.*, 1985; Thompson *et al.*, 1986). To increase the chances of obtaining specific hybridomas, antigen-specific LCL can be selected after EBV transformation and then used for fusion. In addition, fusion of LCL with mouse or human myelomas can lead to loss of the EBV genome (Bron *et al.*, 1984; MacDonald *et al.*, 1987; Pollack *et al.*, 1987).

5.1.7 Humanizing mouse monoclonal antibodies

Chimeric antibodies made by expression in myeloma cells of recombinant mouse variable domains, responsible for antigen binding, and human constant domains, responsible for effector function such as complement-mediated lysis and phagocytosis, have been produced (Boulianne *et al.*, 1984; Morrison *et al.*, 1984; Neuberger *et al.*, 1985). Unfortunately the mouse variable region is recognized as foreign and is immunogenic in humans (Bruggeman *et al.*, 1989).

Insertion of the antigen-binding site of the mouse antibody, rather than the whole variable region directed into the human antibody, has been performed (Verhoeyen *et al.*, 1988) but this is only possible in certain, limited situations (Winter & Milstein, 1991). This approach has been used to 'humanize' a rat mab against mature human leucocytes (Riechmann *et al.*, 1988) which proved clinically effective in destroying lymphoma cells in two patients (Hale *et al.*,

1988). The 'humanization' of mouse monoclonal antibodies (Mumab) is a very useful approach because it allows access to the vast pool of Mumab with good affinity and specificity currently available. The strategies involved in this approach have been recently reviewed by Winter & Milstein (1991) and will not be discussed further (see also Chapters 7 and 8).

5.2   Use of human monoclonal antibodies

Despite the dramatic impact of molecular biology on the understanding of the aetiology and aetiological agents of human disease, the therapeutic potential of Humab is perhaps the most important phenomenon in recent years. This is because Humab offer the means of producing novel specific reagents for the diagnosis and treatment of human diseases. Humab provide the potential for producing tailor-made reagents for the investigation of human immune responses at the single epitope level.

Humab offer several theoretical advantages over Mumab. First, they may interact with important determinants, e.g. Rhesus D, MHC and tumour antigens, not readily recognized by Mumab which tend to be directed against immunodominant epitopes. Furthermore, when Mumab are used to identify and purify candidate antigens for vaccine use, they may fail to recognize epitopes that would provoke protective immunity in humans. Second, *in vivo* administration of Humab would be more effective and less immunogenic. The asparagine-linked carbohydrate sequences of Humab are more compatible with Fc receptors on human effector cells than similar sequences on Mumab. Human anti-mouse Ig responses have limited the effectiveness of Mumab in many diagnostic and therapeutic situations (Shawler *et al.*, 1985; Larrick & Bouria, 1986). Adequate prevention of human anti-mouse Ig responses is not yet possible and high titres of such antibodies are associated with rapid hepatic uptake of the Mumab, resulting in a marked reduction of tumour-imaging quality by immunoscintigraphy. This mab biodistribution alteration is due to the *in vivo* formation of mouse Ig/human antibody complexes (van Kroonenburgh & Pauwels, 1988). Third, Humab can be used to define and probe the human B cell repertoire in health and disease (see reviews by Glassy & Dillman, 1988; Cote, 1989). This last point is perhaps the most fundamental because studies of human immune responses are more relevant to understanding human diseases than comparative studies in experimental animals, even though the latter are often easier to perform.

5.2.1   Human anti-D monoclonal antibodies

The administration of therapeutic anti-D serum postpartum has proved a very effective method of preventing sensitization of Rhesus D-negative mothers, preventing haemolytic disease of the new-born (HDN; Bowman *et al.*, 1978). Initially the anti-D Ig was derived solely from women immunized by pregnancy. The success of this programme so diminished the number of sensitized women that Rhesus D-negative male volunteer blood donors had to be recruited and immunized (Gibson, 1973; Gunsen *et al.*, 1974). Despite this, a U.K. national shortage of immune plasma required to meet the increasing demands for the therapeutic anti-D Ig as well as the considerable demand for an anti-D blood grouping reagent now exists (McCann *et al.*, 1988). The rigorous screening of donor plasma for infectious agents such as hepatitis, cytomegalovirus (CMV) and human immunodeficiency virus (HIV) and the laborious virus-inactivation procedures necessary for the preparation of anti-D Ig has made the development of a Humab-based anti-D preparation highly desirable.

Whereas traditional polyclonal blood grouping reagents with other specificities (e.g. anti-A and anti-B) have been successfully replaced by Mumab, this has not been possible with anti-D because mice tend to respond to the whole Rhesus complex rather than specifically to the D epitope (McCann *et al.*, 1988). A considerable number of human anti-D mab have been generated (see review by McCann *et al.*, 1988). All react specifically with red blood cells (RBC) expressing Rhesus D antigen and have proved useful as blood grouping reagents. Initially these Humab were IgG antibodies and could not directly agglutinate D-positive RBC. Agglutination had to be enhanced by either enzymic treatment of RBC, use of an antiglobulin, reduction and alkylation of the Humab or addition of high albumin concentrations. The development of direct agglutinating saline-reactive IgM anti-D Humab (Thompson *et al.*, 1986; Goosens *et al.*, 1987) has provided a reliable and abundant source of a reagent which otherwise only occurs rarely in serum. One of these mab has been grown on a large scale and marketed in the UK (Thompson *et al.*, 1986).

Other human anti-D mab have been used to type human RBC manually (Bron *et al.*, 1984; Doyle *et al.*, 1985; Foung *et al.*, 1987), in an autogrouper (Lowe *et al.*, 1986), and by flow cytometry (Kornprobst *et al.*, 1986). It has been difficult to assess the relative merits of human anti-D mab as blood group reagents in haemagglutination assays. This is due to the subjective nature and wide variety of haemagglutination techniques and indicator RBC genotypes used (McCann *et al.*, 1988).

As yet, there is no single mab which will detect all D-variant RBC; however, it is feasible that a cocktail of mab will be able to do so. Thus, human anti-D mab are a potential source of reliable blood group reagents which minimize batch to batch variation and would ease the current shortage of anti-D preparations. Unfortunately while IgM anti-D antibodies are good for diagnostic use, they do not prevent HDN, only IgG antibodies can do this.

As the mechanism by which anti-D prophylaxis works has not been elucidated, no clear *in-vitro* biological functional assay which will best predict the *in vivo* efficacy of the therapeutic product has been established. The establishment of such a test to evaluate the polyclonal therapeutic preparations in terms of subclass profile, the Gm allotypes present, monocyte/macrophage binding and phagocyte/monocyte/lymphocyte antibody-mediated cellular cytotoxicity (ADCC), would provide a standard for preparing mab-based products.

It has been found that IgG_3 anti-D mab are up to a 100-fold more potent than IgG_1 mab in many effector assays (Wiener *et al.*, 1987; Kumpel *et al.*, 1988*b*). This has been attributed to the longer more flexible hinge region of IgG_3 rendering the Fc portion more accessible to the effector cells (Pumphery, 1986). Parinaud *et al.* (1985) have reported that fetal haemolysis was more severe with maternal IgG_1 anti-D antibodies of the G1m(3) allotype and this has been confirmed by Kumpel *et al.* (1988*b*) using three IgG_1 mab in *in-vivo* ADCC assays.

Human anti-D mab have proved extremely valuable in characterizing D variant cells (Tippet, 1988), in the investigation of the nature of the Fc–FcR interaction (Kumpel *et al.*, 1988*a*) the biochemical analysis of the D antigen (Paire *et al.*, 1986; Bloy *et al.*, 1987) and in providing new methods for determining the genotype of D-positive cells (Kornprobst *et al.*, 1986).

Humab to other blood group antigens include A, A1, Kell and Rhesus C, G and E (Foung *et al.*, 1986; Goosens *et al.*, 1987). These are proving to be good blood typing reagents and Humab will probably replace rare polyclonal antisera such as anti-C and anti-E (Thompson, 1988).

5.2.2   Human monoclonal antibodies to autoantigens

Many Humabs to autoantigens have been generated from patients suffering from organ-specific autoimmune diseases. A well characterized example is the low affinity IgM anti-insulin mab from a patient suffering from insulin-dependent diabetes which clearly is not representative of the high-affinity IgG antibodies commonly found in the serum of these patients (Livneh *et al.*, 1986). This Humab cross-reacts with insulin from other species but does not bind to isolated A and B insulin chains. Two other IgM mab reactive with pancreatic islet cells have been reported (Eisenbarth *et al.*, 1982; Thivolet *et al.*, 1985).

A Humab identifying a novel thyroid membrane antigen has been described from a patient with Graves' disease (Baker *et al.*, 1988). An IgG anti-thyroid and an IgG anti-TSH receptor Humab which did not react with pancreatic tissue have been generated by Foster *et al.* (1987) from a diabetic patient. Valente *et al.* (1982) have produced two IgG Humab which act as intrinsic thyroid-stimulating factors in experimental animal *in-vivo* and *in-vitro* assays and interact with receptor-associated gangliosides. Another two mab, which inhibit TSH action and bind to the high-affinity glycoprotein receptor component rather than to gangliosides, appear to represent the blocking antibodies found in Graves' disease serum. The report by Rotella *et al.* (1986) that a thyroid-stimulating Humab could increase glycogen synthesis in cultured fibroblasts unequivocally demonstrates the pluritopic nature of antibodies in Graves' disease and suggests that the mechanism for the orbital pathology may be due to shared thyroid/orbital antigens. Kuroki *et al*. (1986) have found cross-reactivity of an anti-thyroglobulin mab with orbital connective tissue membranes.

Garzelli *et al*. (1984, 1986) have generated a series of IgM Humab from diabetic patients, reactive with human pancreatic islet cells and thyroid acinar cytoplasmic antigens with varying degrees of individual tissue specificity. Essani *et al*. (1985) have produced a Humab which recognizes a 35 kDa intracyto-plasmic protein in thyroid, pancreas, stomach and pituitary and which binds to growth hormone. Mouse anti-idiotypic mab which inhibits the binding of this mab has been developed and a rabbit anti-anti-idiotype IgG anti-serum with the same staining pattern as the original human IgM mab has been raised using one of the mouse anti-idiotypes (Essani *et al*., 1985).

An anti-acetyl choline Humab derived from the thymus of a patient with myasthenia gravis has myasthenic properties (Kamo *et al*., 1982) and an IgM, lambda rheumatoid factor Humab, which has certain advantages over conven-tional methods, has been established by Steinitz *et al*. (1980, 1982) as a reagent for the universal detection and quantification of immune complexes.

These examples of organ-specific Humab contrast with the large numbers of mab reactive to a diverse array of antigens, apparently sharing no common epitope, e.g. single-stranded and double-stranded DNA, cytoskeletal proteins, bacterial antigens and chemical haptens (Schwartz, 1987, 1988; Zumla *et al*., 1991). Many of these mab have public idiotypes and sequence homology at the messenger RNA level (Schwartz, 1987, 1988). It has been argued that they are coded for by germline genes that have been conserved during evolution because their products are of some survival value (Sanz & Capra, 1988; Zumla, 1990). Several workers have suggested that their principal physiological role is the clearance of cell debris (Graber, 1983; Logtenberg *et al*., 1987) or as a first line of defence against infection (Nakamura *et al*., 1988). The majority of these antibodies are directed at intracellular antigens and are believed to be pro-duced by a distinct subset of B lymphocytes bearing the CD5[+] marker (Nakamura *et al*. 1988).

There is concensus that these antibodies do not predispose to disease. Schwartz (1988), however, has suggested that antigen-driven mutation or abnormal T cell signal may make them pathogenic. While the sharing of epitopes such as phosphodiester groups might explain the cross-reactivity of certain mab with nucleic acids (Locniskar *et al*., 1988), it cannot account for the polyspecificity of all the mab described. Indeed, some workers (Ghosh & Campbell, 1986; Campbell *et al*., 1987) have suggested that the polyspecific interactions may be artefactual.

5.2.3 *Human monoclonal antibodies to tumour antigens*

The selectivity and specificity of Humab make them promising agents for human cancer therapy. They may be cytotoxic through interaction of their Fc portion with complement or cytotoxic cells. They may inhibit growth by competing at the level of growth factor receptors. Alternatively, mab can act as carriers of cytotoxic agents when linked to radioisotopes, natural toxins, chemotherapeutic agents or cytotoxic cells. The technical difficulties of generating Humab, however, have limited the clinical experience with them. A pilot study using a human IgM mab radiolabelled with [111]Indium to image metastases from breast cancer was performed by Ryan et al. (1988).

One in-vivo trial of Humab for human cancer immunotherapy has shown considerable promise (Irie & Morton, 1986). Intra-tumour injection of an IgM monoclonal antibody to ganglioside GD2, an antigen found on the membrane of 70% of cutaneous melanomas, produced regression in six of the eight patients treated. Complete tumour regression was seen in one patient with no recurrence during 20 months of follow-up. No adverse side-effects were noted and anti-idiotype responses seen in five of the patients did not adversely affect treatment.

Other melanoma-specific Humab have been reported. Gomibuchi et al. (1986) have used an IgM mab to ganglioside GD2 to radioimage human melanoma tumours implanted into nude mice. There was a considerable amount of non-specific hepatic uptake and the mab was susceptible to radiolysis. Imam et al. (1986) have generated two IgG mab from the lymph nodes of a patient with metastatic cutaneous malignant melanoma which distinguishes melanomas from benign naevi and basal/squamous cell carcinomas in fixed tissue sections; something not easy to do using conventional histochemical means.

A major goal has been the production of Humab to carcinoma-associated antigens. Although many mabs have been made, the number of useful products remains small. Antibodies to cytoplasmic antigens far outnumber those to membrane antigens and show varying degrees of cross-reactivity with non-tumour tissues (Cote et al., 1986). After a considerable period of intense investigations using mouse anti-cancer mab, the concensus is that individual mab have limited efficacy and that a cocktail of several mab, each with unique properties, would be more useful (Glassy & Dillman, 1988).

The method known as autologous typing has been used to define three classes of antigen expressed by tumour cells and recognized by the host (Old, 1981). Class 1 antigens are expressed only by autologous tumours. These antigens are not expressed by allogeneic normal/malignant cells or autologous normal cells. Biochemical analysis has indicated that most are proteins/ glycoproteins (Garrett et al., 1977; Albino et al., 1981). Class 2 antigens, which are lipids/glycolipids, are expressed by both autologous and allogeneic tumour cells and are limited to cells of a particular differentiation pathway (Pfreund-schuh et al., 1978; Ueda et al., 1979). Class 3 antigens are expressed by a wide variety of normal and tumour cells and have a varied biochemical composition.

The limited quantities of serum available, containing a heterogeneous mixture of low titre antibodies, has meant that the study of these antigens has strained the limits of conventional serology. The development of Humab reacting with cellular antigens has overcome many of these limitations (Cote *et al.*, 1983, 1984, 1986).

Analysis of 8000 hybridomas derived from lymphocytes of healthy donors and patients with cancers and autoimmune diseases showed that 4000 secreted Ig. A significant number (203; 5–10%) of clones secreted Humab reacting with cellular antigens (Cote, 1989). The majority of these mab (194) were directed against intracellular antigens which were broadly distributed or were epitopes shared by multiple antigens; only nine mab recognized membrane antigens. The paucity of membrane-reactive mab is probably due to immunological tolerance (Nossal, 1983). The cellular antigens recognized by these mab could be divided into three categories; highly restrictive, intermediate or broadly reactive, analogous to the class 1, class 2 and class 3 antigens defined by polyclonal sera (see above).

Although antibodies reactive to cellular antigens have been demonstrated in the sera of patients with malignant and autoimmune diseases as well as patients with monoclonal gammopathies (Old, 1981; Dighiero *et al.*, 1982), these Humab suggested that lymphocytes capable of secreting antibody to cellular antigens comprise a significant proportion of the human repertoire (Cote, 1989). The realization that the majority of these mab react with cytoplasmic rather than membrane antigens (Cote *et al.*, 1983, 1984, 1986) is challenging our current understanding of such basic immunological concepts as the generation of antibody diversity, tolerance and autoimmunity.

As normal individuals have lymphocytes capable of producing similar antibodies, their importance to the development of significant anti-cancer and autoantibody responses in patients with malignant and autoimmune diseases remains unclear. It may be that they simply develop in response to cell lysis (Graber, 1983).

While there has been a failure to develop therapeutically effective anti-cancer Humab, those generated have facilitated the identification and purification of tumour antigens (see review by Smith & Teng, 1987), enabling their quantitation in urine (Huth *et al.*, 1987) and providing valuable information on virus–tumour relationship in humans (Shoenfeld *et al.*, 1987).

5.2.4 Human monoclonal antibodies and transplantation

The belief that mice cannot provide an efficient source of mab against human polymorphisms has been highlighted by the HLA system. Many mouse anti-HLA mab react with monomorphic framework antigens, as distinct from type-specific polymorphisms. Specific human alloreactive immune serum has been used for tissue-typing prior to transplantation. The limited availability of such sera, however, has been a constraint. Hulette *et al.* (1985) have reported a human IgM mab reactive with an HLA framework antigen. Hancock *et al.*

(1986) have had similar success. The value of mab as probes for studying major histocompatibility complex (MHC) antigens, identifying and separating lymphocyte subpopulations is beginning to emerge. The report of Humab recognizing a new MHC antigen (Effros et al., 1986) and recognizing a subpopulation of T cells (Alpert et al., 1987) are good examples of this. Humab have been generated to well-defined MHC products such as HLA B15 (Hansen et al., 1987), HLA DR (Kosinski et al., 1986) and HLA DQ (Kolstad et al., 1987). Pistillo et al. (1985) have reviewed many of these antibodies.

5.2.5   Monoclonal antibodies and infectious diseases

Understandably it is the prophylactic and therapeutic potential of Humab against infectious diseases that has attracted most research. An obvious use is in the passive therapy of infections or in the enhancement of responses to vaccines. This is of considerable importance in cases of resistant infections such as Gram-negative septicaemia (Sawada et al., 1985; Teng et al., 1985a) and falciparum malaria (Schmidt-Ullrich et al., 1986), which are proving increasingly difficult to manage by current therapeutic regimens.

Mab capable of neutralizing Herpes zoster virus in vitro have been prepared which are active at 1–50 μg/ml and have augmented activity in the presence of complement (Foung et al., 1985b; Sugano et al., 1987). Matsumoto et al. (1986) have reported a cytomegalovirus (CMV) neutralizing Humab. An IgM mab reactive with endotoxin lipid A of the J5 mutant of E. coli shows cross-reactivity with other Gram-negative bacteria and protects rabbits against endotoxin (Teng et al., 1985a). This Humab protects mice against bacteraemia at a dose of 2 μg.

Several anti-viral Humab, reactive with both nucleocapsid and envelope antigens, have been reported (see review by O'Hare & Yiu, 1987). These include Humab to measles, influenza virus, Herpes simplex, VZV, CMV, Hepatitis B virus (HBV), EBV, human T-cell lymphotropic virus (HTLV-1) and human immunodeficiency virus (HIV). Some of these Humab react with antigens and epitopes not readily detected by Mumab (Foung et al., 1985b). A few have been shown to be protective in experimental animals (Ostberg & Pursch, 1983), others neutralize virus infection in vitro (Foung et al., 1985b; Koizumi et al., 1986; Matsumoto et al., 1986), the rest are nevertheless of diagnostic value (Emanuel et al., 1984; Stricker et al., 1985). Humab have been used for the mapping of HIV epitopes that evoke neutralizing antibodies (Folks, 1987).

Anti-tetanus toxoid Humab are numerous. In some cases their protective effect following toxin administration has been demonstrated in animal systems (Gigliotti & Insel, 1982; Larrick et al., 1983; Olsson et al., 1984; Tiebout et al., 1984). The usefulness of a mab cocktail was demonstrated by Ziegler-Heitbrock et al. (1986): one mab reactive with the B fragment and another with the C fragment of tetanus toxoid did not separately completely protect mice against tetanus toxoid; however, used together they gave complete protection.

Relatively few Humab to specific bacterial antigens or toxins have been reported other than to tetanus toxoid. One example is the report by Gigliotti *et al*. (1984) of a diptheria toxin neutralizing Humab. Humab reactive with the *H. influenzae* capsular polysaccharide have been shown to protect infant rats (Hunter *et al*., 1982; Gigliotti *et al*., 1984). It is hoped that they will be of prophylactive use in human infants who fail to respond to active *H. influenzae* immunization. Humab against group A streptococcal carbohydrate (Steinitz *et al*., 1979) and pneumococcal capsular polysaccharide type B (Steinitz *et al*., 1984, 1986) have been reported. One, an IgA mab, possessed bacteriocidal activity and opsonized type 8 pneumococci. An IgG, lambda Humab reactive with *Pseudomonas aeruginosa* type 5 lipopolysaccharide protects mice against experimental infection (Sawada *et al*., 1985). Several Humab to various *E. coli* strains have been produced by Bogard *et al*. (1985). Humab to purified protein derivative (PPD) of tuberculin (Garzelli *et al*., 1986) and to various *M. leprae* antigens (Atlaw *et al*., 1985) have also been generated. Rosen *et al*. (1983) have found a Humab to the common genus-specific chlamydial surface antigen to be a useful diagnostic agent.

Humab to protozoa are relatively few in number. Schmidt-Ullrich *et al*. (1986) have produced several IgG_1 and IgG_2 anti-plasmodial mab reactive to the Pf195 schizont/merozoite antigen of *Plasmodium falciparum*, one of which inhibited parasite growth *in vitro*. Other anti-plasmodial Humab, staining schizont/merozoites and trophozoites, inhibit parasite invasion of merozoites (Berzins *et al*., 1985; Udomsangpetch *et al*., 1986). These and other Humab by Monjour *et al*. (1983) and Desgranges *et al*. (1985) have been valuable tools for identifying and characterizing antigenic merozoite peptides and mapping antigenic epitopes for malaria vaccine development.

5.3 Problems with human monoclonal antibody production

After over a decade of laborious endeavour, the successes of the Humab technology have been limited in comparison with the mouse approach. There are many factors responsible for this which will be considered below.

5.3.1 *Screening assays*

There are a number of problem areas in the production of Humab. Initially, extensive screening may be necessary to find suitable donors of immune lymphocytes. Assays are also important for screening immortalized cell lines and can be easily established for solid or particulate antigens using either radioimmunoassay (RIA), enzyme-immunoassay (EIA) or fluoresence-immunoassay (FIA). For a variety of reasons, the non-isotopic EIA and FIA are the most commonly used (Gaffar & Glassy, 1988).

The screening of Humab that recognize cellular antigens is more difficult especially if the antigens are expressed in low density per cell. Screening is often compounded by non-specific binding, cross-reactivity of mab and by the limited specificity of the secondary reagents used to detect the mab. This background immunoreactivity is of particular concern to most laboratories (Imam *et al.*, 1986; Gaffar & Glassy, 1988).

5.3.2   Source of human B lymphocytes

Peripheral blood is undoubtedly the most readily available source of human lymphocytes. Compared with spleens, tonsils or lymph nodes, peripheral blood readily lends itself to repeated sampling from the same individual. Unfortunately, experience in both the mouse and human systems has established that peripheral blood is a suboptimal source of immune B cells (Olsson *et al.*, 1983; Lagace & Brodeur, 1985; Ho, 1987; James & Bell, 1987). Indeed, it has been shown that lymphoid tissues such as spleens, tonsils and lymph nodes are superior at providing B cells for immortalization (Burnett *et al.*, 1985; Ho *et al.*, 1985). Peripheral blood contains insufficient B cells (Cote & Houghton, 1985; Ho *et al.*, 1985) because the majority of lymphocytes are of the non-B variety. The limited B lymphocytes present are small, unstimulated cells that are difficult to fuse (James & Bell, 1987).

5.3.3   Lymphocyte enrichment

For practical and ethical considerations peripheral blood is likely to continue as the main source of lymphocytes for human mab production for the forseeable future. The frequency of antigen-specific B cells in human peripheral blood has been estimated by limiting dilution as 10^{-4} to 10^{-5}, depending on the immune status of the donor (Yarchoan *et al.*, 1981; Carson & Freimark, 1986; Yamaura *et al.*, 1985). A number of strategies to enrich for antigen-specific cells have, therefore, been developed. First, rosetting of lymphocytes with RBC bearing the relevant antigen has been employed by many investigators (Steinitz *et al.*, 1979; Boylston *et al.*, 1980; Doyle *et al.*, 1985). Second, panning on antigen-coated wells has also been successful in this regard (Winger *et al.*, 1983; Cole *et al.*, 1985a). Third, lymphocytes have been mixed with FITC-labelled antigen and the fluorescence-activated cell sorter (FACS) used to identify and select the antigen-reactive cells (Casali *et al.*, 1986). These enrichment procedures are usually only of value when large numbers of B cells are available such as from spleen and other lymphoid tissues. With the relatively low cell numbers available from peripheral blood, insufficient numbers of antigen-specific cells are recovered after selection and these enrichment procedures often damage the cells.

5.3.4 In-vivo *immunization*

Following *in-vivo* immunization, immune B lymphocytes to a wide range of antigens have been obtained from a variety of sources and used to generate Humab. These include B cells from donors actively immunized, using approved immunization schedules, against tetanus toxoid (Boyd *et al.*, 1984*b*), pneumococcal (Schwaber *et al.*, 1984), and Rhesus D antigen (Thompson *et al.*, 1986). Humab have been produced using lymphocytes from patients naturally immunized during the course of acquired diseases such as chlamydial salpingitis (Rosen *et al.*, 1983), malaria (Schmidt-Ullrich *et al.*, 1986) and leprosy (Locniskar *et al.*, 1988).

Investigators have also taken advantage of the inadvertent exposure of people to immunogens such as Rhesus D (Bron *et al.*, 1984), single-stranded DNA (Shoenfeld *et al.*, 1982), colorectal tumours (Borup-Christensen *et al.*, 1986) and haptens (Olsson & Kaplan, 1980) to provide immune B cells for generating Humab. The great majority of mab derived from patients with active disease have been directed to cellular and autoantigens. Although some Humab to bacterial and viral products have been produced following natural infections, most have been generated after active immunization.

Following *in-vivo* immunization antigen-specific B cells appear only transiently in peripheral blood (Burnett *et al.*, 1985). As peripheral blood is the commonest source of immune B cells after *in-vivo* immunization, dynamic studies are necessary to determine the optimum time to bleed donors. Few systems have been studied, however, and intensive investigations following tetanus toxoid immunization have provided conflicting information. It appears that B cells spontaneously secreting anti-tetanus antibody are best drawn 5–8 days after booster immunization (Stevens *et al.*, 1979; Butler *et al.*, 1983; Bogard *et al.*, 1985). A subpopulation of B cells, incapable of spontaneously secreting specific antibody, but which do so on stimulation with antigen or PWM, are best obtained after 2 weeks (Lane & Fauci, 1983). Kozbor & Roder (1981) have found that B cells, transformable with EBV to secrete anti-tetanus toxoid Humab, are best isolated 2–4 weeks after the booster inoculation.

Melamed *et al.* (1987) have reported a similar window of 2–4 weeks for collecting B cells which transform with EBV and secrete anti-Rhesus D antibody after immunization. Our experience with hepatitis B vaccination is that the best time to obtain immune lymphocytes from donors is around 14 days after the third inoculation (unpublished data). With some immunogens, however, lymphocytes obtained 1–3 months after vaccination have generated useful Humab (Boyd *et al.*, 1984*b*; Tiebout *et al.*, 1984; Thompson *et al.*, 1986).

5.3.5 In-vitro *immunization*

In-vitro immunization of lymphocytes followed by fusion to generate hybridomas secreting specific mab was first performed in the mouse system

(Hengartner *et al.*, 1978). Since then, increasing attention has been devoted to methods of *in-vitro* immunization in humans to circumvent the problems of obtaining immune lymphocytes from human donors. The success of *in-vitro* immunization in the mouse system has been more difficult to achieve with human lymphocytes, prhaps because these are derived principally from peripheral blood rather than lymphoid tissues (Reading, 1982; Borrebaeck, 1986). Dorfmann (1985) has said that the lack of well-established techniques for *in-vitro* immunization of human lymphocytes is, perhaps, the most significant obstacle to Humab production.

Studies using hepatitis B surface antigen (HBs) have demonstrated the complexities of *in-vitro* immunization in human systems. Anti-HBs responses are induced in 67% of vaccines when cells are stimulated with PWM but only in 12% when HBsAg stimulation is used (Barnaba *et al.*, 1985; Filion & Saginur, 1987). Filion & Saginur (1987) have reported that the anti-HBs response could be modulated by adding IL-2 (interleukin-2) and removing $CD4^+$ cells, $CD8^+$ cells and complement. They concluded that anti-HBs responses *in vitro* are dependent on the individual and the time peripheral blood is sampled.

Despite these problems it has been possible to generate several Humab following *in-vitro* immunization with autoantigen (Osband *et al.*, 1981), tetanus toxoid (Ho *et al.*, 1985), dinitrophenol (Teng *et al.*, 1985*b*), prostatic acid phosphatase (Yamaura *et al.*, 1985) and *Haemophilus influenzae* (Brodeur *et al.*, 1987). In all cases the lymphocytes have been from seropositive donors; attempts to sensitize cells from sero-negative donors has been singularly unsuccessful (Matsumuto *et al.*, 1986). *In-vitro* immunization has normally been performed with Ficoll gradient separated cells but in a few cases such preparations have been depleted of all T cells or only putative T suppressor subsets (Ho *et al.*, 1985; Teng *et al.*, 1985*a*; Garzelli *et al.*, 1986). Whether such T cell depletion is of any real practical value remains a matter of debate. The success of *in-vitro* immunization is influenced by the dose (Matsumoto *et al.*, 1986), form (Ho *et al.*, 1985) and purity of the antigen. In most cases, non-specific mitogens such as endotoxin, phytohaemagglutinin and Cowan 1 strain of *Staph. aureus* have been used in addition to antigen. While PWM remains the most popular mitogen, Teng *et al.* (1985*b*) have favoured muramyl dipeptide while Olsson & Brams (1985) have advocated the use of antigen–silica complexes. The incorporation of growth factors has been advocated by other workers (Strike *et al.*, 1984; Matsumoto *et al.*, 1986; Brodeur *et al.*, 1987). The majority of workers have successfully used fetal bovine serum, although others claim that human serum is essential, at least during the early stages of *in-vitro* cultivation (Strike *et al.*, 1984; Ho *et al.*, 1985; Teng *et al.*, 1985*b*).

The optimum duration of *in-vitro* culture varies from 3 to 7 days, depending on the donor's immune status and the nature of the antigen (James & Bell, 1987). Prior to immortalization, a period of further culture is favoured by some workers (Teng *et al.*, 1985*b*, Masuho *et al.*, 1986). *In vitro* immunization in the human system has been extensively reviewed by Borrebaeck (1986, 1988, 1989).

5.3.6 Immortalization procedures

Procedures for immortalizing human B lymphocytes need much improvement. For hybridomas, the development of less toxic fusion protocols and better fusion partners are paramount. Although PEG is the most widely used fusion agent, electrofusion techniques are gaining ground. Indeed, hybridomas secreting high-affinity Humab have been generated by antigen-mediated electrofusion (Bischoff *et al.*, 1982; Lo *et al.*, 1984; Wojchowski & Sytkowski, 1986; Ohnishi *et al.*, 1987). There is a concensus, however, that while electrofusion may be superior to PEG for fusing small numbers of lymphocytes (less than a million), the reverse is the case when larger numbers of cells are available.

While the ideal procedure for the production of Humab would be transfection of mouse myeloma cells with specific human antibody genes, one has to first prepare the human cell lines to donate these genes. These lines would be generated by immortalizing human B cells by one of the methods outlined above. Therefore, preparation of Humab by genetic engineering will probably remain dependent on conventional tissue culture techniques, although phage technology is developing rapidly (Chapter 7).

Modulation of mab isotype and affinity is possible using genetic engineering technology. The gene segments coding for the heavy chain constant regions can be changed, switching isotype from IgM to IgG and producing a human/human chimeric mab (Morrison, 1985). Site-directed mutagenesis to the heavy and light chain variable regions of Humab can be used to increase antibody affinity (Roberts *et al.*, 1987).

5.3.7 Human fusion partners

The few myeloma fusion partners developed early in the history of Mumab technology were very effective and became widely available. Most were non-secretors of Ig. In contrast, no satisfactory human fusion partner was developed early in the history of Humab technology and as a result many laboratories spent a great deal of time and effort developing their own. Most were developed from four parent LCL (Table 5.1) and are secretors of Ig. Even those that are non-secretors of Ig may continue to synthesize heavy and/or light chains in the cytoplasm. Fusion often leads to re-secretion of these chains resulting in hybrid Ig molecules which reduce the specific activity of the mab. LCL fusion partners have few polyribosomes, sparse Golgi apparatus and secrete relatively little Ig because they are not in the appropriate differentiation stage to secrete high antibody levels (Kozbor *et al.*, 1983; Kozbor & Croce,

1985). Myelomas, which were used so successfully in the mouse system, are very rarely used in the human system because they grow so poorly in tissue culture.

No human fusion partner has found wide-spread acceptance. A true chain-loss variant of fusion partner incapable of secreting Ig chains after fusion is not currently available, although in fact, hybrid mab have not been too much of a problem in the human system (Glassy & Dillman, 1988). Many of the current LCL are actually renamed lines following cloning or additional selection of the few parent LCL available (see above). In most cases the essential characteristics of the renamed line have changed very little from those of the parent LCL. Although LCL are easier to handle and grow better than human myelomas, they have low fusion frequencies and the resultant hybridomas secrete low levels of mab.

The GM 4672 fusion partner appears to form hybridomas predominantly secreting IgM antibody (Shoenfeld et al., 1982, 1983; Locniskar et al., 1988). The reason for this is not clear but cannot be solely explained by the preponderance of IgM-bearing cells in the peripheral blood (Crawford, 1985) that was the source of the immune lymphocytes used for these fusions. The majority of these human IgM mab have been autoantibodies that react with polyspecific epitopes on a wide variety of antigens (Shoenfeld et al., 1982, 1983; Locniskar et al., 1988).

5.3.8   Mouse fusion partners

In the absence of a suitable human partner, many groups have turned to the available well-characterized mouse fusion partners which do not secrete Ig. In comparable experiments, higher fusion frequency has been observed using mouse myeloma rather than human LCL (Cote et al., 1983, 1984, 1986). The human-mouse heterohybridomas produced grow well in culture, clone easily and produce high amounts of Humab and can be adapted to grow as ascitic tumours in nude mice (Tiebout et al., 1985). A major criticism of this technique is that heterohybridomas are unstable and lose the ability to secrete Humab by preferentially segregating human chromosomes, especially chromosome 2 that codes for kappa light chains (Croce et al., 1980b, Ericson et al., 1981). This tendency has been successfully exploited to assign human genes to particular chromosomes (Ruddle, 1973).

Loss of antibody secretion need not be due to chromosome segregation, it can arise because of a defect in regulatory genes (Raison et al., 1982; Schwaber et al., 1984). At times it seems that Humab secretion is maintained by human genes translocated to mouse chromosomes prior to human chromosome segregation (Yoshikawa et al., 1986). While most workers believe that human-mouse hybridomas are more unstable than mouse-mouse hybridomas (Glassy et al., 1987), Thompson et al. (1986) have remained unconvinced and stressed that these lines can be stabilized by early and repeated cloning.

5.3.9 Heterohybridoma fusion partners

Several groups have attempted to improve the fusion rates and growth characteristics of existing LCL by fusing them with either mouse or human myelomas. Fusion of LCL with mouse myelomas has produced several useful fusion partners (Teng *et al.*, 1983, 1985*a*; Foung *et al.*, 1985*a*) which give greater numbers of stable hybridomas when further fused with immune B cells than do mouse myelomas. Kozbor *et al.* (1984) have used the same principle to improve the growth characteristics of their LCL, KR4, by fusing it with the primate myeloma RPMI 8226 (Stricker *et al.*, 1985). The resultant heterohybridoma fusion partner, KR12, showed improved fusion rates over either of its parent lines and exhibited a myeloma phenotype. Most heterohybridoma fusion partners have better fusion characteristics and growth rates than the original parent lines and have the added advantage of being non-secretors of Ig and being EBNA-negative.

5.3.10 EBV transformation

Following transformation of unfractionated peripheral blood lymphocytes by EBV, cells are subject to regression due to the development of EBV-specific cytotoxic T cells (Moss *et al.*, 1979). This can be minimized either by T cell depletion or by the addition of agents such as phytohaemagglutinin (PHA) (Moss *et al.*, 1979) or cyclosporin A (Bird *et al.*, 1981) which abrogate the T cell effect. The main problem with EBV transformation is the instability and poor cloning ability of the resultant LCL. This instability has been attributed to either overgrowth by non-secreting cells (Olsson *et al.*, 1983) or to terminal differentiation of cells to non-proliferating plasma cell types (Melamed *et al.*, 1985). In some cases, however, cytoplasmic Ig can be demonstrated and a defect in the secretory mechanism is probably responsible for the decline in Ig production (Kozbor *et al.*, 1983; Sikora *et al.*, 1983; McCann *et al.*, 1988).

It is not uncommon for LCL to grow well for 1–2 months before their mab levels suddenly decline. This event is often accompanied by a visible change in cell phenotype from small, highly clumped, irregular shaped cells to large, more uniformly rounded cells which do not grow as quickly. Although early cloning has rescued some mab secreting LCL, many potentially useful lines have been lost due to their extremely poor cloning efficiency. It is interesting that 'cell-driven' transformation appears to lead to LCL which are more stable and secrete higher levels of mab but the mechanism underlying this phenomenon has not been investigated (James & Bell, 1987). It is unfortunate that the plasma cell, the factory for Ig synthesis, cannot be transformed as it lacks the EBV receptor.

5.3.11 Combined EBV/fusion technique

Kozbor *et al.* (1982) have pioneered the technique of using initial EBV transformation prior to fusion to produce what they have termed an 'EBV hybridoma'. This approach was thought to combine the selective advantages of both the EBV transformation and hybridoma methods for producing Humab. Kozbor & Roder (1984) reported that transforming cells with EBV 2–8 weeks before fusion increased the fusion frequency from 20×10^{-7} to over 100×10^{-7}. They attributed the superiority of the 'EBV hybridoma' technique to the more efficient activation and proliferation of B cells by EBV compared with transformation with PWM.

The hybridomas produced by this approach have the same instability problems as any other but undoubtedly clone more readily and produce higher levels of specific antibodies than EBV-transformed LCL. The antibodies secreted are representative of the antibodies being produced by the transformed lines at the time of fusion. As a result, many of the lines produce IgM antibodies although IgG, especially IgG1, antibodies are not uncommon.

5.3.12   Use of feeder cells

A crucial stage in the production of Humab by any of these methods is the selective culture of antigen-specific cells at low cell densities (cloning). Feeder cells have often been used to improve the growth characteristics of cloned cells. They have also been used to improve the growth of newly transformed and fused cell lines. A wide variety of morphologically different cell types have been used as feeder cells in the Humab system, including human fibroblasts (Steinitz *et al.*, 1979; Kozbor & Roder, 1981; Strike *et al.*, 1984), human mononuclear cells (Bischoff *et al.*, 1982; Melamed *et al.*, 1985) and mouse mononuclear cells (Melamed *et al.*, 1985; Thompson *et al.*, 1986; Brodeur *et al.*, 1987). Mononuclear cells may be superior to other cell types because they contain phagocytic cells capable of ingesting cellular debris and contaminating microorganisms. Feeder cells are thought to work by providing essential cellular contact to the developing cell clones as well as by secreting vital growth factors.

Many workers have reported that feeder cells improve the chance of isolating specific antibody secreting cell lines (Tiebout *et al.*, 1984; Crawford, 1985; Teng *et al.*, 1985a). Others feel that they are of limited value (Cote *et al.*, 1983; Strike *et al.*, 1984; Schmidt-Ullrich *et al.*, 1986).

5.3.13   Cloning cell lines

Cloning in soft agar theoretically assures single clone selection but many cells thriving in liquid cultures do not grow well in soft agar. Cell-sorting technology has provided instruments capable of placing a single cell in a single well (Parks *et al.*, 1979) but access to such equipment is limited because of its high cost.

For these reasons, many laboratories still rely on cloning by the technique of 'limiting dilution' (Lefkovits, 1979; Lefkovits & Waldmann, 1980). The statistics for analysing cloning by application of the Poisson distribution has been well worked out (Lefkovits, 1979; Lefkovits & Waldmann, 1980). Goding *et al.* (1980) have used the equation $a = e^{-b}$, where a is the fraction of wells with no growth and b is the number of clones per well. When $b = 1$, $a = 0.37$; therefore, when more than 37% of wells seeded at a given cell concentration show no growth, there is a statistically significant probability that the wells with growth are derived from single cells. We seed wells with 30, 3 or 0.3 cells and perform our cloning procedure at least twice to ensure monoclonality.

LCL can be particularly difficult to clone, even in the presence of feeder cells and/or growth factor, and it is generally accepted that at less than ten cells per well, little or no growth will occur. There have, however, been successes in soft agar containing irradiated human fibroblasts (Hoch *et al.*, 1982; Kosinski & Hammerling, 1986).

5.3.14 Mass production of human monoclonal antibodies

Large supplies of Mumab can be produced by growth of mouse–mouse hybridomas as ascitic tumours in mice, usually after priming the host animals with pristane (Hoogenraad *et al.*, 1983; Brodeur *et al.*, 1984). Similar attempts to grow human–human hybridomas have met with limited success, even in nude mice deficient in T cells (Truitt *et al.*, 1984; Olsson & Brams, 1985; Yoshikawa *et al.*, 1986). Strategies to improve human–human hybridoma uptake include irradiation of pristane treated mice (Bogard *et al.*, 1985; Kozbor *et al.*, 1985), adaptation of the hybridomas by passage as solid subcutaneous tumours (Truitt *et al.*, 1984; Kozbor *et al.*, 1985), mixing the hybridomas with human skin fibroblasts prior to inoculation (Olsson & Brams, 1985) or the use of severe combined immunodeficient (SCID) mice (Ware *et al.*, 1985; Effros *et al.*, 1986).

In contrast, human–mouse heterohybridomas will grow in non-irradiated mice without adaptation (Bron *et al.*, 1984; Insel, 1984; Burnett *et al.*, 1985; Tiebout *et al.*, 1985; Yamaura *et al.*, 1985; Yoshikawa *et al.*, 1986). Failure of rejection is undoubtedly due to lack of expression of surface human leucocyte antigens (HLA) by the heterohybridomas. Attempts to grow EBV-transformed LCL in nude mice have been hampered by infection because of the extreme susceptibility of these animals to EBV.

An alternative approach to producing large quantities of Humab is to use *in-vitro* tissue culture techniques. When relatively small amounts of Humab are required, stationary flask cultures are perfectly adequate. Three litre amounts have been successfully produced in culture suspensions using stirrer flasks (Hunter *et al.*, 1982; Thompson *et al.*, 1986) and roller bottles (Sikora *et al.*, 1983; Thompson *et al.*, 1986). A number of continuous feed systems have been adapted for laboratory use based on the principle of trapping cells in hollow fibres (Feder & Tolbert, 1983; Altschuler *et al.*, 1986) or agarose beads (Schier *et al.*, 1984).

For very large scale production of Humab sufficient for use in mass therapeutic trials, airlift reactors and immobilized cell technologies are probably the
methods of choice (Birch *et al.*, 1985; Duff, 1985; Altschuler *et al.*, 1986). One
of the major headaches of large scale tissue culture production is the requirement for suitable batches of serum, usually fetal bovine serum. Because serum
represents the predominant cost of culture media, there has been an interest in
the development of both serum-free and protein-free media, with the obvious
benefit in batch control and ease of purification of the mab (Cleveman *et al.*,
1983; Cole *et al.*, 1985*b*, 1987).

5.4   Conclusion

Practical problems have hindered the production and dissemination of human
monoclonal antibodies. Human donors can rarely be hyperimmunized, especially to toxic chemicals, pathogenic viruses or cancer cells and peripheral
blood, the primary source of B cells in humans, contains few blast cells that are
actively involved in the immune response. Therefore, antigen-specific B cells
are seldom available in quantity.

EBV transformation does not lead to preferential immortalization of B cell
blasts engaged in antibody responses and leads to lines, secreting low levels of
antibody, which commonly lose the ability to secrete Ig. Human fusion
partners have poor fusion frequency and are secretors of endogenous Ig chains
whereas the use of mouse myeloma fusion partners leads to unstable hybridomas that preferentially lose human chromosomes.

The bulk production of human monoclonal antibodies requires costly cell
culture or passage of heterohybridoma cell lines through immunodeficient
mice. Gradually, however, these problems are being overcome and the production of chimeric mouse–human and human–human antibodies by the genetic
engineering approach holds exciting possibilities for the future (Chapters 7
and 8).

Humab technology has offered novel systems for investigating the generation
of antibody diversity, the control of antibody gene expression and the relationship between antibody structure and function. There are many instances in
which it has improved our understanding, diagnoses, prevention and treatment
of autoimmunity, infection, cancer and transplantation. With greater
intellectual and financial support, the full potential of the Humab technology
will be realized.

5.5   References

Albino, A. P., Lloyds, K. O., Houghton, A. N., Oettgen, H. F. & Old, L. J. (1981).
    Heterogeneity in surface antigen expression and glycoprotein expression of cell
    lines derived from different metastases of the same patient: implications for the
    study of tumour antigens. *Journal of Experimental Medicine*, **154**, 1764–1776.
Alpert, S. D., Turek, P. J., Foung, S. K. H. & Engleman, E. G. (1987). Human

monoclonal anti-T cell antibody from a patient with rheumatoid arthritis. *Journal of Immunology*, **138**, 104–108.

Altschuler, G. L., Dziewulski, D. M., Sowek, J. A. & Belfort, G. (1986). Continuous hybridoma growth and monoclonal production in hollow fiber reactors-separators. *Biotechnology and Bioengineering*, **28**, 646–658.

Aman, P., Ehlin-henrilsson, B. & Klein, G. (1985). Epstein–Barr virus susceptibility of normal human B lymphocyte populations. *Journal of Experimental Medicine*, **159**, 208–220.

Atlaw, T., Kozbor, D. & Roder, J. C. (1985). Human monoclonal antibodies against *Mycobacterium leprae. Infection and Immunity*, **49**, 104–110.

Baker, J. R., Saunders, N. B., Kaulfersch, W. & Burman, K. D. (1988). Development of a human monoclonal antibody from a Graves' disease patient that identifies a novel thyroid membrane antigen. *Journal of Immunology*, **140**, 2593–2599.

Barnaba, V., Valesini, G., Levero, M., Zaccari, M., Van Dyke, A., Falco, M., Musca, A. & Balsano, F. (1985). Immunoregulation of the anti-HBs antibody synthesis in chronic HBsAg carriers and in recently boosted anti-hepatitis B vaccine recipients. *Clinical and Experimental Immunology*, **60**, 259–266.

Berzins, K., Perlmann, H., Udomsangpetch, R., Wahlgren, M., Trorg-Blomberg, M., Carlsson, J., Bjorkman, A. & Perlmann, P. (1985). Pf155, a candidate for blood stage vaccine in *Plasmodium falciparum* malaria. *Developments in Biological Standards*, **62**, 99–106.

Birch, J. R., Borasten, R. & Wood, L. (1985). Bulk production of monoclonal antibodies in fermenters. *Trends in Biotechnology*, **3**, 162–166.

Bird, A. G., McLachan, S. M. & Britton, S. (1981). Cyclosporin A promotes the spontaneous out growth *in vitro* of Epstein–Barr virus-induced B-cell lines. *Nature*, **289**, 300–301.

Bischoff, R., Eisert, R. M., Schedel, I., Vienken, J. & Zimmermann, U. (1982). Human hybridoma cells produced by electro-fusion. *Febs Letters*, **147**, 64–68.

Bloy, C., Blanchard, D., Lambin, P., Goosens, D., Rouger, P., Salmon, C. & Cartron, J.-P. (1987). Human monoclonal antibody against Rh(D) antigen: partial characterization of the Rh(D) polypeptide from human erythrocytes. *Blood*, **69**, 1491–1497.

Bogard, W. C., Hornberger, E. & Kung, P. C. (1985). Production and characterization of human monoclonal antibodies against Gram-negative bacteria. In *Human Hybridomas and Monoclonal Antibodies*, ed. E. G. Engleman, S. K. H. Foung, J. Larrick & A. Raubitschek, pp. 95–112. New York, Plenum Press.

Borrebaeck, C. A. K. (1986). *In-vitro* immunization for the production of murine and human monoclonal antibodies: present status. *Trends in Biotechnology*, **4**, 147–153.

Borrebaeck, C. A. K. (1988). Human mAbs produced by primary *in-vitro* immunization. *Immunology Today*, **9**, 355–359.

Borrebaeck, C. A. K. (1989). Strategy for the production of human monoclonal antibodies using *in-vitro* activated B cells. *Journal of Immunological Methods*, **123**, 157–165.

Borup-Christensen, P., Erb, K., Jensenius, J. C., Nielson, B. & Svehag, S. E. (1986). Human–human hybridomas for the study of anti-tumour immune response in patients with colorectal cancer. *International Journal of cancer*, **37**, 683–688.

Bouhanne, G. L., Hozumi, N. & Shulman, M. J. (1984). Production of functional chimaeric mouse/human antibody. *Nature*, **312**, 643–646.

Bowman, J. M. (1978) Suppression of Rh iso-immunization: a review. *Obstetrics and Gynaecology*, **52**, 385–389.

Boyd, J. E., Hastings, I., Farzad, Z., James, K. & McClelland, D. B. L. (1984*b*).

Experiences in the production of human monoclonal antibodies to tetanus toxoid. *Developments in Biological Standardization*, **57**, 93–98.

Boyd, J. E. & James, K. (1989). Human monoclonal antibodies: their potential, problems and prospects. *Advances in Biotechnological Processes*, **11**, 1–43.

Boyd, J. E., James, K. & McClelland, D. B. L. (1984*a*). Human monoclonal antibodies – production and potential. *Trends in Biotechnology*, **2**, 70–77.

Boylston, A. W., Gardener, B., Anderson, R. L. & Hughes-Jones, N. C. (1980). Production of human IgM anti-D in tissue culture by EB virus-transformed lymphocytes. *Scandinavian Journal of Immunology*, **12**, 355–358.

Brahe, C. & Serra, A. (1981). A simple method for fusing human lymphocytes with rodent cells in monolayer by polyethylene glycol. *Somatic Cell Genetics*, **7**, 109–115.

Brodeur, B. R., Lagace, J., Larose, Y., Martin, M., Joly, J. & Page, M. (1987). Mouse–human myeloma partner for the production of heterohybridomas. In *Monoclonal Antibodies*, ed. B. Schook, pp. 51–63. New York, Marcel Dekker.

Brodeur, B. R., Tsang, P. & Larose, Y. (1984). Parameters affecting ascites tumour formation in mice and monoclonal antibody production. *Journal of Immunological Methods*, **71**, 265–272.

Bron, D., Feinberg, M. B., Teng, N. N. H. & Kaplan, H. S. (1984). Production of human monoclonal IgG antibodies against Rhesus (D) antigen. *Proceedings of the National Academy of Sciences of the U.S.A.*, **81**, 3214–3217.

Bruggeman, M., Winter, G., Waldmann, H. & Neuberger, M. S. (1989). The immunogenicity of chimaeric antibodies. *Journal of Experimental Medicine*, **170**, 2153–2157.

Burk, K. H., Drewinko, B., Trujillo, J. M. & Ahearn, M. J. (1978). Establishment of a human plasma cell line *in vitro*. *Cancer Research*, **38**, 2508–2511.

Burnett, K. G., Leung, J. P. & Martinis, J. (1985). Human monoclonal antibodies to defined antigens: towards clinical application. In *Human Hybridomas and Monoclonal Antibodies*, ed. E. G. Engleman, S. K. H. Foung, J. Larrick & A. Raubitschek, pp. 113–133. New York, Plenum Press.

Butler, J. L., Lane, H. C. & Fauci, A. S. (1983). Delineation of optimal conditions for producing mouse–human heterohybridomas from human peripheral blood B cells of immunized subjects. *Journal of Immunology*, **130**, 165–168.

Campbell, A. M., Whitford, P. & Leake, R. E. (1987). Human monoclonal antibodies and monoclonal antibody multispecificity. *British Journal of Cancer*, **56**, 709–713.

Carson, D. E. & Freimark, B. D. (1986). Human lymphocytes and monoclonal antibodies. *Advances in Immunology*, **38**, 275–311.

Casali, P., Inghirami, G., Akamura, M., Davies, T. F. & Notkins, A. L. (1986). Human monoclonals from antigen specific selection of B lymphocytes and transformation by EBV. *Science*, **234**, 476–479.

Chan, M. A., Stein, L. D., Dosch, H. M. & Sigal, N. H. (1986). Heterogeneity of EBV-transformable human B lymphocyte populations. *Journal of Immunology*, **136**, 106–112.

Cleveman, W. L., Wood, I. & Erlanger, B. F. (1983). Routine large-scale production of monoclonal antibodies in a protein-free culture medium. *Journal of Immunological Methods*, **56**, 221–234.

Cole, S. P. C., Kozbor, D. & Roder, J. C. (1985*a*). The EBV hybridoma technique and its application to human lung cancer. In *Monoclonal Antibodies and Cancer Therapy*, ed. R. A. Reisfeld & S. Sell, pp. 77–96. New York, Alan R. Liss.

Cole, S. P. C., Vreeken, E. H., Mirski, S. E. L. & Campling, B. G. (1987). Growth of human × human hybridomas in protein-free medium supplemented with ethanolamine. *Journal of Immunological Methods*, **97**, 29–35.

Cole, S. P. C., Vreeken, E. H., & Roder, J. C. (1985*b*). Antibody production by human × human hybridomas in serum-free medium. *Journal of Immunological Methods*, **78**, 271–278.

Cote, R. J. (1989). Analysis of the human immune repertoire using human monoclonal antibodies. *The International Journal of Biological Markers*, **4**, 59–64.

Cote, R. J., Morrissey, D. M., Houghton, A. N., Beattie, Jr., E. J., Oettgen, H. F. & Old, L. J. (1983). Generation of human monoclonal antibodies reactive with cellular antigens. *Proceedings of the National Academy of Sciences of the U.S.A.*, **80**, 2026–2030.

Cote, R. J., Morrissey, D. M., Houghton, A. N., Thomson, T. M., Daly, M. E., Oettgen, H. F. & Old, L. J. (1986). Specificity analysis of human monoclonal antibodies reactive with cell surface and intracellular antigen. *Proceedings of the National Academy of Sciences of the U.S.A.*, **83**, 2969–2973.

Cote, R. J., Morrissey, D. M., Oettgen, H. F. & Old, L. J. (1984). Analysis of human monoclonal antibodies derived from lymphocytes of patient with cancer. *Federation Proceedings*, **43**, 2465–2469.

Crawford, D. H. (1985). Production of human monoclonal antibodies using Epstein–Barr virus. In *Human Hybridomas and Monoclonal Antibodies*, ed. E. G. Engleman, S. K. H. Foung, J. Larrick & A. Raubitschek, pp. 37–53. New York, Plenum Press.

Crawford, D. H. & Callard, R. E. (1983). Production of human monoclonal antibody to X31 influenza virus nucleoprotein. *Journal of General Virology*, **64**, 697–700.

Croce, C. M., Linnenbach, A., Hall, W., Steplewski, Z. & Koprowski, H. (1980*a*). Production of human hybridomas secreting antibodies to measles virus. *Nature*, **288**, 488–489.

Croce, C. M., Shander, M., Mortinus, J., Circurel, L., d'Ancona, C. G. & Koprowski, H. (1980*b*). Preferential retention of human chromosome 14 in mouse × human B cell hybrids. *European Journal of Immunology*, **10**, 486–488.

Davidson, R. L. & Gerrard, P. S. (1976). Improved techniques for the induction of mammalian cell hybridization by polyethylene glycol. *Somatic Cell Genetics*, **2**, 165–176.

Desgranges, C., Ploton, I., Paire, J., Dubois, P. & Monjour, L. (1985). Production of human monoclonal antibodies against various antigens of erythrocytic stages of *Plasmodium falciparum*. *Comptes Rendus des Seances de l'Academie des Sciences*, **301**, 219–224.

Dighiero, G., Guilbert, B. & Avraneas, S. (1982). Naturally occurring antibodies against nine common antigens in human sera: ii. High incidence of monoclonal Ig exhibiting antibody activities. *Journal of Immunology*, **128**, 2788–2792.

Dorfmann, N. A. (1985). The optimal technology approach to the development of human hybridomas. *Journal of Biological Response Modifiers*, **4**, 213–239.

Doyle, A., Jones, T. J., Bidwell, J. L. & Bradley, B. A. (1985). *In-vitro* development of human monoclonal antibody-secreting plasmacytomas. *Human Immunology*, **13**, 199–209.

Duff, R. G. (1985). Microencapsulation technology: a novel method for monoclonal antibody production. *Trends in Biotechnology*, **3**, 167–179.

Edwards, P. A. W., Smith, C. M., Neville, A. M. & O'Hare, M. J. (1982). A human/human hybridoma system based on a fast growing mutant of the ARH-77 plasma cell leukemia derived cell line. *European Journal of Immunology*, **12**, 641–648.

Effros, R. B., Hulette, C. M., Ettenger, R., Dillard, L. C., Zeller, E., Duoung, R. & Walford, R. L. (1986). A human–human hybridoma secreting anti-HLA class II antibody. *Journal of Immunology*, **137**, 1599–1603.

Eisenbarth, G. S., Linnenbach, A., Jackson, R., Scearce, R. & Croce, C. M. (1982). Human hybridomas secreting anti-islet auto-antibodies. *Nature*, **300**, 264–267.

Emanuel, D., Gold, J., Calcino, J., Lopez, C. & Hammering, U. (1984). A human monoclonal antibody to cytomegalovirus (CMV). *Journal of Immunology*, **133**, 2202–2205.

Ericson, J., Martinis, J. & Croce, C. M. (1981). Assignment of the genes for human lambda immunoglobulin chains to chromosome 22. *Nature*, **294**, 173–175.

Essani, K., Satoh, J., Prabhakar, B. S., McClintok, P. T., & Notkins, A. L. (1985). Anti-idiotypic antibodies against human multiple organ-reactive autoantibody. Detection of idiotypes in normal individuals and patients with autoimmune disease. *Journal of Clinical Investigation*, **76**, 1649–1656.

Feder, J. & Tolbert, W. R. (1983). The large-scale cultivation of mammalian cells. *Scientific American*, **248**, 36–43.

Filion, I. G. & Saginur, R. (1987). Induction of the *in vitro* anti-HBs response by hepatitis B surface antigen. *Clinical and Experimental Immunology*, **74**, 321–325.

Folks, T. M. (1987). Epitope mapping of human immunodeficiency virus: a monoclonal approach. *Journal of Immunology*, **139**, 3913–3914.

Foster, C. S., Tan, K. S., DeSilva, M., Byfield, P. G., Medlen, A. R., Wright, J. M. & Marks, V. (1987). Human monoclonal antibodies to thyroid antigens derived by hybridization of lymphocytes from a diabetic patient. *Metabolism*, **36**, 327–334.

Foung, S. K. H., Blunt, J., Perkins, S., Winn, L. & Grumet, F. C. (1986). A human monoclonal antibody to Rh G. *Vox Sanguinis*, **50**, 160–163.

Foung, S. K. H., Blunt, J. A., Wu, P. S., Ahern, P., Winn, L. C. & Engleman, E. G. (1987). Human monoclonal antibodies to Rh (D). *Vox Sanguinis*, **53**, 44–47.

Foung, S. K. H., Perkins, S., Arvin, A., Lifson, J., Mohagheghpour, N., Fishwild, D., Grumet, F. C. & Engleman, E. G. (1985*a*). Production of human monoclonal antibodies using a human mouse fusion partner. In *Human Hybridomas and Monoclonal Antibodies*, ed. E. G. Engleman, S. K. H. Foung, J. Larrick & A. Raubitschek, pp. 135–148. New York, Plenum Press.

Foung, S. K. H., Perkins, S., Koropachak, C., Fishwild, D. M., Wittek, I. E., Engleman, E. G., Grumet, F. C. & Arvin, A. M. (1985*b*). Human monoclonal antibody neutralizing varicella-zoster virus. *Journal of Infectious Diseases*, **152**, 280–285.

Frade, R., Barel, M., Ehlin-Henriksson, B. & Klein, G. (1985). gp140, the C3d receptor of human B lymphocytes is also the Epstein–Barr virus receptor. *Proceedings of the National Academy of Sciences of the U.S.A.*, **82**, 1490–1493.

Gaffar, S. A. & Glassy, M. C. (1988). Applications of human monoclonal antibodies in non-isotopic immunoassay. In *Reviews on Immunoassay Technology*, vol. 1, ed. S. B. Pal, pp. 59–94. London, Macmillan Press.

Garrett, T. J., Takahashi, T., Clarkson, B. D. & Old, L. J. (1977). Detection of antibody to autologous human leukemia cells by immune adherence assays. *Proceedings of the National Academy of Sciences of the U.S.A.*, **74**, 4587–4590.

Garzelli, C., Puglisi, C. & Falcone, G. (1986). Human monoclonal antibody to purified protein derivative of tuberculin produced by hybrids constructed with Epstein–Barr transformed B lymphocytes and mouse myeloma cells. *European Journal of Immunology*, **16**, 584–587.

Garzelli, C., Taub, F. E., Scharff, J. E., Prabhakar, B. S., Ginsberg-Fellner, F. & Notkins, A. L. (1984). Epstein–Barr transformed lymphocytes produce monoclonal antibodies that react with antigen in multiple organs. *Journal of Virology*, **52**, 722–725.

Ghosh, S. & Campbell, A. M. (1986). Multispecific monoclonal antibodies. *Immunology Today*, **7**, 217–222.

Gibson, T. (1973). The production of high titre (Rh)D antibody in male volunteers. *Vox Sanguinis*, **24**, 425–431.

Gigliotti, F. & Insel, R. A. (1982). Protective human hybridoma antibody to tetanus toxin. *Journal of Clinical Investigation*, **70**, 1306–1309.

Gigliotti, F., Smith, L. & Insel, R. A. (1984). Reproducible production of protective human monoclonal antibodies by fusion of peripheral blood lymphocytes with a mouse myeloma cell line. *Journal of Infectious Diseases*, **149**, 43–47.

Glassy, M. C. & Dillman, R. O. (1988). Molecular biotherapy with monoclonal antibodies. *Molecular Biotherapy*, **1**, 7–13.

Glassy, M. C., Handley, H. H., Hagiwara, H. & Royston, I. (1983). UC-729-6, a human lymphoblastoid B-cell line useful for generating antibody-secreting human/human hybridomas. *Proceedings of the National Academy of Sciences of the U.S.A.*, **80**, 6327–6331.

Glassy, M. C., Handley, H. H. & Royston, I. (1985). Design and production of human monoclonal antibodies to human cancers. In *Human Hybridomas and Monoclonal Antibodies*, ed. E. G. Engleman, S. K. H. Foung, J. Larrick & A. Raubitschek, pp. 211–225. New York, Plenum Press.

Glassy, M. C., Handley, H. H., Surh, C. S. & Royston, I. (1987). Genetically stable human hybridomas secreting tumour reactive human monoclonal IgM. *Cancer Investigations*, **5**, 449–457.

Goding, J. W. (1980). Antibody production by hybridomas. *Journal of Immunological Methods*, **39**, 285–308.

Gomibuchi, M., Saxton, R. E., Lake, R. R., Katano, M. & Irie, R. F. (1986). Radioimmunodetection of human melanoma tumour xenografts with human monoclonal antibodies. *International Journal of Radiation Applications and Instrumentation*, **13**, 13–19.

Goosens, D., Champomier, F., Rouger, P. & Salmon, C. (1987). Human monoclonal antibodies against blood group antigens: preparation of a series of stable EBV immortalized clones producing high levels of antibody of different isotypes and specificities. *Journal of Immunological Methods*, **101**, 193–200.

Graber, P. (1983). Autoantibodies and the physiological role of immunoglobulins. *Immunology Today*, **4**, 337–340.

Gunsen, H. H., Stratton, F. & Phillips, P. K. (1974). The anti-Rh(D) responses of immunized volunteers following spaced antigen stimuli. *British Journal of Haematology*, **27**, 171–182.

Hale, G., Dyer, M. J. S., Clark, M. R., Phillips, J. M., Marcus, R., Reichmann, L., Winter, G. & Waldmann, H. (1988). Remission induction in non-Hodgkin's lymphoma with reshaped human monoclonal antibody CAMPATH-1H. *Lancet*, **ii**, 1394–1399.

Hancock, R. J. T., Martin, A., Stinchcombe, V., Jones, T. J., Smythe, J., Laundy, G. L. & Bradley, B. A. (1986). *In-vitro* production of anti-HLA-DR antibodies by human B cell lines. *Tissue Antigens*, **28**, 228–232.

Hansen, T., Kolstad, A., Mathisen, G. & Hanvestad, K. (1987). A human–human hybridoma (Tr 7E2) producing cytotoxic antibody to HLA-DQw1. *Human Immunology*, **20**, 307–320.

Hengartner, H., Luzzati, A. L. & Schreier, M. (1978). Fusion of *in-vitro* immunized lymphoid cells with X63.Ag8. *Current Topics in Microbiology and Immunology*, **81**, 92–99.

Ho, M. K. (1987). Production of human monoclonal antibodies by *in-vitro* immunization. In *Human Hybridomas; Diagnostic and Therapeutic Applications*, Immunology Series, vol. 30, ed. A. J. Strelkauskas, pp. 23–57. New York, Marcel Dekker.

Ho, M. K., Rand, N., Murray, J., Kato, K. & Rabin H. (1985). *In-vitro* immunization of human lymphocytes. 1. Production of human monoclonal antibodies against bombesin and tetanus toxoid. *Journal of Immunology*, **135**, 3831–3838.

Hoch, A., Schur, P. H. & Schwaber, J. (1982). Improved method for cloning human B-cell lines. *Cellular Immunology*, **72**, 219–230.

Hoogenraad, N., Helman, T. & Hoogenraad, J. (1983). The effect of preinjection of mice with pristane on ascites tumour formation and monoclonal antibody production. *Journal of Immunological Methods*, **61**, 317–320.

Hulette, C. M., Effros, R. B., Dillard, L. C. & Walford, R. L. (1985). Production of a human monoclonal antibody to HLA by human–human hybridoma technology. *American Journal of Pathology*, **121**, 10–14.

Hunter, Jr., K. W., Fischer, G. W., Hemming, V. G., Wilson, S. R., Hartzman, R. J. & Woody, J. N. (1982). Antibacterial activity of a human monoclonal antibody to *Haemophilus influenzae* type B capsular polysaccharide. *The Lancet*, **ii**, 798–799.

Huth, J. F., Saxton, R. E., Morton, D. L. & Irie, R. F. (1987). A human monoclonal antibody produced by *in-vitro* sensitization of human lymphocytes with an antigen from urine of a sarcoma patient. *Journal of Surgical Research*, **42**, 591–596.

Ichimori, Y., Sasano, K., Itoh, H., Hitotsumachi, S., Kimura, Y., Kaneko, K., Kida, M. & Tsukamoto, K. (1985). Establishment of hybridomas secreting human monoclonal antibodies against tetanus toxin and hepatitis B virus surface antigen. *Biochemical and Biophysical Research Communications*, **129**, 26–33.

Imam, A., Mitchell, M. S., Modlin, R. L., Taylor, C. R., Kemp, R. A. & Ken-Mitchell, J. (1986). Human monoclonal antibodies that distinguish cutaneous malignant melanomas from benign nevi in fixed tissue sections. *Journal of Investigative Dermatology*, **86**, 145–148.

Insel, R. A. (1984). *In-vitro* production of human hybridoma antibody to the *Haemophilus influenzae* B capsule in athymic nude mice. *Journal of Infectious Diseases*, **150**, 959–960.

Irie, R. F. & Morton, D. L. (1986). Regression of cutaneous metastatic melanoma by intralesional injection with human monoclonal antibody to ganglioside GD2. *Proceedings of the National Academy of Sciences of the U.S.A.*, **83**, 8694–8698.

James, K. & Bell, G. T. (1987). Human monoclonal antibody production. Current status and future prospects. *Journal of Immunological Methods*, **100**, 5–40.

Jonak, Z. L., Braman, V. & Kennett, R. H. (1984). Production of continuous mouse plasma cell lines by transfection with human leukemia DNA. *Hybridoma*, **3**, 107–118.

Jondai, M., Klein, G., Oldstone, M. B. A., Bokish, V. & Yefenof, E. (1976). Surface markers on human B and T lymphocytes VIII. Association between complement and Epstein–Barr virus receptors on human lymphoid cells. *Scandinavian Journal of Immunology*, **5**, 401–410.

Kamo, I., Furakawa, S., Tada, A., Mano, Y., Iwasaki, Y., Furuse, T., Ito, N., Hagashi, K. & Satoyashi, E. (1982). Monoclonal antibody to acetylcholine receptor: cell line established from thymus of patient with myasthenia gravis. *Science*, **215**, 995–996.

Koizumi, S., Fujiwara, S., Kikuta, H., Okano, M., Imai, S., Mizumo, F. & Osato, P. T. (1986). Production of human monoclonal antibodies against Epstein-Barr virus-specific antigens by the virus-immortalized lymphoblastoid cell lines. *Virology*, **15**, 161–169.

Kolstad, A., Hansen, T. & Hannestad, K. (1987). A human–human hybridoma antibody (Tr B12) defining subgroups of HLA-DQw1 and −DQw3. *Human Immunology*, **20**, 219–231.

Kornprobst, M., Rouger, P. H., Goosens, D., Champonier, F. & Salmon, C. H. (1986).

Determination of Rh(D) genotype: use of human monoclonal antibodies in flow cytometry. *Journal of Clinical Pathology*, **39**, 1039–1042.

Kosinski, S. & Hammerling, U. (1986). A new cloning method for antibody forming lymphoblastoid cells. *Journal of Immunological Methods*, **94**, 201–208.

Kosinski, S., Hammerling, U. & Yang, S. Y. (1986). A human monoclonal antibody to an HLA-DRw53 (MT3)-like epitope on class II antigens. *Tissue Antigens*, **28**, 150–162.

Kozbor, D., Abramow-Newerly, W., Tripputi, P., Cole, S. P. C., Weibel, J., Roder, J. C. & Croce, C. M. (1985). Specific immunoglobulin production and enhanced tumourgenicity following ascites growth of human hybridomas. *Journal of Immunological Methods*, **8**, 31–42.

Kozbor, D. & Croce, C. M. (1985). Fusion partners for production of human monoclonal antibodies. In *Human Hybridomas and Monoclonal Antibodies*, ed. E. G. Engleman, S. K. H. Foung, J. Larrick & A. Raubitschek, pp. 21–36. New York, Plenum Press.

Kozbor, D., Dexter, D. & Roder, J. C. (1983). A comparative analysis of the phenotypic characteristics of available fusion partners for the construction of human hybridomas. *Hybridoma*, **2**, 7–16.

Kozbor, D., Lagarde, A. & Roder, J. C. (1982). Human hybridomas constructed with antigen-specific Epstein–Barr virus-transformed cell lines. *Proceedings of the National Academy of Sciences of the U.S.A.*, **79**, 6651–6655.

Kozbor, D. & Roder, J. C. (1981). Requirements for the establishment of high titred human monoclonal antibodies against tetanus toxoid using the Epstein–Barr virus technique. *Journal of Immunology*, **127**, 1275–1280.

Kozbor, D. & Roder, J. C. (1983). The production of monoclonal antibodies from human lymphocytes. *Immunology Today*, **4**, 72–79.

Kozbor, D. & Roder, J. C. (1984). *In-vitro* stimulated lymphocytes as source of human hybridomas. *European Journal of Immunology*, **14**, 23–27.

Kozbor, D., Tripputi, P., Roder, J. C. & Croce, C. M. (1984). A human hybrid myeloma for production of monoclonal antibodies. *Journal of Immunology*, **133**, 3001–3005.

Kumpel, B. M., Leader, K. A. & Bradley, B. A. (1988*a*). The relationship between IgG subclass and Gm allotype of monoclonal anti-Rh(D) antibodies and their functional activity. *Biochemical Society Transactions*, **16**, 733–734.

Kumpel, B. M., Wiener, L., Urbaniak, S. J. & Bradley, B. A. (1988*b*). Human monoclonal anti-Rh(D) antibodies. II. The relationship between IgG subclass, Gm allotype and functional activity. *British Society of Haematology*, **71**, 415–420.

Kuroki, T., Kodama, K., Carayou, P., Ruf, J., Miller, A. & Wall J. R. (1986). Use of mouse and human monoclonal antibodies to investigate the immunologic basis of Graves' ophthalmology. *Mount Sinai Journal of Medicine*, **53**, 60–69.

Lagace, J. & Brodeur, B. R. (1985). Parameters affecting *in-vitro* immunization of human lymphocytes. *Journal of Immunological Methods*, **85**, 127–136.

Lane, R. D., Crossman, R. S. & Lachman, M. F. (1984). Comparison of polyethylene glycols as fusogens for producing lymphocyte-myeloma hybrids. *Journal of Immunological Methods*, **72**, 71–76.

Lane, H. & Fauci, A. S. (1983). Hybrid B cell formation. In *Monoclonal Antibodies, Probes for the Study of Autoimmunity and Immunodeficiency*, ed. B. F. Hayes & G. S. Eisenbach, pp. 136–161. New York, Academic Press.

Larrick, J. W. & Bouria, J. M. (1986). Prospects for the therapeutic use of human monoclonal antibodies. *Journal of Biological Response Modifiers*, **5**, 379–393.

Larrick, J. W., Truitt, K. E., Raubitschek, A. A., Senyk, G. & Wang, J. C. N. (1983). Characterization of human hybridomas secreting antibody to tetanus toxoid.

Proceedings of the National Academy of Sciences of the U.S.A., **80**, 6376–6380.

Lefkovits, I. (1979). Limiting dilution analysis. *Immunological Methods*, vol. 1, ed. I. Lefkovits & B. Pernis, pp. 356–370. New York, Academic Press.

Lefkovits, I. & Waldmann, H. (1980). In *Limiting Dilution Analysis of Cells in the Immune System*, London, Cambridge University Press.

Levy, J. A., Virolainen, M. & Defendi, V. (1968). Human lymphoblastoid lines from lymph node and spleen. *Cancer*, **22**, 517–524.

Livneh, A., Avraham, H., Elias, D., Sack, J., Cohen, I. R. & Esshar, Z. (1986). A human monoclonal antibody to insulin. *Diabetes*, **35**, 68–73.

Lo, M. M. S., Tsong, L. Y., Conrad, M. K., Stritmatter, S. M., Hester, L. D. & Snyder, S. H. (1984). Monoclonal antibody production by receptor-mediated electrically induced cell fusion. *Nature*, **310**, 792–794.

Locniskar, M., Zumla, A., Mudd, D. W., Isenberg, D. A., Williams, W. & McAdam, K. P. W. J. (1988). Human monoclonal antibodies to phenolic glycolipid-1 derived from patients with leprosy and production of specific anti-idiotypes. *Immunology*, **64**, 245–251.

Logtenberg, T., Kroon, A., Gmelig-Meyling, F. H. J. & Ballieux, R. E. (1987). Analysis of the human tonsil B cell repertoire by somatic hybridization: occurrence of both 'monospecific' and 'multispecific' (auto)-antibody-secreting cells. *European Journal of Immunology*, **16**, 1497–1501.

Lowe, A. D., Green, S. M., Voak, D., Gibson, T. & Lennox, E. S. (1986). A human–human monoclonal anti-D by direct fusion with a lymphoblastoid line. *Vox Sanguinis*, **51**, 212–216.

MacDonald, G., Primrose, S., Biggins, K., Bowman, J. M., Berczi, I., Friesen, A. D. & Sehon, A. H. (1987). Production and characterization of human–human and human–mouse hybridomas secreting Rh(D)-specific monoclonal antibodies. *Scandinavian Journal of Immunology*, **25**, 477–483.

McCann, M. C., James, K. & Kumpel, B. M. (1988). Production and use of human monoclonal anti-D antibodies. *Journal of Immunological Methods*, **115**, 3–15.

Masuho, Y., Sugano, T., Matsumoto, Y., Sawada, S. & Tomike, K. (1986). Generation of hybridomas producing monoclonal antibodies against herpes simplex virus after *in-vitro* stimulation. *Biochemical and Biophysical Research Communications*, **135**, 495–500.

Matsumoto, Y., Sugano, T., Miyamoto, C. & Masuho, Y. (1986). Generation of hybridomas producing human monoclonal antibodies against human cytomegalovirus. *Biochemical and Biophysical Research Communications*, **137**, 273–280.

Melamed, M. D., Gordon, J., Ley, S. J., Edgar, D. & Hughes-Jones, N. C. (1985). Senescence of a human lymphoblastoid clone producing anti-Rhesus (D). *European Journal of Immunology*, **15**, 724–726.

Melamed, M. D., Thompson, K. M., Gibson, T. & Hughes-Jones, N. C. (1987). Requirements for the establishment of heterohybridomas secreting monoclonal antibody to Rhesus (D) blood group antigen. *Journal of Immunological Methods*, **104**, 245–251.

Miller, G. & Lipman, M. (1973). Release of infectious Epstein–Barr virus by transformed marmoset leukocytes. *Proceedings of the National Academy of Sciences of the U.S.A.*, **70**, 190–194.

Monjour, L., Desgranges, C., Alfred, C., Ploton, I. & Karaninis, A. (1983). Production of human monoclonal antibodies against sexual erythrocytic stages of *Plasmodium falciparum*. *Lancet*, **i**, 1337–1338.

Morrison, S. L. (1985). Transfectomas provide novel chimeric antibodies. *Science*, **229**, 1202–1207.

Morrison, S. L., Johnson, M. J., Herzenberg, L. A. & Oi, V. T. (1984). Chimaeric human antibody molecules: mouse antigen-binding domains with human constant region domains. *Proceedings of the National Academy of Sciences of the U.S.A.*, **81**, 6851–6855.

Moss, D. J., Rickinsen, A. B. & Pope, J. H. (1979). Long-term T cell-mediated immunity to Epstein–Barr virus infected leukocyte cultures. *International Journal of Cancer*, **23**, 618–625.

Nakamura, M., Burastero, S. E., Notkins, A. L. & Casal, P. (1988). Human monoclonal rheumatoid factor-like antibodies from CD5 (Leu-1) + B cells are polyreactive. *Journal of Immunology*, **140**, 4180–4186.

Neuberger, M. S. (1985). Making novel antibodies by expressing transfected immunoglobulin genes. *Trends in Biochemistry*, **10**, 347–349.

Neuberger, M. S., Williams, G. T., Michell, E. B., Jonchal, S. S., Flanagan, J. G. & Rabbitts, T. H. (1985). A hapten-specific chimaeric immunoglobulin E with human physiological effector function. *Nature*, **314**, 268–270.

Nilsson, K., Bennich, H., Johannsson, S. G. O. & Ponten, J. (1970). Established immunoglobulin-producing myeloma (IgE) and lymphoblastoid (IgG) cell lines from an IgE myeloma patient. *Clinical and Experimental Immunology*, **7**, 477–489.

Nossal, G. J. V. (1983). Cellular mechanism of immune tolerance. *Annual Reviews of Immunology*, **1**, 33–62.

O'Hare, M. J. & Yiu, C. Y. (1987). Human monoclonal antibodies as cellular and molecular probes: a review. *Molecular and Cellular Probes*, **1**, 33–54.

Ohnishi, K., Chiba, J., Goto, Y. & Tokunga, T. (1987). Improvement in the basic technology of electrofusion for generation of antibody-producing hybridomas. *Journal of Immunological Methods*, **100**, 181–189.

Oi, V. T. & Morrison, S. L. (1986). Chimeric antibodies. *Biotechniques*, **4**, 214–221.

Old, L. J. (1981). The search for specificity – G. H. A. Clowes Memorial Lecture. *Cancer Research*, **41**, 361–375.

Olsson, L., Andreasen, R. B., Ost, A., Christensen, B. & Biberfeld, P. (1984). Antibody producing human–human hybridomas. II. Derivation and characterization of an antibody specific for human leukemia cells. *Journal of Experimental Medicine*, **59**, 537–550.

Olsson, L. & Brams, P. (1985). Human–human hybridoma technology. Five years of technical improvement and its application in cancer biology. In *Human Hybridomas and Monoclonal Antibodies*, ed. E. G. Engleman, S. K. H. Foung, J. Larrick & A. Raubitschek, pp. 227–244. New York, Plenum Press.

Olsson, L. & Kaplan, H. S. (1980). Human–human hybridomas producing monoclonal antibodies of pre-defined antigenic specificity. *Proceedings of the National Academy of Sciences of the U.S.A.*, **77**, 5429–5431.

Olsson, L., Kronstrom, H., Cambon-de Mouzon, A., Honsik, C., Brodin, T. & Jakobsen, B. (1983). Antibody producing human–human hybridomas. 1. Technical aspects. *Journal of Immunological Methods*, **61**, 17–32.

Osband, M. E., Cohen, E. B., Miller, B. R., Shen, Y. J., Cohen, L., Flesher, L., Brown, A. E. & McCaffrey, R. P. (1981). Biochemical analysis of specific histamine H1 and H2 receptors on lymphocytes. *Blood*, **58**, 87–90.

Ostberg, L. & Pursch, E. (1983). Human X (mouse × human) hybridomas stably producing human antibodies. *Hybridoma*, **2**, 361–367.

Paire, J., Monestier, M., Rigal, D., Martel, F. & Desgranges, C. (1986). Establishment of human cell lines producing anti-D monoclonal antibodies: identification of Rhesus D antigen. *Immunology Letters*, **13**, 137–141.

Parinaud, J., Blaus, M., Grandjean, H., Bienve, S. & Poutonmier, G. (1985). IgG subclasses and Gm allotypes of anti-D antibodies during pregnancy: correlation with the gravity of the fetal disease. *American Journal of Obstetrics and Gynaecology*, **151**, 1111–1115.

Parks, D. R., Bryan, V. M., Oi, V. T. & Herzenberg, L. A. (1979). Antigen-specific identification and cloning of hybridomas with a fluorescence-activated cell sorter. *Proceeding of the National Academy of Sciences of the U.S.A.*, **76**, 1962–1966.

Pfreundschuh, M., Shiku, H., Takahashi, T., Ueda, R., Ransohoff, J., Oettgen, H. F. & Old, L. J. (1978). Serological analysis of cell surface antigens of malignant human brain tumours. *Proceedings of the National Academy of Sciences of the U.S.A.*, **75**, 5122–5126.

Pistillo, M. P., Mazzoleni, O., Tanigaki, N., Hammerlung, U., Lango, A., Frumento, G. & Ferrara, G. B. (1985). Human anti-HLA monoclonal antibodies: production, characterization and application. *Human Immunology*, **21**, 265–278.

Pollack, M., Raubitschek, A. A. & Larrick, J. W. (1987). Human monoclonal antibodies that recognize conserved epitopes in the core-lipid A region of lipopolysaccharides. *Journal of Clinical Investigation*, **70**, 1421–1430.

Pumphery, R. (1986). Computer models of the human immunoglobulins. *Immunology Today*, **7**, 174–178.

Raison, R. L., Walker, K. Z., Halman, C. R. E., Briscoe, D. & Basten, A. (1982). Loss of secretion in mouse–human hybrids need not be due to loss of a structural gene. *Journal of Experimental Medicine*, **136**, 1380–1389.

Reading, C. L. (1982). Theory and methods for immunization in culture and monoclonal antibody production. *Journal of Immunological Methods*, **53**, 261–291.

Redmond, M. J., Leyritz-Wills, M., Winger, L. & Scraba, D. G. (1986). The selection and characterization of human monoclonal antibodies to human cytomegalovirus. *Journal of Virological Methods*, **14**, 9–24.

Riechmann, L., Clark, M., Waldmann, H. & Winter, G. (1988). Reshaping human antibodies for therapy. *Nature*, **332**, 323–327.

Roberts, S., Cheetham, J. C. & Rees, A. R. (1987). Generation of an antibody with enhanced affinity and specificity for its antigen by protein engineering. *Nature*, **328**, 731–734.

Rosen, A. S., Britton, B., Gergegly, P., Jondal, M. & Klein, G. (1977). Polyclonal Ig production after Epstein–Barr virus infection of human lymphocytes *in vitro*. *Nature*, **267**, 52–54.

Rosen, A., Persson, K. & Klein, G. (1983). Human monoclonal antibodies to a genus-specific chlamydial antigen produced by EBV transformed B cells. *Journal of Immunology*, **130**, 2899–2902.

Rotella, C. M., Zonefrati, R., Toccafondi, R., Valente, W. A. & Kohn, L. D. (1986). Ability of monoclonal antibodies to the thyrotropic receptor to increase collagen synthesis in human fibroblasts: an assay which appears to measure exophthalmogenic immunoglobulin in Graves' sera. *Journal of Clinical Endocrinology and Metabolism*, **62**, 357–367.

Ruddle, F. H. (1973). Linkage analysis in man by somatic cell genetics. *Nature*, **242**, 165–169.

Ryan, K. P., Dillman, R. O., DeNardo, S. J., DeNardo, G. L., Beauregard, J., Hagan, P. L., Amox, D. G., Clutter, M. L., Burnett, K. G., Rulot, C. M., Sobol, R. E., Abramson, I., Bartholomew, R. K., Frinche, J. M., Birdwell, C. R., Carlo, D. J., O'Grady, L. F. & Halperm, S. E. (1988). Breast cancer imaging with [111]Indium radiolabelled human IgM monoclonal antibodies: preliminary studies. *Radiology*, **167**, 71–75.

Sanz, I. & Capra, J. D. (1988). The genetic origin of human autoantibodies. *Journal of Immunology*, **140**, 3283–3285.

Sawada, S., Kawamura, T., Masuho, Y. & Tomibe, K. (1985). Characterization of a human monoclonal antibody to lipopolysaccharides of *Pseudomonas aeruginosa* serotype 5: a possible candidate as an immunotherapeutic agent for infection with *P. aeruginosa. Journal of Infectious Diseases*, **152**, 965–970.

Schier, W., Nilsson, K., Merten, D. W., Katinger, H. W. D. & Mosbach, K. (1984). Entrapment of animal cells for the production of biomolecules such as monoclonal antibodies. *Development in Biological Standards*, **55**, 155–161.

Schmidt-Ullrich, R., Brown, J., Whittle, H. & Lin, P.-S. (1986). The human–human hybridomas secreting monoclonal antibodies to the W. M. 195 000 *Plasmodium falciparum* blood stage antigen. *Journal of Experimental Medicine*, **163**, 179–188.

Schwaber, J. F., Posner, M. R., Schlossman, S. F. & Lazarus, H. (1984). Human–human hybrids secreting pneumococcal antibodies. *Human Immunology*, **9**, 137–143.

Schwartz, R. S. (1987). Autoantibodies and normal antibodies: two sides of the same coin. *Harvey Lectures*, **81**, 53–66.

Schwartz, R. S. (1988). Polyvalent anti-DNA auto-antibodies: immunochemical and biological significance. *International Reviews in Immunology*, **3**, 97–115.

Shawler, D. L., Bartholomew, R. M., Smith, L. M. & Dillman, R. D. (1985). Human immune response to multiple injections of murine monoclonal IgG. *Journal of Immunology*, **135**, 1530–1535.

Shoenfeld, Y., Hizi, A., Tal, R., Smorodinsky, N. I., Lavie, G., Mor, C., Schteren, S. & Mammon, Z. (1987). Human monoclonal antibodies derived from lymph nodes of a patient with breast carcinoma react with MUMTV polypeptides. *Cancer*, **59**, 43–50.

Shoenfeld, Y., Hsu-Lin, S. C., Gabriels, J. E., Silberstein, L. E., Furie, B. C., Furie, B., Stollar, B. D. & Schwartz, R. S. (1982). Production of auto-antibodies by human–human hybridomas. *Journal of Clinical Investigation*, **70**, 205–208.

Shoenfeld, Y., Rauch, J., Massicottes, H., Datta, S. K., Andre-Schwartz, J., Stollar, D. B. & Schwartz, R. S. (1983). Polyspecifity of monoclonal lupus auto-antibodies produced by human–human hybridomas. *New England Journal of Medicine*, **308**, 414–420.

Siadak, A. W. & Lostrom, M. E. (1985). Cell-driven viral transformation. In *Human Hybridomas and Monoclonal Antibodies*, ed. E. G. Engleman, S. K. H. Foung, J. Larrick & A. Raubitschek, pp. 167–185. New York, Plenum Press.

Sikora, K., Alderson, T., Ellis, J., Phillips, J. & Watson, J. (1983). Human hybridomas from patients with malignant disease. *British Journal of Cancer*, **47**, 135–145.

Smith, L. H. & Teng, N. N. H. (1987). Applications of human monoclonal antibodies in oncology. In *Human Hybridomas: Diagnostic and Therapeutic Applications*, Immunology Series, vol. 30, ed. A. J. Srelkauskas, pp. 121–141. New York, Marcel Dekker.

Steinitz, M., Izak, G., Cohen, S., Ehrenfeld, M. & Flecher, I. (1980). Continuous production of monoclonal rheumatoid factor by EBV-transformed lymphocytes. *Nature*, **287**, 443–445.

Steinitz, M., Seppala, F., Eichman, K. & Klein, G. (1979). Establishment of a human lymphoblastoid cell line with specific antibody production against group A streptococcal carbohydrate. *Immunobiology*, **156**, 41–47.

Steinitz, M. & Tamir, S. (1982). Human monoclonal antibody produced *in vitro*: rheumatoid factor generated by Epstein–Barr virus-transformed cell line. *European Journal of Immunology*, **12**, 126–133.

Steinitz, M., Tamir, S., Ferne, M. & Goldfarb, A. (1986). A protective human monoclonal IgA antibody produced *in vitro*: antipneumococci antibody engendered by Epstein–Barr virus-immortalized cell line. *European Journal of Immunology*, **16**, 187–93.

Steinitz, M., Tamir, S. & Goldfarb, A. (1984). Human anti-pneumococci antibody produced by an Epstein–Barr virus (EBV)-immortalized cell line. *Journal of Immunology*, **132**, 877–882.

Stevens, R. J., Macy, E., Morrow, C. & Saxson, A. (1979). Characterization of a circulating subpopulation of anti-tetanus toxoid antibody producing B cells following *in-vivo* booster immunization. *Journal of Immunology*, **122**, 2498–2504.

Strelkauskas, A. J., Taylor, C. L., Smith, M. R. & Bear, P. D. (1987). Transfection of human cells. An alternative method for the establishment of human hybrid clones. In *Human Hybridomas: Diagnostic and Therapeutic Applications*, Immunology Series, vol. 30, ed. A. J. Strelkauskas, pp. 95–120. New York, Marcel Dekker.

Stricker, E. A. M., Tiebout, R. F., Lelie, P. N. & Zeijlemarker, W. P. (1985). A human monoclonal IgG, anti-hepatitis B surface antibody: production, properties and applications. *Scandinavian Journal of Immunology*, **22**, 337–343.

Strike, L. E., Devens, B. H. & Lundak, R. L. (1984). Production of human–human hybridomas secreting antibody to sheep erythrocytes after *in-vitro* immunization. *Journal of Immunology*, **132**, 1798–1803.

Sugano, T., Matsumoto, Y. I., Miyamoto, C. & Masuho, Y. (1987). Hybridomas producing human monoclonal antibodies against varicella-zoster virus. *European Journal of Immunology*, **17**, 359–364.

Teng, N. N. H., Kaplan, H. S., Herbert, J. M., Moore, C., Douglas, H., Wunderlich, A. & Braude, A. J. (1985a). Protection against Gram-negative bacteremia and endotoxinemia with human monoclonal IgM antibodies. *Proceeding of the National Academy of Science of the U.S.A.*, **82**, 1790–1794.

Teng, N. N. H., Lam, K. S., Riera, F. C. & Kaplan, H. S. (1983). Construction and testing of mouse–human heteromyelomas for human monoclonal antibody production. *Proceedings of the National Academy of Sciences of the U.S.A.*, **80**, 7308–7312.

Teng, N. N. H., Reyes, G. R., Bieber, M., Fry, K. E., Lam, K. S. & Herbert, J. M. (1985b). Strategies for stable human monoclonal antibody production: construction of heteromyelomas, *in-vitro* sensitization and molecular cloning of human immunoglobulin genes. In *Human Hybridomas and Monoclonal Antibodies*, ed. E. G. Engleman, S. K. H. Foung, J. Larrick & A. Raubitschek, pp. 71–91. New York, Plenum Press.

Thivolet, C., Desgranges, C., Durand, A. & Bertrand, J. (1985). Human monoclonal antibody reacting with islet-cell membrane antigen from immune lymphocytes transformed by Epstein–Barr virus. *Comptes Rendues des Seances de L'Academie des Sciences*, **301**, 611–614.

Thompson, K. M. (1988). Human monoclonal antibodies. *Immunology Today*, **9**, 113–117.

Thompson, K. M., Melamed, M. D., Eagle, K., Gorick, B. D., Gibson, T., Holburn, A. M. & Hughes-Jones, N. C. (1986). Production of human monoclonal IgG and IgM antibodies with anti-D (Rhesus) specificity using heterohybridomas. *Immunology*, **58**, 157–160.

Tiebout, R. F., Stricker, E. A. M., Hagenaars, R. & Zeijlemarker, W. P. (1984). Human lymphoblastoid cell line producing protective monoclonal IgG anti-tetanus toxin. *European Journal of Immunology*, **14**, 399–404.

Tiebout, R. F., Stricker, E. A. M., Oosterhof, F. van Heemstra, D. J. M. & Ziejlemaker, W. P. (1985). Xenohybridization of Epstein–Barr virus-transformed cells for the production of human monoclonal antibodies. *Scandinavian Journal of*

Immunology, **22**, 691–701.

Tippet, P. (1988). Subdivisions of the Rh(D) antigen. *Medical and Laboratory Science*, **45**, 88–93.

Truitt, K. E., Larrick, J. W., Raubitschek, A. A., Buck, D. E. & Jacobson, S. W. (1984). Production of human monoclonal antibody in mouse ascites. *Hybridoma*, **3**, 195–199.

Udomsangpetch, R., Lundgren, K., Berzins, K., Wahlin, B., Perlmann, H., Troye-Blomberg, M., Carlsson, J., Wahlgren, M., Perlmann, P. & Bjorkman, A. (1986). Human monoclonal antibodies to Pf155, a major antigen of malaria parasite *Plasmodium falciparum. Science*, **231**, 57–59.

Ueda, R., Shiku, H., Pfreundschuh, M., Takahashi, T., Li, L. T. C., Whitmore, W. F., Oettgen, H. F. & Old, L. J. (1979). Cell surface antigens of human renal cancer defined by autologous typing. *Journal of Experimental Medicine*, **150**, 564–579.

Valente, W. A., Vitti, P., Yavin, Z., Yavin, E., Rotella, C. M., Grollman, E. F., Toccafondi, R. S. & Kohn, L. D. (1982). Monoclonal antibodies to the thyrotropin receptor: stimulating and blocking antibodies derived from lymphocytes of patients with Graves' disease. *Proceedings of the National Academy of Sciences of the U.S.A.*, **79**, 6680–6684.

Van Kroonenburgh, M. J. & Pauwels, E. K. (1988). Human immunological response to mouse monoclonal antibodies in the treatment or diagnosis of malignant diseases. *Nuclear Medicine Communications*, **9**, 919–930.

Verhoeyen, M., Milstein, C. & Winter, G. (1988). Reshaping human antibodies: grafting an antilysozyme activity. *Science*, **239**, 1534–1536.

Ware, C. F., Donato, N. J. & Dorshkind, K. (1985). Human, rat or mouse hybridomas secrete high levels of monoclonal antibodies following transplantation into mice with severe combined immunodeficiency disease (SCID). *Journal of Immunological Methods*, **83**, 353–361.

Wiener, E., Atwal, A., Thompson, K. M., Melamed, M. D., Garrick, B. & Hughes-Jones, N. C. (1987). Differences between the activities of human monoclonal IgG_1 and IgG_3 subclass of anti-D (Rh) antibody in their ability to mediate red cell binding to macrophages. *Immunology*, **62**, 401–404.

Winger, L., Winger, C., Shastry, P., Russel, A. & Longenecker, M. (1983). Efficient generation *in vitro*, from human peripheral blood cells, of monoclonal EB-virus transformants producing specific antibody to a variety of antigens without prior deliberate immunization. *Proceedings of the National Academy of Sciences of the U.S.A.*, **80**, 4484–4488.

Winter, G. & Milstein, C. (1991). Man-made antibodies. *Nature*, **349**, 293–299.

Wojchowski, D. M. & Sytkowski, A. J. (1986). Hybridoma production by simplified avidin-mediated electrofusion. *Journal of Immunological Methods*, **90**, 173–177.

Yamaura, N., Makino, M., Walsh, L. J., Bruce, A. W. & Choe, B.-K. (1985). Production of monoclonal antibodies against prostatic acid phosphatase by *in-vitro* immunization of human spleen cells. *Journal of Immunological Methods*, **84**, 105–116.

Yarchoan, R., Murphy, B. R., Strober, W., Schneider, H. S. & Nelson, D. L. (1981). Specific anti-influenza virus antibody production *in vitro* by human peripheral blood mononuclear cells. *Journal of Immunology*, **127**, 2588–2594.

Yoshikawa, K., Ueda, R., Obata, Y., Utsumi, K. R., Notake, K. & Takashi, T. (1986). Human monoclonal antibody reactive to stomach cancer produced by mouse–human hybridoma technique. *Japanese Journal of Cancer Research*, **77**, 1122–1133.

Ziegler-Heitbrock, H. W., Reiter, C., Treukman, J., Futtere, A. & Reithmuller, G.

(1986). Protection of mice against tetanus toxin by combination of two human monoclonal antibodies recognizing distinct epitopes on the toxin molecule. *Hybridoma*, **5**, 21–31.

Zumla, A. (1990). Autoantibodies and tropical infections. *Transactions of the Royal Society of Tropical Medicine and Hygiene*, **84**, 197–200.

Zumla, A., Williams, W., Isenberg, D., Locniskar, M., Behrens, R., Mudd, D. & McAdam, K. P. W. J. (1991). Expression of a common idiotype PR4 in the sera of patients with leprosy. *Clinical and Experimental Immunology*, **84**, 522–526.

6

Bispecific monoclonal antibodies

S. SONGSIVILAI and P. J. LACHMANN

6.1 Introduction

Monoclonal antibodies (mab) have been widely used in medicine both in the diagnosis and treatment of disease. Several effector mechanisms are involved in the destruction of target cells by antibodies, namely complement activation, recruitment of cellular effector cells and antibody-dependent cellular cytotoxicity (ADCC). Although these natural effector functions are powerful, the use of mab on their own usually results in the inadequate destruction of target tumour cells. Several efforts have therefore been made to increase their efficiency by attaching antibody molecules to various agents such as bacterial or plant toxins, radionuclides and cytotoxic drugs. These reagents are mainly derived from direct conjugation of antibodies to effector compounds by several distinct methods of covalent coupling (reviewed by Ghose & Blair, 1987; Blakey *et al.*, 1988). Several 'immunoconjugates' are being used for specific diagnosis and therapy and the results are encouraging (reviewed by Goldenberg, 1989).

Direct coupling of antibodies to effector compounds, however, has some major disadvantages. The efficiency of immunoconjugates may be decreased as a result of the chemical manipulation which can inactivate antibody-binding sites and also cause crucial alterations in the effector agents (Hurwitz *et al.*, 1975). Antibody engineering has recently been applied to solve some of these problems by producing fusion proteins that contain both the antigen-binding site of the immunoglobulin molecule and the effector compound, thus avoiding the chemical conjugation process (Neuberger *et al.*, 1984; Chaudhary *et al.*, 1990). Additionally, problems may arise if the covalent bonds between the carrier antibody and effector compound need to be broken for full biological action as such bonds may not be easily split (Raso & Griffin, 1981). Furthermore, the interaction of the Fc domain of immunoconjugates with its receptor on cells of the reticuloendothelial system also results in the undesired accumulation of antibody in some organs, notably the liver and spleen. This high background of labelled antibodies affects the sensitivity of tumour imaging and also leads to non-specific destruction of cells and organs. The use of Fab fragments instead of whole antibody molecules overcomes some of the difficulties but fails to resolve this problem completely (Goldenberg, 1988).

An alternative approach for tumour targeting by a multistage delivery system was proposed, based on the evidence that antibodies which bind non-specifically, probably via their Fc portion, are cleared from the body faster than those that bind specifically to their tumour targets (Henkel *et al.*, 1985; Goldenberg, 1988). This system requires a reagent which can interact specifically with both the target and effector compound. Bispecific antibodies which have two different specific antigen-binding sites, one for tumour-associated antigen (target binding arm) and the other for the effector compounds (effector binding arm) have been developed. For specific targeting, bispecific mab is first targeted to the tumour site by its tumour specificity. After allowing a suitable period of time for the non-specifically bound antibodies to be cleared, the effector compound, which is recognized by the second specificity of the targeted antibody, is then administered separately, leading to its specific localization at the tumour site. As the non-coupled effector compound has a shorter half-life in the body than that of the directly-coupled antibody–effector agent complexes, this system will minimize the toxicity in therapy and maximize the quality of tumour imaging. Bispecific antibodies also have many potential uses ranging from immunodiagnosis to targeted delivery of toxic substances to tumours. They have been studied for targeting effector cells or toxins to tumours and initial results look very promising. Bispecific antibodies also have several advantages over the directly-coupled immunoconjugates. The chemical damage to toxins or cytotoxic drugs during the coupling process can be alleviated and these compounds are released to specific targets without splitting of covalent bonds. Non-specific toxicity from the conjugated immunotoxins may also be reduced. In addition, bispecific antibodies are structurally bivalent but functionally univalent for each antigen-binding site. The mechanism whereby target cells escape killing by redistributing and eventually losing the antigen–antibody complexes from their surface, known as antigenic modulation (Gordon & Stevenson, 1981; Cobbold & Waldmann, 1984), may also be minimized due to the monovalency of the bispecific antibody (Glennie *et al.*, 1988).

Generally, a single antibody-producing cell secretes only one species of mab, consisting of two identical antigen-binding arms, as a result of allelic exclusion. Bispecific mab therefore do not occur naturally. Bispecific antibodies have been produced mainly by two methods: fusion of two different antibody-producing cell lines or chemical linkage of two antibody molecules or their derivatives. Antibodies produced by these two techniques are generally referred to as hybrid antibodies and heteroconjugates, respectively. Recently, another approach for producing bispecific mab by genetic engineering was introduced. The advantages and disadvantages of these approaches will be discussed.

6.2   Production of bispecific monoclonal antibodies

6.2.1   *Somatic cell hybridization*

As a result of allelic exclusion, plasma cells secrete only one set of heavy and light chains of immunoglobulin. Hybridoma cells derived from the fusion of the 'non-secreting' parental myeloma cell line and immune cell also secrete a monospecific mab with two identical antigen-binding arms. Co-dominant expression of both parental immunoglobulin genes occurs in hybrid hybridoma cells derived from the fusion of two myeloma or hybridoma cell lines, each secreting different antibody (Cotton & Milstein, 1973; Schwaber & Cohen, 1974). Two sets of rearranged immunoglobulin genes, one from each parental cell line, can be co-expressed independently in a single cell. The assembly of immunoglobulin molecules allows the formation of both parental antibodies and also the hybrid molecules (Figure 6.1). If random association of heavy and light chains occurs, ten different combinations of immunoglobulin molecules will be generated, only one of which is the desired bispecific antibody. Somatic cell hybridization has successfully been carried out between pairs of existing hybridoma cell lines secreting two distinct mab (Suresh *et al.*, 1986*b*; Tiebout *et al.*, 1987; Urnovitz *et al.*, 1988) or between hybridoma cell lines and immune spleen cells (Kohler & Milstein, 1975; Milstein & Cuello, 1983; Webb *et al.*, 1985). The former approach is preferable because the specificities of the resulting bispecific antibodies are more predictable. The quality and affinity of bispecific antibodies derived from the latter approach remains a matter of

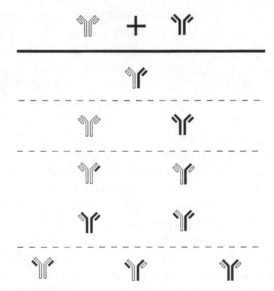

Figure 6.1. Diagram of ten different species of immunoglobulin molecules secreted by a hybrid hybridoma cell as a result of random association of the heavy and light chains from both parental hybridomas.

chance and depends on the contribution of the spleen cell partner, requiring further characterization of the specificity of the hybrid antibodies.

Theoretically, if the rate of production of the two parental pairs of heavy and light chain were the same and the association of heavy and light chains showed no homologous or heterologous preference (therefore the association was totally random), then the yield of the desired bispecific antibody would be 12.5% of the total immunoglobulin secreted by the hybrid cell (Staerz & Bevan, 1986). In practice, the prediction of the yields of bispecific antibody is very difficult as preferential association may occur and thus yields can range from 0 to 50%. The ideal condition for the maximum yield of bispecific antibody should be an absolute homologous preference in heavy–light chain pairing and random pairing of heavy chains, then the yield of the desired bispecific antibody will be 50% of total immunoglobulin (Corvalan & Smith, 1987). On the other hand, the total absence of association between heavy chains of different classes, such as IgM:IgG or IgA:IgG, may prevent the formation of bispecific molecules because of the difference in the position of cysteine residues in the molecules (Zimmerman & Grey, 1971; Takahashi & Fuller, 1988; Urnovitz et al., 1988).

The production of bispecific antibodies by the cell fusion approach has a major advantage in that the resulting bispecific mab are synthesized, assembled and secreted by the same process as that of the native immunoglobulin molecules. Their stability, both in vitro and in vivo, and pharmacokinetics should be thus comparable to those of the normal antibodies. The 'hybrid hybridoma' cell lines, once obtained, will enable the production of an unlimited quantity of bispecific mab in the same way as normal hybridoma cell lines. This cell fusion approach also has some major disadvantages, notably the difficulty in preparing the parental cells, the stability of the resulting hybrid cell lines, low yields and difficulty in purification of the bispecific molecules. Cell fusion is labour intensive, time consuming and may not always succeed with the hybridoma pairs of choice. Not all hybridoma cell lines exhibit good fusion performance (Suresh et al., 1986a). The lack of an easy method for selecting the hybrid hybridoma cells from the non-fused cells results from the fact that most parental hybridomas are derived from the fusion of hypoxanthine aminopterin and thymidine (HAT)-sensitive myeloma fusion partners and immune spleen cells and are thus HAT-resistant. Several approaches have been developed to solve this problem. Parental hybridoma cell lines can be reverted to HAT-sensitivity by selecting the mutants that lack the enzyme hypoxanthine-guanine phosphoribosyltransferase (HGPRT) in a medium containing 8-azaguanine or 6-thioguanine, followed by their fusion with immune spleen cells (Milstein & Cuello, 1983). Hybridoma cells lacking other enzymes such as thymidine kinase or adenosine phosphoribosyltransferase can also be selected in a medium containing bromodeoxyuridine or 6-chloropurine, respectively. Two hybridoma cell lines lacking two independent enzymes can then be fused and the resulting hybrid cells selected in simple HAT-medium (Wong &

Colvin, 1987; Urnovitz *et al.*, 1988). Other selectable markers, such as the resistance to neomycin, methotrexate or actinomycin D, may also be introduced into cells by means of gene transfection (Lanzavecchia & Scheidegger, 1987; Chervonsky *et al.*, 1988; De Lau *et al.*, 1989). Another alternative approach is to use two distinct site-specific irreversible inhibitors of protein synthesis, such as emetine, actinomycin D or iodoacetamide, to inhibit two independent metabolic pathways of each of the two parental cell lines. Fused cells apparently survive by complementing each other (Suresh *et al.*, 1986*b*). This method can be used in combination with HAT selection by fusing a HAT-sensitive hybridoma cell line with a chemically-treated hybridoma (Suresh *et al.*, 1986*a*; Clark & Waldmann, 1987). Alternatively, the parental hybridomas can be labelled with two different vital dyes; hybrid hybridomas may then be selected by a fluorescence-activated cell sorter without relying on drug selection (Karawajew *et al.*, 1987, 1988; Koolwijk *et al.*, 1988).

The resulting hybrid hybridoma cell lines are not stable with regard to the continuing secretion of bispecific antibodies as the chromosomes of these hybrid cells are polyploid, approximately equal to the sum of the chromosomes of both parental hybridomas (Kohler & Milstein, 1975; Koolwijk *et al.*, 1988). Additionally, there is no selective pressure to retain all four functional immunoglobulin genes in the hybrid hybridoma cells. These cells exhibit a higher propensity to lose chromosomes than do the parental hybridomas (Suresh *et al.*, 1986*a*). This was shown in early work on hybridoma technology, prior to the introduction of a non-producing myeloma fusion partner, in which the resulting hybridomas secreted mixed molecules, which at that time was considered to be a disadvantage. Owing to the instability of their chromosomes, mutants which lost immunoglobulin genes from the parental myeloma could easily be cloned and mab-secreting cells selected. For the continuing production of bispecific antibodies, the hybrid hybridoma cell lines may require frequent cloning to maintain the presence of both sets of heavy and light chains.

Isolation of the bispecific antibody from total immunoglobulin secreted from hybrid hybridoma cells can be difficult as a total of ten species of molecules are formed and they may have similar chemical characteristics. Purification has been achieved by several methods such as isoelectric focusing (Wong & Colvin, 1987), hydroxylapatite chromatography (Staerz & Bevan, 1986; Karawajew *et al.*, 1987), ion-exchange chromatography (Suresh *et al.*, 1986*b*) or double affinity chromatography (Corvalan & Smith, 1987).

6.2.2 *Chemical conjugation of antibody molecules or their derivatives*

Antibody molecules can be chemically manipulated *in vitro*. The technique for producing bispecific antibodies by chemical conjugation was pioneered by Nisonoff & Rivers (1961). This approach is less time-consuming than the somatic hybridization approach and the products are also comparatively easy to purify (Karpovsky *et al.*, 1984; Glennie *et al.*, 1987). Chemical coupling can be achieved in two ways: direct coupling of the whole antibody molecules or their derivatives and dissociation and reassociation of heterologous immunoglobulins. Bispecific mab produced by the former approach are usually derived from the coupling of the two antibody fragments using heterobifunctional linkers such as N-succinyl 3-(2-pyridyldithio) proprionate (SPDP). Several techniques can be used to ensure that the majority of the coupled molecules are bispecific antibodies. The latter approach requires chemical manipulation to dissociate immunoglobulins into half molecules without damaging the antigen-binding sites, then to reform the disulphide bonds linking the heavy chains without allowing any interfering side-reactions such as the formation of intrachain or mismatched disulphide bonds.

Bispecific antibodies produced by these approaches are subjected to chemical damage during manipulation processes which may affect the antigen-binding sites of both antigen-binding arms as well as the effector functions of the derived molecules (Webb *et al.*, 1985). Furthermore, the stability of the bispecific antibody molecules is questionable as the chemical bond between the two fragments may easily be cleaved both *in vivo* and *in vitro*. In one study, the yield of heteroconjugate derived from the coupling using SPDP was about 5% of the initial mab used for conjugation and its activity was partially lost 20 days after coupling (Canevari *et al.*, 1988). Physical, chemical and biological properties of the chemical 'heteroconjugates' of mab may also be different from those of the native immunoglobulin molecules, which will affect the function of these molecules *in vivo*. Complete antibody is a large molecule and heteroconjugates derived from direct coupling of two complete antibody molecules may therefore have difficulty penetrating the target site because of their size. Smaller antibody fragments such as Fab or Fv should be used. On the other hand, the lack of Fc of the F(ab')$_2$ heteroconjugates and their small size will also shorten the plasma half-life which may compromise their use as targeting agents; their stability *in vitro* and *in vivo* and their pharmacokinetics have yet to be investigated. Several alternative conjugation techniques are constantly being developed (Karpovsky *et al.*, 1984; Brennan *et al.*, 1985; Liu *et al.*, 1985; Lansdorp *et al.*, 1986; Glennie *et al.*, 1987). Fab fragments were used instead of the whole immunoglobulin molecules, e.g. they can be linked by thioether bonds using *o*-phenylenedimaleimide. The yield and stability of these molecules are better than those of the disulphide-linked molecules (Glennie *et al.*, 1987, 1988).

6.2.3   Genetically engineered bispecific antibodies

The clinical use of xenogeneic mab, mainly produced by mouse hybridoma cell lines, in human is limited partly due to the production of an antiglobulin response to the non-human antibodies (Oldham *et al.*, 1984; Courtenay-Luck *et al.*, 1986). This makes the repeated use ineffective and a severe hypersensitivity reaction may also occur. Xenogeneic antibodies are also not well fitted to destroy human cells *in vivo* because effector cells are not efficiently recruited (Liu *et al.*, 1987; Stevenson *et al.*, 1988). The ideal antibodies for clinical applications should be of human origin. Immortalization of human antibody-secreting cells has, however, been found to be very difficult. Recently, human monoclonal antibodies (Humab) have been produced from Epstein–Barr virus transformation of human B lymphocytes, from heterologous fusion between human B lymphocyte/plasma cells and mouse or rat myeloma cells or from a combination of both techniques. Although the techniques for producing Humab are constantly improving, some problems still remain, notably the low yield of antibody-producing cells from somatic hybridization, difficulties in obtaining high affinity antibodies, low antibody production and instability of the resulting hybridoma cells. Recombinant DNA technology is a powerful alternative technique for producing Humab. Genetically-engineered chimeric human/mouse monoclonal antibodies have been developed by replacing the Fc region of the murine immunoglobulin molecules with the human constant regions (Morrison *et al.*, 1984; Boulianne *et al.*, 1984). Moreover, the framework regions of variable domains of rodent immunoglobulins have also been replaced by their human counterparts (Jones *et al.*, 1986). Fusion proteins between antibody molecules and enzymes or effector molecules have also been genetically constructed and expressed (Neuberger *et al.*, 1984; Schnee *et al.*, 1987). Antibody engineering technology has enormous potential to be used for producing tailor-made antibodies with special physical and functional properties. Another advantage of this technology is that antibody molecules can be designed to have specificity and effector function that may not occur naturally.

The rearranged variable region genes for cloning and expression may be derived from rearranged genomic DNA or from mRNA-derived cDNA. Until recently, the cloning and sequencing of Ig variable regions was time-consuming and was a rate-limiting step in antibody engineering. The standard cloning technique requires a laborious screening of genomic DNA or cDNA libraries using probes specific for the rearranged Ig genes. The cloned genes are then sequenced and recloned for expression. G. Winter and his colleagues in Cambridge have developed a technique based on the polymerase chain reaction (Saiki *et al.*, 1985) for amplifying the Ig variable region genes. Polymerase chain reaction (PCR) technique provides a rapid and facile means of amplifying the sequence of genes; however, it requires the use of sense and antisense oligonucleotide primers from both sides of the target sequence for amplification. For the unknown gene sequence, such as the variable regions of Ig genes, the inability to generate such primers may preclude the use of PCR. The elegant approach by Winter's group relies on the design of oligonucleotide primers corresponding to the relatively-conserved sequences at the 5' and 3' regions of the Ig variable region coding sequences (Orlandi *et al.*, 1989). Restriction sites were incorporated into the primer nucleotide sequences to facilitate cloning into a set of specially-engineered vectors. The amplified genes were sequenced and verified as an error can occur as a result of the amplification. The cloned Ig genes can then be expressed in either a prokaryotic or eukaryotic system (Orlandi *et al.*, 1989; Ward *et al.*, 1989). Recently, oligonucleotide primers for amplification of the heavy and light chain variable region genes of human and mouse have been developed and successfully applied in various systems (Orlandi *et al.*, 1989; Songsivilai *et al.*, 1990; Marks *et al.*, 1991).

Our group has been working on the engineering of bispecific mab molecules. Prior to the work on antibody engineering, attempts were made to generate hybrid hybridoma cell lines by fusing two parental mouse hybridomas of different isotypes, one secreting an IgG1/κ mab against hepatitis B surface antigen (anti-HBsAg) and the other secreting IgG2b/λ antibody against a hapten iodonitrophenylacetyl (anti-NIP). The resulting hybrid hybridomas secreted both parental antibodies but not the bispecific antibody. This is most probably the result of the inability of the two parental heavy chains to form stable hybrid molecules.

Genetic manipulation was therefore employed. In principle, heavy and light chain immunoglobulin genes were cloned from the two mouse hybridomas secreting mab to HBsAg and hapten NIP, by PCR amplification using oligonucleotide primers specific to the variable region genes. The amplified variable region genes were cloned into expression plasmids containing the appropriate constant region genes of human origin, in which the heavy chain genes of both parental antibodies were replaced with the identical human Cγ1 constant region genes. This ensures that stable disulphide bonds between the two heavy chain peptides can be formed. The engineered chimeric heavy and light chain genes of both parental cells were then co-introduced into a non-secreting mouse myeloma cell line (Figure 6.2). Drug selection markers HGPRT and hydromycin were used to select the transfectoma cells from the non-transfected cells. The resulting transfectoma cell lines secreted bispecific monoclonal antibodies with dual specificities to both HBsAg and hapten NIP (Songsivilai *et al.*, 1989).

Genetically-engineered chimeric bispecific mab may overcome three major problems which hamper the applications of mab in clinical medicine, namely, immunogenicity of murine antibodies, rapid serum clearance and non-specific tissue localization. The first two problems are minimized by the use of chimeric immunoglobulin molecules because only the variable regions are derived from mouse antibodies whereas the constant regions are of human origin. Further manipulations can be applied to generate human-like bispecific antibodies (Winter & Milstein, 1991). Bispecific antibodies can alleviate the problem of non-specific tissue localization as the antibodies can be used to prelocalize at the tumour site before the administration of active effector compounds. Chimeric bispecific antibodies will therefore be very useful in clinical applications. This principle could also be applied to produce multimeric bispecific, or even multispecific, antibody molecules. In addition to the approach described,

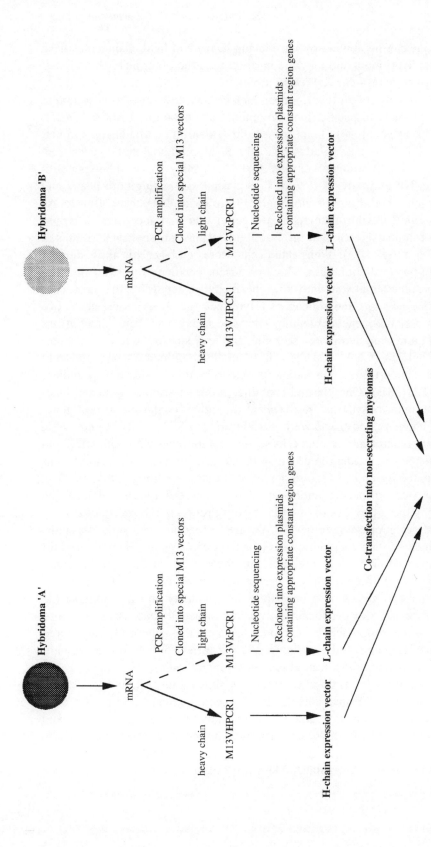

Figure 6.2. Strategy for the cloning and expression of genetically-engineered chimeric bispecific monoclonal antibodies. Heavy and light chain variable region genes of two hybridoma cell lines were amplified using the polymerase chain reaction, cloned into special M13 vectors and sequenced. The V genes were recloned into a set of expression plasmids containing the appropriate constant region genes of human origin. Chimeric constructs were then co-transfected into a non-secreting myeloma cell line NS0. Bispecific antibodies were secreted from the transfectoma cells.

this technique can be applied by introducing heavy and light chain genes from one parental hybridoma into a hybridoma secreting the other mab (S. Songsivilai, unpublished data; Lenz & Weidle, 1990).

To date, at least two other independent groups have also used a similar method to produce bispecific mab by genetic manipulation (Lenz & Weidle, 1990; Phelps *et al.*, 1990). Lenz & Weidle (Boehringer Mannheim GmbH, Germany) cloned the heavy and kappa light chain immunoglobulin genes from an IgG1-secreting hybridoma cell line A20/44 secreting an anti-idiotypic antibody to anti-NP antibody. An expression plasmid containing both heavy and light chain genes and drug selection markers *neo* (bacterial phosphotransferase gene) and *dhfr* (dihydrofolate reductase gene) was introduced into a mouse hybridoma cell line secreting an IgG1 antibody against an isoenzyme of human creatine kinase (CK-MM). Transfected cells expressed bispecific antibodies, as well as both parental antibodies. The introduced specificity was expressed at a lower level in comparison with the specificity secreted by the host cells (anti-CK-MM). Phelps and colleagues (Hybritech Inc, USA) constructed two expression plasmids, one containing chimeric heavy and light chain genes cloned from a murine hybridoma secreting antibody specific to human carcino-embryonic antigen (CEA) and the other containing chimeric heavy and light chain genes cloned from a hybridoma specific to metal chelates such as indium benzyl-EDTA (IBE). One plasmid contained a drug resistance gene xanthine-guanine phosphoribosyltransferase (*gpt*), the other contained a *neo* gene. These two chimeric constructs were introduced into SP2/0 cells by sequential electroporation and transfectoma cells secreting antibodies with both CEA and IBE specificities were identified. Total Ig secreted by the transfectoma cells ranged from 0.6 μg/ml to 25 μg/ml per 10^6 cells. It was estimated that 10–20% of total Ig were bispecific antibodies. The main differences between the researches by these two groups and that by our group are the choice of cloning vectors and selection marker genes. We used separate expression plasmids, each containing either a chimeric heavy or light chain gene, whereas those of other groups contain both heavy and light chain genes in the same plasmid. The results from all three reports, however, have no significant differences. We and the other two groups also envisaged the simplicity and flexibility of the approach, especially for producing therapeutic bispecific mab. Another major advantage of this approach is that once isolated the genetically-engineered immunoglobulin genes can be introduced into a variety of hybridoma cell lines already secreting one of the desired specificity of antibodies.

The yield of bispecific antibodies depends mainly on the affinity between the two parental heavy chains. Genetically-engineered chimeric bispecific antibodies have the same conformation as native immunoglobulin molecules and their yields are subject to the same theoretical principles as those produced by somatic hybridization. By genetically modifying or selecting the heavy chains of the same subclass to allow total random association of each heavy chain, the yield is expected to be only 12.5% of the total antibody secreted from transfectoma cells. The yield may be higher if there is a preferential heavy–light chain pairing of the homologous antibody (Suresh *et al.*, 1986*a*). The total amount of antibodies produced by the genetic engineering approach is relatively small in comparison with hybridoma cells (Winter & Milstein, 1991). This unsatisfactory low yield hampers the use of the engineered monospecific or bispecific antibody in further applications. Another potential problem of the current approach is that each introduced antibody gene is cloned into a separate expression vector. The yield of each chain is different from the others, probably depending on numbers of copies and the location of the gene in the host genome, the choice of promoter/enhancer or other unknown mechanisms. This problem may be ameliorated by cloning all four genes into a single expression plasmid, under the control of the same controlling elements. Development of alternative systems for the high-level expression of the introduced chimeric antibodies is still in an early stage. Introduced immunoglobulin genes could be expressed in plant, insect or COS cells (Hiatt *et al.*, 1989; Hasemann & Capra, 1990; Whittle *et al.*, 1987). To produce large amounts of bispecific antibody for therapeutic purposes, a prokaryotic expression system could be an alternative. This system may not be suitable for the expression of a complete antibody molecule because of the absence of glycosylation and improper folding of Ig in *E. coli* but it may be suitable for producing immunoglobulin fragments (Wetzel, 1988).

One of the interesting designs of bispecific antibodies would be to express them as single-chain bispecific molecules (Songsivilai & Lachmann, 1990). The variable regions of heavy and light chain immunoglobulin genes cloned from each parental hybridoma could be genetically linked together by a polypeptide sequence to form a single-chain antigen-binding complex, utilizing the same principle as that of the genetically engineered single chain Fv antibodies (Huston *et al.*, 1988; Bird *et al.*, 1988). Two sets of the constructs of single chain Fv could then be genetically-linked by a linker sequence, which must ensure free movement of the two antigen-binding complexes. An expression plasmid could contain a cassette for cloning four variable region genes that are designed to have specific restriction sites to allow forced-cloning of each gene into the desired position. Such a construct could be expressed in either eukaryotic or prokaryotic systems. An *E. coli* expression system would be preferable because the handling of bacterial cells is easier and cheaper than mammalian cells, especially when large scale production is required. This design would also ensure that every antibody molecule produced from the cells is a bispecific antibody. The single-chain bispecific antibody fragment will lose the effector functions of the native antibody molecules but these effector functions can later be engineered into the antibody molecules. Its smaller size may increase the penetration of the molecule to its specific target but, on the other hand, may shorten its half-life in the body.

6.3   Applications of bispecific antibodies: current status and future developments

6.3.1   Immunoassays

Bispecific mab can be engineered to have binding specificities to both the antigen and the assay indicators such as a marker enzyme. This construct will enable the design of single-step assay systems without the use of a second antibody and will lead to a simpler method of immunodiagnosis. This can be applied in ELISA or radioimmunoassay (Leong et al., 1986; Karawajew et al., 1988; Takahashi & Fuller, 1988; Tada et al., 1989). In immunohistochemistry, the use of anti-target:anti-peroxidase bispecific antibodies led to an improvement in sensitivity, signal-to-noise ratio and simplification of staining procedures with preservation of fine ultrastructural detail (Milstein & Cuello, 1983; Suresh et al., 1986b; Ribeiro da Silva et al., 1989).

6.3.2   Focusing of effector cell responses to target cells

The use of bispecific antibodies for immunodiagnosis and therapy has shown encouraging results. They have been used for delivering effector substances such as toxins (Corvalan et al., 1987; Webb et al., 1989) and cytotoxic drugs to tumours and some are now in clinical trials (Stickney et al., 1989). Many efforts have been made to use bispecific antibodies to focus cytotoxic effector cell response to tumour cells. This system has been studied in vitro and in vivo, in both animal and human models. Several effector binding specificities were employed. These included antibodies to Fc receptor (Karpovsky et al., 1984; Shen et al., 1986), T cell receptor/CD3 complexes (Perez et al., 1985; Staerz et al., 1985; Jung et al., 1986; Barr et al., 1987; Clark & Waldmann, 1987; Rammensee et al., 1987; Roosnek & Lanzavecchia, 1989) and CD2 molecules (Goedegebuure et al., 1989). Bispecific antibodies which bind to target cells can activate effector cells and crosslink the targets to effector cells. Lysis of virus-infected target cells has also been observed (Staerz et al., 1987). The use of bispecific antibodies may not simply serve to glue the targets and effector cells together but may also trigger the cytolytic process (Karpovsky et al., 1984). Cytotoxicity has been shown not to be due to bystander lysis as direct contact between effector and target cells is required (Barr et al., 1987; Lanzavecchia & Scheidegger, 1987). Most of the experiments on effector cell targeting were performed using homologous effector cell populations such as cloned T cells. The mechanisms of cytotoxicity in vivo may be different and may involve several killing systems. Destruction of the putative effector cells has been observed (Lanzavecchia & Scheidegger, 1987), possibly due to the fact that the bispecific antibody-bound effector cells may themselves serve as targets for antibody-dependent cell-mediated cytotoxicity. It seems that mixed isotype bispecific antibodies, such as rat IgG2b:IgG2c, which can mediate cytotoxicity of target cells by non-ADCC mechanisms, may minimize this problem (Clark & Waldmann, 1987).

6.3.3 *Targeting effector compounds to targets by bispecific antibodies*

A multistage delivery system using bispecific antibodies has an advantage over the system using mab directly coupled to effector compounds. Bispecific antibodies can be administered separately and allowed to concentrate at the target, prior to the injection of functional effector compounds. The combination of the clearance of an uncoupled, less harmful bispecific antibody and a rapid plasma half-life of a functional effector compound will minimize toxicity caused by non-specific binding of antibodies to cells of the reticuloendothelial system and other organs such as liver and spleen. Specific delivery of effector compounds to tumour targets has been investigated by using anti-CEA:anti-vinca alkaloid bispecific antibodies (Corvalan *et al.*, 1987). Radiolabelled vinblastine sulphate was localized at the tumour sites when injected with or after the bispecific antibodies. The background radiation in other organs such as liver and spleen was low compared with the radiolabelled drug alone. Therapeutic data produced in the *in-vivo* mouse xenografted model indicated that this method was more effective in suppressing tumour growth than the vinca alkaloids when given as free drugs (Corvalan *et al.*, 1988). A study using anti-idiotype:anti-saporin heteroconjugates for treatment of lymphoma also showed encouraging results (Glennie *et al.*, 1988). Clinical studies using heteroconjugate bispecific $F(ab)_2$ anti-CEA:anti-BLEDTA IV, an Indium-111 benzyl EDTA derivative of cobalt bleomycin, injected into patients with colon cancer 24–120 h before the injection of [^{111}In] BLEDTA, showed good tumour targeting with low uptake by liver and bone marrow (Stickney *et al.*, 1989). A multistage delivery system using bispecific antibodies, however, may have a disadvantage because its effectiveness relies on the two monovalent antigen–antibody interactions, between two arms of bispecific antibodies and both target and effector molecules. This potential problem may be overcome by the use of high-affinity bispecific mab. The bispecific antibody must also be accessible to the effector molecules on the surface of target cells. This is more likely to be successfull with the bispecific antibodies as their monovalency will alleviate the antigenic modulation mechanism. Bispecific antibodies can also be used to distinguish cells that co-express two different surface antigens. Anti-CD3:anti-CD4 and anti-CD3:anti-CD8 bispecific antibodies were shown to promote complement-mediated lysis of target cells that express both the relevant surface antigens 25–3125 times more efficiently than those expressing only one of the antigens (Wong & Colvin, 1987). Several other systems have also been studied, such as direct targeting of tissue plasminogen activator(tPA) by anti-tPA:anti-fibrin bispecific antibody to enhance thrombolysis (Bode *et al.*, 1989). Anti-interferon (IFN):anti-target cell heteroconjugates have been shown to deliver IFN specifically to target cells and also inhibit their growth *in vitro* (Alkan *et al.*, 1988).

6.3.4   *Mixed-isotype bispecific antibodies*

Mixed-isotype bispecific antibodies, i.e. bispecific antibody molecules containing two different heavy chain isotypes, may have some advantages over normal bispecific antibodies with respect to the mechanisms of cytotoxicity (Clark & Waldmann, 1987). Additionally, purification of the mixed-isotype bispecific antibodies could be carried out readily by a simple separation technique such as ion-exchange chromatography as the different charge characteristics of immunoglobulin are mainly contributed by the two heavy chains (Suresh *et al.*, 1986*a*). Clark & Waldmann (1987) compared two bispecific antibodies against CD3 and Thy-1, one an IgG2b/IgG2b and the other IgG2b/IgG2c; both were produced by somatic hybridization. Both hybrid antibodies were very potent in inducing the killing of Thy-1-positive targets by human T cells. However, only the bispecific IgG2b/IgG2b antibody was able to elicit antibody-dependent cell-mediated cytotoxicity (ADCC). This ADCC could be inhibited by an anti-CD16 mab, which suggests that the effector cells were K cells. The inability of IgG2b/IgG2c mixed-isotype antibody to mediate ADCC may be related to the affinity between its Fc regions and their receptors on the effector cells. In the effector cell retargeting system (ECR), where the putative bispecific antibody-bound effector T cells are also subjected to destruction by ADCC, the mixed-isotype bispecific antibody would have an advantage by exhibiting a better therapeutic ratio of target cell to effector cell cytotoxicity.

It may not be possible to construct some pairs of mixed-isotype antibodies by somatic hybridization or simple gene transfection methods because of the inability of the two heavy chains of different classes/subclasses to form stable disulphide bonds at the hinge region. To date, it is not clearly known about the ability of 'crossed' isotypes to form stable Ig molecules in the cells. Although successful productions of mixed-isotype bispecific antibodies have been reported, the results are still controversial. In a systematic study, Takahashi & Fuller (1988) studied somatic hybridizations between a murine IgG1-secreting hybridoma and either a murine IgM-, IgG1-, IgG2a- or IgG2b-secreting hybridoma. Only the hybrid hybridomas derived from a fusion of the same subclass (IgG1 × IgG1) secreted bispecific antibodies.

Genetic engineering could provide an alternative method for producing mixed-isotype bispecific antibodies. Matched sets of monospecific mab with different isotypes but having the same specificity have already been produced by changing the constant region genes and were used for studying various functional aspects of antibody molecules (Bruggemann *et al.*, 1987; Shaw *et al.*, 1988; Steplewski *et al.*, 1988; Walker *et al.*, 1989). Most of the amino acid residues important for the effector functions of IgG, such as Fc-receptor binding, are located in the carboxy-terminal half of the molecule (Duncan & Winter, 1988; Duncan *et al.*, 1988) and so a bispecific antibody molecule with different CH2 and CH3 domains, but having the same CH1 domains and hinge region, could be produced by a molecular biological approach. Such a design would ensure that the mixed-isotype antibody molecules are formed because both heavy chains have the same hinge regions, thus the ability to form disulphide bonds are not affected. By combining the concepts of bispecific antibody and a matched set of mab, a matched set of mixed-isotype bispecific antibodies with the same specificities could be produced. This set of antibodies would be useful for the study of structure/function relationship of the antibody molecule.

6.3.5   Universal bispecific monoclonal antibodies

For the applications of these antibodies in immunodiagnosis and immuno-therapy, there is a need to produce bispecific antibodies to many specific antigens. The production, however, of so many bispecific antibodies, either by somatic hybridization or chemical conjugation, is still complicated, time con-suming and requires expertise in that system. To avoid the need to create different bispecific antibodies for each target antigen, the idea of a 'universal' bispecific antibody was proposed. Gilliland *et al.* (1988) produced a hybrid bispecific antibody with dual specificities for CD3 and Ig light chain. This bispecific antibody was used in an indirect effector cell retargeting system, in which specific anti-target antibodies were first localized at the target site. The anti-Ig specificity of the bispecific antibody could bind to the target-coating antibody and its anti-CD3 specificity would then activate the effector cells and act as an adaptor between the effector cells and the targets, leading to the destruction of target cells. A single construct of this bispecific antibody, in combination with a panel of specific anti-target mab, could mediate lysis to a wide range of antibody-coated cells. However, clinical applications of this universal bispecific antibody may be limited.

On the other hand, bispecific antibodies with different effector-binding specificities, but having specificity for the same targets, also have a great potential for clinical applications. For example, an anti-tumour bispecific antibody with anti-radionuclide specificity could be used for *in vivo* tumour imaging whereas another with anti-cytotoxic agent specificity could be used for targeted therapy. To avoid generating two bispecific antibodies to two 'effec-tor' antigens, a universal effector-binding antibody may be used. A small hapten such as NIP may be a good choice as the universal 'effector' antigen (Songsivilai & Lachmann, 1990). The hapten NIP can be coupled easily to a wide range of effector compounds and would act as an adaptor between a bispecific antibody and active effector compounds conjugated to NIP. The genetically engineered bispecific antibodies with specificity for target antigens and the hapten NIP would then serve as universal bispecific antibodies for delivering a variety of NIP-coupled effector compounds to the specific target.

A combination of the two approaches, namely a bispecific antibody with dual specificities to a hapten NIP and immunoglobulin molecules together with specific anti-target antibodies and NIP-conjugated effector compounds, may be useful as a method for universal targeting.

6.4   References

Alkan, S. S., Towbin, H. & Hochkeppel, H. K. (1988). Enhanced antiproliferative action of interferon targeted by bispecific monoclonal antibodies. *Journal of Interferon Research*, **8**, 25–33.

Barr, I. G., MacDonald, H. R., Buchegger, F. & von Fliedner, V. (1987). Lysis of tumour cells by the retargeting of murine cytolytic T lymphocytes with bispecific antibodies. *International Journal of Cancer*, **40**, 423–429.

Bird, R. E., Hardman, K. D., Jacobson, J. W., Johnson, S., Kaufman, B. M., Lee, S.-M., Lee, T., Pope, S. H., Riordan, G. S. & Whitlow, M. (1988). Single-chain antigen-binding proteins. *Science*, **242**, 423–426.

Blakey, D. C., Wawrzynczak, E. J., Wallace, P. M. & Thorpe, P. E. (1988). Antibody toxin conjugates: a perspective. *Progress in Allergy*, **45**, 50–90.

Bode, C., Runge, M. S., Branscomb, E. E., Newell, J. B., Matsueda, G. R. & Haber, E. (1989). Antibody-directed fibrinolysis. An antibody specific for both fibrin and tissue plasminogen activator. *Journal of Biological Chemistry*, **264**, 944–948.

Boulianne, G. L., Hozumi, N. & Shulman, M. J. (1984). Production of functional chimaeric mouse/human antibody. *Nature*, **312**, 643–646.

Brennan, M., Davison, P. F. & Paulus, H. (1985). Preparation of bispecific antibodies by chemical recombination of monoclonal immunoglobulin G1 fragments. *Science*, **229**, 81–83.

Bruggemann, M., Williams, G. T., Bindon, C. I., Clark, M. R., Walker, M. R., Jefferis, R., Waldmann, H. & Neuberger, M. S. (1987). Comparison of the effector functions of human immunoglobulins using a matched set of chimeric antibodies. *Journal of Experimental Medicine*, **166**, 1351–1361.

Canevari, S., Menard, S., Mezzanzanica, D., Miotti, S., Pupa, S. M., Lanzavecchia, A. & Colnaghi, M. I. (1988). Anti-ovarian carcinoma anti-T3 heteroconjugates or hybrid antibodies induce tumor cell lysis by cytotoxic T-cells. *International Journal of Cancer*, **2** (Suppl.) 18–21.

Chaudhary, Y. K., Batra, J. K., Gallo, M. G., Willingham, M. C., Fitzgerald, D. J. & Pastan, I. (1990). A rapid method of cloning functional variable-region antibody genes in *Escherichia coli* as single-chain immunotoxins. *Proceedings of the National Academy of Sciences U.S.A.*, **87**, 1066–1070.

Chervonsky, A. V., Faerman, A. I., Evdonina, L. V., Jazova, A. K., Kazarov, A. R. & Gussev, A. I. (1988). A simple metabolic system for selection of hybrid hybridomas (tetradomas) producing bispecific monoclonal antibodies. *Molecular Immunology*, **25**, 913–915.

Clark, M. R. & Waldmann, H. (1987). T-cell killing of target cells induced by hybrid antibodies: comparison of two bispecific monoclonal antibodies. *Journal of the National Cancer Institute*, **79**, 1393–1401.

Cobbold, S. P. & Waldmann, H. (1984). Therapeutic potential of monovalent monoclonal antibodies. *Nature*, **308**, 460–462.

Corvalan, J. R. F. & Smith, W. (1987). Construction and characterisation of a hybrid–hybrid monoclonal antibody recognising both carcinoembryonic antigen (CEA) and vinca alkaloids. *Cancer Immunology and Immunotherapy*, **24**, 127–132.

Corvalan, J. R. F., Smith, W. & Gore, V. A. (1988). Tumour therapy with vinca alkaloids targeted by a hybrid-hybrid monoclonal antibody recognising both CEA and vinca alkaloids. *International Journal of Cancer*, **2** (Suppl.) 22–25.

Corvalan, J. R. F., Smith, W., Gore, V. A. & Brandon, D. R. (1987). Specific *in vitro* and *in vivo* drug localisation to tumour cells using a hybrid-hybrid monoclonal antibody recognising both carcinoembryonic antigen (CEA) and vinca alkaloids. *Cancer Immunology and Immunotherapy*, **24**, 133–137.

Cotton, R. G. H. & Milstein, C. (1973). Fusion of two immunoglobulin-producing myeloma cells. *Nature*, **244**, 42–43.

Courtenay-Luck, N. S., Epenetos, A. A., Moore, R., Larche, M., Pectasides, D., Dhokia, B. & Ritter, M. A. (1986). Development of primary and secondary immune responses to mouse monoclonal antibodies used in the diagnosis and therapy of malignant neoplasms. *Cancer Research*, **46**, 6489–6493.

De Lau, W. B. M., van Loon, A. E., Heije, K., Valerio, D. & Bast, B. J. E. G. (1989). Production of hybrid hybridomas based on HAT^s-neomycin^r double mutants. *Journal of Immunological Methods*, **117**, 1–8.

Duncan, A. R. & Winter, G. (1988). The binding site for C1q on IgG. *Nature*, **332**, 738–740.

Duncan, A. R., Woof, J. M., Partridge, L. J., Burton, D. R. & Winter, G. (1988). Localization of the binding site for the human high affinity Fc-receptor on IgG. *Nature*, **332**, 563–564.

Ghose, T. & Blair, A. H. (1987). The design of cytotoxic-agent-antibody conjugates. *CRC Critical Reviews of Therapeutic Drug Carrier Systems*, **3**, 262–359.

Gilliland, L. K., Clark, M. R. & Waldmann, H. (1988). Universal bispecific antibody for targeting tumour cells for destruction by cytotoxic T cells. *Proceedings of the National Academy of Sciences U.S.A.*, **85**, 7719–7723.

Glennie, M. J., Brennand, D. M., Bryden, F., McBride, H. M., Stirpe, F., Worth, A. T. & Stevenson, G. T. (1988). Bispecific F(ab'γ)$_2$ antibody for the delivery of saporin in the treatment of lymphoma. *Journal of Immunology*, **141**, 3662–3670.

Glennie, M. J., McBride, H. M., Worth, A. T. & Stevenson, G. T. (1987). Preparation and performance of bispecific F(ab'γ)$_2$ antibody containing thioether-linked Fab'γ fragments. *Journal of Immunology*, **139**, 2367–2375.

Goedegebuure, P. S., Segal, D. M., Braakman, E., Vreugdenhil, R. J., van Krimpen, B. A., van de Griend, R. J. & Bolhuis, R. L. (1989). Induction of lysis by T cell receptor $\gamma\delta^+$/CD3$^+$ T lymphocytes via CD2 requires triggering via the T11.1 epitope only. *Journal of Immunology*, **142**, 1797–1802.

Goldenberg, D. M. (1988). Targeting of cancer with radiolabelled antibodies: prospects for imaging and therapy. *Archives of Pathology Laboratory Medicine*, **112**, 580–587.

Goldenberg, D. M. (1989). Targeted cancer treatment. *Immunology Today*, **10**, 286–288.

Gordon, J. & Stevenson, G. T. (1981). Antigenic modulation of lymphocytic surface immunoglobulin yielding resistance to complement-mediated lysis. II. Relationship to redistribution of the antigen. *Immunology*, **42**, 13–17.

Hasemann, C. A. & Capra, J. D. (1990). High-level production of a functional immunoglobulin heterodimer in a baculovirus expression system. *Proceedings of the National Academy of Sciences U.S.A.*, **87**, 3942–3946.

Henkel, R. D., Kennedy, R. C., Sparrow, J. T. & Dressman, G. R. (1985). *In vivo* detection of human hepatoma secreting hepatitis B surface antigen in nude mice with radiolabelled monoclonal antibodies that recognised distinct epitopes. *Clinical Immunology and Immunopathology*, **35**, 146–155.

Hiatt, A., Cafferkey, R. & Bowdish, K. (1989). Production of antibodies in transgenic plants. *Nature*, **342**, 76–78.

Hurwitz, E., Levy, R., Maron, R., Wilchek, M., Arnon, R. & Sela, M. (1975). The covalent binding of daunomycin and adriamycin to antibodies, with retention of both drug and antibody activities. *Cancer Research*, **35**, 1175–1181.

Huston, J. S., Levinson, D., Mudgett-Hunter, M., Tai, M.-S., Novotny, J., Margolies, M. N., Ridge, R. J., Bruccoleri, R. E., Haber, E., Crea, R. & Oppermann, H. (1988). Protein engineering of antibody binding sites: recovery of specific activity in an anti-digoxin single-chain Fv analogue produced in *Escherichia coli*. *Proceedings of the National Academy of Sciences U.S.A.*, **85**, 5879–5883.

Jones, P. T., Dear, P. H., Foote, J., Neuberger, M. S. & Winter, G. (1986). Replacing the complementarity-determining regions in a human antibody with those from a mouse. *Nature*, **321**, 522–525.

Jung, G., Honsik, C. J., Reisfeld, R. A. & Muller-Eberhard, H. J. (1986). Activation of human peripheral blood mononuclear cells by anti-T3: killing of tumour target cells coated with anti-target-anti-T3 conjugates. *Proceedings of the National Academy of Sciences U.S.A.*, **83**, 4479–4483.

Karawajew, L., Behrsing, O., Kaiser, G. & Micheel, B. (1988). Production and ELISA application of bispecific monoclonal antibodies against fluorescein isothiocyanate (FITC) and horseradish peroxidase (HRP). *Journal of Immunological Methods*, **111**, 95–99.

Karawajew, L., Micheel, B., Behrsing, O. & Gaestel, M. (1987). Bispecific antibody-producing hybrid hybridomas selected by a fluoresence activated cell sorter. *Journal of Immunological Methods*, **96**, 265–270.

Karpovsky, B., Titus, J. A., Stephany, D. A. & Segal, D. M. (1984). Production of target-specific effector cells using hetero-cross-linked aggregates containing anti-target cell and anti-Fcγ receptor antibodies. *Journal of Experimental Medicine*, **160**, 1686–1701.

Kohler, G. & Milstein, C. (1975). Continuous cultures of fused cells secreting antibody of predefined specificity. *Nature*, **256**, 495–497.

Koolwijk, P., Rozemuller, E., Stad, R. K., de Lau, W. B. M. & Bast, B. J. E. G. (1988). Enrichment and selection of hybrid hybridomas by Percoll density gradient centrifugation and fluoresence-activated cell sorting. *Hybridoma*, **7**, 217–225.

Lansdorp, P. M., Aalberse, R. C., Bos, R., Schutter, W. G. & van Bruggen, E. F. J. (1986). Cyclic tetramolecular complexes of monoclonal antibodies: a new type of cross-linking reagent. *European Journal of Immunology*, **16**, 679–683.

Lanzavecchia, A. & Scheidegger, D. (1987). The use of hybrid hybridomas to target human cytotoxic T lymphocytes. *European Journal of Immunology*, **17**, 105–111.

Lenz, H. & Weidle, U. H. (1990). Expression of heterobispecific antibodies by gene transfected into producer hybridoma cells. *Gene*, **87**, 213–218.

Leong, M. M. L., Milstein, C. & Pannell, R. (1986). Luminescent detection method for immunodot, Western and Southern blots. *Journal of Histochemistry and Cytochemistry*, **34**, 1645–1650.

Liu, M. A., Kranz, D. M., Kurnick, J. T., Boyle, L. A., Levy, R. & Eisen, H. N. (1985). Heteroantibody duplexes target cells for lysis by cytotoxic T lymphocytes. *Proceedings of the National Academy of Sciences U.S.A.*, **82**, 8648–8652.

Liu, A. Y., Robinson, R. R., Hellstrom, K. E., Murray, E. D. Jr., Chang, C. P. & Hellstrom, I. (1987). Chimeric mouse-human IgG1 antibody that can mediate lysis of cancer cells. *Proceedings of the National Academy of Sciences U.S.A.*, **84**, 3439–3443.

Marks, J. D., Tristem, M., Karpas, A. & Winter, G. (1991). Oligonucleotide primers for polymerase chain reaction amplification of human immunoglobulin variable region genes and design of family-specific oligonucleotide probes. *European Journal of Immunology*, **21**, 985–991.

Milstein, C. & Cuello, A. C. (1983). Hybrid hybridomas and their use in immunohistochemistry. *Nature*, **305**, 537–540.

Morrison, S. L., Johnson, M. J., Herzenberg, L. A. & Oi, V. T. (1984). Chimeric human antibody molecules: mouse antigen-binding domains with human constant region domains. *Proceedings of the National Academy of Sciences U.S.A.*, **81**, 6851–6855.

Neuberger, M. S., Williams, G. T. & Fox, R. O. (1984). Recombinant antibodies possessing novel effector functions. *Nature*, **312**, 604–608.

Nisonoff, A. & Rivers, M. M. (1961). Recombination of a mixture of univalent antibody fragments of different specificity. *Archives of Biochemistry and Biophysics*, **93**, 460–462.

Oldham, R. K., Foon, K. A., Morgan, A. C., Woodhouse, C. S., Schroff, R. W., Abrams, P. G., Fer, M., Schoenberger, C. S., Farrell, M., Kimball, E. & Sherwin, S. A. (1984). Monoclonal antibody therapy of malignant melanoma: *in vivo* localisation in cutaneous metastasis after intravenous administration. *Journal of Clinical Oncology*, **2**, 1235–1244.

Orlandi, R., Gussow, D. H., Jones, P. T. & Winter, G. (1989). Cloning of immunoglobulin variable domains for expression by the polymerase chain reaction. *Proceedings of the National Academy of Sciences U.S.A.*, **86**, 3833–3837.

Perez, P., Hoffman, R. W., Shaw, S., Bluestone, J. A. & Segal, D. M. (1985). Specific targeting of cytotoxic T cells by anti-T3 linked to anti-target cell antibody. *Nature*, **316**, 354–356.

Phelps, J. L., Beidler, D. E., Jue, R. A., Unger, B. W. & Johnson, M. J. (1990). Expression and characterisation of a chimeric bifunctional antibody with therapeutic applications. *Journal of Immunology*, **145**, 1200–1204.

Rammensee, H. G., Julius, M. H., Nemazee, D., Langhorne, J., Lamers, R. & Kohler, G. (1987). Targeting cytotoxic T cells to antigen-specific B lymphocytes. *European Journal of Immunology*, **17**, 433–436.

Raso, V. & Griffin, T. (1981). Hybrid antibodies with dual specificity for the delivery of ricin to immunoglobulin-bearing targets. *Cancer Research*, **41**, 2073–2078.

Ribeiro da Silva, A., Tagari, P. & Cuello, A. C. (1989). Morphological characterisation of substance P-like immunoreactive glomeruli in the superficial dorsal horn of the rat spinal cord and trigeminal subnucleus caudalis: a quantitative study. *Journal of Comparative Neurology*, **281**, 497–515.

Roosnek, E. & Lanzavecchia, A. (1989). Triggering T cells by otherwise inert hybrid anti-CD3/antitumor antibodies requires encounter with the specific target cell. *Journal of Experimental Medicine*, **170**, 297–302.

Saiki, R. K., Scharf, S., Faloona, F., Mullis, K. B., Horn, G. T., Erlich, H. A. & Arnheim, N. (1985). Enzymatic amplification of β-globin genomic sequences and restriction site analysis for diagnosis of sickle cell anemia. *Science*, **230**, 1350–1354.

Schnee, J. M., Runge, M. S., Matsueda, G. R., Hudson, N. W., Seigman, J. G., Haber, E. & Quertermous, T. (1987). Construction and expression of a recombinant antibody-targeted plasminogen activator. *Proceedings of the National Academy of Sciences U.S.A.*, **84**, 6904–6908.

Schwaber, J. & Cohen, E. P. (1974). Pattern of immunoglobulin synthesis and assembly in a human-mouse somatic cell hybrid clone. *Proceedings of the National Academy of Sciences U.S.A.*, **71**, 2203–2207.

Shaw, D. R., Khazaeli, M. B. & LoBuglio, A. F. (1988). Mouse/human chimeric

antibodies to a tumor-associated antigen: biologic activity of the four human IgG
subclasses. *Journal of the National Cancer Institute*, **80**, 1553–1559.

Shen, L., Guyre, P. M., Anderson, C. L. & Fanger, M. W. (1986).
Heteroantibody-mediated cytotoxicity: antibody to the high affinity Fc receptor for
IgG mediates cytotoxicity by human monocytes that is enhanced by interferon-γ
and is not blocked by human IgG. *Journal of Immunology*, **137**, 3378–3382.

Songsivilai, S., Bye, J. M., Marks, J. D. & Hughes-Jones, N. C. (1990). Cloning and
sequencing of human lambda immunoglobulin genes by the polymerase chain
reaction. *European Journal of Immunology*, **20**, 2661–2666.

Songsivilai, S., Clissold, P. M. & Lachmann, P. J. (1989). A novel strategy for
producing chimeric bispecific antibodies by gene transfection. *Biochemical and
Biophysical Research Communications*, **164**, 271–276.

Songsivilai, S. & Lachmann, P. J. (1990). Bispecific antibodies: a tool for diagnosis and
treatment of disease. *Clinical and Experimental Immunology*, **79**, 315–321.

Staerz, U. D. & Bevan, M. J. (1986). Hybrid hybridoma producing a bispecific
monoclonal antibody that can focus effector T-cell activity. *Proceedings of the
National Academy of Sciences U.S.A.*, **83**, 1453–1457.

Staerz, U. D., Kanagawa, O. & Bevan, M. J. (1985). Hybrid antibodies can target sites
for attack by T cells. *Nature*, **314**, 628–631.

Staerz, U. D., Yewdell, J. W. & Bevan, M. J. (1987). Hybrid antibody-mediated lysis of
virus-infected cells. *European Journal of Immunology*, **17**, 571–574.

Steplewski, Z., Sun, L. K., Shearman, C. W., Ghrayeb, J., Daddona, P. & Koprowski,
H. (1988). Biological activity of human-mouse IgG1, IgG2, IgG3 and IgG4
chimeric monoclonal antibodies with antitumor specificity. *Proceedings of the
National Academy of Sciences U.S.A.*, **85**, 4852–4856.

Stevenson, G. T., Glennie, M. J., Hamblin, T. J., Lane, A. C. & Stevenson, F. K.
(1988). Problems and prospects in the use of lymphoma idiotypes as therapeutic
targets. *International Journal of Cancer*, **3** (Suppl.) 9–12.

Stickney, D. R., Slater, J. B. & Fincke, J. M. (1989). Imaging and therapeutic
potential of bifunctional antibody (BFA) in colon carcinoma. In *Fourth
International Conference on Monoclonal Antibody Immunoconjugates for Cancer*
(abstract) p. 29. San Diego, UCSD.

Suresh, M. R., Cuello, A. C. & Milstein, C. (1986a). Bispecific monoclonal antibodies
from hybrid hybridomas. *Methods in Enzymology*, **121**, 210–228.

Suresh, M. R., Cuello, A. C. & Milstein, C. (1986b). Advantages of bispecific
hybridomas in one-step immunochemistry and immunoassays. *Proceedings of the
National Academy of Sciences U.S.A.*, **83**, 7989–7993.

Tada, H., Toyoda, Y. & Iwasa, S. (1989). Bispecific antibody-producing hybrid
hybridoma and its use in one-step immunoassay for human lymphotoxin.
Hybridoma, **8**, 73–83.

Takahashi, M. & Fuller, S. A. (1988). Production of murine hybrid-hybridomas
secreting bispecific monoclonal antibodies for use in urease-based immunoassays.
Clinical Chemistry, **34**, 1693–1696.

Tiebout, R. F., van Boxtel-Oosterhof, F., Stricker, E. A. M. & Zeijlemaker, W. P.
(1987). A human hybrid hybridoma. *Journal of Immunology*, **139**, 3402–3405.

Urnovitz, H. B., Chang, Y., Scott, M., Fleischman, J. & Lynch, R. G. (1988). IgA:IgM
and IgA:IgA hybrid hybridomas secrete heteropolymeric immunoglobulins that are
polyvalent and bispecific. *Journal of Immunology*, **140**, 558–563.

Walker, M. R., Woof, J. M., Bruggemann, M., Jefferis, R. & Burton, D. R. (1989).
Interaction of human IgG chimeric antibodies with the human FcRI and FcRII
receptors: requirement for antibody-mediated host cell-target cell interaction.
Molecular Immunology, **26**, 403–411.

Ward, E. S., Gussow, D., Griffiths, A. D., Jones, P. T. & Winter, G. (1989). Binding activities of a repertoire of single immunoglobulin variable domains secreted from *Escherichia coli*. *Nature*, **341**, 544–546.

Webb, K. S., Poulton, S. H., Liberman, S. N. & Walther, P. J. (1989). Rationale for immunotoxin therapy of metastatic prostate carcinoma formatted as a multi-stage delivery system. *Journal of Urology*, **142**, 425.

Webb, K. S., Ware, J. L., Parks, S. F., Walther, P. J. & Paulson, D. F. (1985). Evidence for a novel hybrid immunotoxin recognizing ricin A-chain by one antigen-combining site and a prostate-restricted antigen by the remaining antigen-combining site: potential for immunotherapy. *Cancer Treatment Reports*, **69**, 663–672.

Wetzel, R. (1988). Active immunoglobulin fragments synthesized in *E. coli* – from Fab to *Sc* antibodies. *Protein Engineering*, **2**, 169–176.

Whittle, N., Adair, J., Lloyd, C., Jenkins, L., Devine, J., Schlom, J., Raubitschek, A., Colcher, D. & Bodmer, M. (1987). Expression in COS cells of a mouse-human chimaeric B72.3 antibody. *Protein Engineering*, **1**, 499–505.

Winter, G. & Milstein, C. (1991). Man-made antibodies. *Nature*, **349**, 293–299.

Wong, J. T. & Colvin, R. B. (1987). Bi-specific monoclonal antibodies: selective binding and complement fixation to cells that express two different surface antigens. *Journal of Immunology*, **139**, 1369–1374.

Zimmerman, B. & Grey, H. M. (1971). Noncovalent interaction between immunoglobulin (Ig) polypeptide chains. II. Absence of hybrid molecule formation between Ig classes. *Journal of Immunology*, **107**, 1788–1790.

7

Production of antibodies using phage display libraries

A. J. T. GEORGE

7.1   Introduction

The description of monoclonal antibody (mab) technology in 1975 by Köhler and Milstein has revolutionized the practice and study of immunology; mab have been produced that are useful in the therapy and diagnosis of a range of diseases and increasingly they are finding industrial applications. In addition, the availability of well-defined antibodies against a wide variety of proteins and other antigens has proved helpful in nearly every aspect of biological science. There are a number of limitations, however, to the current hybridoma-based approach to mab production. First, the production of antibody-producing hybridomas is, on the whole, restricted to the mouse and rat. Some groups have produced mab from other species, including humans, but the low production rates and the inherent instability of the hybridomas has prevented widespread use of such antibodies (Chapter 5). Second, if one wishes to isolate a rare antibody using hybridoma-derived techniques it is necessary to screen a large number of colonies and in many cases this will be prohibitively expensive due to the intensive labour required. Finally, the fact that one has to immunize an animal to produce mab restricts this approach to antibodies that the animal is capable of producing, and it can be difficult to produce antibodies to antigens to which the animal is tolerant.

In recent years a number of techniques have been developed for the production of new mab by recombinant DNA technology (Huse *et al.*, 1989; Clackson *et al.*, 1991). While these approaches are still in their infancy, and far from routine, it is to be expected that they may soon become the favoured approach to the production of certain antibodies. As well as overcoming some of the problems mentioned above they also have the advantage of providing the antibody in a recombinant form, allowing for easy genetic manipulation of the molecule. In this chapter I will discuss one of the more promising of these approaches, the use of filamentous phage expression systems, as well as some of the recombinant antibody molecules that can be produced by these techniques.

142

7.2   Filamentous phage

7.2.1   Filamentous phage: structure

The use of phage display libraries is based on the structure of the filamentous family of phages (Figure 7.1). These phages, which include the popular M13, fd and f1 phages, are single-stranded DNA (ssDNA) bacteriophages (Model & Russel, 1988). The phage particles consist of a long loop of ssDNA (about 6400 nucleotides long in wild type phage) coated with multiple copies (around 2700) of the major coat protein (pVIII, product of gene VIII). The resulting tube is about 1 μm long and 6–7 nm in diameter; however, as the coat is made from multiple subunits of pVIII, it can be lengthened to accommodate more ssDNA. Thus insertion of artificial segments of DNA into the phage genome can be accommodated with little deleterious effect on phage assembly (Sambrook *et al.*, 1989). In addition to the multiple copies of pVIII there are four minor coat proteins on the surface of the phage, present at about five copies each; pVII and pIX located at one tip of the phage and pVI and pIII at the other (Model & Russel, 1988).

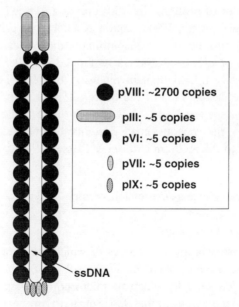

Figure 7.1. Diagrammatic representation of the filamentous phage structure. Filamentous phage contain a long loop of ssDNA surrounded by a tube formed by multiple copies of the major coat protein pVIII. At either end of the phage particle there are minor coat proteins, pIII, pVI, pVII and pIX. The entire structure is about 1 μm long and 6–7 nm in diameter.

7.2.2   Filamentous phage: life cycle

The filamentous phage are capable of infecting only male bacteria that carry the F sex pillus. Infection is initiated by binding of the minor coat protein pIII to the sex pillus, leading to retraction of the pillus and internalization of the phage. Once infected by a phage, bacteria are unable to produce sex pilli, preventing infection of bacteria by more than one phage (Model & Russel, 1988).

Inside the cell the phage is replicated by a complex process that is largely outside the scope of this chapter (Model & Russel, 1988). One important feature, however, of this replication is that it is tightly controlled and infection with filamentous phage does not lead to lysis of the infected bacteria which continue to divide (albeit at a reduced rate) and produce phage on a continual basis at several hundred phage/bacterium/generation (Sambrook *et al.*, 1989).

Assembly of the phage particles does not occur within the cell but proceeds as the phage is extruded through the bacterial wall. The pVIII and pIII coat proteins are made with signal peptides that direct their production to the periplasm of the Gram-negative *E. coli* whereas the other minor coat proteins contain hydrophobic sequences that probably lead to association with the inner membrane of the bacteria (Model & Russel, 1988). (The periplasm lies between the inner and outer membrane of the cell and, unlike the cytoplasm, it is an oxidising environment allowing formation of disulphide bonds. In addition it contains a number of proteins that aid refolding of newly-produced polypeptide chains (Bardwell *et al.*, 1991; Landry & Gierasch, 1991). It is therefore a good site for the production of recombinant molecules, including antibody fragments (Better *et al.*, 1988; Skerra & Plückthun, 1988), as they are more likely to be correctly folded than in inclusion bodies.) The phage ssDNA is carried to the cytoplasmic face of the bacterial inner membrane by one of the phage control proteins (pV) and, as it is goes through the periplasm, it sheds pV and picks up the various coat proteins before being released as the complete virion into the medium (Model & Russel, 1988).

7.3   Filamentous phage as expression vectors

7.3.1   Peptide display by phage

The pIII minor coat protein, five copies of which are expressed at one end of the phage particle, projects from the surface of the phage in a 'ball and stick' manner that can be seen by electron microscopy (Gray *et al.*, 1981). The exposed position of its N-terminal led Smith to propose its use to express proteins that could then be recognized by antibodies. In his initial experiments he inserted a 171 bp fragment from the *Eco*RI endonuclease gene into the 5′ end of the pIII gene of phage (Smith, 1985). The resulting phage particles expressed the endonuclease-derived peptide on their surface where it could be detected with an antibody. In addition it was demonstrated that one could separate the phage bearing the peptide from wild type phage by affinity techniques. The presence of foreign proteins on the pIII has little apparent effect on the phage behaviour although, not surprisingly in view of altered state of the pIII protein, the phage were less infective than wild type phage (Smith, 1985).

7.3.2 Peptide display libraries

These pioneering experiments with peptide display phage led a number of groups to make peptide display libraries, in which a large number of different peptides were displayed as fusion proteins with pIII on the phage surface (Scott, 1992). In two studies, libraries consisting of random hexapeptides on pIII were panned with antibodies, as described above (Cwirla *et al.*, 1990; Scott & Smith, 1990). The antibody-binding phage were eluted and used to infect *E. coli* to amplify the phage. The panning process was repeated a number of times, which generated peptide sequences that were recognized by the antibodies with reasonable affinities (Cwirla *et al.*, 1990; Scott & Smith, 1990). This technique has been exploited to map an epitope, recognized by a mab, that is present on mutant p53 molecules associated with the malignant phenotype of some tumour cells (Stephen & Lane, 1992).

Peptide display libraries have also been used to identify peptides capable of binding to proteins other than antibodies. These have included not only molecules such as the HLA-DR1 class 2 molecule that are expected to bind peptides (Hammer *et al.*, 1992), but also other proteins such as streptavidin (Devlin *et al.*, 1990) and the lectin concanavalin A (Oldenburg *et al.*, 1992; Scott *et al.*, 1992) that are not normally associated with protein or peptide binding.

Some of the advantages of phage display libraries are highlighted by these experiments. First, it is possible to contain representative phage from the entire library in a few microlitres of buffer, ensuring that the number of potential molecules screened is limited only by the size of the initial library. Second, phage binding the desired molecule can be rapidly isolated, using affinity techniques, from non-binding phage. These two factors allow one to rapidly isolate very rare binding molecules from vast numbers of non-binding phage (libraries may contain up to 10^9 different members (Scott, 1992)).

Whereas the majority of work has involved the use of pIII fusion proteins the major coat protein pVIII has been used as a site for peptide display (Felici *et al.*, 1991; Hermes *et al.*, 1989; Ilyichev *et al.*, 1992), and peptides can be selected from random pVIII display libraries in a similar manner to pIII display libraries (Felici *et al.*, 1991). The main difference in this approach is that the major coat protein is present in several thousand copies/phage and so this should lead to many copies of the peptide being displayed, with consequent increases in the avidity of the peptide–antibody interaction. Many of the pVIII fusion proteins, however, are unable to form the phage capsid alone and wildtype pVIII is needed in addition (Felici *et al.*, 1991; Greenwood *et al.*, 1991). The hybrid proteins are therefore dispersed among the wildtype pVIII at a density that, presumably, is dependent on the foreign protein sequence.

7.3.3. Protein display

In addition to peptides a number of other proteins have been displayed on both pIII and pVIII coat proteins. These include both immunoglobulin fragments (7.4), bovine pancreatic trypsin inhibitor (Markland *et al.*, 1991), the human immunodeficiency virus (HIV) *gag* proteins (Tsunetsgu-Yokota *et al.*, 1991) and human growth hormone (Lowman *et al.*, 1991). In the latter case random mutations were introduced at various sites in the growth hormone and a phage display library used to select variants that bound to their receptor with a higher affinity (Lowman *et al.*, 1991). These data demonstrate the ability of the coat proteins to tolerate the fusion of a wide variety of different proteins, with only minimal effects on the assembly and behaviour of the phage.

7.4   Antibody selection on phage

7.4.1   Cloning of antibody V regions by polymerase chain reaction

The ability to express peptides and other proteins as fusion proteins with pIII, and to select binders from a library, led quite naturally to attempts to express antibody fragments on pIII. A prerequisite for such an approach is the ability to isolate and clone the variable (V) region genes from the immunoglobulin heavy and light chains. This has been greatly facilitated with the development of the polymerase chain reaction (PCR) to amplify DNA (Saiki *et al.*, 1985). PCR relies on the use of oligonucleotide primers that bind at the 5' and 3' ends of the target sequence of DNA. A thermostable DNA polymerase (normally *Taq*, although a number of enzymes with improved characteristics are now available) is used to extend the primers, making copies of the target DNA. The reaction is carried out in an automated thermal cycler that cycles between the three temperatures needed for the reaction (denaturation, annealling and extension), making multiple copies of the DNA fragment. Theoretically, the number of copies increases exponentially with each cycle, as the copies themselves become templates for further copies.

A number of strategies exist for the PCR amplification of immunoglobulin V region genes. In the first reports of PCR amplification, degenerate oligonucleotide primers were described that were derived from relatively conserved sequences present at the 5' and 3' ends of the rearranged V region gene (the 3' primer binds to the part of the gene that is derived from the J region) (Orlandi *et al.*, 1989). One can use panels of primers derived from families of V region genes, from the constant regions of the immunoglobulin gene, and from signal peptides (Larrick & Fry, 1991; Sastry *et al.*, 1989; Ward *et al.*, 1989). Primers are now described that are suitable for the amplification of human (Dübel *et al.*, 1992; Larrick & Fry, 1991; Marks *et al.*, 1991*b*), as well as murine, V regions.

The most common source of V region DNA for PCR amplification is cDNA derived from mRNA from a suitable B cell source. If the primers used, however, react with sequences within the V region it is possible to use genomic DNA as starting material for the PCR, relying on the apposition of the various variable region genes (V, D, J in heavy chain and V, J in light chains) to bring the primers close enough to allow amplification of the intervening sequences.

7.4.2 Antibody fragments on phage

In an initial set of experiments, a single chain antibody (sFv) directed against lysozyme was expressed as a fusion with pIII (McCafferty *et al.*, 1990) (Figure 7.2). An sFv molecule, which consists of the V_L and V_H domains of an immunoglobulin linked by a peptide spacer, contains the minimal antigen-binding domains of an antibody (Bird *et al.*, 1988; Huston *et al.*, 1988) (see 7.5.2 for a full discussion). Phage expressing the anti-lysozyme sFv on pIII could be selected from phage not bearing the antibody by passing them down a lysozyme-Sepharose column. This resulted in more than 1000-fold purification of the desired sFv bearing phage on each pass down the column, demonstrating the feasibility of isolating antigen-binding sFv from a phage display library (McCafferty *et al.*, 1990).

The major pVIII coat protein has also been used as a site for attachment of antibody fragments (Kang *et al.*, 1991) (Figure 7.3). This allows multivalent interaction of the antibody fragments with their antigen. As will be discussed below it has been suggested that pVIII fusion proteins may be useful for low-affinity antibodies, mimicking to some extent the predominance of IgM in the early phase of the immune response.

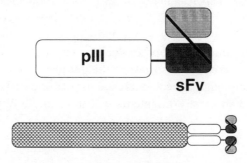

Figure 7.2. Expression of sFv on the surface of phage. Fusion proteins between sFv (see 7.5.2 and Figure 7.6) and the pIII minor coat protein allows expression of the sFv on the surface of the phage, where it is available to bind antigen. Five copies of pIII are expressed on the surface of the phage (in this figure only two are shown). It is possible, therefore, to express up to five sFv on the phage. For technical reasons, however, some vectors often only lead to the expression of one or two sFv on the phage.

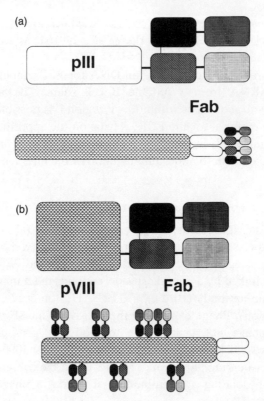

Figure 7.3. Expression of Fab fragments on filamentous phage. Fab fragments of anti-bodies can be expressed on the surface of phage either as fusion proteins with pIII (a) or with the pVIII major coat protein (b). In the latter case multiple copies of the antibody fragment will be expressed along the length of the phage particle, which may be useful in the isolation of low affinity antibodies.

In addition to sFv, Fab fragments of antibodies may also be expressed on phage (Barbas *et al.*, 1991; Garrad *et al.*, 1991; Hoogenboom *et al.*, 1991; Kang *et al.*, 1991) (Figure 7.3). The V_H and C_{H1} domains and the light chains are produced as separate polypeptide chains, with one fused to the pIII or pVIII protein. The two chains associate in the periplasm and are expressed as a functional antigen-binding molecule attached to pIII or pVIII. At this stage it is not clear whether Fab or sFv fragments will have any advantages over each other.

7.4.3   *Selection of novel antibodies from phage expression libraries*

The first attempts to produce novel antibodies from a phage antibody system utilized mice that had been immunized with the antigen phenyloxazolone (Clackson *et al.*, 1991). Spleen cells from these animals were used as a source of immunoglobulin cDNA and the antibody V regions isolated by PCR. The V regions were spliced together with an appropriate oligonucleotide linker into sFv constructs and a library of sFv fusion proteins on pIII was made. Phage-bearing sFv were isolated by several rounds of affinity purification on a phenyloxazolone affinity column and amplification in *E. coli*. Antibodies were selected using this technique that bound the hapten with high affinity, demonstrating for the first time that it is possible to isolate novel antibodies using the phage display technology (Clackson *et al.*, 1991) (Figure 7.4).

Phage display libraries have also been made from humans immunized with tetanus toxoid, hepatitis B surface antigen (Barbas *et al.*, 1991; Zebedee *et al.*, 1992) or infected with HIV (Burton *et al.*, 1991). Panning of the libraries on the appropriate antigens led to isolation of antibodies of the desired specificities.

These examples demonstrate some of the advantages of the phage antibody approach. The ability to screen large numbers of different sFv allows selection of rare antibody specificities. Selection strategies can be tailored to obtain useful antibodies, for example selecting on a different antigen from that used to immunize the animal may allow isolation of cross-reactive antibodies. The use of human as well as murine antibodies has obvious advantages and it should prove possible to isolate antibodies of other species, such as rabbits. It has also been suggested that phage display libraries could be made from memory B cells, helping capture the 'fossil record' of an individual's antibody response against an infectious agent (Lerner *et al.*, 1991).

A potential disavantage of the approach is that the libraries produced by the PCR will contain random combinations of V_H and V_L genes. This means that the chances of isolating a V_H and V_L combination found in nature is low. In addition, pairs of V regions that may be deleted *in vivo*, owing to autoreactivity, can be present in the library. One potential solution to this problem is to do 'in-cell PCR' in permeabilized B cells. Diffusion of the oligonucleotide primers and other PCR reagents into the cell allows amplification of the V region genes, and their assembly, within individual cells – thereby preventing formation of random combinations (Embleton *et al.*, 1992).

7.4.4   *Tapping the primary immune response*

The above results still draw on the secondary immune response, using an immunized donor (either animal or human) as a source of V region sequences. It may be of advantage, where immunization is not practical or desirable, to bypass this step and use the phage display system to tap the primary, naïve, immune response. Peripheral blood B cells from unimmunized humans have been used to produce phage display libraries (Marks *et al.*, 1991a). Rare phage with antigen-binding activities were selected by panning on either bovine serum albumin, turkey egg lysozyme or phenyloxazolone. Two libraries were produced, one derived from μ heavy chain mRNA representing the primary response and the other from γ heavy chain mRNA from antigen selected IgG

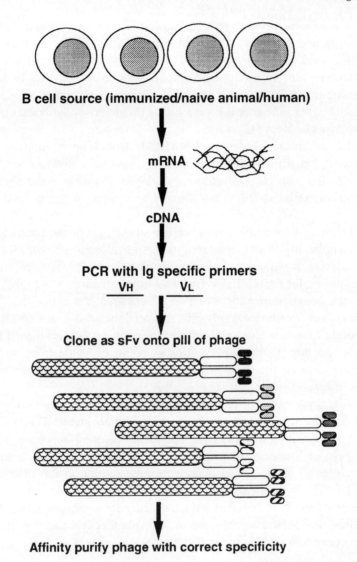

B cell source (immunized/naive animal/human)

mRNA

cDNA

PCR with Ig specific primers
V_H   V_L

Clone as sFv onto pIII of phage

Affinity purify phage with correct specificity

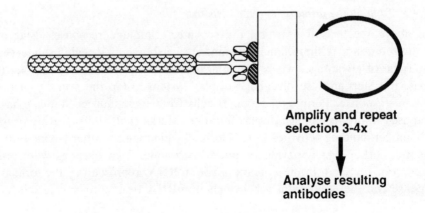

**Amplify and repeat
selection 3-4x**

**Analyse resulting
antibodies**

antibodies. Interestingly, the IgM-derived library produced more antigen-reactive clones, possibly because it contained a higher diversity of V_H genes than the IgG-derived library, which is more representative of the individuals' memory B cells (Marks *et al.*, 1991*a*).

Similar naïve libraries (displayed on pVIII) have been derived from murine B cells and used to obtain antibodies reactive with progesterone (Gram *et al.*, 1992). Together with affinity maturation of the antibodies (discussed below) the availability of these libraries should allow us to circumvent the need for immunization totally. Indeed, the need to use V region sequences derived from animals may be totally obviated: recently two groups have described phage display libraries in which the third hypervariable region of the V_H domain is totally artificial, produced by use of random oligonucleotides (Barbas *et al.*, 1992; Hoogenboom & Winter, 1992). Antibodies could be isolated from these libraries that bind to a variety of haptens with high affinity, demonstrating that it may prove possible to construct totally artificial antibodies using synthetic hypervariable regions.

7.4.5   Affinity maturation of phage antibodies

The antibodies produced in such a system would be expected to be of relatively low affinity as they represent IgM-derived low-affinity antibodies. In the course of a normal immune response somatic mutations increase the affinity of the antibodies, producing the high-affinity IgG antibodies needed for most purposes. The ability to increase the affinity of the recombinant phage antibodies is therefore essential if one is to make useful antibodies by this route. Several strategies have been used to do this, some of which mimic the natural somatic mutation, followed by selection, of B cells. Others are artificial methods not normally seen in the immune response. All the methods use phage display systems to select antibodies which have increased affinity for their antigen (Garrad *et al.*, 1991).

One artificial methods for increasing the affinity of an antibody is by chain shuffling. This relies on the supposition that the particular H and L chain combination that has been selected may not be optimal. If this were the case, one can take the selected antibody, cut out the light or heavy chain V region

Figure 7.4. Scheme of the method for isolating antibodies using phage technology. B cells from a variety of sources can be used as a source of mRNA, as described in the text. The mRNA is reverse transcribed into cDNA and amplified using primers specific for the V_H and V_L genes. The amplified variable regions are then cloned as appropriate antibody constructs fused to the gene encoding for the pIII coat protein. A library is then produced of phage which display the antibody fragment on their surface. This allows affinity purification of the phage with antigen, selecting phage displaying (and containing the appropriate genes for) an antibody of the desired specificity. After several rounds of amplification and repeated selection the resulting antibodies can be further analysed for specificity and other properties.

and clone in random V regions to form a secondary library (Clackson *et al.*, 1991; Kang *et al.*, 1991). This ability to shuffle the V_H and V_L regions is a reflection of the promiscuity of H and L chain pairings and the capability of antibodies with suboptimal pairing to bind antigen. In one example low affinity anti-hapten (phenyloxazol) antibodies derived from a human naïve library had their affinities increased by about 300-fold, to the levels seen in conventional mab derived from immunized mice, by a combination of inserting random V_L chains and also shuffling the first two heavy chain hypervariable regions (Marks *et al.*, 1992), demonstrating the applicability of this approach to the production of high-affinity antibodies typical of the secondary immune response.

Perhaps the most intellectually satisfying approach is to mimic the immune response and introduce random mutations, followed by selection of better binders. Error-prone PCR has been used to introduce such mutations in antibodies (Gram *et al.*, 1992; Hawkins *et al.*, 1992), phage can then be selected which display antibodies with a higher affinity for their antigen. In one elegant study, anti-progesterone Fab fragments were selected from a naïve library using a multivalent pVIII expression system, which should be better at picking up low-affinity antibodies. The selected antibody was then transferred to a pIII expression system for mutation and selection of high-affinity Fab fragments (Gram *et al.*, 1992). While it is not yet clear that the use of the pVIII has any advantages (it should be noted that, depending on the vector used, it is theoretically possible to express up to five antibody fragments on the pIII of one phage), the mimicry of the immune response seen in this example is attractive. In addition to error-prone PCR it is theoretically possible to use 'spiked' PCR (Hermes *et al.*, 1989) or to propagate the antibody constructs in a mutating strain of *E. coli* (Schaaper, 1988).

A final approach to producing high-affinity human antibodies is to allow the affinity maturation to occur *in vivo*. This has been accomplished by reconstituting severe combined immunodeficient (SCID) mice, which lack B and T cells, with human peripheral blood lymphocytes. Immunization of these hu-PBL-SCID animals leads to the production of human antibodies, which can then be 'captured' and immortalized using the phage systems described above (Duchosal *et al.*, 1992). While the return to an animal might be viewed as a retrograde step it is possible that in some circumstances the ability to produce antibodies in an animal environment, with all the accessory cells and immune architecture, may be useful.

7.4.6 *Bacterial display systems*

In addition to the phage display libraries there have been initial reports of an sFv antibody fragment, directed against lysozyme, expressed as fusion proteins with peptidoglycan-associated lipoprotein, a surface protein on *E. coli* (Fuchs *et al.*, 1991). Functional lysozyme-binding antibody could be detected on the surface of intact bacteria. It may, therefore, be possible to use such a system as a bacterial expression system and select bacteria that bind antigen. While such an approach is likely to be technically more difficult, it is possible that it will be useful for selection of some antibodies that cannot be isolated on phage display libraries.

7.4.7 Phage antibodies: summary

The use of phage antibodies offers an attractive alternative to hybridoma technology. It provides a method for making antibodies from human and other non-murine species. In addition, the ability to rapidly select antigen-binding phage from many irrelevant phage (up to 10^9 different phages can be panned in one experiment, with multiple rounds of selection and amplification taking a week or two to perform) contrasts with the screening of hybridomas where testing more than 10^4 clones becomes laborious and the whole process of producing a characterized mab may take several months. It must be admitted that the phage technology is far from routine at present and many of the parameters have yet to be worked out. It should be remembered that it took several years for hybridoma technology to become widely used, as the expertise and techniques developed, so we should not be surprised if the phage approach has a similar lag period.

At present we can see that it may be possible to recapitulate the entire humoral immune response using the phage system, with the selection of low-affinity antibodies from libraries of V_H and V_L domains from naïve animals, followed by further rounds of mutation and selection to obtain higher

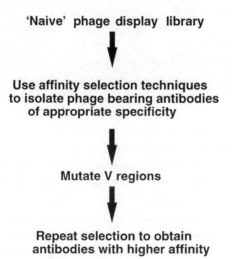

'Naive' phage display library

**Use affinity selection techniques
to isolate phage bearing antibodies
of appropriate specificity**

Mutate V regions

**Repeat selection to obtain
antibodies with higher affinity**

Figure 7.5. Recapitulation of the immune response *in vitro*. It is possible to mimic several aspects of the natural antibody response *in vitro*, selecting low-affinity antibodies from a naïve library (in a similar manner to the antigen-driven selection of antibodies in the primary immune response), and then mutating the variable regions and selecting antibodies of higher affinity (thereby mimicking the somatic mutation found in the secondary immune response).

affinity antibodies (Figure 7.5). In the future we may also make totally artificial antibodies, by introducing random sequences into the hypervariable regions, thereby bypassing any bias introduced by the evolutionary selection of V region genes.

7.5   Recombinant antibody fragments

7.5.1   *Production of recombinant antibody fragments*

Once an antibody fragment has been produced using the phage technology, or has engineered an antibody to have a desired characteristic, there are a number of ways of producing soluble molecules. The appropriate method depends on the nature of the recombinant species produced, including the need for glycosylation or other post-translational processing, and the desired yields. Recombinant antibodies and their derivatives have been produced in myeloma cells (Shin & Morrison, 1989), in non-lymphoid mammalian cell lines (de Waele *et al.*, 1988), in baculovirus systems (Hasesmann & Capra, 1990), in yeast (Horwitz *et al.*, 1988), in plants (Hiatt *et al.*, 1989), in bacteria (Huston *et al.*, 1988; Plückthun, 1991*a,b*) and also totally *in vitro* using rabbit reticulocyte lysates (Nicholls *et al.*, 1993).

The most common method of producing sFv antibodies is probably in bacterial expression systems. These have the advantages that they are relatively cheap, quick and allow facile genetic manipulation of the construct. There are two major categories of expression systems: those that produce the recombinant protein without a leader peptide, leading to accumulation of the antibody within the cell (Huston *et al.*, 1988, 1991), normally in insoluble inclusion bodies, and those that use a leader peptide to cause the protein to be secreted into the periplasmic space of the bacteria (Better *et al.*, 1988; Skerra & Plückthun, 1988). In the former method the molecules need to be refolded, which can be a laborious process; however, the yields of protein can be very high (Huston *et al.*, 1991). In the periplasmic expression system the proteins are produced in an oxidising environment, in the presence of a number of molecules that aid refolding of newly-produced polypeptide chains, and so they can be produced in a refolded state. In some cases the antibodies are found in a soluble form in the bacterial growth medium, presumably because of leakage through the outer membrane of dead or dying bacteria (Ward *et al.*, 1989). It is frequently necessary, however, especially if high yields are needed, to solubilize the protein from insoluble aggregates that form in the periplasm (Johnson & Bird, 1991; Plückthun, 1991*b*; Whitlow & Filpula, 1991). This is a simpler task than refolding from inclusion bodies.

The yields from bacterial systems can be high; in one report, in which the conditions were carefully optimized, a F(ab')$_2$ antibody was produced at several grammes/litre of bacterial culture (Carter *et al.*, 1992). This, combined with the rapid growth of bacteria, makes the bacterial systems very attractive. In some circumstances, however, the other methods of production mentioned above will be better.

7.5.2   *Nature of antibody fragments produced from phage libraries*

All the antibody fragments so far produced using phage expression systems have been either Fab or sFv molecules. The Fab fragment of IgG consists of four of the immunoglobulin domains, the V_H and C_{H1} from the heavy chain and the V_L and C_L of the light chain, linked by a disulphide bond between the two constant domains. The resulting molecule has a molecular weight of approximately 50 000. The sFv fragment of an antibody contains just the Fv portion of the molecule (the two V region domains) stabilized by a linker peptide that joins the N-terminus of one chain with the C-terminus of the other (Figure 7.6). The sFv has a molecular weight of 25 000–30 000. Both Fab and sFv contain the variable domains that determine the antigen-binding properties of the antibody, without the effector functions associated with the constant region of the molecule (while some effector functions are associated with the C_{H1} and C_L domains of the Fab fragment, most of them are associated with the Fc portion of the molecule).

In some situations the unmodified molecule may be useful. One example of this is in tumour imaging in which radiolabelled antibodies are used to detect tumour *in vivo* (discussed in Chapter 10B). In these circumstances the small size of the antibody fragments (in particular the sFv) leads to better penetration of solid tumours and rapid clearance of unbound antibody from the circulation, allowing the tumours to be visualized more quickly (Colcher *et al.*, 1990; Milenic *et al.*, 1991; Yokota *et al.*, 1992). The removal of the highly immunogenic Fc portion of the antibody should also reduce the induction of human anti–mouse antibodies (HAMA) that prevents repeated imaging with murine antibodies. In animal studies, sFv have been shown to be effective at imaging more rapidly than conventional antibody fragments (including Fab) (Colcher *et al.*, 1990; Milenic *et al.*, 1991; Yokota *et al.*, 1992).

A second situation in which the effector functions of antibodies are not required is in catalytic antibodies, in which the antigen-binding site can catalyse chemical reactions. Such catalytic antibodies have been produced as recombinant sFv and Fab molecules (Gibbs *et al.*, 1991) and phage display libraries may be useful in isolating novel catalytic antibodies (Barbas *et al.*, 1992).

Finally, recombinant antibodies which lack Fc regions can still be effective at blocking the interaction of ligands with their receptors. For example recombinant Fab and sFv molecules have been used to block infection of cultured cells with human rhinovirus (Condra *et al.*, 1990) and the improved pharmacokinetics and low immunogenicity of these molecules may be important in a number of similar applications.

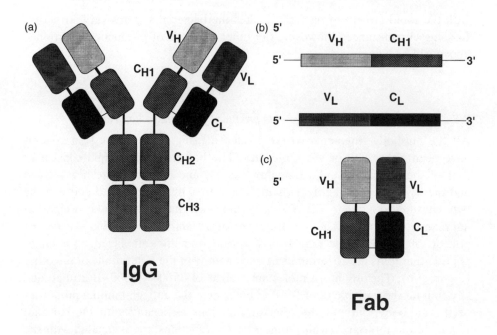

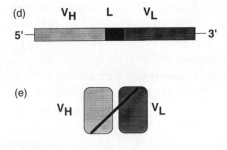

Figure 7.6. Comparative structure of IgG, Fab and sFv molecules. The structure of the IgG molecule is shown in (a) with the domains indicated by blocks. The disulphide bonds between the various chains are represented by thin lines and the various types of domain by different shading of the blocks. The continuous polypeptide chain that links the domains and forms the hinge region is shown by the heavier lines. Fab fragments of IgG, which consist of the variable domains and their two proximal constant domains linked by a disulphide bridge (c), can be produced by recombinant methods, the two chains of the molecule are encoded on separate gene constructs (b) and the separate chains must recombine to form the complete Fab molecule. The sFv molecule, on the other hand, is produced by a single gene construct (d), which codes for the two variable domains and their joining linker peptide (e), with the entire molecule being formed from a single polypeptide chain.

7.5.3   Engineering of effector functions

As mentioned above, the sFv and Fab fragments have no effector functions on their own. Whereas antigen binding properties alone may be useful for such tasks as *in-vivo* imaging and blocking of binding of various molecules, for most purposes it will be necessary to alter the antibody obtained by the phage approach. In this section I will discuss a few of the possible molecules that have been, or might be, made.

7.5.3.1 Immunoglobulin-like molecules

One obvious way to give sFv or Fab molecules effector functions is to incorporate them into a recombinant immunoglobulin-like molecule. It is possible when doing this to specify the species and class or subclass of the immunoglobulin molecule, thereby influencing such factors as the immunogenicity, half-life and effector functions. If a human antibody is desired, and the sFv or Fab are derived from a murine source, then one could make either a chimeric antibody, where the entire molecule except for the V regions is of human origin (Shin & Morrison, 1989) or a humanized antibody where the hypervariable regions are from the mouse and the framework part of the V domains is human (Reichmann *et al.*, 1988). These approaches are described in Chapter 8.

7.5.3.2 Fusion proteins

The production of antibody fragments as fusion proteins with other molecules is a popular method of conferring new functions on the antibodies (Neuberger *et al.*, 1984). The sFv molecule has particular advantages in making such fusion proteins as it is encoded on a single strand of DNA which can be easily spliced with a gene encoding for a second protein (Figure 7.7).

The second protein can be linked to either the N- or C-terminus of the sFv molecule and the use of a peptide between the two proteins can help space them, preventing them from sterically blocking each other's function (Batra *et al.*, 1991; Tai *et al.*, 1990).

Fusion proteins have been made between sFv and a range of other proteins, including protein A (Tai *et al.*, 1990), enzymes (Holvoet *et al.*, 1991; Wels *et al.*, 1992), cytokines (Savage *et al.*, 1993), CD4 (Traunecker *et al.*, 1991) and toxins (Chaudhary *et al.*, 1989; Nicholls *et al.*, 1993; Pastan *et al.*, 1992). This allows the function of the partner protein to be targeted to cells or antigens by the sFv. Thus, fusion proteins formed between sFv and toxins are highly specific cytotoxic agents, killing cells bearing the appropriate antigen but not antigen-negative cells (Chaudhary *et al.*, 1989; Nicholls *et al.*, 1993; Pastan *et al.*, 1992). Other bifunctional molecules may be useful at targeting cytotoxic effector cells; anti-tumour sFv linked to interleukin-2 may be useful in recruiting T lymphocytes to kill the neoplastic cells (Savage *et al.*, 1993) and hybrid

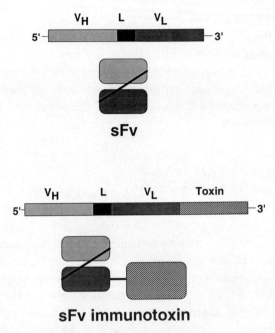

Figure 7.7. sFv fusion proteins. Fusion of a gene encoding a protein, such as a toxin, to either the 5' or 3' end of an sFv gene construct leads to the production of a hybrid protein (in this case an immunotoxin) which combines the antigen-binding (or targeting) functions of the sFv and the properties of the second molecule.

molecules (termed Janusins) containing both an anti-CD3 sFv and CD4 have been generated that allow targeting of T cells (via anti-CD3 sFv) to gp120-expressing HIV-infected cells (via CD4) (Traunecker *et al.*, 1991). Antibody–enzyme molecules may prove useful immunocytochemical reagents (Wels *et al.*, 1992) and may also find a use in prodrug therapy, in which an enzyme targeted to the tumour site converts a harmless prodrug into a cytotoxic agent (Bagshawe, 1989). Such conjugates may also prove useful in other situations where the localization of an enzymatic activity is needed, such as the targeting of urokinase to blood clots (Holvoet *et al.*, 1991).

The use of sFv fusion proteins has a number of advantages over conventional immunoconjugates produced by chemical means. They are capable of being produced in large amounts using suitable expression systems, as described above. There is no requirement for chemical modifications that can be deleterious to the molecules. It is also possible to alter the fusion protein to decrease unwanted properties (for example removing cell binding properties of a toxin (Nicholls *et al.*, 1993)). In addition, fusion proteins will be smaller than most conventional immunoconjugates, thereby improving pharmacokinetic properties.

7.5.4   Bivalent antibody fragments

The sFv and Fab fragments isolated by the phage methodology are univalent, having only one binding site. For many circumstances it would be desirable to produce bivalent antibodies as the gain in avidity from having two antigen-binding sites can raise the functional affinity of an antibody (Chapter 3). This may be especially important if one wants the antibody to bind a cell surface in the face of soluble blocking antigen. The ability of bivalent antibodies to promote modulation and endocytosis of cell surface antigens may also help in the internalization of some molecules, for example toxins. In addition, if the two antigen-binding arms have different specificities, it is possible to form bispecific antibodies that can be used to target either cytotoxic cells or toxins and other noxious molecules to kill unwanted neoplastic or virally infected cells (Segal *et al.*, 1992, 1993).

Two major methods have been described for the production of bivalent Fab or sFv molecules. One is simply to incorporate a cysteine in the molecule, allowing the disulphide bond to form between the two molecules. While the disulphide bond can form in the bacterial periplasm, for the most efficient production it is necessary to mildly reduce the fragments and allow the mixture to oxidize *in vitro* (Carter *et al.*, 1992; Shalaby *et al.*, 1992). Alternatively, one can use the cysteines to link the two molecules with stable thioether bonds, using a *bis* maleimide reagent (Cumber *et al.*, 1992).

An elegant method has recently been described that relies on the formation of dimers between amphiphilic helices (Kostelny *et al.*, 1992; Pack & Plück-thun, 1992). A number of such helices, including those derived from leucine zippers, can be fused to sFv or Fab molecules, allowing formation of strong inter-molecular associations, which can be further stabilized by incorporation of cysteine residues. The resulting molecules have the avidity and properties expected of $F(ab')_2$ fragments, although, in the case of 'miniantibodies' formed from sFv molecules they can be approximately half the size (Pack & Plückthun, 1992). The use of leucine zippers which prefer heterologous association (such as the jun/fos combination) can be used to promote the formation of bispecific antibodies (Kostelny *et al.*, 1992) (Figure 7.8).

7.6   Conclusion

We are now in a very exciting phase of antibody engineering, which may have as big an impact on immunological research as the advent of monoclonal antibodies less than two decades ago. The potential for producing antibodies *de novo*, using the phage display systems or similar techniques, may yield a new generation of antibodies with improved specificities and properties. In addition, the ability to engineer novel effector functions means that we are no longer constrained by what is provided by nature for us but rather by our imaginations.

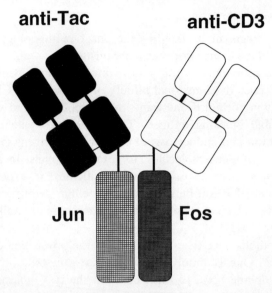

anti-Tac   anti-CD3

Jun   Fos

Figure 7.8. Production of a bispecific antibody using leucine zippers. Both sFv and Fab fragments can be joined to form bivalent molecules using amphiphilic helices, as discussed in the text. In the example shown here, taken from Kostelny *et al.* (1992), Fab′ fragments of anti-CD3 and anti-Tac antibodies are linked to fos and jun, two transcription control proteins which form a tight leucine zipper, bringing the two Fab′ fragments together to form a bispecific antibody. The molecule is further stabilized by hinge region disulphide bonds. The preference of jun and fos for heterologous pairing, rather than homologous pairing, ensures that the majority of the bivalent molecules produced are bispecific.

7.7   References

Bagshawe, K. D. (1989). Towards generating cytotoxic agents at cancer sites. *British Journal of Cancer*, **60**, 275–281.

Barbas, C. F., III, Bain, J. D., Hoekstra, D. M. & Lerner, R. A. (1992). Semisynthetic combinatorial antibody libraries: a chemical solution to the diversity problem. *Proceedings of the National Academy of Sciences U.S.A.*, **89**, 4457–4461.

Barbas, C. F., III, Kang, A. S., Lerner, R. A. & Benkovic, S. J. (1991). Assembly of combinatorial antibody libraries on phage surfaces: the gene III site. *Proceedings of the National Academy of Science U.S.A.*, **88**, 7978–7982.

Bardwell, J. C. A., McGovern, K. & Beckwith, J. (1991). Identification of a protein required for disulfide bond formation *in vivo*. *Cell*, **67**, 581–589.

Batra, J. K., FitzGerald, D. J., Chaudhary, V. K. & Pastan, I. (1991). Single-chain immunotoxins directed at the human transferrin receptor-containing *Pseudomonas* exotoxin A or diptheria toxin: anti-TFR(Fv)-PE40 and DT388-anti-TFR(Fv). *Molecular and Cellular Biology*, **11**, 2200–2205.

Better, M., Chang, C. P., Robinson, R. R. & Horwitz, A. H. (1988). *Escherichia coli* secretion of an active chimeric antibody fragment. *Science*, **240**, 1041–1043.

Bird, R. E., Hardman, K. D., Jacobson, J. W., Johnson, S., Kaufman, B. M., Lee, S.-M., Lee, T., Pope, S. H., Riordan, G. & Whitlow, M. (1988). Single-chain antigen-binding proteins. *Science*, **242**, 423–426.

Burton, D. R., Barbas, C. F., III, Persson, M. A. A., Koenig, S., Chanock, R. M. &

Lerner, R. A. (1991). A large array of human monoclonal antibodies to type 1 human immunodeficiency virus from combinatorial libraries of asymptomatic seropositive individuals. *Proceedings of the National Academy of Sciences U.S.A.*, **88**, 10134–10137.

Carter, P., Kelly, R. F., Rodrigues, M. L., Snedecor, B., Covarrubias, M., Velligan, M. D., Wong, W. L. T., Rowland, A. M., Kotts, C. E., Carver, M. E., Yang, M., Bourell, J. H., Shepard, H. M. & Henner, D. (1992). High level *Escherichia coli* expression and production of a bivalent humanized antibody fragment. *Bio/ Technology*, **10**, 163–167.

Chaudhary, V. K., Queen, C., Junghans, R. P., Waldmann, T. A., FitzGerald, D. J. & Pastan, I. (1989). A recombinant immunotoxin consisting of two antibody variable domains fused to *Pseudomonas exotoxin*. *Nature (London)*, **339**, 394–397.

Clackson, T., Hoogenboom, H. R., Griffiths, A. D. & Winter, G. (1991). Making antibody fragments using phage display libraries. *Nature (London)*, **352**, 624–628.

Colcher, D., Bird, R. Roselli, M., Hardman, K. D., Johnson, S., Pope, S., Dodd, S. W., Pantoliano, M. W., Milenic, D. E. & Schlom, J. (1990). *In vivo* tumor targeting of a recombinant single-chain antigen-binding protein. *Journal of the National Cancer Institute*, **82**, 1191–1197.

Condra, J. H., Sardana, V. V., Tomassini, J. E., Schlabach, A. J., Davies, M.-E., Lineberger, D. W., Graham, D. J., Gotlib, L. & Colonno, R. J. (1990). Bacterial expression of antibody fragments that block human rhinovirus infection of cultured cells. *Journal of Biological Chemistry*, **265**, 2292–2295.

Cumber, A. J., Ward, E. S., Winter, G., Parnell, G. D. & Wawrzynczak, E. J. (1992). Comparative stabilities *in vitro* and *in vivo* of a recombinant mouse antibody FvCys fragment and a bisFvCys conjugate. *Journal of Immunology*, **149**, 120–126.

Cwirla, S. E., Peters, E. A., Barrett, R. W. & Dower, W. J. (1990). Peptides on phage: a vast library of peptides for identifying ligands. *Proceedings of the National Academy of Sciences U.S.A.*, **87**, 6378–6382.

De Waele, P., Feys, V., van de Voorde, A., Molemans, F. & Fiers, W. (1988). Expression in non-lymphoid cells of mouse recombinant immunoglobulin directed against the tumour marker human placental alkaline phosphatase. *European Journal of Biochemistry*, **176**, 287–295.

Devlin, J. J., Panganiban, L. C. & Devlin, P. E. (1990). Random peptide libraries: a source of specific protein binding molecules. *Science*, **249**, 404–406.

Dübel, S., Breitling, F., Seehaus, T. & Little, M. (1992). Generation of a human IgM expression library in *E. coli*. *Methods in Molecular and Cellular Biology*, **3**, 47–52.

Duchosal, M. A., Eming, S. A., Fischer, P., Leturcq, D., Barbas, C. F., III, McConahey, P. J., Caothien, R. H., Thornton, G. B. Dixon, F. J. & Burton, D. R. (1992). Immunization of hu-PBL-SCID mice and the rescue of human monoclonal fab fragments through combinatorial libraries. *Nature (London)*, **355**, 258–261.

Embleton, M. J., Gorochov, G., Jones, P. T. & Winter, G. (1992). In-cell PCR from mRNA: amplifying and linking the rearranged immunoglobulin heavy and light chain V-genes within single cells. *Nucleic Acids Research*, **15**, 3831–3837.

Felici, F., Castagnoli, L., Musacchio, A., Jappelli, R. & Cesareni, G. (1991). Selection of antibody ligands from a large library of oligopeptides expressed on a multivalent exposition vector. *Journal of Molecular Biology*, **222**, 301–310.

Fuchs, P., Breitling, F., Dübel, S., Seehaus, T. & Little, M. (1991). Targeting recombinant antibodies to the surface of *Escherichia coli*: fusion to a peptidoglycan associated lipoprotein. *Bio/Technology*, **9**, 1369–1372.

Garrad, L. S., Yang, M., O'Connell, M. P., Kelley, R. F. & Henner, D. J. (1991). F$_{AB}$ assembly and enrichment in a monovalent phage display system. *Bio/Technology*, **9**, 1373–1377.

Gibbs, R. A., Posner, B. A., Filpula, D. R., Dodd, S. W., Finkelman, M. A. J., Lee, T. K., Wroble, M., Whitlow, M. & Benkovic, S. J. (1991). Construction and characterization of a single-chain catalytic antibody. *Proceedings of the National Academy of Sciences U.S.A.*, **88**, 4001–4004.

Gram, H., Marconi, L.-A. & Barbas, C. F., III (1992). *In vitro* selection and affinity maturation of antibodies from a naive combinatorial immunoglobulin library. *Proceedings of the National Academy of Sciences U.S.A.*, **89**, 3576–3580.

Gray, C. W., Brown, R. S. & Marvin, D. A. (1981). Adsorption comples of filamentous fd virus. *Journal of Molecular Biology*, **146**, 621–627.

Greenwood, J., Willis, A. E. & R. N. Perham (1991). Multiple display of foreign peptides on a filamentous bacteriophage. Peptides from *Plasmodium falciparum* circumsporozoite protein as antigens. *Journal of Molecular Biology*, **220**, 821–827.

Hammer, J., Takacs, B. & Sinigaglia, F. (1992). Identification of a motif for HLA-DR1 binding peptides using M13 display libraries. *Journal of Experimental Medicine*, **176**, 1007–1013.

Hasesmann, C. A. & Capra, J. D. (1990). High-level production of a functional immunoglobulin heterodimer in a baculovirus expression system. *Proceedings of the National Academy of Sciences U.S.A.*, **87**, 3942–3946.

Hawkins, R. E., Russell, S. J. & Winter, G. (1992). Selection of phage antibodies by binding affinity. Mimicking affinity maturation. *Journal of Molecular Biology*, **226**, 889–896.

Hermes, J. D., Parekh, S. M., Blacklow, S. C., Koster, H. & Knowles, J. R. (1989). A reliable method for random mutatagenesis: the generation of mutant libraries using spiked oligodeoxyribonucleotide primers. *Gene*, **84**, 143–151.

Hiatt, A., Cafferkey, R. & Bowdish, K. (1989). Production of antibodies in transgenic plants. *Nature (London)*, **342**, 76–78.

Holvoet, P., Laroche, Y., Lijnen, H. R., Cauwenbere, R. V., Demarsin, E., Brouwers, E., Matthyssens, G. & Collen, D. (1991). Characterization of a chimeric plasminogen activator consisting of a single-chain Fv fragment derived from a fibrin fragment D-dimer-specific antibody and a truncated single-chain urokinase. *Journal of Biological Chemistry*, **266**, 19717–19724.

Hoogenboom, H. R., Griffiths, A. D., Johnson, K. S., Chiswell, D. J., Hudson, P. & Winter, G. (1991). Multi-subunit proteins on the surface of filamentous phage: methodologies for displaying antibody (Fab) heavy and light chains. *Nucleic Acids Research*, **19**, 4133–4137.

Hoogenboom, H. R. & Winter, G. (1992). By-passing immunisation. Human antibodies from synthetic repertoires of germline V_H gene segments rearranged *in vitro*. *Journal of Molecular Biology*, **227**, 381–388.

Horwitz, A. H., Chang, C. P., Better, M., Hellstrom, K. E. & Robinson, R. R. (1988). Secretion of functional antibody and Fab fragment from yeast cells. *Proceedings of the National Academy of Sciences U.S.A.*, **85**, 8678–8682.

Huse, W. D., Sastry, L., Iverson, S. A., Kang, A. S., Alting-Mees, M., Burton, D. R., Benkovic, S. J. & Lerner, R. A. (1989). Generation of a large combinatorial library of the immunoglobulin repertoire in phage lambda. *Science*, **246**, 1275–1281.

Huston, J. S., Levinson, D., Mudgett-Hunter, M., Tai, M.-S., Novotny, J., Margolies, M. J., Ridge, R. J., Bruccoleri, R. E., Haber, E., Crea, R. & Oppermann, H. (1988). Protein engineering of antibody binding sites: recovery of specific activity in an anti-digoxin single-chain Fv analogue produced in *Escherichia coli*. *Proceedings of the National Academy of Sciences U.S.A.*, **85**, 5879–5883.

Huston, J. S., Mudgett-Hunter, M., Tai, M.-S., McCartney, J., F. Warren, Haber, E. & Oppermann, H. (1991). Protein engineering of single-chain Fv analogs and fusion proteins. *Methods in Enzymology*, **203**, 46–88.

Ilyichev, A. A., Minenkova, O. O., Kishchenko, G. P., Tat'kov, S. I., Karpishev, N. N., Eroshkin, A. M., Ofitzerov, V. I., Akimenko, Z. A., Petrenko, V. A. & Sandakhchiev, L. S. (1992). Inserting foreign peptides into the major coat protein of bacteriophage M13. *FEBS Letters*, **301**, 322–324.

Johnson, S. & Bird, R. E. (1991). Construction of single-chain Fv derivatives of monoclonal antibodies and their production in *Escherichia coli*. *Methods in Enzymology*, **203**, 88–98.

Kang, A. S., Barbas, C. F., Janda, K. D., Benkovic, S. J. & Lerner, R. A. (1991). Linkage of recognition and replication functions by assembling combinatorial antibody Fab libraries along phage surfaces. *Proceedings of the National Academy of Sciences U.S.A.*, **88**, 4363–4366.

Kang, A. S., Jones, T. M. & Burton, D. R. (1991). Antibody redesign by chain shuffling from random combinatorial immunoglobulin libraries. *Proceedings of the National Academy of Sciences U.S.A.*, **88**, 11120–11123.

Köhler, G. & Milstein, C. (1975). Continuous cultures of fused cells secreting antibody of predefined specificity. *Nature (London)*, **256**, 495–497.

Kostelny, S. A., Cole, M. S. & Tso, J. Y. (1992). Formation of a bispecific antibody by the use of leucine zippers. *Journal of Immunology*, **148**, 1547–1553.

Landry, S. J. & Gierasch, L. M. (1991). Recognition of nascent polypeptides for targeting and folding. *Trends in Biochemical Sciences*, **16**, 159–163.

Larrick, J. W. & Fry, K. E. (1991). PCR amplification of antibody genes. *Methods: A Companion to Methods in Enzymology*, **2**, 106–110.

Lerner, R. A., Barbas, C. F., III, Kang, A. S. & Burton, D. R. (1991). On the use of combinatorial antibody libraries to clone the 'fossil record' of an individual's immune response. *Proceedings of the National Academy of Sciences U.S.A.*, **88**, 9705–9706.

Lowman, H. B., Bass, S. H., Simpson, N. & Wells, J. A. (1991). Selecting high-affinity binding proteins by monovalent phage display. *Biochemistry*, **30**, 10832–10838.

McCafferty, J., Griffiths, A. D., Winter, G. & Chiswell, D. J. (1990). Phage antibodies: filamentous phage displaying antibody variable domains. *Nature (London)*, **348**, 552–554.

Markland, W., Roberts, B. L., Saxena, M. J., Guterman, S. K. & Ladner, R. C. (1991). Design, construction and functional of a multicopy display vector using fusions to the major coat protein of bacteriophage M13. *Gene*, **109**, 13–19.

Marks, J. D., Griffiths, A. D., Malmqvist, M., Clackson, T. P., Bye, J. M. & Winter, G. (1992). By-passing immunization: building high-affinity human antibodies by chain shuffling. *Bio/Technology*, **10**, 779–783.

Marks, J. D., Hoogenboom, H. R., Bonnert, T. P., McCafferty, J., Griffiths, A. D. & Winter, G. (1991a). By-passing immunization. Human antibodies from V-gene libraries displayed in phage. *Journal of Molecular Biology*, **222**, 581–597.

Marks, J. D., Tristem, M., Karpas, A. & Winter, G. (1991b). Oligonucleotide primers for polymerase chain reaction amplification of human immunoglobulin variable genes and design of family-specific oligonucleotide probes. *European Journal of Immunology*, **21**, 985–991.

Milenic, D. E., Yokota, T., Filpula, D. R., Finkelman, M. A. J., Dodd, S. W., Wood, J. F., Whitlow, M., Snoy, P. & Schlom, J. (1991). Construction, binding properties, metabolism and tumor targeting of a single-chain Fv derived from the pancarcinoma monoclonal antibody CC49. *Cancer Research*, **51**, 6363–6371.

Model, P. & Russel, M. (1988). Filamentous bacteriophage. In *The Bacteriophages*, vol. 2, ed. R. Calendar, pp. 375–456. New York, Plenum Press.

Neuberger, M. S., Williams, G. T. & Fox, R. O. (1984). Recombinant antibodies possessing novel effector functions. *Nature (London)*, **312**, 604–608.

Nicholls, P. J., Johnson, V. G., Andrew, S. M., Hoogenboom, H. R., Raus, J. C. M. & Youle, R. J. (1993). Characterization of single-chain antibody (sFv)-toxin fusion proteins produced *in vitro* in rabbit reticulocyte lysate. *Journal of Biological Chemistry*, **268**, 5302–5308.

Oldenburg, K. R., Longanathan, D., Goldstein, I. J., Scholtz, P. G. & Gallop, M. A. (1992). Peptide ligands for a sugar-binding protein isolated from a random peptide library. *Proceedings of the National Academy of Sciences U.S.A.*, **89**, 5395–5397.

Orlandi, R., Güssow, D. H., Jones, P. T. & Winter, G. (1989). Cloning immuno-globulin variable domains for expression by the polymerase chain reaction. *Proceedings of the National Academy of Sciences U.S.A.*, **86**, 3833–3837.

Pack, P. & Plückthun, A. (1992). Miniantibodies: use of amphipathic helices to produce functional, flexibly linked dimeric F_V fragments with high avidity in *Escherichia coli*. *Biochemistry*, **31**, 1579–1584.

Pastan, I., Chaudhary, V. & FitzGerald, D. J. (1992). Recombinant toxins as novel therapeutic agents. *Annual Review of Biochemistry*, **61**, 331–354.

Plückthun, A. (1991*a*). Antibody engineering. *Current Opinion in Biotechnology*, **2**, 238–246.

Plückthun, A. (1991*b*). Strategies for the expression of antibody fragments in *Escherichia coli*. *Methods: A Companion to Methods in Enzymology*, **2**, 88–96.

Reichmann, L., Clark, M., Waldman, H. & Winter, G. (1988). Reshaping human antibodies for therapy. *Nature (London)*, **322**, 323–327.

Saiki, R. K., Scharf, S., Faloona, F., Mullis, K. B., Horn, G. T., Erlich, H. A. & Arnheim, N. (1985). Enzymatic amplification of β-globin genomic sequences and restriction site analysis for diagnosis of sickle cell anemia. *Science*, **230**, 1350–1354.

Sambrook, J., Fritsch, E. F. & Maniatis, T. (1989). *Molecular Cloning: a Laboratory Manual*. New York, Cold Spring Harbor Laboratory Press.

Sastry, L., Alting-Mees, M., Huse, W. D., Short, J. M., Sorge, J. A., Hay, B. N., Janda, K. D., Benkovic, S. J. & Lerner, R. A. (1989). Cloning of the immunoglobulin repertoire in *Escherichia coli* for generation of monoclonal catalytic antibodies: construction of a heavy chain variable region-specific cDNA library. *Proceedings of the National Academy of Sciences U.S.A.*, **86**, 5728–5732.

Savage, P., So, A., Spooner, R. A. & Epenetos, A. A. (1993). A recombinant single chain antibody interleukin-2 fusion protein. *British Journal of Cancer*, **67**, 304–310.

Schaaper, R. M. (1988). Mechanisms of mutagenesis in the *Escherichia coli* mutator mutD5: role of DNA mismatch repair. *Proceedings of the National Academy of Sciences U.S.A.*, **85**, 8126–8130.

Scott, J. K. (1992). Discovering peptide ligands using epitope libraries. *Trends in Biological Sciences*, **17**, 241–245.

Scott, J. K., Loganathan, D., Easley, R. B., Gong, X. & Goldstein, I. J. (1992). A family of concanavalin A-binding peptides from a hexapeptide epitope library. *Proceedings of the National Academy of Sciences U.S.A.*, **89**, 5398–5402.

Scott, J. K. & Smith, G. P. (1990). Searching for peptide ligands with an epitope library. *Science*, **249**, 386–390.

Segal, D. M., Jost, C. R. & George, A. J. T. (1993). Targeted cellular cytotoxicity. In *Cytotoxic Cells: Generation, Recognition, Effector Functions, Methods*, ed. M. V. Sitkovsky & P. A. Henkart. Boston, Birhäuser, 96–110

Segal, D. M., Urch, C. E., George, A. J. T. & Jost, C. R. (1992). Bispecific antibodies in cancer treatment. In *Biologic Therapy of Cancer Updates*, vol. 2, ed. V. T. deVita Jr., S. Hellman & S. A. Rosenberg, pp. 1–12. Philadelphia, Lippincott.

Shalaby, M. R., Shephard, M. H., Presta, L., Rodrigues, M. L., Beverly, P. C. L., Feldmann, M. & Carter, P. (1992). Development of humanized bispecific antibodies reactive with cytotoxic lymphocytes and tumor cells overexpressing the HER2 protooncogene. *Journal of Experimental Medicine*, **175**, 217–225.

Shin, S.-U. & Morrison, S. L. (1989). Production and properties of chimeric antibody molecules. *Methods in Enzymology*, **178**, 459–476.

Skerra, A. & Plückthun, A. (1988). Assembly of a functional immunoglobulin Fv fragment in *Escherichia coli*. *Science*, **240**, 1038–1041.

Smith, G. P. (1985). Filamentous fusion phage: novel expression vectors that display cloned antigens on the virion surface. *Science*, **228**, 1315–1317.

Stephen, C. W. & Lane, D. P. (1992). Mutant conformation of p53. Precise epitope mapping using a filamentous phage epitope library. *Journal of Molecular Biology*, **225**, 577–583.

Tai, M.-S., Mudgett-Hunter, M., Levinson, D., Wu, G.-M., Haber, E., Oppermann, H. & Huston, J. S. (1990). A bifunctional fusion protein containing Fc-binding fragment B of staphylococcal protein A amino terminal to antidigoxin single-chain Fv. *Biochemistry*, **29**, 8024–8030.

Traunecker, A., Lanzavecchia, A. & Karjalainen, K. (1991). Bispecific single chain molecules (Janusins) target cytotoxic lymphocytes on HIV infected cells. *EMBO Journal*, **10**, 3655–3659.

Tsunetsgu-Yokota, Y., Tatsumi, M., Robert, V., Devaux, C., Spire, B., Chermann, J. C. & Hirsch, I. (1991). Expression of an immunogenic region of HIV by a filamentous bacteriophage vector. *Gene*, **99**, 261–265.

Ward, E. S., Güssow, D., Griffiths, A. D., Jones, P. T. & Winter, G. (1989). Binding activity of a repertoire of single immunoglobulin variable domains secreted from *Escherichia coli*. *Nature (London)*, **341**, 544–546.

Wels, W., Harwerth, I.-M., Zwickl, M., Hardman, N., Groner, B. & Hynes, N. E. (1992). Construction, bacterial expression and characterization of a bifunctional single-chain antibody-phosphatase fusion protein targeted to the human erbB-2 receptor. *Bio/Technology*, **10**, 1128–1132.

Whitlow, M. & Filpula, D. (1991). Single-chain Fv proteins and their fusion proteins. *Methods: A Companion to Methods in Enzymology*, **2**, 97–105.

Yokota, T., Milenic, D. E., Whitlow, M. & Schlom, J. (1992). Rapid tumor penetration of a single-chain Fv and comparison with other immunoglobulin forms. *Cancer Research*, **52**, 3402–3408.

Zebedee, S. L., Barbas, C. F., III, Hom, Y.-L., Caothien, R. H., Graff, R., DeGraw, J., Pyati, J., LaPolla, R., Burton, D. R., Lerner, R. A. & Thornton, G. B. (1992). Human combinatorial antibody libraries to hepatitis B surface antigen. *Proceedings of the National Academy of Sciences*, *U.S.A.*, **89**, 3175–3179.

8

Genetic manipulation of monoclonal antibodies

N. S. COURTENAY-LUCK

8.1 Introduction

Although monoclonal antibodies (mab) have found widespread application in science and diagnostic medicine, such as *in-vitro* assay kits based on both enzyme-linked immunosorbent assays (ELISA) and radioimmunoassays (RIA), the purification and characterization of antigens, cytology and histology, the expectations of their *in-vivo* clinical application have, on the whole, not been realized due to a number of factors. These include: immunogenicity because most mab used *in vivo* are of mouse origin and therefore xenogeneic; the size of the intact immunoglobulin molecule which is responsible for poor tissue penetration and therefore low uptake in the targeted organ; and also their mouse origin diminishes their ability to elicit effector mechanisms such as complement-mediated lysis or antibody-dependent cell-mediated cytotoxicity (ADCC).

With knowledge of these limitations, a whole area of research emerged to create a new generation of structurally predetermined molecules, or recombinant molecules as they are more commonly known. Advances in molecular biology over the past decade have enabled researchers to exploit not only the binding specificity of mab but also the ever expanding knowledge of lymphokines and their interactions in the regulation of the immune system.

This chapter will attempt to give an overview of these advances and the role that these recombinant molecules are playing in the diagnosis and therapy of human diseases.

8.2 Humanization

The clinical use of xenoantibodies in human patients has proven to be severely limiting owing to their being seen as foreign proteins by the patients immune system. To overcome this problem, a number of strategies have been used to increase the human content of antibodies which have proven clinical application. Such strategies include producing human mab, replacing the constant regions of murine monoclonals with those of human antibodies, yielding

166

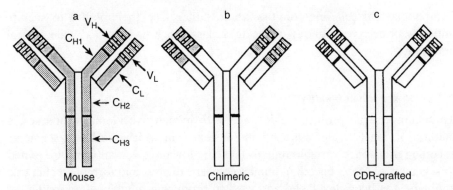

Figure 8.1. How a murine monoclonal antibody (a) can be humanized by replacement of all its constant regions with those of a human antibody resulting in a chimeric antibody (b) or by insertion of the mouse antibody's CDRs into a human antibody by CDR grafting (c).

chimeric antibodies and, more recently, replacing the complementarity-determining regions (CDRs) of a human antibody with those of a clinically useful murine antibody by a process known as CDR grafting (Figure 8.1).

8.2.1 Human monoclonal antibodies

Various strategies have been used to generate human antibodies. These include the fusion of human lymphoid cells with mouse myeloma cells to create chimeric hybridomas, Epstein–Barr virus (EBV) transformation of human B lymphocytes, the fusion of human B lymphocytes with EBV-transformed B lymphoblastoid cell lines, the fusion of human myeloma cell lines with B lymphocytes and the expression of human monoclonal antibody (Humab) genes in mouse myeloma cells.

Owing to the selective loss of human chromosomes from chimeric hybridomas (Bron *et al.*, 1985) which are derived by fusion between human lymphoid cells and mouse myeloma cells, very few antibodies with long-term use have been generated.

Numerous groups have produced Humab using the immortalization of human immunoglobulin-producing cells by fusion with mouse myeloma cells. The antibodies generated have been against a large number of different antigens, such as tetanus toxoid.

Other attempts to produce stable long-term secreting hybridomas have included the fusion of human lymphoid cells with human myelomas (Olsson & Kaplan, 1980); however, the level of antibody production is nearly always too low for any practical application. EBV immortalization of peripheral B-cells has been used to generate a number of lymphoblastoid cell lines secreting antibody to antigens found on tumours such as those of neuroectodermal origin (Irie *et al.* 1982; Katano *et al.*, 1984), and colorectal origin (Steis *et al.*, 1990).

Lymphoblastoid cell lines on the whole either lose their ability to secrete antibody or secrete antibody of the IgM class which has not had wide clinical application.

8.2.2   Chimeric antibodies

To circumvent the problems associated with human hybridoma techniques, a method of constructing immunoglobulin genes, in which the DNA segments encoding the mouse variable regions (specific for any given antigen) are joined to segments of DNA encoding human constant regions and forming a chimeric antibody, has been developed and used to produce a number of antibodies of clinical use (Figure 8.1).

In an early report (Boulianne *et al.*, 1984), a chimeric antibody with specificity for the hapten trinitrophenol (TNP) was secreted due to the successful expression of chimeric genes.

To introduce the chimeric genes into cells, plasmid vectors, such as pSVgpt and pSVneo, are used to transform mouse myeloma cells, e.g. X63Ag8.653. These transformants have been shown to produce 10–30 μg/ml of chimeric antibody which is comparable to that made by murine hybridomas secreting mouse antibodies. Examples of such chimeric antibodies have included those generated to acute lymphoblastic leukaemia antigens (Nishimura *et al.*, 1987), carcinoma-associated antigen 17-1A (Sun *et al.*, 1987), colorectal carcinoma (Brown *et al.*, 1987) and melanoma antigens (Liu *et al.*, 1987).

The advantages of using chimeric antibodies are that stable mouse myeloma cell lines can be used to produce the transformants (also known as 'transfectomas') and that the chimeric antibody has both the binding specificities of a well-characterized mouse monoclonal antibody (Mumab) and tumouricidal activity in the presence of human effector cells due to CDC and antibody-dependent cellular cytotoxicity (ADCC) by virtue of having human constant regions.

Expression of such chimeric constructs in stable cell lines overcomes the problem of instability of the cell lines used to generate human antibodies. Chimeric antibodies, however, whose variable regions are murine, are still potentially immunogenic when used *in vivo*.

To increase the humanization of chimeric antibodies, a number of groups replaced not only the constant regions of mouse antibodies with human equivalents but also the framework regions of the variable domains. This left only the complementarity-determining regions being of mouse origin. The process is now known as CDR grafting (Figure 8.1).

8.2.3   CDR grafting

Sequence comparisons among heavy and light chain variable domains (V_H and V_L) show that each domain has three complementarity-determining regions which are flanked by four relatively conserved regions, known as framework regions. These framework regions form the majority of the beta-sheet which, with the CDRs, forms the antigen-binding site. Using antibodies whose crystallographic structure is known, Jones and colleagues were able to substitute the CDRs from the heavy chain variable region of a human myeloma protein NEWM with the CDRs of a Mumab B1–8, which binds the hapten NP-cap (4-hydroxy-3-nitrophen-acetyl caproic acid). When the new variable heavy chain was combined with the B1–8 light chain, the hapten affinity was found to be comparable to that of the mouse B1–8 (Jones *et al.*, 1986).

Using an antibody raised to a large protein antigen (lysozyme) Verhoeyen and co-workers were able to demonstrate that CDR grafting could result in functional variable regions recognizing not only small haptens but also large protein antigens (Verhoeyen *et al.*, 1988).

In both the above examples of CDR grafting, only the heavy chain CDRs were replaced. In a study of Reichmann *et al.* (1988) all six CDRs from the heavy and light chain variable domains of a rat antibody, directed against human lymphocytes, were grafted into a human IgG1 antibody.

In this study, Reichmann used a rat antibody with therapeutic potential as a source of CDRs and grafted them into a human IgG1 antibody which was selected as being the best isotype for complement and cell-mediated lysis. The antigen, recognized by both the rat antibody and the reshaped human antibody, is the Campath-I antigen that is strongly expressed on human lymphocytes and monocytes but is absent from other blood cells including the haemopoietic stem cells (Hale *et al.*, 1988).

The reshaped antibody was shown by *in-vitro* experiments to be identical to other antibodies in complement lysis and more effective than the parent rat antibody in cell-mediated lysis. Similar results were obtained when target and effector cells were obtained from three different donors; the antibody Campath-IH was also shown to be effective in killing leukaemic cells obtained from three patients with B cell lymphocytic leukaemia.

Following these *in-vitro* studies, Campath-IH was used to treat two patients with non-Hodgkins lymphoma. Intravenous doses of 1–20 mg were given daily for up to 43 days (Hale *et al.*, 1988). In this first clinical study using a reshaped (CDR-grafted) human IgG1 antibody, very encouraging results were obtained. These results included the clearing of lymphoma cells from both patients' blood and bone marrow, resolving splenomegaly and, in one patient, lymphadenopathy. These effects were all achieved without myelosuppression.

The results obtained in the above study showed that tumour treatment by passive immunotherapy, using reshaped human antibodies, was both viable and effective, and that antibodies could be specifically selected to exploit the most potent physiological effector mechanisms.

This ability to modify, at will, both variable and constant domains by means of genetic engineering procedures is currently being exploited by a number of groups using antibodies of varied clinical relevance including anti-Rh antibodies which when directed against the Rh(D) antigen can be used in the prophylaxis of blood transfusion accidents and haemolytic disease of the new-born.

The *in-vivo* use of antibodies such as Campath-IH should greatly reduce the human antiglobulin response due to the antibody being virtually of human origin. Few data are available at present on the generation of anti-idiotypic responses generated to human antibodies.

In the case of the Campath-IH trial, such responses would not be expected due to the immunosuppressive nature of the disease and the fact that Campath-IH is probably immunosuppressive itself. Only large clinical trials using escalating doses of human or humanized mab will provide us with data regarding their immunogenicity and its restriction, in terms of anti-constant region versus anti-idiotypic.

Even with the advent of human or humanized mab of acceptably low immunogenicity, their size, just as with their murine counterparts, is likely to be restrictive in that only low amounts will penetrate into the tumour. To overcome the problem of size-related distribution, recent approaches have been used to genetically engineer new antigen-binding fragments (Winter & Milstein 1991). The advantages of these fragments (such as single chain or single domain antibodies) over intact immunoglobulins will now be discussed.

8.3   Recombinant antibody fragments

One of the main disadvantages to the production of human, chimeric or CDR-grafted antibodies is the stability of the mammalian cell expressing the immunoglobulin and the drop in levels of secreted product with time. Recent approaches have been proposed with the potential to bypass hybridoma technology. These approaches involve the cloning of antibody genes directly from hybridomas or B lymphocytes expressing antibody of desired specificity.

Antibody engineering, as it is now known, has enabled the construction of a wide range of antibody fragments, all of which can be expressed in an active form from genes introduced into mammalian (Neuberger *et al.*, 1984) or bacterial cells (Skerra & Plückthun, 1988). These fragments, as shown in Figure 8.2, include Fv fragments, which are non-covalently associated hetero-dimers of V_H and V_L domains.

To stabilize these Fv fragments, a flexible hydrophilic linker can be engineered to link the two domains, forming what is known as a single chain Fv fragment (sFv) (Huston *et al.*, 1988).

Single domain antibodies, which consist of only the V_H or V_L domain, have been expressed and shown to bind antigen (Ward *et al.*, 1989). The major drawback to the use of single domain antibodies is their 'stickiness' due to an exposed hydrophobic surface, which normally interacts with its complementary domain. The smallest of all antibody fragments is known as a minimal recognition unit (MRU) (Williams *et al.*, 1989). An example of an MRU is a single CDR which can be shown to retain antigen-binding activity.

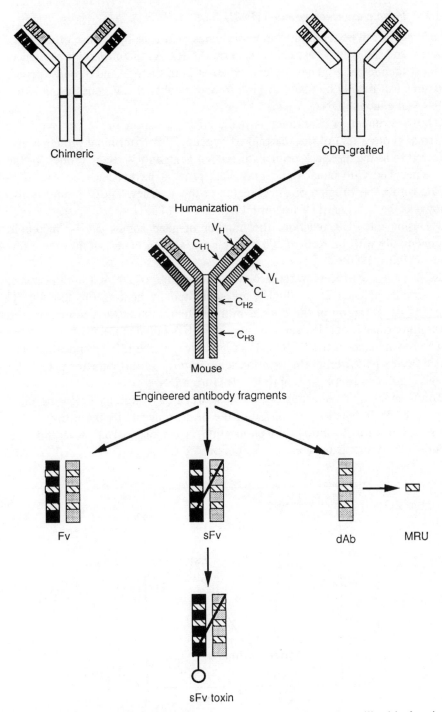

Figure 8.2. How the binding domains of a murine antibody can be utilized in forming a chimeric or CDR-grafted antibody and the various recombinant binding units that can be produced using genetic engineering. These binding units include the dAb (V_H or V_L), Fv (V_H and V_L), sFv (V_H + V_L + peptide linker) and a small minimal recognition unit that could be derived from the peptide sequence of a single CDR.

8.3.1   Polymerase chain reaction (PCR)

The V genes can be rescued from hybridomas or B cells by the use of universal primers and the polymerase chain reaction (PCR). As the nucleotide sequences of most families of V genes are conserved at both their 5' and 3' ends, primer mixtures can readily be made to bind to and amplify the V genes using either mRNA or genomic DNA.

The N-terminal or 5' primer is made to bind within the signal sequence (Larrick *et al.*, 1989) of the rearranged V gene. This N-terminal primer is also referred to as the V_H Back primer for the V_H gene and V_L Back primer for the V_L gene. The C-terminal or 3' end PCR primers have been constructed to locate within the J region or the C region of the V genes. The 3' primer is also known as the V forward (V for) primer.

By using the PCR reaction, the number of gene copies can be increased exponentially with more than 100 billion copies being made within only a few hours (Mullis, 1990).

PCR is a cyclic process, with each cycle the number of DNA strands doubles. The strands in each DNA duplex are separated by heating (at about 95 °C allowing denaturation of the double-stranded template) in the presence of the extension primers, dNTPs, and a heat stable DNA polymerase.

The second step of the PCR reaction is known as the primer annealing step which occurs by lowering the reaction temperature. In this annealing step, the 5' and 3' primers simply anneal to the denatured DNA.

For V genes, this annealing occurs at between 55 °C and 65 °C. In the third step of the PCR reaction, extension of the primers occurs by the action of the DNA polymerase, resulting in a duplication of the original DNA strand (see Figure 8.3). Primer extension occurs at about 72 °C.

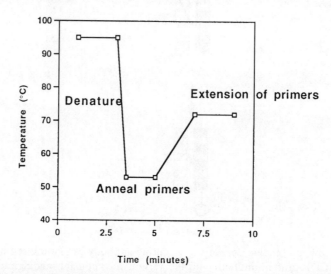

Figure 8.3. Temperatures and periods of time for the three steps of a PCR cycle: the template denaturation step, the primer annealing step and the primer extending step.

Amplification of DNA by PCR is a highly efficient and relatively cheap technique. The specificity of the PCR reaction is dictated by the oligonucleotide primers which are usually 15–25 bases in length.

When designing primers, it is important that the 3′ end of the primer pairs does not contain complementary bases, as this often results in the formation of 'primer-dimer'. It has also been found that primers with a high GC content generally require a higher reannealing and extension temperature (Bell, 1989).

The amount of DNA product obtained by PCR can be varied by alteration of the cycle number, temperature and magnesium concentration.

When designing primers, it is normal to build in restriction sites (Orlandi *et al.*, 1989) which can be cut by unique restriction enzymes. This allows the amplified DNA to be cloned directly into an expression vector for expression in bacterial or mammalian cells.

8.3.2 *Expression of Fv, single chain and single domain antibodies*

Over the past few years, a large number of groups have been working on the optimization of bacterial expression systems, such as *E. coli* (Field *et al.*, 1990). *E. coli* has been used for a number of reasons, which include ease of genetic manipulation, rapid growth, ease of transformation, cost and prior knowledge of growth requirements.

Although there are a large number of plasmids which can be used as expression vectors, some of the most utilized are those from the pUC family of plasmids (Sambrook *et al.*, 1989). The plasmid carries an antibiotic resistance gene, which allows easy identification of transformed colonies, when grown on ampicillin-containing agar. A colony can be picked from the agar plate and grown up as a 'Maxi-prep' providing large amounts of plasmid containing the immunoglobulin variable light and heavy genes for expression. Expression of the desired molecules is attained by addition to the medium of isopropyl β-D-thiogalactoside (IPTG), when the plasmid contains a lac promoter-operator ($\text{lac}^{p/o}$).

It has recently been shown that functional Fv proteins can be obtained due to the synthesis of approximately equal amounts of heavy and light chains, transport of both precursor proteins to the bacterial periplasmic space, correct processing of both signal sequences and correct folding of the proteins to yield both globular and soluble domains with intramolecular disulphide bonds resulting in a heterodimer (Skerra & Plückthun, 1988).

In this study the affinity of the recombinant Fv fragment was identical to that of the native mab when assayed under the same conditions.

Other studies, which have focused on the use of *E. coli* to obtain recombinant binding units where the heavy and light chains are held together by a polypeptide linker to form a single chain Fv (sFv), have also shown that the binding specificity and affinity of the recovered proteins are similar to those of the parent mab molecule (Huston *et al.*, 1988).

Escherichia coli has also been used for the expression of mouse–human chimeric Fab fragments, where the variable regions are from a Mumab and the C_H1 and C_K constant regions from a human IgG1 antibody (Better *et al.*, 1988). The expressed chimeric Fab was shown to specifically bind to its antigen expressed by a human carcinoma cell line.

Single chain antigen-binding proteins, where the carboxy terminus of the V_L is linked to the amino terminus of the V_H by a peptide linker, have now been produced against a large number of targets which include growth hormones, fluorescein (Bird *et al.*, 1988) and ovarian cancer cells (Chaudhary *et al.*, 1990).

In a recent study, the stability of immunoglobulin Fv molecules, where various strategies to stabilize them had been used (Glockshuber *et al.*, 1990), showed that of three types of linker used (peptide linker, chemical crosslinking and intermolecular disulphide bond), the disulphide-linked Fv fragment was the most thermally stable. This study also showed that all three strategies dramatically improved the thermal stability of Fv fragments when compared with Fv fragments that had no linker.

The first report on the *in-vivo* targeting of a recombinant single chain antibody showed stability and potential for their use in diagnostic and therapeutic applications (Colcher *et al.*, 1990). The single chain antibody was derived from a mab, B6.2, which recognizes a 90 kDa glycoprotein found on a number of human carcinomas. This study also provided data regarding the pharmacokinetics and renal accumulation. The sFv was shown to clear rapidly from the central blood pool but not so rapidly that binding could not occur. Unlike Fab' and F(ab')2 fragments which accumulate in the kidneys, and when radio-labelled cause renal toxicity, the sFv was excreted.

This study, although in athymic mice, did demonstrate uptake in a human tumour xenograft and therefore their potential clinical application. What we will have to await are data regarding their immunogenicity in humans.

Antigen binding has also been demonstrated in a study using a V_H domain alone, which is referred to as a single domain antibody (dAb). In this study (Ward *et al.*, 1989), the V_H of an anti-lysozyme antibody was expressed and secreted from *E. coli* and bound to its target antigen, lysozyme, with an affinity only tenfold lower than that of the parent antibody.

Although this study clearly demonstrated antigen binding by a V_H single chain antibody domain, it also demonstrated the 'sticky' nature of such constructs, which is due to an exposed hydrophobic surface normally capped by the V_κ or V_λ domains. This stickiness results in non-specific binding which would be unacceptable for *in-vivo* use. Further work on dAb will be required if they are to find clinical application.

8.3.3   *Minimal recognition unit (MRU)*

Although the dAb is the smallest antigen-binding unit to be cloned and expressed in *E. coli*, it is not believed to be the smallest antigen-binding protein obtainable. Research is ongoing into the production of minimal recognition units (MRUs). MRUs are small peptides which correspond to a CDR or other antigen recognition sites located within the variable domain of an antibody.

In a recent study, a peptide derived from the amino acid sequence of the second CDR of a mab, raised against the cell attachment site of retrovirus type 3, has been shown to downregulate the receptor after binding. This down regulation of the receptor was seen in conjuction with the inhibition of DNA synthesis in the cells bound by the peptide (Williams *et al.*, 1989). These effects are the same as those observed when the intact antibody binds to the receptor.

Another study has shown that when all six CDRs of an antibody specific for the platelet fibrinogen receptor were sequenced, five were germline sequences, whereas one, CDR3, of the V_H domain, mimicked the receptor recognition domain of fibrinogen (Taub *et al.*, 1989). In-depth studies of the CDR3 revealed a short sequence (RYD) which, if in the right conformation, could behave like the RGD sequence of fibrinogen. Substitutions of the tyrosine within this RYD sequence were found to increase or decrease the affinity of a 21 amino acid peptide which encompassed the CDR3 region.

Using computer modelling to determine active and inactive peptide analogues of the second CDR of an anti-reovirus type 3 cell surface receptor mab, researchers from the University of Pennsylvania have synthesized an organic compound, known as a mimetic, which mimicked the binding properties of the parent mab (Saragovi *et al.*, 1991). The authors claim that the mimetic, being synthetic, is resistant to protease activity, is possibly non-immunogenic and could permeate the blood-brain barrier (because of its solubility and size) all of which would be in contrast to a peptide-binding unit. The authors conclude that the mimetic should have an increased half-life in the blood and 'thus should be useful for the development of new pharmaceutical, therapeutic, diagnostic and receptor-binding agents'.

8.4   Discussion

Immunotherapy, dismissed by many because of the failure of early clinical trials involving poorly defined polyclonal antibodies, has now emerged as one of the most advancing fields in medicine. Immunotherapeutics are now being developed and used in various clinical applications, including the treatment of cancer. Much of the renewed interest in immunotherapy arose out of the development of mab secreted from stable mouse hybridomas (Kohler & Milstein, 1975). Mab of desired specificity and affinity could be produced in large quantities over long periods without variation from batch to batch.

The availability of mab has enabled an in-depth study of antigen-binding sites. Our understanding of what does and does not constitute a binding site changes as rapidly as the advances being made in crystallography and molecular biology.

As described in this chapter, the results of research over the past decade has enabled binding units to be reduced in size from a large glycoprotein antibody molecule to a small organic molecule. With this increase in understanding of antibody binding has come the potential to design molecules for specific purposes.

Where intact immunoglobulin molecules are required, it is possible to substitute constant regions for those known to be optimal for desired effector functions, such as complement lysis or antibody-dependent cell cytotoxicity. Novel effector functions can also be recruited by fusing gene segments encoding antigen-binding sites to genes coding for toxins (Chaudhary et al., 1989) or enzymes (Neuberger et al., 1984).

Recombinant antibody molecules allow a high degree of flexibility; genes encoding both variable domains or one variable domain can be joined recombinantly to genes encoding molecules such as IL-2, toxins or hormones.

The fact that the fusion protein is designed from the outset allows humans and not nature to determine its in-vivo specificity. Affinity can be altered by site-directed mutagenesis, amino acid substitution or by recombining heavy and light chains of different antibodies with the same specificity (Clackson et al., 1991).

Diverse libraries of antibody fragments expressed on the surface of phage can be screened rapidly for both specificity and affinity using hapten columns or antigen-impregnated nitrocellulose (Huse et al., 1989). Using phage screening systems millions of different peptides can be expressed and screened in a very short period (Cwirla et al., 1990).

Advances over the past decade have provided the potential to bypass hybridoma technology. The advent of PCR enables the isolation and amplification of relevant genes. Rather than having to obtain large numbers of cells in order to isolate sufficient immunoglobulins or receptors, as few as 100 cells can provide sufficient mRNA or genomic DNA for PCR amplification, yielding large quantities of the relevant gene for use in sequencing and expression studies. The ability to obtain sufficient genetic material from a few cells will enable the isolation of antibodies directly from B cells present in the peripheral blood of patients and thereby will circumvent the problem of establishing cell lines, which are all too often unstable (Songsivilai et al., 1990).

Rather than fuse B cells from an immunized animal with myeloma cells and establish a hybridoma cell line by time-consuming limiting dilution, the spleen cells can be used to obtain large combinatorial libraries of immunoglobulin which will allow rapid and easy identification of antibody-binding sites that can then be used for genetic manipulation.

The advances in genetic and protein engineering outlined in this chapter should yield a new generation of molecules for use in the diagnosis and therapy of human diseases. What is not yet clear are the possible problems associated with the in-vivo use of recombinant molecules, for example, their pharmacokinetics. Will they be cleared too rapidly? Will they be immunogenic? To what degree will they be toxic? Whatever the outcome of early clinical trials, recombinant molecules will form a foundation on which to build a generation of new and novel designer molecules.

8.5   References

Bell, J. (1989). The polymerase chain reaction. *Immunology Today*, **10**, 351–355.

Better, M., Chang, C. P., Robinson R. R. & Horwitz A. H. (1988). *Escherichia coli* secretion of an active chimeric antibody fragment. *Science*, **240**, 1041–1043.

Bird, R. E., Hardman, K. D., Jacobson, J. W., Johnson, S., Kaufman, B. M., Lee, S. M., Lee, T., Pope, S. H., Riordan G. S. & Whitlow, M. (1988). Single-chain antigen-binding proteins. *Science*, **242**, 423–426.

Boulianne, G. L., Hozumi, N. & Shulman, M. J. (1984). Production of functional chimeric mouse/human antibody. *Nature (London)*, **312**, 643–646.

Bron, D., Delforge, A. & Stryckmans, P. (1985). Human monoclonal antibodies: new approaches and perspectives in cancer. *European Journal of Cancer and Clinical Oncology*, **21**, 283–285.

Chaudhary, V. J., Batra, J. K., Gallo, M. G., Willingham, M. C., Fitzgerald, D. J. & Pastan, I. (1990). A rapid method of cloning functional variable-region antibody genes in *Escherichia coli* as single-chain immunotoxins. *Proceedings of the National Academy of Sciences U.S.A.*, **87**, 1066–1070.

Clackson, T., Hoogenboom H. R., Griffiths, A. D. & Winter, G. (1991). Making antibody fragments using phage display libraries. *Nature*, **352**, 624–628.

Colcher, D., Bird, R., Roselli, M., Hardman, K. D., Johnson, S. Pope, S., Dodd, S., Pantoliano, M. W., Milenic, D. E. & Schlom, J. S. (1990). *In vivo* tumour targeting of a recombinant single-chain antigen-binding protein. *Journal of the National Cancer Institute*, **82**, 1191–1197.

Cwirla, S. E. Peters, E. A., Barret, R. W. & Dower, W. J. (1990). Peptides on phage: a vast library of peptides for identifying ligands. *Proceedings of the National Academy of Sciences U.S.A.*, **87**, 6378–6382.

Field, H., Yarranton, G. T. & Rees, A. R. (1990). Expression of mouse immunoglobulin light and heavy chains. Variable regions in *Escherichia coli* and reconstitution of antigen binding activity. *Protein Engineering*, **3**, 641–647.

Glockshuber, R., Malia, M., Pfitzinger, I. & Plückthun, A. (1990). A comparison of strategies to stabilise immunoglobulin Fv fragments. *Biochemisty*, **29**, 1362–1367.

Hale, G., Clark, M. R., Marcus, R., Winter, G., Dyer, M. J. S., Phillips, J. M., Riechmann, L. & Waldmann, H. (1988). Remission induction in non-Hodgkin's lymphoma with reshaped human monoclonal antibody Campath-IH. *Lancet*, **2** (8625), 1394–1399.

Huse, W. D., Sastry, L., Iverson, S. A., Kang, A. S., Alting-Mees, M., Burton, D. R., Benkovic, S. J. & Lerner, R. A. (1989). Generation of a large combinatorial library of the immunoglobulin repertoire in phage lambda. *Science*, **246**, 1275–1281.

Huston, J. S., Levinson, D., Mudgett-Hunter, M., Tai, M.-S., Novotny, J., Margolies, M. N., Ridge, R. J., Bruccoleri, R. E., Haber, E., Crea, R. & Oppermann, H. (1988). Protein engineering of antibody binding sites: recovery of specific activity in an anti-digoxin single-chain Fv analogue produced in *Escherichia coli*. *Proceedings of the National Academy of Sciences U.S.A.*, **85**, 5879–5883.

Irie, R. F., Sze, L. L. & Saxton, R. E. (1982). Human antibody to OFA-1, a tumor antigen produced *in vitro* by Epstein–Barr virus-transformed human B lymphoid cell lines. *Proceedings of the National Academy of Sciences U.S.A.*, **79**, 5666–5670.

Jones, P. T., Dear, P. H., Foote, J., Neuberger, M. S. & Winter, G. (1986). Replacing the complementarity determining regions in a human antibody with those from a mouse. *Nature (London)*, **321**, 522–525.

Katano. M., Saxton, R. E. & Irie, R. F. (1984). Human monoclonal antibody to tumor associated ganglioside GD2. *Journal of Clinical Laboratory Immunology*, **15**, 119–126.

Kohler, G. & Milstein, C. (1975). Continuous cultures of fused cells secreting antibody of predefined specificity. *Nature*, **256**, 495–497.

Larrick, J. W., Danielsson, L., Brenner, C. A., Abrahamson, M., Fry, K. E. & Borrebaeck, C. A. (1989). Rapid cloning of rearranged immunoglobulin genes from human hybridoma cells using mixed primers and the polymerase chain reaction. *Biochemical Biophysical Research Communications*, **160**, 1250–1255.

Liu, A. Y., Robinson, R. R., Hellström, K. E., Murray, E. D., Jr., Chang, C. P. & Hellström, I. (1987). Chimeric mouse-human IgG1 antibody that can mediate lysis of cancer cells. *Proceedings of the National Academy of Sciences U.S.A.*, **84**, 3439–3443.

Mullis, K. B. (1990). The unusual origin of the polymerase chain-reaction. *Scientific American*, **262**, 36–43.

Neuberger, M. S., Williams, G. T. & Fox, R. O. (1984). Recombinant antibodies possessing novel effector functions. *Nature (London)*, **312**, 604–608.

Nishimura, Y., Yokoyama, M., Araki, K., Ueda, R., Kudo, A. & Watanabe, T. (1987). Recombinant human-mouse chimeric monoclonal antibody specific for common acute lymphocytic leukaemia antigen. *Cancer Research*, **47**, 999–1005.

Olsson, L. & Kaplan, H. S. (1980). Human hybridomas producing monoclonal antibodies of predefined antigenic specificity. *Proceedings of the National Academy of Sciences U.S.A.*, **77**, 5429–5431.

Orlandi, R., Güssow, D. H., Jones, P. T. & Winter, G. (1989). Cloning immunoglobulin variable domains for expression by the polymerase chain reaction. *Proceedings of the National Academy of Sciences U.S.A.*, **86**, 3833–3837.

Riechmann, L., Clark, M., Waldmann, H. & Winter, G. (1988). Reshaping human antibodies for therapy. *Nature*, **332**, 323–327.

Sambrook, J., Fritsch, E. F. & Maniatis T. (1989). *Molecular Cloning: a Laboratory Manual*. New York, Cold Spring Habor Laboratory Press.

Saragovi, H. U., Fitzpatrick, D., Raktabutr, A., Nakanishi, H., Kahn, M. & Greene, M. I. (1991). Design and synthesis of a mimetic from an antibody complementarity determining region. *Science*, **253**, 792–795.

Skerra, A. & Plückthun, A. (1988). Assembly of a functional immunoglobulin Fv fragment in *Escherichia coli*. *Science*, **240**, 1038–1040.

Songsivilai, S., Bye, J. M., Marks, J. D. & Hughes-Jones, N. C. (1990). Cloning and sequencing of human lambda immunoglobulin genes by the polymerase chain reaction. *European Journal of Immunology*, **20**, 2661–2666.

Steis, R. G., Carrasquillo, J. A., McCabe, R., Bookman, M. A., Reynolds, J. C., Larson, S. M., Smith, J. W. II, Clark, J. W., Dailey, V., Del Vecchio, S., Shuke, N., Pinsky, C. M., Urba, W. J., Haspel, M., Perentesis, P., Paris, B., Longo, D. L., & Hanna, M. G. Jr. (1990). Toxicity, immunogenicity and tumor radioimmuno-detecting ability of two human monoclonal antibodies in patients with metastatic colorectal carcinoma. *Journal of Clinical Oncology*, **8**, 476–490.

Sun, L. K., Curtis, P., Rakowicz-Szulczynska, E., Ghrayeb, J., Chang, N., Morrison, S. L. & Koprowski, H. (1987). Chimeric antibody with human constant regions and mouse variable regions directed against carcinoma-associated antigen 17-1A. *Proceedings of the National Academy of Sciences U.S.A.*, **84**, 214–218.

Taub, R., Gould, R. J., Garsky, V. M., Ciccarone, T. M., Hoxie, J., Friedman, P. A.

& Shattil, S. J. (1989). A monoclonal antibody against the platelet fibrinogen receptor contains a sequence that mimics a receptor recognition domain in fibrinogen. *Journal of Biological Chemistry*, **264**, 259–265.

Verhoeyen, M., Milstein, M. & Winter, G. (1988). Reshaping human antibodies. Grafting antilysozyme activity. *Science*, **239**, 1534–1536.

Ward, E. S., Güssow, D., Griffiths, A. D., Jones, P. T. & Winter, G. (1989). Binding activities of a repertoire of single immunoglobulin variable domains secreted from *Escherichia coli. Nature*, **341**, 544–546.

Williams, W. V., Moss, D.A., Kieber-Emmons, T.,Cohen, J. A., Myers, J. N., Weiner, D. B. & Greene, M. I. (1989). Development of biologically active peptides based on antibody structure. *Proceedings of the National Academy of Sciences U.S.A.*, **86**, 5537–5541.

Winter, G. & Milstein, C. (1991). Man-made antibodies. *Nature*, **349**, 293–299.

9

Monoclonal antibodies in diagnostic immunoassays

D. B. COOK and C. H. SELF

9.1 Introduction

The term immunochemistry was conceived by Arrhenius in 1907 but the use of immunochemical analytical and diagnostic techniques can be traced to the previous century[1]. Among the most significant advances relevant to the present discussion, however, was the introduction of the radioimmunoassay by Yalow & Berson (1959) for the estimation of insulin. This technique was based on the general competitive principle of saturation analysis (Ekins, 1960) and was undoubtedly the factor which permitted the enormous growth of discovery in endocrinology that occurred in the following years. It is incredible to immunoassayists of the present era that Yalow and Berson's original attempt to publish the crucial finding that insulin-treated diabetics produced antibodies specific for the insulin, the landmark observation in the development of our subject, was rejected on the grounds that it was considered impossible that antibodies could be produced to a molecule as small as insulin. Subsequently a learned journal in which their work did appear could not go so far as to permit the use of the expression 'insulin antibody' – at least in the title (Yalow & Berson, 1971). Nonetheless, the technique very quickly reached beyond the borders of endocrinology as a general analytical method.

By the mid-1970s it was realized that radioisotopes were far from ideal tracers for the technique and that improved signal could theoretically be obtained with alternatives. An editorial comment in *The Lancet* in 1976 predicted the demise of radioimmunoassay 'within a few years' in the context of enzymes being used in place of radioisotopes. Great emphasis at the time, often unjustifiably, was placed on the potential hazards of radioisotopes which the use of enzymes could circumvent but, more importantly, it was realized theoretically that greater sensitivity would eventually be achieved by the use of enzymes rather than with isotopes such as ^{125}Iodine. Thus it can be reflected

---

[1] Gruber & Durham (1896), Widal & Sicard (1896) and Kraus (1897) published some of the earliest immunological diagnostic techniques. Paul Ehrlich, however, has been described as the first immunochemist although his 1897 paper on the measurement of diphtheria antitoxin preceded the coining of the word by a decade.

that 10^7 molecules of ^{125}Iodine will yield only about 10 dpm (disintegrations per min), detectable with about 70% efficiency on the typical gamma counters available in diagnostic laboratories. Development of assays with much greater sensitivity depended on the use of tracers with lower detection limits. The use of enzymes with their potential for amplifying the signal was immediately attractive. Since that time a substantial number of alternative techniques with the potential of improved sensitivity of detection have been applied.

It had also become clear that the saturation principle employing a labelled analyte as applied by Berson & Yalow (and others) was inferior in many aspects to the use of the labelled reagent methodology (Miles & Hales, 1968). Thus the use of the tracer on the reagent antibody (originally again ^{125}Iodine) theoretically provided potential for assays with sensitivities several orders of magnitude greater than with the saturation principle and with a much wider working range (Ekins, 1987). Very quickly, the labelled reagent methodology became consolidated for practical purposes as the two-site immunometric assay, depending on excess reagent; first described by Addison & Hales in 1971, it is today very familiar to analysts (Figure 9.1).

The use of radioisotopes, however, has persisted for very much longer than forecast and the immunoradiometric assay is still widely encountered in analytical and diagnostic laboratories throughout the world. The competitive

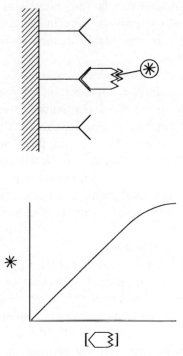

Figure 9.1. Principle of the two-site immunometric assay as often employed. Capture antibody is bound to a solid phase and the signal from the marker antibody (*) is proportional to the concentration of analyte.

radioimmunoassay itself is still used even in situations where the application of the two-site principle would appear to be the technique demanded by the standards of the 1990s if not the 1980s. What then have been the impediments to progress towards the establishment even of radioassays with improved sensitivity, the establishment of theoretical optimal sensitivity with alternative labels and the long-predicted demise of the radioisotope as a tracer in routine analytical and diagnostic use?

It has to be remembered that in practice, laboratories throughout the world, up to about 1980, were almost universally using expensive equipment designed to detect the signal from radioisotopes. As a result there was bound to be resistance on economic grounds to 'alternative' assays, at least until their equipment required replacing. Nonetheless, even the immunoradiometric assay (IRMA) was more limited in its application than it might have been, although it was used for example in hospital laboratories particularly for the assay of thyroid-stimulating hormone (TSH).

A more obvious restraint was the limited availability of antisera prepared with the technology of the day. Thus suitable immunochemical reagents in terms of affinity and specificity would only be available in milligram quantities at the most, even if the host animal had been a large species such as the sheep or goat. There was the need for at least one available antibody to be highly purified from serum as a requirement for labelling. The excess reagent principle required the use of relatively large quantities of reagent antibodies and whatever drawbacks could already be seen in the competitive radioimmunoassay principle, at least it was highly economical in its use of precious antibodies at great dilutions.

Thus where immunoradiometric analysis was employed, reagents inevitably quickly became exhausted and any organization providing reagents in the form of kits had necessarily to be in a continuous process of producing and evaluating quantities of antisera in new animals for the requirements of their kit production. This would have been especially difficult in the case of very weak antigens. When different antisera were introduced into kits as old bleeds became exhausted, there was of course no guarantee that the properties of the new material would be the same, with potentially ominous implications for future comparison with all the research and routine work that had depended on it. The more successful and widespread the procedures became, as was inevitable, the worse the problem became.

The achievement of Köhler & Milstein (1975), therefore, in the discovery of the principle of producing monoclonal antibodies on an industrial scale removed this barrier to progress and over the decade of the 1980s resulted in the availability of monoclonal antibodies (mab) in unlimited amounts to a vast range of antigens of importance and interest and across widely diverse fields of routine and research work. Thus, without shortage of antibody with which to work, it became possible to develop and optimize the variety of alternatives to radioisotopes.

The ready availability of better assays quickly demanded their introduction in terms of improved sensitivity, precision, speed and the ability to use ever smaller samples whether this was of importance *per se* as in paediatrics or continuous monitoring or whether it enabled analysis at greater dilution thereby negating the effects of potentially non-specific interfering material in the sample. Thus by 1984, the first such sensitive assays (reviewed by Woodhead & Weeks, 1985) for the pressing diagnostic problem of the estimation of TSH were introduced into routine clinical biochemistry. Even the use of radioisotope labels provided for the first time the means to assess the lowered serum TSH concentrations encountered in hyperthyroidism; this was a most significant diagnostic advance.

It might be reflected that this single application introduced to technologists by the thousand, almost overnight, the advantages of sensitivity, stability and other benefits of the new technology. It could not have occurred on this scale without the development of the techniques of manufacture of mab.

It is less than 20 years since Köhler and Milstein's paper was published, yet the worldwide immunoassay diagnostic industry could not exist without monoclonal antibodies. Many analytical techniques already regarded as routine in hospital biochemistry depend absolutely upon it. Apart from their uses in diagnostic clinical biochemistry, important applications can be found in most clinical disciplines as well as in agriculture and the food industry.

9.2 Advantages and pitfalls in using monoclonal antibodies

Production of mab has ensured a continuous supply of antibodies of defined characteristics that can be selected and extensively characterized from perhaps hundreds of clones of a given fusion. The appropriate clone, once selected, can be cultured continuously and the invaluable antibody it produces can be obtained, theoretically, without limit. In particular, specificity is a property that can be selected in this manner which is enhanced by the use of the two-site technique employing two separate highly specific antibodies to the same peptide or protein. The problem of exhaustion of invaluable reagents, once chosen, has now been circumvented. Of enormous importance, furthermore, is that there is no need for the immunogen employed to be pure because specificity is determined by the cloning process.

First, it is undoubtedly the absolute specificity of a given mab for a defined epitope that offers the major advantage to their use. For a polyclonal system a variety of antibodies will be encountered in a given antiserum which will have specificities for different epitopes in a protein sequence. One or more of these may predominate but a substantial population of antibodies may be expected, even if of low affinity, which almost certainly will recognize different epitopes.

An advantage is that such a mixture of components may permit measurement of proteins which exhibit heterogeneity, although heterogeneity may be unrelated to the recognition of the different epitopes, for example post-translational glycosylation. A potential danger, however, of this type of reaction is immediately apparent when in a two-site system a situation arises where a labelled mab (as in Figure 9.1) recognizes an epitope that has already been occupied by a component of a polyclonal mixture. To avoid this with polyclonal antibodies it would be necessary either to absorb out the immunoreactivity of certain antibody components with specified peptides or to employ protein or peptide fragments to raise antisera (e.g. PTH, ACTH), at some risk of compromising the secondary structure and subsequent immunoreactivity of the molecule.

One way round this problem has been to construct assays in which the labelled mab is incubated with the sample first in a sequential system, before the addition of the unlabelled polyclonal mixture, as a slurry on a solid phase such as cellulose which, as well as shortening the incubation time, circumvents the potential problem of masking an epitope. It is not an approach that lends itself easily to the use of the coated microtiter plate that has become so predominant in immunoassay in the 1980s and particularly it largely excludes the use of the 'alternative technologies' to radioisotopes for many practical and most routine diagnostic purposes.

A mab on the other hand has selected and characterized specificity and provides confidence that the immunochemical reaction is only obtained in the presence of a defined epitope. If, in practice, protein heterogeneity does become a problem, as indicated below in the case of luteinizing hormone (LH), it may be advantageous and possibly mandatory to introduce mixtures of monoclonal antibodies to allow for different epitopes, although unlike the polyclonal system, this is done in a defined and controllable manner (Ehrlich & Moyle, 1986). Whether the usual pair of mab are used in a sandwich assay or a limited mixture has been employed, there can be no danger of minor, perhaps unrecognized, components of a polyclonal mixture interfering with the binding of the labelled antibody that is subsequently added. The use of mixtures of different labelled mab recognizing different epitopes has also been used as a means of increasing the signal attached to the antigen of interest (Rattle *et al.*, 1984).

It should be noted that mixtures of mab often prove to exhibit greater affinity for protein detection on account of cooperativity between antibody-binding sites in a manner which may help to account for the greater affinity characteristic of a typical polyclonal antiserum compared with an equivalent monoclonal system (Ehrlich *et al.*, 1982).

As affinity constants of mab are often lower than it has been possible to achieve with polyclonal antibodies this may be disadvantageous when a relatively insensitive detection method is employed. Particularly, this may render mab less valuable than polyclonal antibodies in competitive techniques.

In considering the choice of mab or polyclonal antibody it is necessary to take into account the time, facilities and expertise required to generate the antibodies. It is not difficult or expensive to produce polyclonal antibodies by traditional procedures. When a fusion to produce hybrid cells is made, however, over 99.99% of the antibody-producing spleen cells do not survive, thus reducing by a considerable factor the range of potentially useful antibodies that may be eventually derived. On the other hand, a good polyclonal antibody can be relatively easily purified by affinity chromatography. Thus the worker is faced with a choice of reagent: polyclonal or monoclonal?

9.3   Specificity

Antibody recognition may be so specific as to be affected by a single hydroxyl group, for example on a steroid. Thus it has proved possible to obtain antibodies to oestradiol which do not recognize oestriol (Dray *et al.*, 1971). In using traditional antisera availability of such reagents is largely a matter of luck and might require immunoadsorption of antibodies reacting with potentially cross-reacting steroids. By using the techniques of production of mab, such antibody-producing clones may be selected and once produced are available in unlimited quantities without fear of the inevitable rapid exhaustion of supply.

Parvaz *et al.* (1989) produced mab against a dehydroepiandrosterone (DHEA)-bovine serum albumin conjugate in this way with the aim of producing antibodies specific for DHEA-sulphate. Similarly, Ghosh (1988) selected a mab with high specificity for oestriol. De Lauzon *et al.* (1989) described a mab against oestradiol with less than 1% cross-reactivity to oestrone or oestriol. Lewis *et al.* (1992) obtained an antibody against cortisol which did not react significantly with progesterone or 17α-hydroxyprogesterone with a remaining 19% cross-reactivity with 11-deoxycortisol. This ability to select mab for specific small ligands can thus be seen to be a major feature of importance in the application of mab, particularly in the case of steroids where there are so many potential cross-reactants. No doubt in the next few years a wide range of highly specific antibodies to steroids and other small molecules will become available with a goal of ever increasing specificity.

The same situation applies with drugs, small peptides and situations where glycosylation affects the reactivity of otherwise identical epitope structures, i.e. that antibodies may be selected which react with particular glycosylated forms and are thus available in unlimited quantity. An important exploitation of the phenomenon of specificity in relation to glycosylation is the introduction of assays for glycated haemoglobin A_{1c} and their use in the monitoring of diabetic control. Mab have been selected for this purpose which detect the glycated form specifically and do not react with other haemoglobins. In view of the many hundreds of clones that have had to be screened for the selection of a single antibody with such specificity (Zeuthen, 1988), it can readily be understood why such a diagnostic test would have been virtually impossible to devise without mab technology. It is barely conceivable that a specific antibody could have been raised by polyclonal methods. This test is available in commercial kit form (e.g. Dako Diagnostics Ltd, Bio-Rad).

Glycosylation is proving particularly problematical in the field of tumour-associated antigens but major progress is being made in the development of assays to a variety of tumour markers using the availability of mab (reviewed in Reckel, 1989). At the present time most of these markers have overlapping clinical specificity and the problem has not been helped by the fact that many of the mab employed in their detection have been raised against impure or uncharacterized preparations, including cell membranes and tumour cells themselves (Hakomori, 1989). Thus searches have been instituted for antigens reacting with mab produced in this way. Furthermore, the epitopes detected may be present on a number of apparently biologically different molecules (Nilsson et al., 1988). Undoubtedly rapid progress will be made in the selection of monoclonal antibodies which will clarify this important diagnostic application.

An important example of a mab-dependent immunoassay for a specific condition which is finding widespread use in routine diagnostic laboratories is provided by the example of the Prostate-Specific Antigen (PSA): an important new analyte for monitoring patients after treatment for prostate cancer (Armbruster, 1993). The antigen is a single chain glycoprotein not present in other tissues or apparently in non-prostate cancers. The rate of change in PSA concentration may be a sensitive and early indicator of prostate cancer (Carter et al., 1992) or its recurrence (Stamey et al., 1993). As the patients' PSA will require to be monitored over many years the importance of mab technology in providing long-term consistency of specificity, ultrasensitivity and precision over such a period is evident.

As a result of the high incidence of carcinoma of the prostate, it has also been suggested that the technique be employed for screening men over 50 years of age for prostate cancer (Catalona et al., 1991; Brawer et al., 1992).

Reports of work exploiting the ability to select among antibody clones for desired specificity are appearing with increasing frequency. Choi et al. (1991) have reported a system involving a common catching antibody for both the whole chorionic gonadotrophin molecule and its free beta-subunit. By selecting appropriate mab from the clones produced, they were then able to employ either an antibody specific for the whole molecule or a third antibody specific for the beta-subunit. By labelling these detecting antibodies with different enzymes, they were able to construct a simultaneous assay for the two molecules, depending on the substrate employed for measurement of the enzyme. The assay was used to investigate the ratios of the two analytes in women with abnormal pregnancies or tumours of the reproductive system.

Zegers et al. (1991) have been able to study genetic variation in the α_1-antitrypsin molecule. Mab were selected with different specificities for the 342 region, where the Z mutation occurs, the ZZ genotype being associated with severe alpha$_1$-antitrypsin deficiency. Z homo- and heterozygotes could be detected in rapid simple immunoblot assays. The authors comment that the detection procedure itself is both sensitive and very easy and represents a rapid and straightforward tool for the diagnosis of alpha$_1$-antitrypsin deficiencies, allowing early treatment and advice on lifestyle. It is highly unlikely that the work would have been possible, or even envisaged, if mab technology had not been developed as an alternative to the production of polyclonal antisera. As the authors point out, variant-specific polyclonal antibodies are not easy to produce as they would have to recognize a difference of only one amino acid. Purified alpha$_1$-antitrypsin from either MM or ZZ origin does not generate antibodies specific for the 342 region when injected into animals.

Examples of more widespread routine diagnostic applications include the determination of isoenzymes which has hitherto depended on electrophoresis and visual staining resulting from enzyme activity. Many enzymes are now being subjected to immunometric analysis and some such techniques have already been introduced into diagnostic practice. Superior procedures to differentiate between bone and liver alkaline phosphatase, for example, have been developed by exploiting the specificity of mab. Bone and liver isoenzymes differ only in their glycosylation and so the development of immunoassays specific for either isoenzyme depends on mab technology for selection of specificity. Hill & Wolfert (1989) investigated 20,441 clones and selected just 5 showing differences in response between bone and liver enzyme. A sandwich assay has been devised which is specific for the skeletal isoenzyme (Price *et al.*, 1993). The investigation is of value in disorders of bone metabolism such as osteoporosis, bone tumours, Paget's disease, primary hyperparathyroidism and in renal disease.

Similarly, in the investigation of the cardiovascular system, immunoassays depending on highly specific mab technology are being introduced for the estimation of the CK-MB form of creatine phosphotransferase (creatine kinase) which predominates in cardiac muscle and is indicated in the investigation of myocardial infarction (Collins *et al.*, 1993). Additionally, an immunoassay depending on mab technology has been proposed for the estimation of myosin heavy chain fragments after acute myocardial infarction (Larue *et al.*, 1991). Myosin is the major structural protein of the myocardium and the assay may well improve diagnostic specificity in myocardial infarction by detecting the myosin heavy chain fragments liberated into plasma after the infarction. The test may also indicate the degree of damage to tissue. The importance of using mab arises because myosin is rapidly proteolysed into fragments in the circulation. Only antibodies specific for the fragments most resistant to proteolysis are useful and these are most readily selected by mab technology.

A final example of this type of exploitation is provided by an assay for glycocalicin, a proteolytic fragment of platelet membrane glycoprotein 1b (Kunushima *et al.*, 1991). This substance has been measured by the classical competitive radioimmunoassay methods but glycocalicin is degraded by proteolytic enzymes in the blood. These authors found lower values for glycocalicin in plasma than previously reported, attributable to the use of two mab with differing specificities which they were able to select from the clones produced.

The single-site assays are of course subject to cross-reaction with the contaminating degraded fragments in plasma. Using the two-site assay, Kunushima *et al.* confirmed reports that the plasma glycocalicin concentration is useful in classifying the mechanism of thrombocytopenia.

This last assay is reminiscent of the well-recognized problems in the assay of parathyroid hormone (PTH), where degraded fragments seriously interfere with one-site assays and give a false impression of the amount of circulating intact PTH. The situation has been resolved by choosing antibodies recognizing different ends of the molecule, thus enabling the sandwich to be formed only in the presence of the intact peptide sequence. As it happens many such assays for intact PTH have been performed with affinity-purified polyclonal antibodies and as such are commercially available. The availability of appropriate mab ensures a greater and continued supply of reproducible reagents. Whereas fragments of the PTH peptide have long been widely available and consequently have been employed in several centres for raising polyclonal antibodies against specific regions of the whole molecule, this is not the case with glycocalicin. Hence there is the necessity to produce mab using the whole molecule and select the specificity. This situation will apply to a wide number of proteins and peptides which are in short supply and for which fragments are not available and we can expect to see a great increase in the exploitation of this feature in the very near future.

The high specificity achievable, however, must be carefully used. A given antibody system may, for example, be too specific for the detection of a protein that exhibits even a small degree of heterogeneity. An example of this problem has recently been highlighted in the case of LH. Pettersson & Söderholm (1991) have demonstrated at least ten distinct epitopes on LH and that genetic variants also exist. A specific mab may fail to recognize one or more of these epitopes, generating a different result for a sample of LH containing that epitope compared with another mab. The problem appears to be particularly troublesome with the pituitary glycoprotein hormones, especially LH. Pettersson *et al.* (1991) have demonstrated a normal subject with no LH detectable in one such highly specific assay method. Demers (1991) has predicted that manufacturers may find it necessary to produce mixtures of antibodies, thus returning to a poly/monoclonal system, so that predictable epitopes will be recognized and genetic variants, especially, do not escape detection in a particular system (see note on p. 208).

The application of mab in relation to the measurement of chemically closely-related hormones (e.g. glycoprotein hormones, proinsulin family) is discussed in Chapter 14.

9.4   Small molecular weight analytes

There is no doubt that the two-site sandwich immunometric approach has benefited from the availability of mab; however, it can be seen that in many cases equally useful assays could have been constructed with polyclonal anti-sera. This technique, however, depends on two spatially separate sites on the analyte and breaks down with analytes of low molecular size, such as the majority of therapeutic drugs, drugs of abuse, environmental toxins and pollutants, small peptides and other metabolic products.

Valentine & Green (1967) showed simultaneous binding of anti-dinitrophe-nol antibodies to a structure only 25 nm long and more recently Jackson *et al.* (1988) demonstrated simultaneous binding of two mab to epitopes separated in sequence by only three amino acid residues but the simultaneous separate high-affinity binding of analytes of very low molecular size by two antibodies, required for practical useful immunoassays, has not been reported. The competitive immunoassay approach has continued to provide the basis of most assays.

The use of mab in this regard has been twofold. First, they have been used simply to replace the polyclonal antibody with the advantages of constant supply of defined reagent discussed above. Second, because of their homogen-eous nature, it has been more practicable to raise anti-idiotypic antibodies against them to use instead of analyte-analogue-conjugates in the assays (Potocnjak *et al.*, 1982). As these authors point out, this approach brought the distinct advantage of not needing to purify and label analyte. Indeed, as long as the assay can be related to something such as a clinical finding it is not even necessary to know what the analyte is. The approach has been used for the assay of both large molecular analytes such as adenosine deaminase-binding protein (Thompson *et al.*, 1985) and small molecular antigens such as thyroxine (Gorman & Daiss, 1991) and oestradiol (Altamirano-Bustamante *et al.*, 1991). They all represent, however, the direct application of competitive immuno-assay methods in which the number of binding sites *not bound* by the analyte is determined by the addition of labelled component (Figure 9.2). This raises a fundamental problem with these assays, especially when low concentrations of

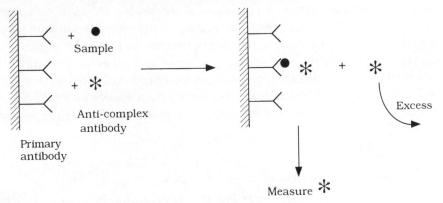

Figure 9.2. Anti-Immune Complex Immunoassay for a small analyte. The analyte binds to primary antibody causing it to bind labelled anti-complex antibody. Excess label is removed and remaining label is determined.

analyte need to be determined. In such situations a large amount of labelled component is bound which is difficult to distinguish from the large amounts bound at other low analyte concentrations. The sensitivity is restricted with competitive methods that measure analyte *unbound* sites. In addition, in competitive immunoassays the concentration of the reagents involved in the competition (the antibody and labelled component) need to be precisely controlled. Changes, for example due to imprecision of reagent addition or decay of reagent, are reflected in the operation of the assay to an extent not seen in reagent excess assays. In competitive immunoassays there is a strong association between reducing the amounts of labelled component and increase in sensitivity, unlike that in reagent excess assays. This may be understood by considering that at a low concentration of analyte a substantial concentration of the labelled component will compete with it to such an extent that it will not be measured.

The drawbacks of competitive systems are the focus of two new immuno-assay systems which allow the determination of *analyte-bound* sites in excess-reagent systems.

In the first system, 'Anti-Immune Complex Immunoassay' (Self, 1985*a*), a secondary mab is raised which can specifically bind a receptor (such as a primary mab against a small molecular analyte) once it has bound the small molecule. As this secondary anti-complex antibody does not bind the analyte or primary antibody alone it can be employed to directly determine the primary antibody analyte-bound sites as in Figure 9.2. The resulting immunoassay system provides highly sensitive, precise, specific and extremely rapid assays as shown by clinical application in the determination of digoxin (C. H. Self, J. L. Dessi and L. A. Winger, submitted for publication).

The second system, is the 'Selective Antibody' system (Self, 1989). This is based on preparing a secondary antibody which can selectively bind a primary receptor (such as a mab against a small molecular analyte) bound with the small analyte but which cannot bind that receptor bound with a specific blocking substance such as a conjugate of the analyte or an anti-idiotypic antibody. The blocker thus prevents binding of the selective antibody which might occur with analyte-unbound primary receptor and thus allows the direct measurement of analyte-bound primary receptor sites as shown in Figure 9.3. As with the anti-complex approach, the general system is of very wide potential applicability (Self, 1989) and indeed has already been applied by others to give rise to an impressive immunometric assay for oestradiol (Barnard & Kohen, 1990).

9.5   Endogenous interference in immunoassays

It should be noted that notwithstanding the very high specificity selectable for mab, there is one troublesome feature of any two-site system that must not be overlooked: that of recognition of the antibody reagent components of the

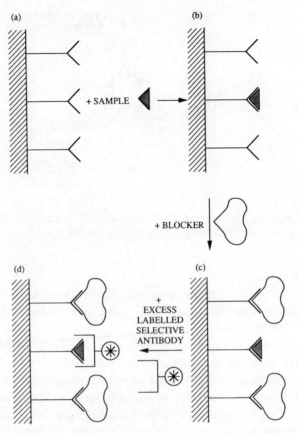

Figure 9.3. Selective antibody immunometric assay for a small analyte. (a) and (b) Analyte binds to antibody binding sites, (c) specific blocking agent saturates remaining sites, (d) labelled selective antibody binds to small analyte-bound sites.

system by broadly specific antibodies to non-human immunoglobulins (hetero-philic antibodies) in the samples under investigation. Such antibodies are capable of linking the detecting antibodies together (Figure 9.4) and as a result producing a signal which may be misinterpreted as that of the specific analyte. Conversely, if the reagent antibodies were from different species the interfering antibodies would be capable of binding to only one of them. A negative bias rather than a positive effect would be obtained if this binding, in addition, prevents reaction with a specific analyte and the excess of reagent antibody is not sufficient to overcome both analyte and interfering antibody.

It has been proposed that such effects may be reduced by employing antibody fragments, such as Fab fragments, instead of the intact immuno-globulin (Schroff *et al.*, 1985; Clark & Price, 1987). While certainly useful, such an approach is not always successful. As well as heterophilic antibodies having broad specificities, interfering antibodies have been found which bind to

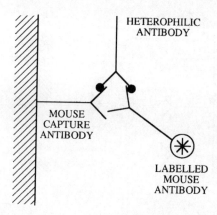

Figure 9.4. Capture and marker antibodies (mouse IgG) become linked by heterophilic, or specific anti-mouse, antibodies in a sample, giving rise to a false positive signal.

F(ab')$_2$ (Wolfe *et al.*, 1984), lactoperoxidase (Ericson & Larsson, 1984), agarose (Hamilton & Adkinson, 1985) and analyte itself (Braunstein *et al.*, 1983).

In current practice, however, it remains essential to counter anti-antibody effects by the inclusion in the incubation buffers of immunoglobulin of one or both of the detecting antibodies (for example mouse IgG in a mab system) so that any such antibody present is overwhelmed by the additional immuno-globulin and thus rendered incapable of reacting with the specific mononclonal immunoglobulins of the system. There is a report of the existence of hetero-philic antibodies in up to 40% of an Australian population (Boscato & Stuart, 1986). Bovine immunoglobulin or serum is often more efficient than mouse in eliminating the interference, supporting the view proposed by Hunter & Budd (1980) that the antibodies result from immunization against dietary components such as meat and milk. Specific anti-mouse antibodies can, however, arise in cases of therapeutic or diagnostic use *in vivo* of mouse mab.

Rheumatoid factors, mostly IgM autoantibodies, are capable of similar interference. Their affinity for the labelled antibodies in solution may not be sufficiently great for them to be as serious a problem as the heterophilic antibodies noted above. Mouse IgG rarely binds human rheumatoid factor and some authorities consider that the high frequency of interference observed in rheumatoid patients is in fact due to a concomitant high prevalence of antibodies directed against dietary immunoglobulins.

Autoantibodies are a further problem for certain specific analytes, the commonest causes for concern probably relating to analyses of thyroglobulin and insulin. In the latter case, antibodies can arise not only spontaneously but as a result of insulin treatment.

The problems of endogenous interference in the new generation of immuno-metric assays has recently been reviewed by Weber *et al.* (1990).

9.6   High-dose hook phenomenon

The phenomenon of the high-dose hook must always be borne in mind. This effect occurs at high antigen concentration where, apparently paradoxically, the signal rather than increasing with antigen concentration first exhibits a plateau and then actually begins to decrease (Figure 9.5) when the antigen is in excess. The explanation is that the amount of solid-phase 'catching' antibody is limiting. Thus at very high concentrations, antigen first having saturated the solid phase causing the plateau, eventually also saturates the labelled antibody and free antigen then begins to compete with the labelled antibody-antigen complex for the solid phase, resulting in the inversion.

In a clinically useful assay the hook region needs to be fixed at a level well in excess of the range expected to be encountered in practice but there are still situations where the range met may be so wide as to encompass the hook area. An example is with prolactinomas when the circulating concentrations of prolactin may be many hundreds of times higher than the values encountered in normal subjects. In such cases the danger is that such a high concentration may be disastrously misinterpreted as being normal if the concentration were sufficiently high for the inversion to have reached a signal representing normal values. Sequential addition of reagents so that unreacted antigen is removed by washing between steps will usually restrict the problem to that of a plateau, thus removing the danger of ambiguity. Samples giving a signal in the plateau region are thus indicated as needing repeating at dilution for absolute concentrations to be determined. The only absolutely reliable countermeasure is to assay all samples at two dilutions to check that on dilution the signal is not, apparently paradoxically, unchanged or higher.

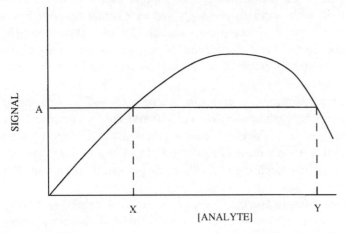

Figure 9.5. High-dose hook phenomenon (see text). The signal A may be interpreted as analyte concentration X or Y.

9.7   Use of established labelling technology

The initial applications of mab depended on the use of techniques which had
largely been developed for use with polyclonal antibodies involving some form
of labelling. Thus use of detection techniques involving radioisotopes (Butt,
1984), enzymes and enzyme amplification (Ishikawa, 1987), chemiluminescence (Weeks & Woodhead, 1984), enhanced chemiluminescence (Thorpe *et
al.*, 1985), fluorescence, (Hemmilä, 1985), time resolution fluorimetry (Diamandis, 1988) and avidin/biotin (Wilchek & Bayer, 1990) have been adequately reviewed. For a fully comprehensive account of immunoassay developments over the decade of the 1980s, the reader is referred to Gosling (1990).

In this chapter we discuss some exciting topics regarding 'ultrasensitivity', the
study of electrochemical labels and non-labelling procedures and methods that
will enable bedside and general practitioner estimations.

9.8   Sensitivity

Twenty-five years ago, microanalysis in clinical biochemistry might well have
meant the use of a 2 ml plasma sample for a non-specific estimation, for
example of a plasma steroid (Wootton, 1964). Simple and specific protein
analysis was for the most part merely a dream, still more so in the case of
peptide hormones. Nowadays, highly specific assays for a myriad of proteins,
peptides, steroids, drugs, etc. with immunochemical techniques are routine to
the District General Hospital laboratory and even a 100 μl sample can be
considered extravagant. Techniques have emerged for specific measurement of
protcins and peptides with sensitivity reported as high as 10^{-21} and 10^{-22}
moles.

Theoretical considerations of assay design and sensitivity have been the
subject of much controversy over the years. It is clear that the predicted
theoretical limits of immunoassay technology (Jackson & Ekins, 1986) are close
to being achieved both with competitive assays and excess reagent techniques
(in practice almost always the two-site approach). In the latter case the
sensitivity of a given analysis ultimately depends largely on the sensitivity of the
detection technique employed rather than on the characteristics of the antibodies used (Ekins, 1987).

The fact that pure preparations of mab can be characterized so well makes
them particularly useful for high sensitivity applications. This is important, for
example, in the preparation of labelled antibody conjugates of high specific
activity. Also the ability to obtain a constant supply of the defined reagent
means that, once developed, such high sensitivity assays can be reproduced at
will.

There are numerous reasons for the development of immunoassays of very
high sensitivity. The prime reason is of course to be able to detect materials
which would otherwise be undetectable. With high sensitivity immunoassays
new analytes may be studied and low concentrations of sub-populations of

existing analytes detected. The particular advantages in this respect can easily be imagined in the assessment of tumour markers, an expanding field of investigation (see Reckel, 1989), where perhaps earlier indicators may be vital in signalling the need for treatment.

In clinical practice it is not only the ability to detect analytes which is important but also the ability to investigate them at the 'lower limit of normal' and beyond. This reason was the force behind the development of highly sensitive immunoassays for TSH – the ability to measure down to the lower limit of normal concentration and distinguish those hyperthyroid individuals producing TSH at a level below this.

Clinically, there is also a clear requirement for highly sensitive methods which allow small sample volumes (ideally a capillary sample) to be sufficient and, where feasible, to use samples obtained by less invasive methods, such as saliva and urine where the concentration of analyte may be lower than that in the serum. For example using a mab-based procedure, it has recently been possible to determine HIV antibodies in urine: a far less hazardous sampling procedure than blood (Connell *et al.*, 1990).

The need for small samples is particularly important when there is a demand for frequent blood sampling or continuous monitoring (e.g. pulsatile hormone investigations). Multiple sampling of small quantities inevitably adds up to a much greater sum of blood required; this is an especial problem in small children. The availability of ultramicroanalysis, in modern terms, avoids the danger of relatively large blood sampling requirements from small children, even neonates, not to mention adults! Biosensor technology points towards new possibilities of chemical monitoring by sensors without the need for sampling.

The precision of assays may also be increased with increases in sensitivity. This may be a consequence of the assay no longer running at the limit of its sensitivity, removal of the need to concentrate or extract a sample before analysis or, conversely, the ability to dilute the sample thus reducing non-specific effects. Moreover, it becomes possible to analyse multiple samples from small animals such as mice which could be of enormous benefit to research and veterinary medicine.

9.9 Speed

Mab have been important in meeting the extremely urgent need for faster immunoassays. Not only is this important with respect to obtaining results more quickly but also in reducing the chance of analyte decay and thus imprecision during the analytical procedure. The excess antibody methods, which the availability of mab have made so popular, may be designed to run quickly because of the relatively high concentration of reagents in them causing antibody–antigen reactions to proceed more quickly than in competitive equilibrium methods. In addition, with a highly sensitive immunoassay, it is often possible to accept some reduction in sensitivity for an increase in speed, most notably in neonatal screening for congenital hypothyroidism using a TSH assay. Fast assays may be very important, for example as an aid in monitoring surgical removal of tumours or endocrine tissue during operation.

9.10   Convenience

Covenience is, in reality, a central requirement for immunoassays. They lend themselves to it and it is on this basis that they are often chosen in preference to other methods. Mab have helped greatly in this regard. Excess reagent assays have been shown to have extremely good precision, apparently more resistant than competitive formats to uncontrolled variation of concentration of the reagents during storage or performance of the assay. The consistency of reagents also allows ready comparison between different assay batches. In addition, mab lend themselves to the development of easy to use formats such as the liquid circuit immunoassay device (Bunce *et al.*, 1991).

Reliable and sensitive 'over the counter' pregnancy tests (for human chorionic gonadotrophin, hCG) are another example. In the latter case the 'hands-on' technology has of necessity become so simple, with visual endpoints, as to be operable by the general public. One frequently hears anecdotal evidence that these techniques may be more reliable than those used in some hospital laboratories who have not overcome their inertia to replacing the previous generation of technology!

One method employs polystyrene latex microparticles having a high anti-body-binding capacity agglomerated around the fibres of a glass membrane (Brown, 1987). The microparticles can be applied to the membrane in any shaped design. In the test pack the membrane contains two crossed 'lines' of immobilized reagents. The vertical line is prepared by covalently coupling an hCG-specific mab to the microparticles and applying a line of microparticles onto the membrane. The horizontal line also contains microparticles but with hCG immobilized on their surface. The patient's urine is added to a disposable reaction disc whereby the flow of specimen onto the reaction membrane is controlled. The assay is completed by the addition of enzyme-conjugated antibody, wash solution and substrate. This always results in the formation of a sandwich complex along the horizontal axis with the hCG already present (acting as a built-in procedural control). If the specimen contains hCG within the detection limit of the assay, a second complex is formed along the vertical axis resulting in a '+' sign and a '−' sign for negative specimens, negative specimens always producing this control result. The test can be completed in less than 4 min, typical of this type of over-the-counter technology.

These techniques have become so robust and reliable at these ultrasensitive levels that commercial procedures have even been introduced for LH so that mid-cycle fertility peaks can be determined on a 'home monitoring' basis, picking up the mid-cycle surge of LH for prediction of ovulation and the most fertile 2–3 days of the menstrual cycle (Unipath Ltd, Bedford, U.K.)

Quality control of this type of usage is often lacking and it is difficult to imagine how it could be done, although many 'over-the-counter' pregnancy test kits do include some form of check procedure.

9.11 Methods of detection

Speed, sensitivity and convenience have been important features in the development of methods of detection of antibodies. Many of these methods have found particular application with respect to mab. Rather than provide a comprehensive review of this large area we have concentrated on particular methods indicating what is possible to be achieved with mab given suitable methods of detection.

9.11.1 Enzyme labels

Initially, the direct application of enzyme labels to immunoassays was not as successful as had been expected. With improvements of materials, however, including solid phases on which to conduct the assays and labelling techniques, impressive sensitivities have been achieved with direct labels in the hands of dedicated workers (Ishikawa, 1987). It was, however, apparent that the activity of the enzyme label itself was often lacking and that if this could be increased then not only more sensitive but also more rapid immunoassays could be constructed. The need for assays with these characteristics plus convenience led to the development of enzyme amplification (Self, 1981). The method is based on causing the enzyme which is to be detected to make a substance which itself is catalytic for a secondary reaction. Thus the enzyme catalyst gives rise to another catalyst and amplification is achieved. This concept gave rise to extremely sensitive assays for alkaline phosphatase based on the enzyme dephosphorylating NADP to NAD which is then locked in a redox cycle. While the NAD co-factor is alternately reduced and then reformed to its original state by oxidation in the cycle, the activity of the cycle is monitored by measuring an irreversible reaction accompanying the cycle's operation. The most widely used configuration is shown in Figure 9.6. A colourless tetrazolium (iodonitrotetrazolium) is reduced to an intensely red coloured formazan; it is also conducted by entering the cycle from the other end as a result of allowing the enzyme to convert NADPH to NADH.

It was demonstrated that this method could be employed both with alkaline phosphatase as a label in an immunoassay or for the direct quantification of the enzyme as the analyte itself (Self, 1985b). This latter use was made particularly effective by means of first capturing the enzyme with a specific monoclonal antibody against the isoenzyme of interest before its assay by enzyme

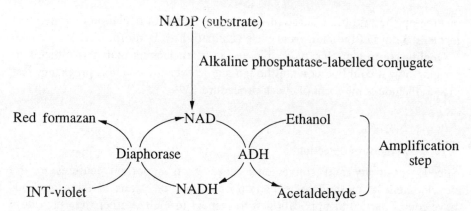

Figure 9.6. Principle of enzyme amplification in detection of alkaline phosphatase label and production of red formazan.

amplification. Warren *et al.* (1985) exploited this approach in a chorionic villus sampling diagnostic test for the severe infantile form of hypophosphatasia. The method has been found to be very effective when used in conjunction with monoclonal antibodies in immunometric assays. Johannsson *et al.* (1986) have demonstrated that the system allows the detection of 0.01 attomole of alkaline phosphatase and when employed in a mab-based assay for TSH the assay was shown to have a detection limit of 1.3 μ units/l (0.43 amol). Recently Cook and Self (1993) have demonstrated even greater sensitivity by employing fluorimetric detection (Figure 9.7). One-thousandth of an attomole (350 molecules) of alkaline phosphatase has been measured in a non-optimized system, enabling a mab-based immunoassay for proinsulin to be built with a sensitivity of 0.017 pmole/l (Cook & Self, 1993).

Colorimetric detection systems have a distinct advantage in terms of convenience: colorimeters are relatively simple and inexpensive and may even be dispensed with in certain applications where a visual recording suffices. They are, however, more restricted in their range of measurement than fluorimeters or electrochemical systems. This fact has led to applications of the amplification technology to include an electrochemical means to oxidise and measure the co-factor. Stanley *et al.* (1988) have employed a conducting salt electrode or potassium ferricyanide as an electron carrier from the cycle to a platinum electrode. An alternative application was made by Athey *et al.* (1991) who employed an NADH oxidase to produce hydrogen peroxide which was measured electrochemically. When applied to a mab-based TSH assay, a sensitivity of 0.4 mU/l was obtained. While the combination of these technologies still has some way to go their potential is clear.

Chemiluminescent detection methods for alkaline phosphatase have been described resulting in a TSH assay with a sensitivity of 4.5 μU/l (Bronstein *et al.*, 1989). A suitable reagent is available commercially under the trade name LUMI-PHOS (Schaap *et al.*, 1989).

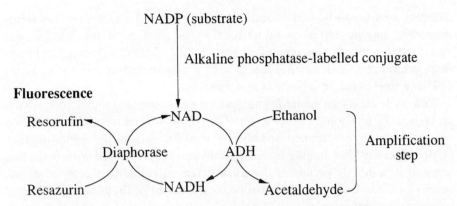

Figure 9.7. Fluorescence-amplified enzyme-linked immunoassay principle. The resorufin produced is quantified fluorimetrically at activation wavelength of about 560 nm and emission wavelength of about 580 nm.

9.11.2 *Ultrasensitivity with non-enzyme labels*

There are some other approaches that have permitted significant improvements in the sensitivity of detection. Notable among these are applications of chemiluminescence and fluorescence.

The most successful of the chemiluminescent compounds employed as labels has been the acridinium esters which react with hydrogen peroxide and require no catalyst. Some applications have been described by Weeks & Woodhead (1984). Again these labels provide more sensitive detection than ^{125}I and permit an assay for TSH that is capable of distinguishing the low levels found in hyperthyroidism from levels found in euthyroid individuals.

Time resolution fluorimetry has also proved to be an important technology. The process takes advantage of the fluorescence properties of lanthanide ion chelates (used as labels) which have a relatively long-lived fluorescence permitting them to be detected by time resolution techniques that distinguish the fluorescence produced in the test from the short-lived interfering background biological fluorescence. The large Stokes shift also leads to increased sensitivity of detection by permitting irradiation of the sample with a wide spectrum of light without the requirement to isolate narrow wavelengths, losing light intensity in the process.

An assay format that depends particularly on ultrasensitivity is the Ambient Analyte Immunoassay (Ekins & Chu, 1991). These authors have shown both theoretically and practically that fractional antibody occupancy (the key factor on which immunoassays depend) is independent of antibody concentration and sample volume *provided that* the antibody concentration used is 'vanishingly small'. From these principles Ekins has envisaged and developed the multi-analyte microspot assay which depends on a 'sensor' antibody (preferably monoclonal) deposited on a microspot of area approximately 100 μm^2. Such small areas of deposition permit arrays of microspots, each directed against a different analyte, to be accommodated within areas of about 1 cm². A signal depending on the ratios of fluorescent signal from both the 'sensor' and 'developing' antibodies is quantified with a dual channel scanning-laser confocal microscope. A demonstration of such a 'ratiometric' microspot assay for TSH as a single analyte is given as an example.

With such ability to quantify multiple analytes simultaneously, the advantages of mab technology become obvious, when several very closely related epitopes can be determined specifically and simultaneously. Ekins & Chu (1991) point out that finding immunoassays can be performed with these tiny amounts of antibody permitted the construction of antibody microspot arrays, enabling theoretically the simultaneous measurement of thousands of different substances in 1 ml samples.

9.11.3 Evanescent wave immunoassay

The evanescent wave technique depends on total internal reflection of a light beam within an optical waveguide, either a quartz slide or a fibre optic (Sutherland *et al.*, 1984*a*, *b*) to monitor immunological reaction at the quartz-liquid interface. The authors have exploited the principle to detect a fluorescent label.

9.11.4 Non-labelling detection of immunochemical reactions

Surface plasmon oscillation is a total internal reflection technique related to the evanescent wave technology used to study surface chemistry (Liedberg *et al.*, 1983). A similar application of the principle has also been described by Mayo & Hallock (1989). It has the entirely novel advantage of monitoring antibody–antigen reactions without the requirement for the use of a label. It depends on total internal reflection at an interface to monitor antigen–antibody reaction in a layer absorbed to the reflecting surface. Surface plasmon oscillations (resonances) are stimulated by the evanescent wave associated with total internal reflection.

For a specific wavelength of light there is an incident angle at which the beam of light hits the glass metal interface where light energy is maximally transferred to the metal layer thus causing a marked reduction in the measured reflection. This 'resonance angle' changes quantitatively with the deposition of protein on the metal surface and it can thus be used, for example, to follow the combination of antibody with its metal-associated antigen.

While the method suffers from relatively low sensitivity it has the advantage of not requiring a labelled component and allowing the interactions to be studied as they occur in 'real time'. This is particularly useful in establishing kinetic properties of mab such as association and dissociation constants (VanCott *et al.*, 1992).

Commercial equipment exploiting the phenomenon of surface plasmon resonance has already been introduced (BIAcore, Pharmacia) using a gold film which is more stable to buffer solutions (Liedberg *et al.*, 1983). It appears to be particularly valuable for epitope mapping of mab (Fägerstam *et al.*, 1990). An immunometric procedure for the clinical analysis of $beta_2$-microglobulin over the range 10–1000 $\mu g/l$ has been described (Pharmacia Biosensor AB, 1991). The technique is also applicable in competitive formats for the assay of small molecules, as exemplified by a BIAcore assay for theophylline (Pharmacia Biosensor AB, 1991).

9.12 Fibre optic sensors

One of the more attractive applications of the new technologies is the adaptation of biosensors for use as probes. The fluorescence energy transfer technique has been adapted to fibre optic technology (Anderson & Miller, 1988) in an assay for phenytoin where a reaction chamber is constructed of cellulose dialysis tubing cemented to an optical fibre. B-phycoerythrin-labelled phenytoin and Texas Red-labelled antibody to phenytoin were sealed inside the dialysis tubing. When the phenytoin reacts with the antibody, the B-phycoerythrin and Texas Red are brought into close proximity and non-radiative transfer of energy from B-phycoerythrin and Texas Red occurs, producing a quenching of B-phycoerythrin fluorescence. When the sensor is placed in a sample containing phenytoin, unlabelled drug diffuses into the reaction chamber and displaces the labelled phenytoin from the antibody thus causing an increase in B-phycoerythrin fluorescence which is monitored remotely with a fibre optic fluorimeter.

The sensor could apparently be used for about 30 single measurements. It is small enough to fit through a 23-gauge needle giving the intriguing potential for applications *in vivo* once problems of biocompatibility, stability and calibration have been solved. Such a design of course has the potential for the measurement of any small molecule for which an antibody is available and appears to be a highly practical alternative to electrochemical sensors presently being developed.

9.13 Future of monoclonal antibodies in diagnostics

The fact that mab are homogeneous characterizable populations opens up many chemical and genetic possibilities to change them in highly specific and controlled ways. For example, bispecific antibodies may be obtained by using heterobifunctional crosslinkers to simply crosslink the antibodies (Staertz *et al.*, 1985; Percz *et al.*, 1985). Alternatively, hybridomas may be fused with another cell line capable of giving rise to another antibody: the progeny producing a mixture of the various light and heavy chains in different associations (Milstein & Cuello, 1983). While the utility of this approach has been demonstrated with respect to somatostatin immunoassay it requires separation of the various species produced. It also provides an important tool for assessing the contribution of chain diversity to antibody characteristics and already appears to confirm the dominant role of heavy chain in antibody specificity (Hudson *et al.*, 1987).

The potential for changing mab at the genetic level to fit them for particular diagnostic applications is clearly very great. This includes being able to change specificity and association and dissociation rate constants. This may be achieved by subtle approaches such as variable region point mutation (Schildbach *et al.*, 1991). Gene transfection (Winter & Milstein, 1991) opens the possibility of being able to change and select suitable antibodies and then obtain them from a cellular source easier to grow and manipulate than hybridomas. Such manipulation may include the ability to genetically graft onto the antibody, during its biosynthesis, a label such as an enzyme that is to be detected in a subsequent immunoassay (Neuberger, 1985; Williams & Neuberger, 1986; Chapters 7 and 8).

Many antigens remain problematical in terms of having toxicity or low immunoreactivity. Direct injection of antigen into lymph nodes and the spleen was successfully introduced in the 1960s to counter the difficulties of raising polyclonal antisera against weakly antigenic small peptides, for example angiotensin (Boyd *et al.*, 1967). Sometimes the antigens were injected adsorbed to microfine carbon particles. The technique enabled the use of small quantities of antigen (20 μg), vital in cases where material was in very short supply. Clearly the technique lends itself to mab production. Spitz *et al.* (1984) described the production of mab from mice and rats which had received intrasplenic injections, again with small amounts of immunogen.

A further step possible, however, with mab production is the use of immunization *in vitro* (van Ness *et al.*, 1984) whereby additional advantages are obtained. Van Ness *et al.* employed antigen adsorbed to fumed silica microparticles for the presentation of both soluble and insoluble antigens. An important application of this approach may well be in the production of antibodies against toxic materials.

There is no doubt that there is an increasing momentum in the application of mab; the emergence of technologies dependent upon them and the introduction of methods involving them in routine clinical biochemistry will without doubt accelerate.

9.14   References

Addison, G. M. & Hales, C. N. (1971). Two site assay of human growth hormone. *Hormone and Metabolic Research*, **3**, 59–60.

Altamirano-Bustamante, A., Barnard, G. & Kohen, F. (1991). Direct time-resolved fluorescence immunoassay for serum oestradiol based on the idiotypic anti-idiotypic approach. *Journal of Immunological Methods*, **138**, 95–101.

Anderson, F. P. & Miller, W. G. (1988). Fiber optic immunochemical sensor for continuous, reversible measurement of phenytoin. *Clinical Chemistry*, **34**, 1417–1421.

Anon. (1976). Editorial. ELISA: a replacement for radioimmunoassay? *Lancet*, **2**, 406–407.

Armbruster, D. A. (1993). Prostate-specific antigen; Biochemistry, analytical methods and clinical application. *Clinical Chemistry*, **39**, 181–195.

Arrhenius, S. (1907). The employment of physical chemistry in the theory of immunity. *Hygeia*, **2**, 1–11.

Athey, D., McNeil, C. J. & Cooper, J. M. (1991). Enzyme amplified electrochemical immunoassay using thermostable NADH oxidase. *Proceedings of the Association of Clinical Biochemists National Meeting*, Glasgow 13–17 May, p. 112 (abstract).

Barnard, G. & Kohen, F. (1990). Idiometric assay; noncompetitive immunoassay for small molecules typified by the measurement of estradiol in serum. *Clinical Chemistry*, **36**, 1945–1950.

Boscato, L. M. & Stuart, M. C. (1986). Incidence and specificity of interference in two-site immunoassays. *Clinical Chemistry*, **32**, 1491–1495.

Boyd, G. W., Landon, J. & Peart, W. S. (1967). Radioimmunoassay for determining plasma-levels of angiotensin II in man. *Lancet*, **2**, 1002–1005.

Braunstein, G. D., Bloch, S. K., Rasor, J. L. & Winikoff, J. (1983). Characterisation of antihuman chorionic gonadotropin serum antibody appearing after ovulation induction. *Journal of Clinical Endocrinology and Metabolism*, **57**, 1164–1172.

Brawer, M. K., Chetner, M. P., Beatie, J., Buchner, D. M., Vessella, R. L. & Lange, P. H. (1992). Screening for prostatic carcinoma with prostate-specific antigen. *Journal of Urology*, **147**, 841–845.

Bronstein, I., Voyta, J. C., Thorpe, G. H. G., Kricka, L. J. & Armstrong, G. (1989). Chemiluminescent assay of alkaline phosphatase applied in an ultrasensitive enzyme immunoassay for thyrotropin. *Clinical Chemistry*, **35**, 1441–1446.

Brown, W. E. (1987). Microparticle-capture membranes: application to testpack hCG-urine. *Clinical Chemistry*, **33**, 1567–1568.

Bunce, R., Thorpe, G. & Keen, L. (1991). Disposable analytical devices permitting automatic, timed, sequential delivery of multiple reagents. *Analytica Chimica Acta*, **249**, 263–269.

Butt, W. R. (1984). Problems of iodination. In *Practical Immunoassay, The State of the Art*, ed. W. R. Butt, pp. 19–35. New York & Basel, Marcel Dekker.

Catalona, W. J., Smith, D. S., Ratliff, T. L., Dodds, K. M., Coplen, D. E., Yuan, J. J. J., Petros, J. A. & Andriole, G. L. (1991). Measurement of prostate-specific antigen in serum as a screening test for prostate cancer. *New England Journal of Medicine*, **324**, 1156–1161.

Carter, H. B., Pearson, J. D., Mettler, J., Brant, L. J., Chan, S. W., Andres, R., Fozard, J. L. and Walsh, P. C. (1992). Longitudinal evaluation of prostate-specific antigen levels in men with and without prostate disease. *Journal of the American Medical Association*, **267**, 2210–2215.

Choi, M. J., Choe, I. S., Kang, H. K., Lee, J. S. & Chung, T. W. (1991). Simple enzyme immunoassay for the simultaneous measurement of whole choriogonado-tropin molecules and free β-subunits in sera of women with abnormal pregnancies or tumours of the reproductive system. *Clinical Chemistry*, **37**, 673–677.

Clark, P. M. S. & Price, C. P. (1987). Removal of interference by immunoglobulins in an enzyme-amplified immunoassay for thyrotropin in serum. *Clinical Chemistry*, **33**, 414.

Collins, D. R., Wright, D. J., Rinsler, M. G., Thomas, P., Bhattacharya, S. & Raftery, E. B. (1993). Early diagnosis of acute myocardial infarction with use of a rapid immunochemical assay of creatine kinase MB isoenzyme. *Clinical Chemistry*, **39**, 1725–1728.

Connell, J. A., Parry, J. V., Mortimer, P. P., Duncan, R. J. S., McClean, K. A., Johnson, A. M., Hambling, M. H., Barbara, J. & Farrington, C. P. (1990). Preliminary report: accurate assays for anti-HIV in urine. *Lancet*, **335**, 1366–1369.

Cook, D. B. & Self, C. H. (1993). Determination of one-thousandth of an attomole (1 zeptomole) of alkaline phosphatase: application in an immunoassay of proinsulin. *Clinical Chemistry*, **39**, 965–971.

De Lauzon, S., El Jabri, J., Desfosses, B. & Cittanova, N. (1989). Improvement of estradiol enzymoimmunoassay, using a monoclonal antibody and an avidin/biotin amplification system. *Journal of Immunoassay*, **10**, 339–357.

Demers, L. M. (1991). Monoclonal antibodies to lutropin: are our immunoassays too specific? (Editorial). *Clinical Chemistry*, **37**, 311–312.

Diamandis, E. P. (1988). Immunoassays with time-resolved fluorescence spectroscopy: principles and applications. *Clinical Biochemistry*, **21**, 139–150.

Dray, F., Terqui, M., Desfosses, B., Chauffornier, J. M., Mowszowicz, I., Kahn, D., Rombauts, P. & Jayle, M. F. (1971). Propriétés d'immusérums anti 17β-oestradiol obtenus chez différentes espèces animales avec l'antigène 17β-oestradiol-6-0-carboxyméthoxime-sérum albumin de boeuf. *Comptes Rendus hebdomadaires des Séances de l'Académie des Sciences de Paris, Série D*, **273**, 2380–2383.

Ehrlich, P. (1897). Die Wertbemessung des Diphtherieheilserums und deren theoretische Grundlagen. *Klinische Jahrbuch*, **60**, 299–314.

Ehrlich, P. & Moyle, W. R. (1986). Ultrasensitive cooperative immunoassays with mixed monoclonal antibodies. *Methods in Enzymology*, **121**, 695–707.

Ehrlich, P., Moyle, W. R., Moustafa, Z. A. & Canfield, R. E. (1982). Mixing two monoclonal antibodies yields enhanced affinity for antigen. *Journal of Immunology*, **128**, 2709–2713.

Ekins, R. P. (1960). The estimation of thyroxine in human plasma by an electrophoretic technique. *Clinica Chimica Acta*, 453–459.

Ekins, R. P. (1987). An overview of present and future ultrasensitive non-isotopic immunoassay development. *Clinical Biochemistry Reviews*, **8**, 12–23.

Ekins, R. P. & Chu, F. W. (1991). Multianalyte microspot immunoassay – microanalytical 'compact disk' of the future. *Clinical Chemistry*, **37**, 1955–1967.

Ericsson, U. B. & Larsson, I. (1984). Interference of endogenous lactoperoxidase antibodies in a solid-phase immunosorbent radioassay for antibodies to protein hormones. *Clinical Chemistry*, **30**, 1836–1838.

Fägerstam, L. G., Frostell, Å., Karlsson, R., Kullman, M., Larsson, A., Malmqvist, M. & Butt, H. (1990). Detection of antigen-antibody interactions by surface plasmon resonance. Application to epitope mapping. *Journal of Molecular Recognition*, **3**, 208–214.

Ghosh, S. K. (1988). Production of monoclonal antibodies to estriol and their application in the development of a sensitive nonisotopic immunoassay. *Steroids*, **52**, 1–14.

Gorman, K. M. & Daiss, J. L. (1991). Antiidiotypic antibodies as alternative labels in competitive immunoassays for thyroxine. *Clinical Chemistry*, **37**, 1034 (abstract).

Gosling, J. P. (1990). A decade of development in immunoassay methodology. *Clinical Chemistry*, **36**, 1408–1427.

Gruber, M. & Durham, H. E. (1896). Eine neue Methode zur raschen Erkennung des Choleravibrio und des Typhusbacillus. *Münchener Medicinische Wochenschrift*, **43**, 285–286.

Hakomori, S.-I. (1989). Abberrant glycosylation in tumours and tumour-associated carbohydrate antigens. *Advances in Cancer Research*, **52**, 257–331.

Hamilton, R. G. & Adkinson, N. F. (1985). Naturally occurring carbohydrate antibodies: interference in solid-phase immunoassays. *Journal of Immunological Methods*, **77**, 95–108.

Hemmilä, I. (1985). Fluoroimmunoassays and immunofluorimetric assays. *Clinical Chemistry*, **31**, 359–370.

Hill, C. S. & Wolfert, R. L. (1989). The preparation of monoclonal antibodies which react preferentially with human bone alkaline phosphatase and not liver alkaline phosphatase. *Clinica Chimica Acta*, **186**, 315–329.

Hudson, N. W., Mudgett-Hunter, M., Panka, D. J. & Margolies, M. N. (1987). Immunoglobulin chain recombination among antidigoxin antibodies by hybridoma-hybridoma fusion. *Journal of Immunology*, **139**, 2715–2723.

Hunter, W. M. & Budd, P. S. (1980). Circulating antibodies to ovine and bovine immunoglobulin in healthy subjects: a hazard for immunoassays. *Lancet*, **2**, 1136.

Ishikawa, E. (1987). Development and clinical applications of sensitive enzyme immunoassays for macromolecular antigens – a review. *Clinical Biochemistry*, **20**, 375–385.

Jackson, T. M. and Ekins, R. P. (1986). Theoretical limitations on immunoassay sensitivity. Current practice and potential advantages of fluorescent Eu^{3+} chelates as non-radioisotopic tracers. *Journal of Immunological Methods*, **87**, 13–20.

Jackson, D. C., Poumbourios, P. & White, D. O. (1988). Simultaneous binding of two monoclonal antibodies to epitopes separated in sequence by only three amino acid residues. *Molecular Immunology*, **25**, 465–471.

Johannsson, A., Ellis, D. H., Bates, D. L., Plumb, A. M. and Stanley, C. J. Enzyme amplification for immunoassays. Detection limit of one hundredth of an attomole. *Journal of Immunological Methods*, **87**, 7–11, 1986.

Köhler, G. and Milstein, C. Continuous cultures of fused cells secreting antibody of predefined specificity. *Nature*, **256**, 495–497, 1975.

Kraus, R. (1897). Ueber specifische Reactionen in keimfreien Filtraten aus Cholera, Typhus und Pestbouillonculturen, erzeugt durch homologes Serum. *Wiener Klinische Wochenschrift*, **10**, 736–738.

Kunushima, S., Hayashi, K., Kobayashi, S., Naoe, T. and Ohno, R. (1991). New enzyme-linked immunosorbent assay for glycocalicin in plasma. *Clinical Chemistry*, **37**, 169–172.

Larue, C., Calzolari, C., Léger, J., Léger, J. & Pau, B. (1991). Immunoradiometric assay of myosin heavy chain fragments in plasma for investigation of myocardial infarction. *Clinical Chemistry*, **37**, 78–82.

Lewis, J. G., Manley, L., Whitlow, J. C. & Elder, P. A. (1992). Production of a monoclonal antibody to cortisol: application to a direct enzyme-linked immunosorbent assay of plasma. *Steroids*, **57**, 82–85.

Liedberg, B., Nylander, C. & Lundström, I. (1983). Surface plasmon resonance for gas detection and biosensing. *Sensors and Actuators*, **4**, 299–304.

Mayo, C. S. & Hallock, R. B. (1989). Immunoassay based on surface plasmon oscillations. *Journal of Immunological Methods*, **120**, 105–114.

Miles, L. E. M. & Hales, C. N. (1968). Labelled antibodies and immunological assay systems. *Nature*, **219**, 186–189.

Milstein, C. & Cuello, A. C. (1983). Hybrid hybridomas and their use in immuno-histochemistry. *Nature*, **305**, 537–540.

Neuberger, M. S. (1985). Making novel antibodies by expressing transfected immunoglobulin genes. *Trends in Biochemical Science*, **10**, 347–349.

Nilsson, O., Bæckström, D., Johannsson, C., Karlsson, B. & Lindholm, L. (1988). CA-50 and related tumour-associated antigens. *Scandinavian Journal of Clinical and Laboratory Investigation*, **48** (Suppl. 190) S3 41–44.

Parvaz, P., Mathian, B., Patricot, M. C., Garcia, I., Revol, A., Mappus, E. Grenot, C. & Cuilleron, C. Y. (1989). Production of monoclonal antibodies to dehydro-epiandrosterone-sulphate after immunization of mouse with dehydroepian-drosterone-bovine serum albumin conjugate. *Journal of Steroid Biochemistry*, **32**, 553–558.

Perez, P., Hoffman, W. R., Shaw, S., Bluestone, A. J. & Segal, D. M. (1985). Specific targeting of cytotoxic T cells by anti-T3 linked to anti-target cell antibody. *Nature*, **316**, 354–356.

Pettersson, K., Ding, Y.-Q. & Huhtaniemi, I. (1991). Monoclonal antibody based discrepancies between two-site immunometric tests for lutropin. *Clinical Chemistry*, **37**, 1745–1748.

Pettersson, K. S. I. & Söderholm, J. R.-M. (1991). Individual differences in lutropin immunoreactivity revealed by monoclonal antibodies. *Clinical Chemistry*, **37**, 333–340.

Pharmacia Biosensor AB. (1991). *Application notes 201 and 202*. Pharmacia Biosensor AB, Milton Keynes MK5 8PH, U.K.

Potocnjak, P., Zavala, F., Nussenzweig, R. & Nussenzweig, V. (1982). Inhibition of idiotypic-anti-idiotype interaction for detection of a parasite antigen: a new immunoassay. *Science*, **215**, 1637–1639.

Price, C. P., Mitchell, C. & Noonan, K. (1993). Validation of an immunoradiometric assay for skeletal alkaline phosphatase. *Proceedings of the ACB National Meeting*, Association of Clinical Biochemists, Birmingham, 19–23 April 1993, p. 78 (abstract).

Rattle, S. J., Purnell, D. R., Williams, P. I. M., Siddle, K. & Forrest, G. C. (1984). New separation method for monoclonal immunoradiometric assays and its application to assays for thyrotropin and human chorionic gonadotropin. *Clinical Chemistry*, **27**, 1797–1806.

Reckel, R. (1989). Monoclonal antibodies: clinical applications. *Advances in Clinical Chemistry*, **27**, 355–415.

Schaap, A. P., Akhavan, H. & Romano, L. J. (1989). Chemiluminescent substrates for alkaline phosphatase: application to ultrasensitive enzyme-linked immunoassays and DNA probes. *Clinical Chemistry*, **35**, 1863–1864.

Schildbach, J. F., Panka, D. J., Parks, D. R., Jager, G. C., Novotny, J., Herzenberg, L. A., Mudgett-Hunter, M., Bruccoleri, R. E., Haber, E. & Margolies, M. N. (1991). Altered hapten recognition by two anti-digoxin hybridoma variants due to variable region point mutations. *Journal of Biological Chemistry*, **266**, 4640–4647.

Schroff, R. W., Foon, K., Beatty, S. M., Oldham, R. K. & Morgan, A. C. (1985). Human anti-murine immunoglobulin responses in patients receiving monoclonal antibody therapy. *Cancer Research*, **45**, 879–885.

Self, C. H. (1981). Assay method using enzymes as labelling substances. *European Patent Publication* number 0027036.

Self, C. H. (1985*a*). Antibodies, manufacture and use. *World Intellectual Property Organisation International Publication* number 85/04422, 1985.

Self, C. H. (1985*b*). Enzyme amplification – a general method applied to provide an immunoassisted assay for placental alkaline phosphatase. *Journal of Immunological Methods*, **76**, 389–393.

Self, C. H. (1989). Method, use and components. *World Intellectual Property Organisation International Publication*, number 89/05453.

Spitz, M., Spitz, L., Thorpe, R., & Eugui, E. (1984). Intrasplenic primary immunization for the production of monoclonal antibodies. *Journal of Immunological Methods*, **70**, 39–43.

Staertz, U. D., Kanagawa, O. & Bevan, M. J. (1985). Hybrid antibodies can target sites for attack by T cells. *Nature*, **314**, 628–631.

Stamey, T. A., Graves, H. C. B., Wehner, N., Ferrari, M. & Freiha, F. (1993). Early detection of residual prostate cancer after radical prostatectomy by an ultrasensitive assay for prostate-specific antigen. *Journal of Urology*, **149**, 787–792.

Stanley, C. J., Cox, R. B., Cardosi, M. F. & Turner, A. P. F. (1988). Amperometric enzyme-amplified immunoassays. *Journal of Immunological Methods*, **112**, 153–161.

Sutherland, R. M., Dähne, C., Place, J. F. & Ringrose, A. R. (1984*a*). Immunoassays at quartz-liquid interface: theory, instrumentation and preliminary application to the fluorescent immunoassay of human immunoglobulin G. *Journal of Immunological Methods*, **74**, 253–256.

Sutherland, R. M., Dähne, C., Place, J. F. & Ringrose, A. R. (1984*b*). Optical detection of antibody-antigen reactions at a glass-liquid interface. *Clinical Chemistry*, **30**, 1533–1538.

Thompson, R. E., Hewitt, C. R., Piper, D. J., Hanse, W. P., Rubin, R. H., Tolkoff-Rubin, N. E., Barrett, M. C. & Nelles, M. J. (1985). Competitive idiotype-anti-idiotype immunoassay for adenosine deaminase binding protein in urine. *Clinical Chemistry*, **31**, 1833–1837.

Thorpe, G. H. G., Kricka, L. J., Moseley, S. B. & Whitehead, T. P. (1985). Phenols as enhancers of the chemiluminescent horseradish peroxidase-luminol-hydrogen peroxide reaction: application in luminescence-monitored enzyme immunoassays. *Clinical Chemistry*, **31**, 1335–1341.

Valentine, R. C. & Green, M. M. (1967). Electron microscopy of an antibody-hapten complex. *Journal of Molecular Biology*, **27**, 615–617.

Van Ness, J., Laemmli, U. K. & Pettijohn, D. E. (1984). Immunization *in vitro* and production of monoclonal antibodies specific to insoluble and weakly immunogenic proteins. *Proceedings of the National Academy of Sciences U.S.A.*, **81**, 7897–7901.

VannCott, T. C., Loomis, L. D., Redfield, R. D. & Birx, D. L. (1992). Real-time biospecific interaction analysis of antibody reactivity to peptides from the envelope glycoprotein, gp160 of HIV-1. *Journal of Immunological Methods*, **146**, 163–176.

Warren, R. C., Rodeck, C. H., Brock, D. J. H., McKenzie, C. F., Moscoso, G. & Barron, L. (1985). First trimester diagnosis of hypophosphatasia with a monoclonal antibody to the liver/bone/kidney isoenzyme of alkaline phosphatase. *Lancet*, **2**, 856–858.

Weber, T. H., Käpyaho, K. I. & Tanner, P. (1990). Endogenous interference in immunoassays in clinical chemistry. A review. *Scandinavian Journal of Clinical and Laboratory Investigation*, **50** (Suppl. 201), 77–82.

Weeks, I. & Woodhead, J. S. (1984). Chemiluminescence immunoassay. *Journal of Clinical Immunoassay*, **7**, 82–89.

Widal, G. F. I. & Sicard, A. (1896). Recherche de la réaction agglutinante dans le sang et le sérum desséchés des typhiques et dans la sérosité des vésicatoires. *Bulletins et Mémoires de la Société Médicale des Hôpitaux de Paris*, **13**, 681–682.

Wilchek, M. & Bayer, E. A. (eds). (1990). Avidin-biotin technology. *Methods in Enzymology*, **184**,

Williams, G. T. & Neuberger, M. S. (1986). Production of antibody-tagged enzymes by myeloma cells: application to DNA polymerase I Klenow fragments. *Gene*, **43**, 319–324.

Winter, G. & Milstein, C. (1991). Man-made antibodies. *Nature*, **349**, 293–299.

Wolfe, L. D., Abruzzo, J. L. & Heimer, R. (1984). Specificity of IgM antibodies to pooled human F(ab′)$_2$ fragments. *Immunological Communications*, **13**, 15–27.

Woodhead, J. S. & Weeks, I. (1985). Circulating thyrotrophin as an index of thyroid function. *Annals of Clinical Biochemistry*, **22**, 455–459.

Wootton, I. D. P. (1964). *Micro-Analysis in Medical Biochemistry*, London, Churchill. pp. 177–183.

Yalow, R. S. and Berson, S. A. (1959). Assay of plasma insulin in human subjects by immunological methods. *Nature*, **185**, 1648–1649.

Yalow, R. S. and Berson, S. A. (1971). In *Principles of Competitive Protein-Binding Assays*, ed. W. D. Odell & W. H. Daughaday, pp. 1–24. Philadelphia, Lippincott.

Zegers, N. D., Claasen, E., Gerritse, K., Deen, C. & Boersma, W. J. A. (1991). Detection of genetic variants of α_1-antitrypsin with site-specific monoclonal antibodies. *Clinical Chemistry*, **37**, 1606–1611.

Zeuthen, J. (1988). Applications of monoclonal antibodies in clinical chemistry. *Scandinavian Journal of Clinical and Laboratory Investigation*, **S9** (Suppl. 190), 110–113.

Note added in proof

Since this chapter went to press, a new variant haemoglobin, Hb TYNE has been identified following an observation of an unexpectedly low result in a frankly diabetic patient using a mab based enzyme immunoassay for glycated haemoglobin. Evidence suggests that Hb TYNE differs by only one amino acid from normal haemoglobin, in that the single proline residue in the βT1 peptide is replaced by serine. This single substitution results in the inability of the mab used in the assay to recognize it. This is a further example of such a potential pitfall in the use of mab; users must be alert to the implications of unexpected results in routine diagnostic situations.

Gibb, I., Williamson, D., Pulman, G. & Barker, J. (1994). Identification of a new haemoglobin variant; Hb TYNE (β5(A2)Pro→Ser). *Proceedings of the Association of Clinical Biochemists National Meeting*, Brighton, 9–13 May 1994, p. 56 (abstract).

10A

Monoclonal antibodies in oncology: diagnostic pathology

A. COLFOR and P. A. HALL

10A.1 Introduction

For more than a century histopathological diagnosis has been based on the morphological analysis of tissue sections stained with a range of tinctorial reagents. More recently, the availability of electron microscopy added a further dimension to pathological studies. These morphological methods for defining the phenotype of cells and tissues have in the past decade been revolutionized by the ability to define the presence or absence of particular antigens using immunohistological methods. The use of immunohistological methods is now widespread for the resolution of differential diagnoses in many areas of diagnostic pathology, in particular in cancer diagnosis. In addition, there is increasing evidence that the definition of phenotypes may be of prognostic value, at least in some tumours. Furthermore, the use of immunohistological methods has been a great impetus to investigative studies. In this brief review the scope of such approaches will be summarized and the advantages and limitations will be addressed. Finally, possible future developments will be discussed.

10A.2 Genotype and phenotype

With the exception of those cells that rearrange their antigen receptor genes (B and T lymphocytes), it is widely held that all somatic cells in an organism possess the same complement of genes or genotype. In contrast, it is evident that the pattern of expression of that genotype (i.e. phenotype) differs radically between cells of different tissues and often within a tissue. For example, in humans there are estimated to be about 10^5 genes encoded by about 6×10^9 nucleotides. While there will be a subset of 'housekeeping' genes whose expression is common to many cell types, other genes will be expressed in a spatially and temporally regulated manner: this defining both the process and state of differentiation.

The practice of pathology has in the past relied heavily on the characterization of phenotype or state of differentiation using morphological methods (morphophenotype). This is now often supplemented by the use of objective antibody markers of specific gene products (immunophenotype). Consequently, when considering the value of immunophenotype in pathology, it is self-evident that this is an adjunct to conventional morphological diagnosis: providing a further insight into the phenotype of a cell, not replacing the insight provided by conventional morphological analysis. Perhaps the greatest value of immunohistochemistry is the bringing to pathology of the specificity of antigen–antibody interactions with the preservation of those facets of conventional pathology, cellular and tissue architecture which are central to conventional diagnosis.

10A.3   Use of immunohistochemistry in diagnostic pathology

Evidence for the rapid increase in use of immunohistochemistry in pathology comes from several sources. An analysis of the proportion of research papers in British pathology journals during the 1980s shows the rapid rise in the use of antibodies for demonstration of antigens in tissue sections and cytological material (Hall *et al.*, 1987). But the use of immunohistochemistry has not merely been a research tool! Surveys of the use of immunohistochemistry in diagnostic pathology laboratories revealed that by 1986, nearly all surgical pathology departments had available to them some level of immunohistochemistry, while 7 years earlier the figure was less than 10% (Hall *et al.*, 1987; Angel *et al.*, 1989). Identical trends have been observed elsewhere in Europe and North America.

   This rapid impact in day-to-day routine surgical pathology has been for two principal reasons. First, important early studies from several groups but notably Gatter and Mason in Oxford (Gatter *et al.*, 1982, 1985) demonstrated the value of antibodies that allow the distinction of lymphoid and epithelial phenotypes in morphologically undifferentiated neoplasms. This was of particular note because of the existence of therapeutic regimens suitable for successfully treating high grade lymphomas. The second major reason was the relative cheapness and robustness of the technique. One estimate suggested that the total cost of immunohistochemistry in diagnostic pathology for England and Wales was less that £5 000 000 in 1988 (Gatter, 1989). While the relevance of such data are questionable (do they really include all costs, such as staff salaries and capital charges?), they do indicate the relative cheapness of diagnostic immunohistochemistry compared with for example radiology.

10A.4   Use of immunohistochemistry in diagnosis

In histopathology, it is generally the case that the majority of diagnoses can be made using haematoxylin and eosin stained sections in the light of the relevant clinical data. There exists a residue of cases (principally tumours), however, where there are real diagnostic difficulties, usually as a consequence of there being a limited number of differential diagnoses for a given case. In the past the primary means of resolving such diagnostic dilemmas was the use of electron microscopy or conventional histochemical techniques. These techniques still have considerable use in carefully selected cases and their application should not be abandoned. Nevertheless, it is clear that immunohistochemistry has in many situations supplanted these conventional diagnostic strategies. In some situations they are inferior to immunohistochemistry. For example in the identification of endocrine cells and their hormonal contents, the use of silver stains and the argentaffin reaction have largely been replaced by immunostaining using antibodies to components of neurosecretory granules including hormones and their precursors. In addition to being more specific, immunological methods may actually be cheaper, quicker and more reproducible than capricious and costly silver-based histochemical methods.

The range of antibodies that are now available for use in resolving differential diagnostic problems is large (see other chapters in this volume) and will not be reviewed here. We will focus, however, on practical and theoretical problems in the use of such reagents. A frequently overlooked area, in busy surgical pathology laboratories, is the importance of meticulous quality control over the technical aspects of immunohistochemistry whether they relate to factors prior to immunostaining such as fixation, processing or section heating or to the immunostaining procedure itself. Poor audit of technical quality of immunohistochemistry will inevitably lead to incorrect diagnoses being made.

In the early days of diagnostic immunohistochemistry the majority of antibodies available only recognized antigens that were sensitive to fixation and embedding in conventional histological practice; thus most immunostaining was performed on cryostat sections. Indeed there was for many years a suspicion that much of immunohistochemistry was based in some 'black art'. Over the past decade immunohistochemistry has become progressively easier, particularly with the availability of very well standardized and robust commercial kit-based detection systems. In addition, there are now very many antibodies that recognize fixation and processing resistant epitopes and are thus (at least in theory) ideal for use in surgical pathology.

A number of important caveats remain. First, while immunohistochemistry has become easier, the production of reproducible, high quality preparations still depends on high technical standards (details of buffer composition are of particular note) and the obligatory use of appropriate technical controls. A second point relates to the question of fixation. Certainly it is true that many antibodies recognize fixation-resistant epitopes; however, in many cases the resistance of epitopes to fixation is *relative* and not *absolute*. For example, proliferating cell nuclear antigen (PCNA) can be recognized by a number of antibodies in fixed and wax-embedded material (Waseem & Lane, 1990). Prolonged fixation, however, can dramatically reduce immunoreactivity (Hall *et al.*, 1990). Furthermore, different fixatives and variation in a range of ambient conditions (especially temperature) can significantly alter detectable antigen. Another significant parameter is the practice of baking wax sections onto glass: many antigens do not survive this well, again PCNA is an example (Wakins et al., 1991)[1]. With every antibody employed in a diagnostic laboratory the operating characteristics of the reagent should be well documented by experimentation in that setting.

An important, but under-investigated, aspect of immunohistochemistry in clinical practice is the objective assessment of its true value. Dogma states that immunohistochemistry is of great value in resolving differential diagnostic problems: this is certainly true . . . in some situations . . . some of the time! A study reported by d'Ardenne et al. (1986) indicated that in tumour pathology immunohistochemistry was of objective value in 72% of cases whereas in 28% it did not provide information of discriminant value. Similar data was obtained from a survey of British pathologists (Hall et al., 1987). The cynic might argue that it is not uncommon for surgical pathologists to request immunohistological studies on difficult cases, then only to ignore results that do not fit with the previously favoured differential: if the data don't fit . . . discard the data! Is it not possible that immunohistochemistry is sometimes ordered in a particular case as a delaying tactic? Obviously these are extreme situations. It must be recognized that it is often those cases that give the most diagnostic difficulty using conventional morphological criteria that are the most difficult to interpret when immunohistological methods are used. A particular component of this problem is the truism that when antibodies are assessed for their value in some differential diagnostic problem, then the range of samples of a given condition studied are usually selected as being representative clear-cut examples. Under such circumstances it may appear that immunoreactivity with this antibody is a good operational marker of the disease in question. This is fine, but we must ask as to how relevant such data are in the context of 'the difficult case'. Clearly, any immunohistological marker (or panel of markers, as there is general agreement that panels of antibodies are often more informative than the use of a single reagent) should be tested in a truly representative group of cases (typical of the kind of cases for which the antibody is being proposed as a marker) and independently confirmed. Only then can the value of the antibody (or panel) be truly assessed.

The use of some form of meta-analysis has been advocated as a means of generating useful data on the value of antibodies, singly and in panels. For example, Hall & d'Ardenne (1987) reported a detailed analysis of studies using antibodies of the CD15 cluster in the diagnosis of Hodgkin's disease. Such an analysis led to the proposal that CD15 immunostaining was neither a sensitive nor specific marker of Sternberg–Reed cells. Similar strategies have been employed by a number of groups and some have incorporated this strategy into computer-based systems for determining the most informative groups of antibodies in particular diagnostic settings (Harkin et al., 1990). Most of the data

---

[1] Note: why section heating should be so damaging when the tissue block is similarly heated in the embedding phase is unclear but may relate to oxidation events being possible on the exposed surface of sections which are not possible in solid tissue blocks.

employed in these analyses are based on 'good' examples, as argued above, and so it is difficult to accept that conclusions drawn are necessarily relevant to diagnostically difficult cases. A successful scheme has been described by Reynolds (1989).

A further aspect of the same problem relates to quality control in the interpretation of immunohistochemistry. This is an aspect of the subject to which far too little attention has been paid in the past. There is considerable scope for prospective studies of the reproducibility of performance and interpretation of immunohistochemistry and an assessment of its real objective value in diagnostic pathology. Given the large amount of immunohistochemistry being performed and the public funds used it behoves us to perform this audit.

10A.4.1 Benign versus malignant

By way of an illustrative example, we shall consider perhaps the most thorny issue in surgical immunohistopathology: the distinction of benign from malignant cellular proliferations. In some cell types there exist objective markers which can be employed to infer neoplasia. The best known of these is the demonstration of light chain restriction in B cell lymphoproliferations; however, there are problems: both theoretical and practical. Light chain restriction is not necessarily synonymous with clonality because it is theoretically possible for an immune response to be predominantly composed of one light chain type (as has been described in experimental animals and in autoimmunity) (Jasani, 1988). Demonstration of light chain restriction remains one of the most demanding immunohistological techniques, particularly in fixed and wax-embedded material. Similar strategies may be used to demonstrate restricted T cell receptor beta chain V region usage (Clark *et al.*, 1986): again this may occur in the context of certain non-neoplastic immune responses. Finally, lymphomas without detectable gene rearrangements are being described (Nakamura & Suchi, 1991) and thus the absence of demonstrable clonality may not preclude a diagnosis of neoplasia.

In the early 1980s, McGee and co-workers made remarkable claims for an antibody designated Ca1 (McGee *et al.*, 1982). In particular, it was proposed that this reagent would facilitate the distinction of benign (no Ca1 immunoreactivity) from malignant (Ca1 positive). In fact the antibody Ca1 recognizes a mucin molecule which is certainly expressed by (at least some) neoplastic epithelia but is also widely present in a range of non-neoplastic epithelia (and other tissues). This rapidly became well known and remains a caution to all who seek the ideal 'tumour marker'. How could this occur? The reasons are complex but perhaps the most persuasive and significant is the relatively limited number of cases studied.

More recently it has become clear that the tumour suppressor gene p53 is a frequent target for molecular alteration (either by mutation or by allelic deletion) in a wide range of neoplasms (Lane & Benchimol, 1990; Levine *et al.*, 1991). A particular property of the p53 protein is its very short half-life such that it is undetectable in normal cells. The presence of mutations in the p53 gene may lead to protein with altered conformation and half-life. This leads to the accumulation of protein to levels detectable by conventional immunohistological methods. Consequently it has been proposed that detection of p53 protein may indicate neoplasia. Until recently this was the generally accepted dogma and indeed we reported the possible diagnostic utility of p53 staining in cytopathology as an adjunct to conventional morphology (Hall *et al.*, 1991). As with Ca1, there may be exceptions. p53 immunoreactivity can be detected in normal thymocytes (B. Ansari *et al.*, unpublished data), in UV exposed human keratinocytes (Hall *et al.*, 1993) and in heat shocked or mitomycin treated normal human peripheral blood lymphocytes (Hall *et al.*, 1993). It may be that there are a number of situations where p53 protein accumulates, including situations associated with DNA damage (UV irradiation, mitomycin) and apoptosis (thymocytes). Again this points to the need for careful analysis of large numbers of cases from a very wide range of conditions before absolute reliance is placed on an immunohistological technique. It emphasizes that immunohistological data cannot be interpreted in isolation: it is an adjunct to other diagnostic processes and data have to be interpreted cautiously.

Another approach to the identification of malignancy has been the proposal that aberrant phenotype may be associated with neoplasia. This has most frequently been reported in lymphoid tissues (Picker *et al.*, 1987) but may occur in other cell populations.

10A.5   Immunohistochemistry as an educational aid

One possible role for immunohistochemistry, which should not be underestimated, is as an aid in the training of neophyte microscopists. Trainee pathologists may test their skills in assessing morphological appearances against a 'benchmark' of immunohistochemistry, thus building knowledge and experience of diagnosis and developing confidence. For example, although the distinction of low and high-grade non-Hodgkin's lymphoma can usually be made by examination of conventional fixed histological sections, the use of antibodies that recognize proliferation associated antigens (see below) may aid this therapeutically vital decision and make it more objective, particularly helping those pathologists with relatively limited experience in lymphoma pathology.

10A.6   Use in prognosis

One of the great hopes for immunohistochemistry has been the possibility that objective definition of antigen expression might provide prognostic information either for the individual patient and (or) for patient subgroups who might be given different therapies. With notable exceptions this hope has not yet been fulfilled but important exceptions are worthy of mention.

On the basis of a small series of cases, Salmon *et al*. (1987) reported that amplification of the *c-erb*B-2 gene is associated with an adverse prognosis in breast cancer. Identification of overexpression of the oncoprotein *c-erb*B-2, which is associated with gene amplification (Venter *et al*., 1987), has since been shown in several large series to be an adverse prognostic factor in breast cancer. Prognostic relevance in other tumour types is much less well established at present. Prognostic significance for expression of other growth factor receptors, such as the EGF receptor, has been claimed in a number of settings (Sainsbury *et al*., 1985, 1987). In addition, recent data point to expression of the p53 tumour suppressor gene as an adverse prognostic factor in several tumour types. The possibility that these, and related, gene products (which are associated either with early events in neoplasia and/or with tumour progression) may be of prognostic significance is very attractive, particularly given the relative ease with which they can be demonstrated. Identification of expression of molecules associated with tumour spread, whether metastasis gene products (e.g. nm23) or adhesion molecules (e.g. LFA-1) are other potential immunohistological targets which may provide prognostic information.

In the majority of cases, however, there are still insufficient data on which to decide the truth of any claims made. How should potential claims be assessed? There are three steps in assessing the value of a potential prognostic marker. First, there should be some good rational reason for the clinical association: ideally the function of the target molecule should be understood (at least in part). Second, there should be data from a large clinical study indicating the prognostic value and the types of parameter that should be quantified. Of particular note here is that the study should be of sufficient size to give it significant statistical power. It should be remembered that even small differences may be important in some clinical groups, but must be tested in appropriate multivariate models (e.g. the Cox proportional hazards model). The patient population studied should be well-defined and documented. Finally, the significance of any potential clinical difference must be tested in a second, independent, data set.

10A.6.1 Markers of cell proliferation

An attractive application of immunohistochemistry which may have prognostic significance is the definition of levels and distribution of antigens with clear functional relevance to aspects of cellular proliferation. Pathologists have for some time recognized the possible diagnostic and prognostic value of assessing cell proliferation (Hall & Levison, 1990). A range of methods exists for assessing proliferation (Hall *et al*., 1992), all of which have technical and other disadvantages. The identification of specific proliferation-associated antigens has led to the extensive use of immunohistochemistry in studying proliferation (Hall & Woods, 1990). Particular advantages of this approach are the relative ease of the technique and the retention of the spatial relationships of the cells and tissue, which is not seen with flow cytometric methods for example.

In some tumours evidence has accrued that indices of proliferation can provide prognostically relevant data. For example, Hall *et al.* (1988) showed that the use of the mab Ki67 (which recognizes a nuclear antigen expressed in all phases of the cell cycle except G_0) could distinguish between low-grade (relatively indolent) and high-grade (aggressive) forms of non-Hodgkin's lymphoma. Furthermore, within the high-grade tumours enumeration of the number of Ki67 immunoreactive cells could identify a subgroup with a particularly bad outlook. Similar studies have been reported using a range of parameters of cellular proliferation in histological material in non-Hodgkin's lymphoma and a range of other tumour subtypes (Hall & Levison, 1990).

While immunocytochemical methods have notable advantages (reviewed in Hall & Woods, 1990), currently available antibodies such as Ki67 are only active in snap-frozen material and thus require special specimen handling. Finally, the information provided by these methods is limited in that it (1) provides information about the state of cell proliferation rather than rate, and (2) fails to provide information about the number and distribution of growth-arrested cells or those cells committed to or undergoing programmed cell death (apoptosis). Using recombinant DNA technology mabs have been generated that recognize PCNA (proliferating cell nuclear antigen) in fixed and wax-embedded material (Waseem & Lane, 1990, Hall *et al.*, 1990). The spatial distribution of PCNA immunoreactivity correlates very well with other parameters of cell proliferation in normal tissues; PCNA immunoreactivity parallels that of Ki67 in phorbol ester-treated HL60 cells and with bromodeoxyuridine incorporation in peripheral blood mononuclear cells. The simple enumeration of PCNA immunoreactive cells in non-Hodgkin's lymphoma, gastric carcinomas and in a subclass of soft tissue tumours (haemangiopericytomas) can provide prognostically relevant information. The third phase, however, must now involve the establishment in second data sets of the veracity of these preliminary observations.

10A.7 Histogenesis versus differentiation

Throughout tumour pathology the confusion between the terms histogenesis and differentiation persists. By histogenesis is meant the cell or tissue of origin of a tumour. The phenotype of a tumour resembles some normal tissue to a greater or lesser degree; therefore the tumour arose in the cells of that normal tissue. Such a histogenetic argument based on phenotypic similarities is not unreasonable in many situations but cannot be considered proof of the hypothesis (Gould, 1986; reviewed in Hall, 1991). Perhaps the most common misuse of immunohistochemistry is the extension of this confusion of the difference between histogenesis and differentiation. The published record is full of statements (many ludicrous in their naivity) suggesting that the expression in neoplastic cells of some marker or other indicates that the tumour arose in some normal tissue which expresses the same antigen. Almost invariably the data presented does not allow rigourous distinction between the hypothesis that tumour X expressed antigen Y, normally expressed on tissue Z, therefore tumour X arose in tissue Z and the alternative possibility that tumour X is differentiating towards the phenotype typical of tissue Z.

As an example of the difficulties of the histogenetic view, consider pancreatic cancer. On the basis of morphological and immunophenotypic studies it is widely held that ductal carcinoma looks like (to greater or lesser extents) normal pancreatic ducts and therefore must arise in those cells. This may be true but there are some conflicting data. Acinar cell abnormalities have been described in human pancreas in association with ductal tumours (Longnecker *et al*., 1980). Ultrastructural studies suggest that the earliest lesions in the hamster model involve the centro-acinar cells (Pour, 1988) or cells of acinar origin (Flaks, 1984). More convincing evidence that tumours with a ductal phenotype do not necessarily originate from ductal cells comes from studies of transgenic animals. In transgenic mice the expression of an elastase promoter-TGF-alpha construct by acinar cells leads to acinar-ductal transformation (Jhappen *et al*., 1990; Sandgren *et al*., 1990). Transgenic mice in which *c-myc* expression is targeted to pancreatic acinar cells develop tumours with a ductal phenotype (Sandgren *et al*., 1991). These studies point to the phenotypic plasticity of pancreatic acinar cells but might be explained by the possible leaky expression of acinar promoters in ductal epithelial cells. Cultured normal human pancreas may undergo rapid transdifferentiation from an acinar to a ductal phenotype (Hall & Lemoine, 1992). DeLisle & Logsdon (1990) have recently reported very similar observations in an *in-vitro* murine pancreas culture system. Consequently it can no longer be simply held that the phenotypic similarity of established pancreatic cancer to normal pancreatic ducts indicates the origin of the tumour in duct cells. The possibility that the tumour arises in a related, but distinct population, and undergoes differentiation towards a ductal phenotype is equally tenable. This example indicates the danger in making histogenetic statements on the basis of phenotypic data.

These arguments should not be taken as indicating any opposition to the use of antibodies to define phenotype. On the contrary, such approaches are valuable and potentially very interesting. The example of malignant fibrous histiocytoma (MFH) indicates this well. While argued by many to represent a specific tumour, MFH has been shown to be a remarkably heterogenous group of tumours all with a common growth pattern and morphology (Fletcher, 1992). Some examples show evidence of muscle differentiation, others neural and yet others adipose differentiation. Some carcinomas and even melanoma can take on an 'MFH'-like appearance. It is only by the careful use of immunohistological methods as an adjunct to conventional morphology that the heterogeneity of this 'entity' became apparent. Whether this has anything other than academic significance, however, remains to be determined.

10A.8   Future prospects

It is perhaps worth speculating on the future development of immunohisto-chemistry in the context of diagnostic pathology and neoplasia. One area that is already bearing fruit is the identification of molecules that function in cell adhesion (Clayburger *et al.*, 1987). In the future such reagents could prove of value, for example in defining the possible sites of spread of lymphomas. The ability to recognize transcriptional regulators may be of value in defining the various factors that regulate phenotype. Indeed, it might be that this is of more interest than looking at the phenotypic markers themselves. In this vein, it may be that the family of transcriptional regulators that can define developmental fate such as the products of the homeobox genes could be valuable targets for antibodies.

Quantification immunohistochemistry remains a difficult area and there has still been little of value for the surgical pathologist although there are clear research uses. In the same context while image analysis methods have been advocated, for example in the enumeration of proliferating cells, this has still had relatively little general use. Development of expert systems and computer-aided diagnosis may revolutionize the use of immunohistochemistry, although the cynic might suggest that the human brain is a more flexible (albeit fallible) 'expert' system than has hitherto been invented. Certainly the use of Bayesian analysis and meta-analysis might be a simpler way of getting the most out of the available panels of antibodies.

10A.9   Conclusion

It is important to realize that immunohistochemistry has revolutionized the practice of histopathology, particularly in the context of tumour pathology, with our enhanced ability to make objective diagnoses. The ability to object-ively define phenotype is of great value, although we would argue that it does not enhance our abilities to define histogenesis per se (Hall, 1991). In the context of sarcomas it is clear that this enhanced objectivity can alter our perspective of some tumour categories, as has recently been shown with the dismantelling of malignant fibrous histiocytoma (sic) and its replacement with more specific diagnoses (Fletcher, 1992). There are important limitations in immunohistological methods and these have frequently been compounded by an unrigorous attitude to application of antibodies and many unrealistic claims for specificity. There is a clear need, we believe, for more direct assessment of the true value of immunohistochemistry in surgical pathology using prospective studies with clearly-defined parameters and external reference points. Never-theless, the use of antibodies in diagnosis is now very widespread and is probably very cost-effective in comparison with the expense of many imaging and other diagnostic modalities currently used in medicine. Our goal in this review has been to take a slightly iconoclastic viewpoint, playing devil's advocate, our primary objective being to improve the rigour with which we all use immunohistochemistry in diagnostic pathology.

10A.10 References

Angel, C., Heyderman, E. & Lauder, I (1989). Use of immunochemistry in Britain: EQA forum antibody usage questionnaire. *Journal of Clinical Pathology*, **42**, 1009–1011.

Clark, D. M., Boylston, A. W., Hall, P. A. & Carrel, S. (1986). Antibodies to T cell antigen receptor β chain families detect monoclonal T cell proliferations. *Lancet*, **2**, 835–837.

Clayburger, C., Wright, A., Medeiros, L. J., Koller, T. D., Link, M. P., Smith, S. D., Warnke, R. A. & Krensky, A. M. (1987). Absence of cell surface LFA-1 as a mechanism of escape from immunosurveillance. *Lancet*, **2**, 533–536.

d'Ardenne, A. J., Butler, M. G., Hall, P. A. & Stearn, P. M. (1986). The role of immunocytochemistry in routine tumour diagnosis. *Journal of Pathology*, **149**, 213.

DeLisle, R. C. & Logsdon, C. D. (1990). Pancreatic acinar cells in culture: expression of acinar and ductal antigens in a growth related manner. *European Journal of Cell Biology*, **51**, 64–75

Flaks, B. (1984). Histogenesis of pancreatic carcinogenesis in the hamster. Ultrastructural evidence. *Environmental Health Perspectives*, **56**, 187–203.

Fletcher, C. D. M. (1992) Pleomorphic malignant fibrous histocytoma: fact or fiction? A critical reappraisal based on 159 tumours diagnosed as pleomorphic sarcoma. *American Journal of Surgical Pathology*, **16**, 213–228.

Gatter, K. C. (1989). Diagnostic immunocytochemistry: achievements and challenges. *Journal of Pathology*, **159**, 183–190.

Gatter, K. C., Abdullaziz, Z., Beverley, P. C. L., Corvalan, J. R. F., Ford, C., Lane, E. B., Mota, M., Nash, J. R. G., Pulford, K. A., Stein, H., Taylor-Papadimitriouu, J., Woodhouse, C. & Mason, D. Y. (1982). Use of monoclonal antibodies for the histopathological diagnosis of malignancy. *Journal of Clinical Pathology*, **35**, 1253–1267.

Gatter, K. C., Alcock, C., Heryet, A & Mason, D. Y., (1985). Clinical importance of analysing tumours of uncertain origin with immunohistochemical techniques. *Lancet*, **1**, 1302–1305.

Gould, V. E. (1986). Differentiation and histogenesis: a re-evaluation of concepts. *Human Pathology*, **17**, 212–215.

Hall, P. A. (1991). Stem cells, histogenesis and differentiation. In *Recent Advances in Histopathology*, Vol. 15, ed. R. M. N. MacSween & P. P. Anthony pp. 1–15.

Hall, P. A. & d'Ardenne, A. J. (1987). Value of CD15 immunostaining in diagnosing Hodgkin's disease: a review of published reports. *Journal of Clinical Pathology*, **40**, 1299–1304.

Hall, P. A., Domizio, P., Slavin, G. & Levison, D. A. (1987). Immunohistochemistry in District General Hospitals in England and Wales. *Journal of Clinical Pathology*, **40**, 1306–1309

Hall, P. A., Gregory, W., Richards, M. A., d'Ardenne, A. J., Lister, T. A. & Stansfeld, A. G. (1988). The prognostic significance of Ki67 immunostaining in non-Hodgkin's lymphoma. *Journal of Pathology*, **154**, 223–235.

Hall, P. A. & Lemoine, N. R. (1992). Rapid transdifferentiation of pancreatic ductal to acinar phenotype. *Journal of Pathology*, **166**, 97–103.

Hall, P. A. & Levison, D. A. (1990). Assessment of cell proliferation in histological material. *Journal of Clinical Pathology*, **43**, 184–192.

Hall, P. A., Levison, D. A., Lane, D. P., Gillett, C. E., Camplejohn, R., Dover, R., Waseem, N. H., Woods, A. L., Yu, C. C.-W., Kellock, D. B., Watkins, J. A. & Barnes, D. M. (1990). Proliferating cell nuclear antigen (PCNA) immunolocalisation in paraffin sections. An index of cell proliferation with evidence of deregulated expression in some neoplasms. *Journal of Pathology*, **162**, 285–294.

Hall, P. A., Levison, D. A. & Wright, N. A. (eds). (1992). *Assessment of Cell Proliferation in Clinical Practice*, p. 215. London, Springer.

Hall, P. A., McKee, P. H., Menage, H. D., Dover, R. & Lane, D. P. (1993). High levels of p53 protein in UV-irradiated normal human skin. *Oncogene*, **8**, 203–207.

Hall, P. A., Ray, A., Midgley, C., Lemoine, N. R., Krausz, T. & Lane, D. P. (1991). p53 immunostaining in diagnostic cytopathology. *Lancet*, **338**, 513.

Hall, P. A. & Woods, A. L. (1990). Immunohistological markers of cell proliferation. *Cell and Tissue Kinetics*, **23**, 531–549.

Harkin, P. J., Kelly, S. A. & Jack, A. S. (1990). Computer assisted selection and assessment of antibodies in the diagnosis of lymphomas. *Journal of Clinical Pathology*, **43**, 740–843.

Jasani, B. (1988). Immunohistologically definable light chain restriction in autoimmune disease. *Journal of Pathology*, **154**, 1–5.

Jhappen, C., Stahle, C., Harkins, R. N. Fausto, N., Smith, G. H. & Merlino, G. T. (1990). TGFα overexpression in transgenic mice induces liver neoplasia and abnormal development of the mammary gland and pancreas. *Cell*, **61**, 1137–1146.

Lane, D. P. & Benchimol, S. (1990). p53: oncogene or anti-oncogene? *Genes & Development*, **4**, 1–8.

Levine, A. J., Momand, J. & Finlay, C. A. (1991). The p53 tumour suppressor gene. *Nature*, **351**, 453–456.

Longnecker, D. S., Shinozuka, H. & Dekker, A. (1980). Focal acinar cell dysplasia in human pancreas. *Cancer*, **45**, 534–540.

McGee, J. O., Woods, J. C., Ashall, F., Bramwell, M. E. & Harris, H. (1982). A new marker for human cancer cells. 2. Immunohistochemical detection of the Ca antigen in human tissues with the Ca1 antibody. *Lancet*, **2**, 7.

Nakamura, S. & Suchi, T. (1991). Angioimmunoblastic lymphoma, T-zone lymphoma and lymphoepithelioid lymphoma. *Cancer*, **67**, 2565–2578.

Picker, L. J., Weiss, L. M., Medeiros, L. J., Wood, G. S. & Warnke, R. A. (1987). Immunophenotypic criteria for the diagnosis of non-Hodgkin's lymphoma. *American Journal of Pathology*, **128**, 181–201.

Pour, P. M. (1988). Mechanism of pseudoductular (tubular) formation during pancreatic carcinogenesis in the hamster model. An electron microcopic and immunohistochemical study. *American Journal of Pathology*, **130**, 335–344.

Reynolds, G. J. (1989). External quality assurance and assessment in immunocytochemistry. *Histopathology*, **15**, 627–633.

Sainsbury, J. R. C., Farndon, J. R., Needham, G. K., Malcolm, A. J. & Harris, A. L. (1987). Epidermal-growth-factor receptor status as predictor of early recurrence of and death from breast cancer. *Lancet*, **1**, 1398–1402.

Sainsbury, J. R. C., Malcolm, A. J., Appleton, D. R., Farndon, J. R. & Harris, A. L. (1985). Presence of epidermal growth factor receptor as an indicator of poor prognosis in patients with breast cancer. *Journal of Clinical Pathology*, **38**, 1225–1228.

Slamon, D. J., Clark, G. M., Wong, S. G., Levin, W. J., Ullrich, A. & McQuire, W. L.

(1987). Human breast cancer: correlation of relapse and survival with amplification of the HER-2/*neu* oncogene. *Science*, **235**, 177–182.

Sandgren, E. P., Luettke, N. C., Palmiter, R. D., Brinster, R. L. & Lee, D. C. (1990). Overexpression of TGFα in transgenic mice: induction of epithelial hyperplasia, pancreatic metaplasia and carcinoma of the breast. *Cell*, **61**, 1121–1135.

Sandgren, E. P., Quaife, C. J., Paulovich, A. G., Palmiter, R. D. & Brinster, R. L. (1991). Pancreatic tumour pathogenesis reflects the causative genetic lesion. *Proceedings of the National Academy of Sciences U.S.A.*, **88**, 93–97.

Venter, D. J., Tuzi, N. L. Kumar, S. & Gullick, W. J. (1987). Overexpression of c-erbB 2 oncoprotein in human breast carcinomas: immunohistological assessment correlates with gene amplification. *Lancet*, **1**, 69–72.

Waseem, N. H. & Lane, D. P. (1990). Monoclonal antibody analysis of the proliferating cell nuclear antigen (PCNA). Structural conservation and the detection of a nucleolar form. *Journal of Cell Science*, **96**, 121–129.

Wakins, J., Kellock, D., Gillet, C., Egan, M., Pontin, J. E., Millis, R. R. & Levinson, D. A. (1991). Enhancement of immunostaining. *Histopathology*, **17**, 185.

10B

Monoclonal antibodies in oncology: in-vivo targeting for immunoscintigraphy and therapy of human malignancies

A. BAMIAS and A. A. EPENETOS

10B.1 Introduction

The idea of targeting human tumours with antibodies is not new. In fact, it appeared towards the end of the last century (Hericourt & Richet, 1895) and it was renewed by Paul Ehrlich's concept of the 'magic bullet' (Himmelweit, 1957). Since then, many clinical studies using polyclonal antisera have been performed (Bale et al., 1955; Mach et al., 1980; Goldenberg et al., 1980). Successful imaging can be achieved but the use of polyclonal antisera has certain limitations. It consists of antibodies of various specificities and affinities. The specificity of affinity-purified antibodies is not usually higher than 20% (Mach et al., 1974). Additionally, only limited quantities can be obtained from animals.

Hybridoma technology has enabled the creation of monoclonal antibodies (mab) of unique specificities and potential large-scale production (Köhler & Milstein, 1975). Hundreds (if not thousands) of mab recognizing various known or unknown epitopes have been reported. Recently, the production of chimeric or humanized mab has also been achieved (Verhoeyen et al., 1988).

Mab are widely used in immunocytochemistry for the differential diagnosis of malignant effusions (Epenetos et al., 1982a) and immunohistochemistry of benign and malignant diseases (Callard et al., 1981; Crawford et al., 1981). Their contribution in the study and cell typing of haemopoietic malignancies has been of major importance (Beverley, 1980).

The production of mab has renewed the interest in targeting of human tumours for diagnosis and therapy. The detection of tumour-associated antigens, i.e. antigens present in high amounts in tumours but absent or weakly expressed in normal tissues (Taylor-Papadimitriou et al., 1981; Spurr et al., 1986) offered an attractive target for radioisotopes or other toxic substances which could be carried to the tumours by means of mab recognizing such antigens.

222

10B.2 Immunoscintigraphy

Radioimmunoscintigraphy represents one of the earliest applications of mab in medicine and especially in clinical oncology. Clinical studies have been ongoing for over a decade but there is still controversy regarding the usefulness of this approach.

10B.2.1 Animal studies

Nude mice bearing human or animal tumours have long been used as models for the study of various substances including antibodies as a first step before their application in clinical trials (Quinones *et al.*, 1971). This model does not always resemble the human situation although it can be useful in the study of mab both for imaging and therapy.

In 1981, Mach *et al.* reported the biodistribution of an anti-CEA mab after intravenous (i.v.) administration in mice bearing human colon carcinoma xenografts (Mach *et al.*, 1981). This was the first evidence that localization of an antibody in the tumour was the result of specific antigen–antibody interaction and not due to non-specific uptake observed after administration of control IgG.

Since then, several studies have demonstrated successful imaging using tumour-associated mab labelled with radioiodines (Epenetos *et al.*, 1982*b*) or metals (Gerretsen *et al.*, 1991). The smallest tumour detected was about 1 mm in diameter. Tumours could be visualized at early time points after the injection depending on the size of the tumours and the blood supply of the surrounding tissues. Simultaneous administration of a non-specific antibody labelled with a different isotope revealed a significant difference between the specific and non-specific tumour uptake. Furthermore, autoradiography confirmed specific antigen–antibody interaction *in vivo*.

Animal models have been used for the study of antibody fragments for immunoscintigraphy (Gerretsen *et al.*, 1991). It has been shown that their clearance is more rapid than that of intact antibodies resulting in more favourable tumour:tissue ratios and improved imaging.

The stability and degradation of radioantibodies has been tested in animal models (Hnatowich *et al.*, 1983; Fritzberg *et al.*, 1988; Zalutsky *et al.*, 1989) prior to clinical studies addressing questions regarding different isotopes and their fate, i.e. dehalogenation and thyroid uptake for radioiodines, high liver and spleen uptake for metals such as ^{111}In and early imaging with short-lived isotopes such as ^{99m}Tc. More recently, two-step strategies involving separate administration of antibodies and radionuclides have been studied in nude mice (Pimm *et al.*, 1988; Paganelli *et al.*, 1990) prior to clinical applications.

10B.2.2 Clinical studies

Historically, imaging of human tumours with polyclonal antibodies had been reported well before the production of mab (Bale *et al.*, 1955). Successful localization was reported in some studies (Goldenberg *et al.*, 1974) although other investigators questioned the utility of immunoscintigraphy in cancer diagnosis (Mach *et al.*, 1978).

With the use of mab, immunoscintigraphy appears to be a sensitive and specific method, useful in the diagnosis of metastatic disease (Epenetos *et al.*, 1985; Kalofonos *et al.*, 1989*a*; Griffin *et al.*, 1991). The question of specificity (Kalofonos *et al.*, 1988) and the role of circulating antigens (Griffin *et al.*, 1991) are some of the issues addressed by previous studies. In this chapter, we will focus on certain issues which may improve the clinical usefulness of mab: (1) choice of radioisotope, (2) intact antibodies versus fragments, (3) routes of administration, and (4) two or more step strategies.

10B.2.2.1 Choice of radioisotope

Table 10B.1 shows some of the isotopes used in many clinical studies. There has been a progressive movement from iodines to radiometals, such as ^{111}In and more recently to ^{99m}Tc, which is both suitable for present day gamma camera use and relatively inexpensive.

Iodines were the first isotopes used in clinical studies because of the ease of availability and simplicity of protein iodination. Many methods of iodination are available but the iodogen technique is one of the most popular (Fracker & Speck, 1978). This introduces an iodine atom mainly into a tyrosine ring. The use of 'mild' conditions can preserve immunological integrity of the antibodies, although differences in the sensitivity among different antibodies have been observed (Matzku *et al.*, 1985). ^{123}I and ^{131}I have been used clinically (Epenetos *et al.*, 1986; Reiners *et al.*, 1986; Kalofonos *et al.*, 1989*b*) and useful results have been reported. With ^{123}I successful imaging of diverse solid tumours can be achieved within 24 h after the administration of the radiolabelled mab (Bamias *et al.*, 1991). In certain cases the presence of the antibody at tumour sites was confirmed by immunohistochemistry and autoradiography (Epenetos *et al.*, 1982*c*). Primary and metastatic lesions can be detected in many cases even when conventional radiology has failed (Riva *et al.*, 1988). On the other hand, administration of radiolabelled non-specific mab can sometimes result in successful imaging, particularly of large primary tumours in the lungs (Kalofonos *et al.*, 1988*b*). Radioiodinated mab can undergo deiodination *in vivo*, resulting in accumulation of radioactivity in the stomach and thyroid. This problem can be circumvented by the administration of potassium iodide (Reiners *et al.*, 1986). Recently a new iodination method, which results in improved stability *in vivo*, has been described (Zalutsky *et al.*, 1989). Preliminary studies have shown that it can decrease dehalogenation 40–100 times and

Table 10B.1. *Radioisotopes as potential agents in immunoscintigraphy*

Radionuclide	Maximum γ-energy (keV)	$T_{\frac{1}{2}}$	Advantages	Disadvantages
[131]I	364	8 days	Availability Labelling method	High β-energy Unstable *in vivo*
[123]I	159	13 h	Optimal energy Labelling method	Availability Expensive Unstable *in vivo* Short $T_{\frac{1}{2}}$
[111]In	173 247	68 h	Availability Optimal energy	Liver uptake
[99m]Tc	140	6 h	Availability Optimal energy	Short $T_{\frac{1}{2}}$

increase 12-fold tumour radioactivity. Its superiority in clinical trials remains to be seen.

The use of diethylenetriaminepentaacetic acid (DTPA), a bifunctional agent for the labelling of mab with [111]In (Hnatowich *et al*., 1983), resulted in the production of stable radioantibodies. ^{111}In-labelled mab have been used extensively during the past 5 years for the detection of human tumours (Epenetos *et al*., 1985; Siccardi *et al*., 1989; Griffin *et al*., 1991). In certain cases lesions not detectable with other methods could be visualized by immunoscintigraphy (Epenetos *et al*., 1985). Although improved tumour:tissue ratios can be achieved in animal models by ^{111}In compared with [131]I (Hnatowich *et al*., 1983), this has not always been the case in clinical studies (Reiners *et al*., 1986; Riva *et al*., 1988). High liver uptake is the most serious disadvantage of ^{111}In immunoscintigraphy (Halpern *et al*., 1985; Murray *et al*., 1987). This can impair the detection of liver metastases which is a common site of metastasis in many human carcinomas.

Both ^{131}I and ^{111}In have long half-lives of 8 days and 68 h, respectively. When antibody fragments are used, tumour uptake and blood clearance occur more rapidly, allowing the application of shorter half-life radionuclides such as [99m]Tc. This is near the ideal radioisotope for diagnostic purposes with 6 h half-life, 140 keV radiation, no particulate radiation and convenient availability and cost. Despite these advantages, problems related to the chemistry of antibody-labelling with ^{99m}Tc did not allow, until recently, the production of ^{99m}Tc-labelled mab which could be used in clinical studies (Fritzberg *et al*., 1988; Mather & Ellison, 1990). Direct labelling of antibodies could result in poor *in-vivo* stability while 'pre-tinning' of the antibody, which increases the stability of the complex, results in fragmentation of the antibody with preferential labelling of Fab fragments and may impair the immunoreactivity of the antibody (Patik *et al*., 1985a; Rhodes *et al*., 1986). The use of bifunctional

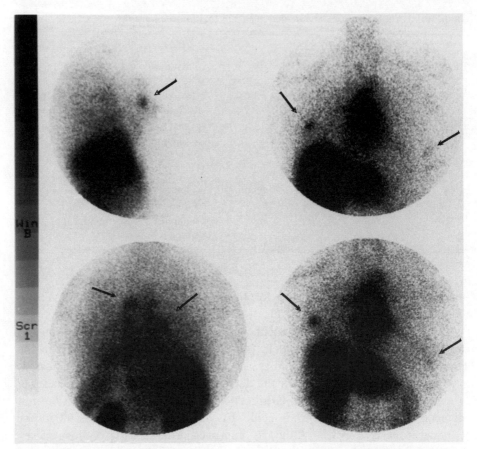

Figure 10B.1. Antibody scan of a patient with carcinoma of the right breast. HMFG1-^{99m}Tc was administered i.v. and scans were taken immediately and at 24 h after the injection. The arrows show high accumulation of radioactivity 24 h after the injection in the left breast and the lumbar spinal cord. Biopsies revealed metastases in both areas. Additionally, there was a lower accumulation of radioactivity in the right breast (arrows) which proved to be a recurrence at the site of the mastectomy.

agents such as DTPA has not been as successful for ^{99m}Tc as for ^{111}In (Patik et al., 1985b). Encouraging results have been reported recently (Granowska & Britton, 1991; Gooden et al., 1991) but further clinical studies are needed to address the utility of ^{99m}Tc-labelled mab in immunoscintigraphy (Figure 10B.1).

10B.2.2.2 Use of antibody fragments

When intact radiolabelled mab are administered i.v. the elimination of radioactivity from the circulation is slow with a half-life of 30–40 h (Sharkey et al., 1990; Griffin et al., 1991). The clearance depends on many factors such as the molecular size and the radioisotope used. It may also be dose-dependent (Sharkey *et al.*, 1990) but this has not been confirmed by all investigators (Griffin *et al.*, 1991). The clearance of blood radioactivity is more rapid when antibody fragments are used (Kalofonos *et al.*, 1988*a*; Siccardi *et al.*, 1989). The whole body radiation half-life is 9 h and differs significantly from intact IgG. Animal and clinical studies have shown that favourable tumour:tissue ratios can be obtained by $F(ab')_2$ fragments (Kalofonos *et al.*, 1988*a*; Gerretsen *et al.*, 1991). The smaller molecules, Fab fragments, are cleared more rapidly than $F(ab')_2$ fragments (Delaloye *et al.*, 1986) with a half-life of whole body radiation of less than 5 h. Tumour uptake of Fab fragments, however, is considerably less than that of IgG or $F(ab')_2$ fragments (Durbin *et al.*, 1988). This can result in lower tumour:tissue ratios (Riva *et al.*, 1988; Siccardi *et al.*, 1989).

10B.2.2.3 *Routes of administration*

In systemic therapy, i.v. administration of mab usually results in low absolute amounts of antibody in the tumour and unacceptable systemic toxicity (Epenetos *et al.*, 1986). Regional administration such as intraperitoneally (i.p.), intrapleurally or intrathecally may have therapeutic advantages. A small number of studies using regional administration of antibodies for tumour localization has produced impressive results (Pectasides *et al.*, 1986).

Intralymphatic administration can be used for the detection of involved lymph nodes (Athanassiou *et al.*, 1988; Mulshine *et al.*, 1991). The staging of patients with cutaneous T cell lymphomas was altered after antibody scans were performed (Mulshine *et al.*, 1991). Intraperitoneal administration of radiolabelled B.72.3 mab, which recognizes a glycoprotein expressed by colorectal carcinomas and other human malignancies, resulted in positive scans in cases where conventional radiology had previously failed to detect peritoneal lesions (Colcher *et al.*, 1987). In spite of these encouraging results it seems unlikely that regional administration of radiolabelled mab will be used widely for radioimmunoscintigraphy, although it may be advantageous for immunotherapy.

10B.2.2.4 *Two-step strategies*

Tumour:blood and tumour:tissue ratios can be improved if the clearance of the radiolabelled antibody is enhanced or the radioisotope is administered separately from the antibody at a time when antibody had cleared from the circulation and normal tissues and had localized in the tumour. This would enable successful imaging soon after administration of the radioisotope. Several approaches have already been described. They have been mostly applied in animal models but promising results have also been obtained in clinical studies.

Administration of anti-antibodies

Most of the mab used in clinical studies are of murine origin. The administration of anti-mouse antibodies could enhance their clearance from the blood. This has been confirmed by studies in animal models (Goldenberg et al., 1987). Encouraging results were obtained with anti-IgG antibodies following the administration of anti-CEA antibodies in patients with carcinomas (Goldenberg et al., 1987). Radioactivity in the liver was increased during the first 2 h but this dissipated by 24 h after the injection. Liposomally-entrapped anti-antibodies had been used previously for the clearance of antibodies from the circulation with encouraging results (Begent et al., 1982). Tumour:non-tumour ratios could increase tenfold and successful imaging was observed at 24 h after the injection of the second antibody.

Bifunctional haptens

Bispecific antibodies are monoclonal antibodies with specificity for two different antigens. They can be produced either by fusing two hybridomas and then selecting for antibodies with dual specificity or by chemically conjugating two fragments of such antibodies (see also, Chapter 6). Bispecific antibodies recognizing a tumour-associated antigen and a hapten which can be radiolabelled (such as DTPA) have been described for imaging purposes (Goodwin et al., 1988). The antibody is administered as a first step and is allowed to localize to the tumour. After it is cleared from the circulation, a radiolabelled hapten is administered as a second step. Before doing so, an unlabelled 'chase' can be administered as an intermediate step. This clears the antibody from the circulation rapidly so that when the hapten is administered the antibody concentration on the tumour is high but low in the circulation (Goodwin et al., 1988). It has been shown that the administration of a radiolabelled-hapten after the injection of an anti-hapten antibody could result in reduction of 20–60% in whole body radiation and 85% in blood radioactivity within 3 h after administration.

Avidin–biotin systems

In this system the extremely high affinity of biotin for avidin or streptavidin ($kDa = 10^{-15}$ M) (Green, 1975) is exploited to deliver radioisotopes or other substrates to tumour cells. Biotin (formerly called vitamin H) is a small molecule that can be chemically attached to proteins by its carboxyl end while its binding to avidin remains relatively unaffected.

As in the previous two-step methods, avidin or biotin-conjugated mab are administered first. After a predetermined interval, which allows for the clearance of the antibody from the circulation and its targeting to the tumour, radiolabelled biotin or avidin is administered, respectively. Avidin–biotin systems have been used for imaging human tumours in clinical studies (Kalofonos et al., 1990). Streptavidin-labelled HMFG1 mab was administered in patients with lung carcinomas, followed by ^{111}In-labelled biotin 1–3 days later.

Table 10B.2. *Applications of mono-clonal antibodies in cancer therapy*

Unconjugated monoclonal antibodies
Complement-mediated toxicity
Cell-mediated toxicity
Anti-idiotypic antibodies

Conjugated monoclonal antibodies
Radioisotopes
Chemotherapeutic agents
Toxins
Amplification systems
 Avidin–biotin
 Prodrug–enzyme

Pharmacokinetics and distribution data showed that endogenous biotin is not likely to interfere with the administered streptavidin-conjugated antibody. In other studies, biotinylated mab were followed by ^{111}In-streptavidin in patients with ovarian carcinomas. Both agents were administered i.p. Tumours could be visualized at 30 min after injection. Normal organ uptake, such as liver activity, was lower than those expected from i.v. administration (Paganelli *et al.*, 1991).

10B.3 Immunotherapy

The concept of treating human malignancies with antibodies was first reported in the last century (Hericourt & Richet, 1895). Mab have replaced polyclonal antisera in the last 15 years for use either alone or as specific transmitters of cytotoxic agents to tumour sites (Table 10B.2). Recently, the progress in protein engineering enabled the creation of chimeric and humanized mab as well as of single chain antibodies. Technical details and future prospects of these products are analysed in detail elsewhere (chapters 7 and 8). Although the principle of immunotherapy is the same as in immunoscintigraphy, the parameters which are important differ between the two approaches.

10B.3.1 Unconjugated monoclonal antibodies

The two most widely recognized mechanisms of antibody-mediated toxicity are: (1) complement-mediated cytotoxicity (CMC), where antibody binding results in the fixation of complement onto the target cell (Kohler & Milstein, 1975), and (2) antibody-dependent cell-mediated cytotoxicity (ADCC), where the antibody attracts cytotoxic cells by means of their Fc receptors (FcR) (Henney

& Gillis, 1984). Recently, bispecific mab, with specificity for both tumour-associated antigens and the FcR of cytotoxic cells, have been produced that can attract the cytotoxic cells through antigen–antibody interactions (De Palazzo *et al.*, 1990). Both mechanisms depend on the subclass of the antibody as certain subclasses can fix complement (human IgG1, IgG3 and IgM) or attract cytotoxic cells (IgG2a and IgG3) more successfully than others (Herlyn & Koprowski, 1982). The idea, theoretically, is correct and these systems can be cytotoxic *in vitro* (De Palazzo *et al.*, 1990), it has not proved successful, however, when applied in patients and the antibodies used so far were ineffective in fixing human complement *in vivo* (Pukel *et al.*, 1982; Cheresch *et al.*, 1985). Many questions remain unanswered, such as the correlation of dose escalation and the responses or the kinetics of the antibodies; additionally, human anti–mouse antibody (HAMA) responses represent a serious limitation when mouse antibodies are used.

Unconjugated mouse monoclonal antibodies (Mumab) have been used in patients with acute (Ball *et al.*, 1983) and chronic leukaemias (Dillman *et al.*, 1982; Capone *et al.*, 1983) and B and T cell lymphomas (Miller & Levy, 1981). Responses were poor and transient and serious adverse effects were observed when high antibody doses were administered. Clinical studies in patients with solid tumours have been even more restricted. Anti-ganglioside mab have been used in patients with melanomas (Houghton *et al.*, 1985; Cheung *et al.*, 1986). Some IgG3 antibodies produced encouraging results probably because of their greater activity in CMC and ADCC than other antibodies used. Recently, a genetically reshaped Humab was used for the treatment of two patients with non-Hodgkin's lymphoma (Hale *et al.*, 1988). This antibody was constructed by the transplantation of the DNA encoding the hypervariable regions of a rat mab, which recognizes an antigen present on human lymphocytes and monocytes (Hale *et al.*, 1983), into normal human immunoglobulin genes (Riechmann *et al.*, 1988). Human IgG1 was chosen because of its greater activity than other human isotypes both in CMC and ADCC (Bindon *et al.*, 1988). Both patients showed impressive responses and they restored their haemopoiesis during the therapy. No anti-antibody response was detected in either patient.

Jerne's idiotypic hypothesis offers an interesting avenue of tumour therapy (Jerne, 1984). This hypothesis views the immune system as a collection of elements, each capable of binding an antigenic determinant through its combining site, designated as paratope, and each capable of being recognized by other elements because it displays one or more paratopes. This theory has raised controversy and it is not the aim of this chapter to analyse it in detail. It is feasible that the administration of mab recognizing an idiotope on the surface of malignant B cells could affect the dynamic balance of the immune system towards the supression of the malignant B cell clone to its premalignant state (Geha, 1981). Pilot clinical studies have also shown that administration of anti-idiotypic mab can result in antigen-specific immune responses in patients with solid tumours (Tsujisaki *et al.*, 1991).

Anti-idiotypic mab were used for the treatment of 11 patients with B cell lymphomas (Meeker *et al.*, 1985). Five patients showed partial and one showed a complete remission of the disease. Unfortunately, these responses were only of short durability.

10B.3.2 Conjugated monoclonal antibodies

10B.3.2.1 Radioisotopes

Radiotherapy is widely used for the therapy of human malignancies with success in many cases. Nevertheless, irradiation of normal tissues can result in considerable toxicity which is dose-dependent. The radiosensitivity of human tumours is variable and in many cases only suboptimal doses can be given in order not to exceed the maximal tolerable toxicity. The delivery of radiation specifically to tumour sites represents the ideal form of radiotherapy. Mab were considered as the agents that could make this form of selective radio-therapy possible. There are two important factors related to the effectiveness of this approach: (1) a sufficient amount of the radioisotope must reach the tumour, which means that the *antibody uptake by the tumour* should reach a certain level, and (2) the dose needed to eradicate the tumour mass should not exceed the maximal tolerable *toxicity* in the normal organs.

Several animal studies have shown that administration of radiolabelled-mab can result in tumour uptake ranging from 5 to 20% of the injected dose per gram (i.d./g) of tumour tissue. The antibody uptake by normal organs is usually lower than that of the tumour with tumour:normal tissue ratios being higher than 2 at 24 h or later after administration. The radioactivity in tumours usually reaches a maximum point at 2–4 days and in many cases there is retention of radioactivity for up to 1–2 weeks after administration (Colcher *et al.*, 1984). These results are promising because they show that successful tumour irradiation is achievable. Unfortunately, clinical studies have shown that in most cases the tumour uptake after i.v. administration of a radiolabelled mab will not exceed 0.01% of the injected dose per gram although good tumour:normal tissue ratios can be obtained (Esteban *et al.*, 1987). This level of tumour uptake does not allow the delivery of cytotoxic doses of radiation to the tumour without exceeding the maximal tolerable dose (Epenetos *et al.*, 1986). The great difference between the results in animals and in humans is intriguing and can be attributed to many factors but primarily to the different tumour:blood volume ratios.

The absolute antibody uptake by the tumour can be theoretically improved using various approaches. Combinations of mab have been used to avoid the antigenic heterogeneity (Epenetos *et al.*, 1987) which is a common feature of many human tumours and can also be the cause of failure when one mab is used (Esteban *et al.*, 1991). It has also been shown that the binding of certain mab can be augmented when they are used in combination with each other *in*

Table 10B.3. *Radioisotopes as potential therapy agents in radioimmunotherapy*

Isotope	Emission	Energy (keV)	$T_{\frac{1}{2}}$	Advantages	Disadvantages
^{131}I	β	600	8 days	Availability	High energy γ-ray
	γ	364		Labelling method	Unstable *in vivo*
^{90}Y	β	2200	65 h	Availability	Unstable *in vivo*
				Labelling method	Accumulation in bones
^{188}Re	β	2120		Availability	Inadequately studied
	γ	155		Labelling method	
^{32}P	β		14.3 days	Availability	Inadequately studied
				Labelling method	Unstable *in vivo*
^{211}At	α	5900	7.2 h	High linear energy transfer	Volatile Radiation safety
				Long $t_{\frac{1}{2}}$ for an α	Availability Labelling method
^{212}Bi	α	8800 2250 727	1 h	High linear energy Not volatile	Short $T_{\frac{1}{2}}$ Availability
^{125}I	Auger	36	60 days	Availability Labelling method	Low energy

vitro (Mulshine *et al.*, 1991) but this has not been proved in clinical studies. Autoradiographic and immunohistochemical studies have shown that i.v. administration of radiolabelled mab in nude mice bearing human tumour xenografts results in poor penetration (Pervez *et al.*, 1988*a, b*) restricted in depth to a few cells at the periphery of the tumour. The central portion of a large tumour, therefore, will be inadequately irradiated. Use of smaller size fragments results in better penetration (Pervez *et al.*, 1988*a*) and could lead to higher tumour uptake. Animal and clinical studies using antibody fragments, however, failed to confirm this (Kalofonos *et al.*, 1989*a*; Gerretsen *et al.*, 1991) probably because fragments are cleared faster than intact IgG.

The use of suitable isotopes may compensate for the poor penetration of the antibody (Table 10B.3). By using isotopes with long range, a proportion of the tumour cells located towards the centre of the tumour will be irradiated from the peripheral portion of the tumour where the antibody is bound.

When a tumour is located in a cavity of the human body it seems reasonable that a mab administered into the cavity will localize more successfully in the tumour than when it is administered i.v. Regional administration (intraperitoneal, intrapleural, intra-arterial, intrapericardial, intralymphatic, intrahepatic, intravesical, intratumour) of radiolabelled mab has been used to overcome the problem of low tumour uptake (Epenetos, 1984; Delaloye *et al.*, 1985; Pectasides *et al.*, 1986; Epenetos *et al.*, 1987: Zalutsky *et al.*, 1990;

Mulshine *et al.*, 1991; Bamias *et al.*, 1991; Rowlinson-Busza *et al.*, 1991*a*). Animal studies have shown that i.p. administration of ^{125}I-labelled mab increases the tumour uptake up to 50-fold compared with i.v. administration (Rowlinson *et al.*, 1987). Intratumour administration results in high accumulation of radioactivity in the tumour with minimal circulating radioisotope (Rowlinson-Busza *et al.*, 1991*a*). Dosimetric calculations showed that a dose sufficient for radioimmunotherapy can be delivered. Biodistribution studies have confirmed the superiority of regional administration in clinical studies (Colcher *et al.*, 1987; Mulshine *et al.*, 1991; Bamias *et al.*, 1991) although this was not the case in all the studies (Zalutsky *et al.*, 1990). Phase I–II clinical studies have shown that in certain cases useful clinical responses can be obtained (Kalofonos *et al.*, 1988*a*). Regional administration of mab represents the most widely studied and currently the most promising application of radioimmunotherapy for the treatment of cancer.

The use of mab for targeting human tumours has several potential advantages although there are at least two major problems that need to be overcome: systemic irradiation and human anti–mouse Ig antibody (HAMA).

Intravenously administered mabs are cleared slowly from the circulation (Frodin *et al.*, 1990) with most of the radioactivity remaining in the body 24 h after administration (Siccardi *et al.*, 1989). The circulating radioisotope can irradiate normal tissues with the bone marrow being the organ that suffers the most severe toxicity, resulting in myelosuppression. Another cause of systemic toxicity is the instability of the radioimmunoconjugates currently used in radioimmunotherapy. ^{131}I was the first radioisotope employed in radioimmunotherapy (Larsson *et al.*, 1985; Epenetos *et al.*, 1987) because of the well-studied chemistry of antibody labelling and the availability of this isotope. It is far from ideal, nevertheless, mainly because of its low beta energy ($\beta_{max} = 0.6$ MeV) and the instability of the conjugates. Doses over 150 mCi can cause myelosuppression (Epenetos *et al.*, 1987) with high accumulation of the isotope in the thyroid and excretion of more than 50% in the urine as free iodine (Stewart *et al.*, 1988). ^{90}Y is more suitable for radioimmunotherapy than ^{131}I. It is a pure beta emitter with a high beta energy ($\beta_{max} = 2.2$ MeV) and thus can penetrate deeper into the tumour mass. DTPA has been used as a bifunctional chelate for the labelling of antibodies with ^{90}Y (Vaughan *et al.*, 1985). It was found that such radioantibodies localize to tumours but they also sequestred to bone, resulting in high radioactivity doses to the marrow (Vaughan *et al.*, 1985). Clinical studies defined that ^{90}Y-labelled mab are limited to doses of less than 30 mCi because of myelotoxicity (Stewart *et al.*, 1990*a*). The administration of chelating agents such as EDTA can remove free yttrium from the circulation and cause its excretion in the urine resulting in reduced myelotoxicity (Stewart *et al.*, 1990*a*).

Bone marrow toxicity and HAMA reactions can occur even when regional administration is applied although only a proportion of the administered dose enters the circulation (Stewart *et al.*, 1988). Two approaches to improve therapeutic efficacy include the accelerated clearance of the circulating radio-antibodies (for ^{131}I conjugates) and the production of more stable radioimmu-noconjugates (especially when ^{90}Y is used). Anti-mouse antibodies have been used to remove circulating radiolabelled antibodies by the formation of im-mune complexes. Liposomally entrapped anti-antibodies were initially used to clear antibodies from the circulation with encouraging results (Begent *et al.*, 1982). Tumour:non-tumour ratios could increase ten-fold. Similar results were obtained with anti-IgG antibodies following the administration of anti-CEA antibodies to patients with carcinomas (Goldenberg *et al.*, 1987). Radioactivity in the liver was increased during the first 2 h but this dissipated by 24 h after injection. We developed a modification of the above method by increasing the clearance of ^{131}I-labelled mab administered i.p. in patients with ovarian carci-nomas (Stewart *et al.*, 1990*b*). HAMA isolated from patients who had previ-ously received mouse monoclonal antibodies were administered to other pa-tients treated with the same mab. We showed that the administration of anti-mouse antibodies could increase the clearance of the mab from the circulation with a four-fold lower irradiation to the bone marrow. Nevertheless, all patients developed HAMA responses indicating that despite the exogenous administration of HAMA, the patients developed their own HAMA in res-ponse to circulating mouse antibodies.

Significant progress in the chemistry of antibody labelling using bifunctional chelates has been achieved over the last few years. The use of site-specific agents for the labelling of mab with ^{90}Y resulted in reduced myelotoxicity compared with the conventional DTPA technique (Lee *et al.*, 1990). Addition-ally, [188]Re-labelled mab have shown adequate stability *in vitro* and successful localization in human tumour xenografts (Griffiths *et al.*, 1991). Recently, improved therapeutic efficacy has also been reported using a bifunctional agent for the labelling of mab with [131]I (Schuster *et al.*, 1991). The superiority of these conjugates remains to be confirmed by clinical studies.

Ovarian carcinoma has been extensively studied by our own group at the Hammersmith Hospital, using mab labelled with ^{131}I or [90]Y (Epenetos, 1984; Epenetos *et al.*, 1987; Stewart *et al.*, 1990*a*). Initially, a panel of tumour-associated mab (AUA1, HMFG1, HMFG2, H17E2), labelled with ^{131}I, were administered i.p. in patients with residual disease after cytoreductive surgery and chemotherapy for advanced ovarian carcinoma (stages III and IV) (Table 10B.4). Patients with malignant nodules of more than 2 cm did not respond to therapy whereas the best results were obtained in patients with microscopic disease (positive washings only) (Kalofonos *et al.*, 1988*a*). Dosimetric studies showed that, in patients with nodules of more than 2 cm, high amounts of radioactivity could be delivered to tumour cells. The dose would be cor-respondingly less in patients with larger nodules (Epenetos *et al.*, 1987). Doses higher than 100 mCi resulted in reversible thrombocytopenia (nadir at 30 days) and neutropenia (nadir at 42 days). From March 1987 to March 1988, 25 patients with stage III ovarian carcinoma were treated with ^{90}Y-labelled HMFG1 mab. Patients with microscopic disease benefited most.

Table 10B.4. *Responses of patients with ovarian carcinomas treated with intraperitoneal administration of ^{131}I-labelled monoclonal antibodies*

Disease status	No.	Response	Local recurrence	Dead
Nodules > 2 cm	7	0	7	7
Nodules < 2 cm	14	1PR, 1NED	12	9
Microscopic disease	6	3CR, 2NED	1	1

PR, partial response; NED, no evidence of disease; CR, complete response.

One of the earliest applications of radiolabelled mab was in the palliation of malignant effusions (Epenetos, 1984). Intrapleural and intrapericardial administration of HMFG2 mab labelled with ^{131}I delivered 50–70 Gy to tumour sites with only 10–25 cGy whole body radiation. More recently our group showed that administration of various mab in patients with malignant effusions could result in resolution of the effusions for prolonged periods of time in many cases (Pectasides *et al.*, 1986).

In brain tumours, H17E2 and EGFR1 mab were labelled with 40–140 mCi of ^{131}I and administered i.v. or in the carotid artery in 10 patients with grade III or IV relapsed gliomas following surgery, radiotherapy and/or chemotherapy (Kalofonos *et al.*, 1989a). Three patients responded initially but only one maintained a long-term remission. Other studies have shown that there is no advantage in intra-arterial over i.v. administration (Zalutsky *et al.*, 1990).

Intrahepatic administration of radiolabelled mab has been used by our group for the management of liver metastases secondary to colonic adenocarcinoma (Pawlikowska *et al.*, 1986). ^{131}I-labelled anti-CEA F(ab′)$_2$ was administered into the hepatic artery simultaneously with degradable microspheres which can achieve reversible embolization causing temporary blood flow stasis. There was marked improvement in the clinical condition of one patient. CEA levels fell to normal and a subsequent laparotomy showed considerable diminution of the metastases. Mild leukopenia and thrombocytopenia were observed.

10B.3.2.2 Antibody–drug conjugates

Chemotherapeutic agents represent the conventional treatment of cancer either in metastatic disease or in an adjuvant or primary setting. Toxicity and side-effects of chemotherapy are related to its relative absence of selectivity, as it is toxic to normal cells as well as to the cancer. Tumour-associated mab have been used as selective carriers of chemotherapeutic drugs to tumour cells. Studies *in vitro* and *in vivo* using animal models have been carried out during the past decade but only a few clinical studies have been performed.

Table 10B.5 shows some of the chemotherapeutic agents used up to now in clinical trials. The drug can be delivered to the tumour either by chemical

Table 10B.5. *Chemotherapeutic*
agents used for antibody-guided
therapy of cancer

Vinca alkaloids
Methotrexate
Daunorubicin
Doxorubicin
Cisplatin

conjugation to the antibody (Kanellos *et al.*, 1985) or by the use of bispecific antibodies which recognize both a tumour-associated antigen with one antigen-combining site and the drug with the other (Pimm *et al.*, 1990). The specificity and the efficacy of such systems have been studied in both *in vitro* and *in vivo* models. This is a promising avenue for therapy and in many cases the conjugate proved to be more toxic than the unconjugated drug (Greenfield *et al.*, 1990; Braslawsky *et al.*, 1990).

In one clinical study, 791T/36 mab conjugated with methotrexate was given to 16 patients with colorectal carcinoma (Ballantyne *et al.*, 1988) and was found to localize successfully to tumours. In another study (Oldham, 1987) 10 patients were treated with mab conjugated with adriamycin (doxorubicin hydrochloride). Toxicity was significantly lower than that of adriamycin alone but no clinical responses were noted.

10B.3.2.3 Antibody–toxin conjugates

Natural toxins are considered to be some of the most potent cytotoxic agents. Only one to two molecules of toxin are needed to kill a tumour cell once they have reached their target. Mab have been used to direct their cytotoxic potential selectively to tumour cells. This can be achieved either by chemical linking (Thorpe *et al.*, 1985) by means of a bispecific antibody (Embleton *et al.*, 1991) or by recombinant DNA techniques (Spooner & Lord, 1991). Table 10B.6 shows the toxins that have been used thus far. Studies *in vitro* and *in vivo* have shown that antibody–toxin conjugates can be extremely toxic to tumour cells (Roffler *et al.*, 1991; Embleton *et al.*, 1991). Rapid catabolism of immunotoxins and the fact that many toxins need to be internalized before they can kill a cell represent the important problems of this approach.

Fab fragments of an anti-CD22 mab coupled with ricin A chain were administered i.v. to 15 patients with refractory B cell lymphoma (Vitetta *et al.*, 1991). The maximum tolerated toxin dose was 75 mg/m^2. Toxicity was observed in all patients but it was transient and reversible within 2 weeks of treatment in most of the cases. Responses correlated with antigen expression of the malignant cells; however, they were generally transient lasting between 1 and 4 months.

Table 10B.6. *Toxins used for antibody-guided therapy of cancer*

Ricin
Abrin
Pseudomonas toxin
Amantin
Gelonin
Trichosanthin
Diptheria toxin
Staphylococcus exotoxin

10B.3.2.4 Amplification systems

The localization of a cytotoxic agent at tumour sites can be amplified by two or more step approaches. Some amplification systems include avidin–biotin and enzyme–prodrug systems.

Avidin–biotin

The rationale of this system has already been discussed. Studies performed in animal models showed that both approaches can result in higher tumour-:normal tissue ratios compared with the administration of radiolabelled mab but in certain cases the absolute amount of the antibody in the tumour decreased (Paganelli *et al.*, 1990; Rowlinson-Busza *et al.*, 1991*a*). High accumulation of avidin in kidneys and liver are a disadvantage when biotinylated antibodies are used.

Enzyme–prodrug

The activation of inactive prodrugs at tumour sites represents a promising new approach in the use of mab for cancer treatment. Tumour-associated antibodies could be conjugated with enzymes and delivered to tumour sites. Subsequently, an inactive prodrug is administered. This can be converted into an active cytotoxic agent by the enzyme. The interval between the two administrations can be optimized to achieve satisfactory accumulation of the drug in the tumour with minimal toxicity. As a third step, an anti-enzyme antibody can be used to facilitate the clearance of the conjugate. This approach has two goals: (1) the safe release of a cytotoxic agent selectively at tumour sites, and (2) to overcome the problem of low absolute amount of antibody in the tumour, because one molecule of enzyme can potentially activate many prodrug molecules. The enzyme–prodrug systems studied are shown in Table 10B.7.

In most cases the prodrug is a modified chemotherapeutic agent that can be converted into the native active form by means of the enzyme used in the system (Bagshawe *et al.*, 1988; Senter *et al.*, 1988). Our group has developed a different approach where cyanide is released as a result of hydrolysis of amygdalin (Rowlinson-Busza *et al.*, 1991*b*). Studies *in vitro* and *in vivo* have

Table 10B.7. *Enzymes used in enzyme-prodrug systems*

Carboxypeptidase
Alkaline phosphatase
Penicillin-V amidase
Cytosine deaminase
β-glucosidase
Lactoperoxidase
Thymidine kinase
Peroxidase

===

shown that antibody–enzyme conjugates can successfully localize at tumour sites although tumour uptake can be lower than that of the unconjugated antibody (Melton *et al*., 1990; Senter *et al*., 1988). These approaches have great cytotoxic potential (Bagshawe *et al*., 1988; Senter *et al*., 1989) but systemic toxicity can also occur. Preliminary clinical studies have been performed and results show that clinical responses can be achieved with acceptable toxicity (K. D. Bagshawe, personal communication).

10B.4   Conclusion

During the past 15 years mab have been used widely to target human tumours. Imaging can be successful in many cases although immunoscintigraphy has not become a routine method for screening cancer patients. Nevertheless, there has been considerable progress in the chemistry of labelling antibodies with various isotopes which could prove useful in the future. Systemic administration of mab does not seem promising for cancer therapy. Regional administration has given promising results in selected cases but systemic toxicity remains a serious limitation. Recently, amplification systems have been developed. They represent a new promising avenue which may overcome certain problems related to the use of mab in cancer therapy. These sytems, together with the progress in protein engineering and the production of chimeric antibodies and fragments employing genetic manipulations (see Chapters 7 and 8), may lead the way to a new exciting decade for the applications of mab in clinical oncology.

10B.5   References

Athanassiou, A., Pectasides, D., Pateniotis, K., Tzimis, L., Natsis, P., Lafi, A.,
   Arapantoni, P., Koutsiouba, P., Taylor-Papadimitriou, J. & Epenetos, A. (1988).
   Immunoscintigraphy with ^{131}I-labelled HMFG2 and HMFG1 F(ab')2 in the
   pre-operative detection of clinical and subclinical lymph node metastases in breast
   cancer patients. *International Journal of Cancer*, **3** (Suppl.), 89–95.

Bagshawe, K. D., Springer, C. J., Searle, F., Antoniw, P., Sharma S., Melton, R. G. & Sherwood, R. P. (1988). A cytotoxic agent can be generated selectively at cancer sites. *British Journal of Cancer*, **58**, 700–703.

Bale, W. F., Sparl, F., Goodland, R. L. & Wolfe, D. E. (1955) *In-vivo* and *in-vitro* studies of labelled antibodies against rat kidney and Walker carcinoma. *Proceedings of the Society of Experimental Biology and Medicine*, **89**, 564–568.

Ball, E. D., Bernier, G. M., Cornwell, G. G. III, McIntyre, D. R., O'Donnell, J. F. & Fanger, M. W. (1983). Monoclonal antibodies to myeloid differentiation antigens. *In-vivo* studies of three patients with acute myelogenous leukemia. *Blood*, **62**, 1203–1210.

Ballantyne, K. C., Perkins, A. C., Pimm, M. V., Garnett, M. C., Clegg, J. A., Armitage, N. C., Baldwin, R. W. & Hardcare, J. D. (1988). Biodistribution of a monoclonal antibody–methotrexate conjugate (791T/36-MTX) in patients with colorectal cancer. *International Journal of Cancer*, **42** (Suppl. 2), 103–108.

Bamias, A., Keane, P., Krausz, T., Williams, G. & Epenetos, A. A. (1991). Intravesical administration of radiolabelled antitumour monoclonal antibody in bladder carcinoma. *Cancer Research*, **51**, 724–728.

Begent, R. H., Keep, P. A., Green, A. J., Searle, F., Bagshawe, K. D., Jewks, R. F., Jones, B. E., Barratt, G. N. & Rymans, B. E. (1982). Liposomally entrapped second antibody improves tumour imaging with radiolabelled (first) antitumour antibodies. *Lancet*, **2**, 739–742.

Beverley, P. C. L. (1980). Transplantation and clinical immunology. *XI Excerpta Medica*, Amsterdam, p. 87.

Bindon, C. I., Hale, G., Bruggemann, M. & Waldmann, H. (1988). Human monoclonal IgG antibodies differ in complement activation function at the level of C4 as well as C1q. *Journal of Experimental Medicine*, **268**, 127–152.

Braslawsky, G. R., Edson, M. A., Pearce, W., Kaneko, T. & Greenfield, R. S. (1990). Antitumor activity of adriamycin (hydrazone-linked) immunoconjugates compared with free adriamycin and specificity of tumour cell killing. *Cancer Research*, **50**, 6608–6614.

Callard, R. E., Smith, C. M., Worman, C., Linch, D., Cawley, J. C. & Beverley, P. C. (1981). Unusual phenotype and function of an expanded subpopulation of T cells in patients with haemopoietic disorders. *Clinical and Experimental Immunology*, **43**, 497–505.

Capone, P. M., Papsidero, L. D., Crogham, G. & Ming Chu, T. (1983). Experimental tumouricidal effects of monoclonal antibody against solid breast tumours. *Proceedings of the National Academy of Sciences U.S.A.*, **80**, 7328–7334.

Cheresch, D., Honsilla, C. J., Staffileno, L. K., Juny, G. & Reisfeld, R. A. (1985). Disialoganglioside GD3 on human melanoma serves as a relevant target antigen for monoclonal antibody-mediated tumour cytolysis. *Proceedings of the National Academy of Sciences U.S.A.*, **82**, 5155–5159.

Cheung, N. K., Berger, N., Coccia, P., Kallick, S., Lazarus, H., Milardi, F., Savaridus, U. & Standjord, S. (1986). Murine monoclonal antibody specific for GD2 ganglioside: a phase I trial in patients with neuroblastoma, melanoma and osteogenic sarcoma. *Proceedings of the American Association for Cancer Research*, **27**, 318–322.

Colcher, D., Esteban, J., Carrasquillo, J. A., Sugarbaker, P., Reynolds, J. C., Bryant, G., Larson, S. M. & Schlom, J. (1987). Complementation of intracavitary and intravenous administration of a monoclonal antibody (B72.3) in patients with carcinoma. *Cancer Research*, **47**, 4218–4224.

Colcher, D., Keenan, A. M., Larson, S. M. & Schlom, J. (1984). Prolonged binding of a radiolabelled monoclonal antibody (B72.3) used for the *in-situ* radioimmunodetection of human colon carcinoma xenografts. *Cancer Research*, **44**, 5744–5751.

Crawford, D. H., Brickell, P. & Tidmann, N. (1981). Increased numbers of cells with supressor T cell phenotype in the peripheral blood of patients with infectious mononucleosis. *Clinical and Experimental Immunology*, **43**, 291–297.

De Palazzo, I. J., Gercel-Taylor, C., Kitson, J. & Weiner, L. M. (1990). Potentiation of tumour lysis by a bispecific antibody that binds to Ca 19-9 antigen and the Fcγ receptor expressed by large granular lymphocytes. *Cancer Research*, **50**, 7123–7128.

Delaloye, B., Bischoff-Delaloye, A., Buchegger, F., Fliender, V., Grob, J.-P., Volant, J.-C., Pettavel, J. & Mach, J.-P. (1986). Detection of colorectal carcinoma by emission computerised tomography after injection of ^{123}I-labelled Fab and F(ab')$_2$ fragments from monoclonal anti-carcinoembryonic antigen antibodies. *Journal of Clinical Investigations*, **7**, 301–306.

Delaloye, B., Bischoff-Delaloye, A., Volant, J.-C., Grob, J.-P., Pettavel, J. & Mach, J.-P. (1985). First approach to therapy of liver metastases in colorectal carcinoma by intrahepatically infused ^{131}I labelled monoclonal anti-CEA antibodies. *European Journal of Nuclear Medicine*, **11**, 37–41.

Dillman, R. O., Shawler, D. L. & Sobol, R. E. (1982). Murine monoclonal antibody therapy in two patients with chronic lympholytic leukemia. *Blood*, **59**, 1036–1045.

Durbin, H., Milligan, E. M., Mather, S., Tucker, D. F., Raymond, R. & Bodmer, W. F. (1988). Monoclonal antibodies to placental alkaline phosphatase: preclinical evaluation in a human xenograft tumour model of F(ab')$_2$ and Fab fragments. *International Journal of Cancer*, **42** (Suppl. 2), 59–66.

Embleton, M. J., Charlewston, A., Robins, R. A., Pimm, M. V. & Baldwin, R. W. (1991). Recombinant ricin A chain cytotoxicity against carcinoembryonic antigen-expressing tumour cells mediated by a bispecific monoclonal antibody and its potentiation by ricin B chain. *British Journal of Cancer*, **63**, 670–674.

Epenetos, A. A. (1984). Antibody-guided irradiation of malignant lesions. *Lancet*, **2**, 1441–1443.

Epenetos, A. A., Britton, K. E. & Mather, S. (1982*b*). Targeting of iodine-123-labelled tumour-associated monoclonal antibodies to ovarian, breast and gastrointestinal tumours. *Lancet*, **2**, 999–1003.

Epenetos, A. A., Ganti, G., Taylor-Papadimitriou, J., Curling, M. & Bodmer, W. F. (1982*a*). Use of two epithelial specific monoclonal antibodies for diagnosis of malignancy in serous effusions. *Lancet*, **2**, 1004–1006.

Epenetos, A. A., Munro, A. J., Stewart, S., Rampling, R., Lambert, H. E., McKenzie, C. G., Soutter, P., Rahemtulla, A., Hooker, G., Sivolapenko, G. B., Snook, D., Dhokia, B., Krausz, T., Taylor-Papadimitriou, J., Durbin, H. & Bodmer, W. F. (1987). Antibody-guided irradiation of advanced ovarian cancer with intraperitoneally administered radiolabelled monoclonal antibodies. *Journal of Clinical Oncology*, **5**, 1890–1899.

Epenetos, A. A., Nimon, C. C., Arklie, J., Elliott, A. T., Hawkins, L. A., Knowles, R. W., Britton, K. E. & Bodmer, W. F. (1982*c*). Detection of human cancer in an animal model using radiolabelled tumour-associated monoclonal antibodies. *British Journal of Cancer*, **46**, 1–8.

Epenetos, A. A., Snook, D., Durbin, H., Johnson, P. M. & Taylor-Papadimitriou, J. (1986). Limitations of radiolabelled monoclonal antibodies for localisation of human neoplasms. *Cancer Research*, **46**, 3183–3191.

Epenetos, A. A., Snook, D., Hooker, G., Begent, R., Durbin, H., Oliver, R. T. D., Bodmer, W. F. & Lavender, J. P. (1985). Indium-111-labelled monoclonal antibody to placental alkaline phosphatase in the detection of neoplasms of testis, ovary and cervix. *Lancet*, **2**, 350–353.

Esteban, J. E., Colcher, D., Subarger, P., Carrasquillo, J. A., Bryant, G., Thor, A.,

Reynolds, J. L., Larson, S. M. & Schlom, J. (1987). Quantitative and qualitative aspects of radiolocalisation in colon cancer patients of intravenously administered MAb B72.3. *International Journal of Cancer*, **39**, 50–59.

Esteban, J. E., Kuhn, J. A., Felder, B., Wong, J. Y. C., Battifora, H., Beatty, J. D., Waneck, P. M. & Shivery, J. E. (1991). Carcinoembryonic antigen expression of resurgent human colon carcinoma after treatment with therapeutic doses of ^{90}Y-a-carcinoembryonic antigen monoclonal antibody. *Cancer Research*, **51**, 3802–3806.

Fracker, P. J. & Speck, J. C. (1978). Protein and cell membrane iodination with a sparingly soluble chloramine 1,3,4,6,tetrachloro-5,6-diphenyl-glycoril. *Biochemical and Biophysical Research Communications*, **80**, 849–854.

Fritzberg, A. R., Abrams, P. G. & Beaumier, P. L. (1988). Specific and stable labelling of antibodies with technetium-99m with a diamide dithiolate chelating agent. *Proceedings of the National Academy of Sciences U.S.A.*, **85**, 4025–4032.

Frodin, J.-A., Karri, A. & Mellstedt, H. (1990). Pharmacokinetics of the mouse monoclonal antibody 17-1A in cancer patients receiving various treatment schedules. *Cancer Research*, **50**, 4866–4871.

Geha, R. S. (1981). Regulation of the immune response by idiotype anti-idiotype interaction. *New England Journal of Medicine*, **305**, 25–35.

Gerretsen, M., Quak, J. J., Suh, J. S., van Walsum, M., Meijer, C. J. L. M., Snow, J. B. & van Dongen, G. A. M. S. (1991). Superior localisation and imaging of radiolabelled monoclonal antibody E48 F(ab')$_2$ fragment in xenografts of human squamous cell carcinoma of the head and neck and the vulva as compared to monoclonal antibody E48 IgG. *British Journal of Cancer*, **63**, 37–44.

Goldenberg, D., Kim, E., Deland, F., Spanelli, E. & Primus, F. J. (1980). Clinical studies on radioimmunodetection of tumours containing alphafoetoprotein. *Cancer*, **45**, 2500–2505.

Goldenberg, D., Preston, D. F. & Primus, F. J. (1974). Photoscan localisation of GW-39 tumours in hamsters using radiolabelled anticarcinoembryonic antigen immunoglobulin. *Cancer Research*, **34**, 1–9.

Goldenberg, D. M., Sharkey, R. M. & Ford, E. (1987). Anti-antibody enhancement of iodine-131 anti-CEA radioimmunodetection in experimental and clinical studies. *Journal of Nuclear Medicine*, **28**, 1604–1610.

Gooden, K., Snook, D., Henderson, B. Lavender, J. P. & Epenetos, A. A. (1991). Analysis of quality of technetium-99m-labelled monoclonal antibodies. In *Advances in the applications of monoclonal antibodies in clinical oncology*. Eighth International Hammersmith Meeting. Porto Carras, Halkidiki, Greece, 8–13 May 1991.

Goodwin, D. A., Meares, C. F., McCall, M. J., McTigue, M. & Chaovapony, W. (1988). Pre-targeted immunoscintigraphy of murine tumours with Indium-111-labelled bifunctional haptens. *Journal of Nuclear Medicine*, **29**, 226–234.

Granowska, M. & Britton, K. E. (1991). ^{99m}Tc-labelled antibodies for radioimmunoscintigraphy. In *Advances in the applications of monoclonal antibodies in clinical oncology*. Eighth International Hammersmith Meeting, Porto Carras, Halkidiki, Greece, 8–13 May 1991.

Green, N. M. (1975). Avidin. *Advances in Protein Chemistry*, **29**, 85–133.

Greenfield, L., Bloch, W. & Moreland, M. (1990). Thiol-containing cross-linking agent with enhanced steric hindrance. *Bioconjugate Chemistry*, **1**, 400–410.

Griffin, T. W., Brill, A. B., Stevens, S., Collins, J. A., Bokhari, F., Bushe, H., Stochl, M. C., Gionet, M., Rusckowski, M., Stroupe, S. P., Kieter, H. C., Sumerdom, G. A., Johnson, D. K. & Hnatowich, D. J. (1991). Initial clinical study of indium-111-labelled clone 110 anticarcinoembryonic antigen-antibody in patients with colorectal cancer. *Journal of Clinical Oncology*, **9**, 631–640.

Griffiths, G. L., Goldenberg, D. M., Knapp, F. F., Callahan, A. P., Chang, C.-H. & Hansen, H. J. (1991). Direct radiolabelling of monoclonal antibodies with generator-produced rhenium-188 for radioimmunotherapy: labelling and animal biodistribution studies. *Cancer Research*, **51**, 4594–4602.

Hale, G., Dyer, M. J. S., Clark, M. R., Phillips, J. M., Marcus, R., Riechmann, L., Winter, G. & Waldmann, H. (1988). Remission induction in non-Hodgkin's lymphoma with reshaped human monoclonal antibody Campath-1H. *Lancet*, **2**, 1394–1399.

Hale, G., Swisky, D. M., Hayhoe, F. G. J. & Waldmann, H. (1983). Effects of monoclonal anti-lymphocyte antibodies *in vivo* in monkeys and human. *Molecular Biology and Medicine*, **1**, 321–324.

Halpern, S., Hagan, P., Witztum, K. F. & Dillman, R. O. (1985). Radioimmunoscintigraphy using ^{111}In-labelled monoclonal antibodies and the case for immunotherapeutics. *Journal of Medical Technology*, **2**, 301–305.

Henney, C. S. & Gillis, S. (1984). Cell-mediated cytotoxicity. In *Fundamental Immunology*, ed. W. E. Paul, pp. 193–217. New York, Raven Press.

Hericourt, J. & Richet, C. (1895). Traitment d'un cas de sarcome par la serotherapie. *Compte rendu hebdomadaire des sceances de l'Academie des sciences*, **120**, 948–952.

Herlyn, D. & Koprowski, H. (1982). IgG2a monoclonal antibodies inhibit human tumour growth through interaction with effector cells. *Proceedings of the National Academy of Science U.S.A.*, **79**, 4761–4765.

Himmelweit, F. (ed.) (1957). The collected papers of Paul Ehrlich. *Immunology and Cancer Research*, vol. 2, London, Pergamon Press.

Hnatowich, D. J., Leigne, W. W. & Childs, R. L. (1983). Radioactive labelling of antibody: a simple and efficient method. *Science*, **235**, 613–615.

Houghton, A. N., Mintzer, D., Cordon-Cardo, C., Welt, S., Fliegel, B., Vadhan, S., Carswell,E., Melamed, M. R., Oettgen, H. F. & Old, L. J. (1985). Mouse monoclonal IgG3 antibody detecting GD3 ganglioside: a phase I trial in patients with malignant melanoma. *Proceedings of the National Academy of Sciences U.S.A.*, **85**, 1242–1246.

Jerne, N. K. (1984). Towards a network theory of the immune system. *Annals of Immunology*, **125C**, 373–381.

Kalofonos, H. P., Pawlikowska, T. R., Hemingway, A., Courtenay-Luck, N., Dhokia, B., Sivolapenko, G. B., Hooker, G., McKenzie, C. G., Lavender, P. J., Thomas, D. G. T. & Epenetos, A. A. (1989*a*). Antibody-guided diagnosis and therapy of brain gliomas using radiolabelled monoclonal antibodies against epidermal growth factor receptor and placental alkaline phosphatase. *Journal of Nuclear Medicine*, **30**, 1636–1645.

Kalofonos, H. P., Rusckowski, M., Siebecker, D. A., Sivolapenko, G. B., Snook, D., Lavender, J. P., Epenetos, A. A. & Hnatowich, D. J. (1990). Imaging of tumour in patients with indium-111-labelled biotin and streptavidin-conjugated antibodies: preliminary communication. *Journal of Nuclear Medicine*, **31**, 1791–1796.

Kalofonos, H. P., Sackier, J. M., Hatzistylianou, M., Pervez, S., Taylor-Papadimitriou, J., Waxman, J. H., Lavender, J. P., Wood, C. & Epenetos, A. A. (1989*b*). Kinetics, quantitative analysis and radioimmunolocalisation using indium-111-HMFG1 monoclonal antibody in patients with breast cancer. *British Journal of Cancer*, **59**, 939–942.

Kalofonos, H. P., Sivolapenko, G. B., Courtenay-Luck, N. S., Snook, D., Hooker,G., Winter, R., McKenzie, C. G., Taylor-Papadimitriou, J. J., Lavender, P. J. & Epenetos, A. A. (1988*a*). Antibody-guided targeting of non-small cell lung cancer using ^{111}In-labelled HMFG1 F(ab')$_2$ fragments. *Cancer Research*, **48**, 1977–1981.

Kalofonos, H. P., Stewart, S. & Epenetos, A. A. (1988*b*). Antibody-guided diagnosis and therapy of malignant lesions. *International Journal of Cancer*, **42** (Suppl. 2), 74–80.

Kanellos, J., Pietersz, G. A. & McKenzie, L. F. C. (1985). Studies of methotrexate-monoclonal antibody conjugates for immunotherapy. *Journal of the National Cancer Institute*, **75**, 319–328.

Köhler, G. & Milstein, C. (1975). Continuous culture of fused cells secreting antibody of predefined specificity. *Nature*, **256**, 1197–1203.

Larsson, S. M., Carrasquillo, J. A., Krohn, K. A., Brown, J. P., McGruffin, R. W., Ferens, J. M., Grahams, M. M., Hill, L. D., Beaumier, P. L., Hellstrom, K. E. & Hellstrom, I. (1985). Localisation of ^{131}I-labelled specific Fab fragments in human melanomas as a basis for radiotherapy. *Journal of Clinical Investigations*, **72**, 2101–2104.

Lee, Y. C. C., Washburn, L. C., Sun, T. T. H., Byrd, B. L., Crook, J. E., Holloway, E. C. & Steplewski, Z. (1990). Radioimmunotherapy of human colorectal carcinoma xenografts using ^{90}Y-labelled monoclonal antibody CO17-1A prepared by two bifunctional chelate techniques. *Cancer Research*, **50**, 4546–4551.

Mach, J. P., Buchegger, F., Forni, M., Ritchard, J., Berche, C., Lumbroso, J. D., Schreyer, M., Girardet, C., Accola, R. S. & Carrel, S. (1981). Use of radiolabelled monoclonal anti-CEA antibodies for the detection of human carcinomas by external photoscanning and tomoscintigraphy. *Immunology Today*, **10**, 239–248.

Mach, J. P., Carrel, S., Forni, M., Ritchard, J., Dunath, A. & Alberto, P. (1980). Tumour localisation of radio labelled-antibodies against carcinoembryonic antigen in patients with carcinoma. *New England Journal of Medicine*, **303**, 5–10.

Mach, J. P., Carrel, S., Merenda, C., Sordat, B., Cerottini, J.-C. (1974). *In-vivo* localision of radiolabelled antibodies to carcinoembryonic antigen in human colon carcinoma grafted into nude mice. *Nature*, **248**, 704–706.

Mach, J. P., Vienny, H., Jaeger, P., Haldemann, B., Egely, R. & Pettavel, J. (1978). Long-term follow-up of colorectal carcinoma patients by repeated CEA radioimmunoassay. *Cancer*, **42** (Suppl.), 1439–1447.

Mather, S. J. & Ellison, D. (1990). Reduction-mediated technetium-99m labelling of monoclonal antibodies. *Journal of Nuclear Medicine*, **31**, 692–697.

Matzku, S., Kirchgessner, H., Dippold, W. G. & Bruggen, J. (1985). Immunoreactivity of monoclonal antimelanoma antibodies in relation to the amount of radioactive iodine substituted to the antibody molecule. *European Journal of Nuclear Medicine*, **11**, 260–264.

Meeker, T. C., Lowder, J., Maloney, D., Miller, R. A., Thielemans, K., Warnke, R. & Levy, R. (1985). A clinical trial of anti-idiotype therapy for B cell malignancy. *Blood*, **65**, 1349–1370.

Melton, R. G., Searle, F., Sherwood, R. F., Bagshawe, K. D. & Boden, J. A. (1990). The potential of carboxypeptidase G2:antibody conjugates in a xenograft model. *British Journal of Cancer*, **61**, 420–424.

Miller, R. A. & Levy, R. (1981). Response of cutaneous T cell lymphoma to therapy with hybridoma monoclonal antibody. *Lancet*, **2**, 226–230.

Mulshine, J. L., Carrasquillo, J. A. Weinstein, J. N., Keenan, A. M., Reynolds, J. C., Herdt, J., Bunn, P. A., Sansville, E., Eddy, J., Cotelingam, A., Parentesis, P., Pinsky, C. & Larson, S. M. (1991). Direct intralymphatic injection of radiolabelled ^{111}In-T101 in patients with cutaneous T-cell lymphoma. *Cancer Research*, **51**, 688–695.

Murray, J. L., Rosenblum, M. G., Lamki, L., Haynie, T. P., Glenn, H. J. & Plager, C. E. (1987). Radioimmunoimaging in malignant melanoma patients with the use of indium-111-labelled antimelanoma monoclonal antibody (ZME-018) to high molecular weight antigen. *NCI-Monograph*, **3**, 3–9.

Oldham, R. K. (1987). Immunoconjugates. In *Principles of Cancer Biotherapy*, ed. R. K. Oldham. New York, Raven Press.

Paganelli, G., Magnani, P., Zitto, F., Villa, E., Sudati, F., Lopalco, L., Rosetti, C., Malcovati, M., Chiolerio, F., Seccamani, E., Siccardi, A. G. & Fazio, F. (1991). Three-step monoclonal antibody tumour targeting in carcinoembryonic antigen-positive patients. *Cancer Research*, **51**: 5960–5966.

Paganelli, G., Pervez, S., Siccardi, A. G., Rowlinson, G., Deleide, G., Chiolerio, F., Malcovati, M., Scassellati, G. A. & Epenetos, A. A. (1990). Intraperitoneal radiolocalisation of tumours pre-targeted by biotinylated IgG after infusion of avidin. *International Journal of Cancer*, **45**, 1184–1189.

Patik, C. H., Hong, J. J., Ebbert, M. A., Heald, S. C. & Eckelman, W. C. (1985b). Relative reactivity of DTPA immunoreactive antibody-DTPA conjugates and non-immunoreactive antibody-DTPA conjugates toward indium-111. *Journal of Nuclear Medicine*, **26**, 482–487.

Patik, C. H., Phan, L. N. B. & Hong, J. J. (1985a). The labelling of high affinity binding sites of antibodies with Tc. *Journal of Nuclear Medicine and Biology*, **12**, 3–8.

Pawlikowska, T. R. B., Hooker, G., Myers, M. & Epenetos, A. A. (1986). Treatment of tumours with radiolabelled antibodies. *Clinics in Oncology*, **5**, 93–107.

Pectasides, D., Stewart, S., Courtenay-Luck, N., Rampling, R., Munro, A. J., Krausz, T., Dhokia, B., Snook, D., Hooker, G., Durbin, H., Taylor-Papadimitriou, J., Bodmer, W. F. & Epenetos, A. A. (1986). Antibody-guided irradiation of malignant, pleural and pericardial effusions. *British Journal of Cancer*, **53**, 727–731.

Pervez, S., Epenetos, A. A., Mooi, J., Evans, D. J., Rowlinson, G., Dhokia, B. & Krausz, T. (1988a). Localisation of monoclonal antibody AUA1 and its F(ab')$_2$ fragments in human tumour xenografts: an autoradiographic and immunohistochemical study. *International Journal of Cancer*, **42** (Suppl. 3), 23–29.

Pervez, S., Paganelli, G., Epenetos, A. A., Mooi, J., Evans, D. J. & Krausz, T. (1988b). Localisation of biotinylated monoclonal antibody in nude mice bearing subcutaneous and intraperitoneal human tumour xenografts. *International Journal of Cancer*, **42** (Suppl. 3), 30–33.

Pimm, M. V., Fells, H. F., Perkins, A. C. & Baldwin, R. W. (1988). Iodine-131 and indium-111 labelled avidin and streptavidin for pre-targeted immunoscintigraphy with biotinylated anti-tumour monoclonal antibody. *Nuclear Medicine Communications*, **9**, 931–941.

Pimm, M. V., Robin, R. A., Embleton, M. J., Jacobs, E., Markham, A. J., Charleston, A. & Baldwin, R. W. (1990). A bispecific monoclonal antibody against methotrexate and a human tumour-associated antigen augments cytotoxicity of methotrexate-carrier conjugate. *British Journal of Cancer*, **61**, 508–513.

Pukel, C. S., Lloyd, K. O., Travassos, L. R., Dippold, W. G., Oetgen, H. F. & Old, L. I. (1982). GD3, a prominent ganglioside of human melanoma. *Journal of Experimental Medicine*, **155**, 1133–1136.

Quinones, J., Mizejewski, G. & Beierwaltes, W. H. (1971). Choriocarcinoma scanning using radiolabelled antibody to chorionic gonadotrophin. *Journal of Nuclear Medicine*, **12**, 69–75.

Reiners, C., Eilles, C., Spiegel, W., Becker, W. & Borner, W. (1986). Immunoscintigraphy in medullary thyroid cancer using an [123]I- or ^{111}In-labelled monoclonal anti-CEA antibody fragment. *Nuclear Medicine*, **25**, 227–231.

Rhodes, B. A., Zamora, P. O., Newell, K. D. & Valdez, E. F. (1986).

Technetium-99m-labelling of murine monoclonal antibody fragments. *Journal of Nuclear Medicine*, **27**, 685–689.

Riechmann, L., Clark, M. R., Waldmann, H. & Winter, G. (1988). Reshaping human antibodies for therapy. *Nature*, **332**, 323–327.

Riva, P., Moscatelli, G., Paganelli, G., Benini, S. & Siccardi, A. (1988). Antibody-guided diagnosis: an Italian experience on CEA-expressing tumours. *International Journal of Cancer*, **42** (Suppl. 2), 114–120.

Roffler, S. R., Yu, M. H., Chen, B. M., Tung, E. & Yeh, M. Y. (1991). Therapy of human cervical carcinoma with monoclonal antibody-*Pseudomonas* exotoxin conjugates. *Cancer Research*, **51**, 4001–4007.

Rowlinson, G., Snook, D., Busza, A. & Epenetos, A. A. (1987). Antibody-guided localization of intraperitoneal tumours following intraperitoneal or intravenous antibody administration. *Cancer Research*, **47**, 6528–6531.

Rowlinson-Busza, G., Bamias, A., Krausz, T. & Epenetos, A. A. (1991*a*). Uptake and distribution of specific and control monoclonal antibodies in subcutaneous xenograft following intratumour injection. *Cancer Research*, **51**, 3251–3256.

Rowlinson-Busza, G., Bamias, A., Krausz, T., Evans, D. J. & Epenetos, A. A. (1991*b*). Cytotoxicity following specific activation of amygdalin. In *Monoclonal Antibodies: Applications in Clinical Oncology*, ed. A. A. Epenetos, pp. 179–183. London, Chapman & Hall Medical.

Schuster, J. M., Garg, P. K., Bigner, D. D. & Zalutsky, M. R. (1991). Improved therapeutic efficacy of a monoclonal antibody radioiodinated using N-succinimidyl-3-(tri-n-butylstannyl)benzoate. *Cancer Research*, **51**, 4164–4169.

Senter, P, D., Saulnier, M. G., Schreiber, G. L., Hirschberg, D. L., Brown, J. P., Hellstrom, I. & Hellstrom, K. E. (1988). Anti-tumour effects of antibody-alkaline phosphatase conjugates in combination with etoposide phosphate. *Proceedings of the National Academy of Sciences U.S.A.*, **85**, 4842–4846.

Senter, P. D., Schreiber, G. L., Hirschberg, D. L., Ashe, S. A., Hellstrom, K. E. & Hellstrom, I. (1989). Enhancement of *in vitro* and *in vivo* anti-tumour activities of phosphorylated mitomycin C and etoposide derivatives by monoclonal antibody alkaline phosphatase conjugates. *Cancer Research*, **49**, 5789–5792.

Sharkey, R. M., Goldenberg, D. M., Goldenberg, H., Lee, R. E., Ballance, C., Pawlyk, D., Varga, D. & Hansen, H. J. (1990). Murine monoclonal antibodies against carcinoembryonic antigen: immunological, pharmacokinetic and targeting properties in humans. *Cancer Research*, **50**, 2823–2831.

Siccardi, A. G., Buraggi, G. L., Callergo, L., Centi Colella, A., De Filippi, P. G., Galli, G., Mariani, G., Masi, R., Palumbo, R., Riva, P., Salvatore, M., Scassellati, G. A., Scheidhauer, K., Turco, G. L., Zaniol, P., Benini, S., Deleide, G., Gasparini, M., Lastoria, S., Mansi, L., Paganelli, G., Salvischianni, E., Seregni, E., Viale, G. & Natali, P. G. (1989). Immunoscintigraphy of adenocarcinomas by means of radiolabelled F(ab')$_2$ fragments of an anti-carcinoembryonic antigen monoclonal antibody: a multicenter study. *Cancer Research*, **49**, 3095–3103.

Spooner, R. A. & Lord, J. M. (1991). Expression of antibody-ricin A chain fusion in mammalian cells. In *Monoclonal Antibodies: Applications in Clinical Oncology*, ed. A. A. Epenetos, pp. 65–77. London, Chapman & Hall Medical.

Spurr, N. K., Durbin, H., Sheer, D., Parkar, M., Bobrow, L. & Bodmer, W. F. (1986). Characterization and chromosomal assignment of a human cell surface antigen defined by the monoclonal antibody AUA1. *International Journal of Cancer*, **38**, 631–636.

Stewart, J. S. W., Hird, V., Snook, D., Dhokia, B., Sivolapenko, G. B., Hooker, G., Taylor-Papadimitriou, J., Sullivan, M., Lambert, H. E., Coulter, C., Mason, W. P., Soutter, W. P. & Epenetos, A. A. (1990*a*). Intraperitoneal Yttrium-90-labelled monoclonal antibody in ovarian cancer. *Journal of Clinical Oncology*, **8**, 1941–1950.

Stewart, J. S. W., Hird, V., Snook, D., Sullivan, M., Myers, M. J. & Epenetos, A. A. (1988). Intraperitoneal [131]I- and ^{90}Y-labelled monoclonal antibodies for ovarian cancer: pharmacokinetics and normal tissue dosimetry. *International Journal of Cancer*, **42** (Suppl. 3), 71–76.

Stewart, J. S. W., Sivolapenko, G. B., Hird, V., Davies, K. A. A., Walport, M., Ritter, M. A. & Epenetos, A. A. (1990*b*). Clearance of [131]-I-labelled murine monoclonal antibody from patients blood by intravenous human anti-murine immunoglobulin antibody. *Cancer Research*, **50**, 563–567.

Taylor-Papadimitriou, J. T., Peterson, J. A. & Arklie, J. (1981). Monoclonal antibodies to epithelium specific components of the human milk fat globule membrane: production and reaction with cells in culture. *International Journal of Cancer*, **28**, 17–19.

Thorpe, P. E., Detre, S. I., Foxwell, B. M. J., Brown, A. N. F., Skilleter, D. N., Wilson, G., Forrester, J. A. & Stirpe, F. (1985). Modification of the carbohydrate in ricin with metaperiodate-cyanoborohydride mixtures: effector toxicity and *in vivo* distribution. *European Journal of Biochemistry*, **147**, 197–209.

Tsujisaki, M., Imai, K., Tokuchi, S., Hanzawa, Y., Ishida, T., Kitagawa, H., Hinoda, Y. & Yachi, A. (1991). Induction of antigen-specific immune response with the use of anti-idiotypic monoclonal antibodies to anti-carcinoembryonic antigen antibodies. *Cancer Research*, **51**, 2599–2604.

Vaughan, A. T. M., Keeling, A. & Yankuba, S. C. S. (1985). The production and biological distribution of yttrium-90-labelled antibodies. *International Journal of Applied Radiation and Isotopes*, **36**, 803–806.

Verhoeyen, M., Milstein, G. & Winter, G. (1988). Reshaping human antibodies: grafting an anti-lysozyme activity. *Science*, **239**, 1534–1536.

Vitetta, E. S., Stone, M., Amlot, P., Fay, J., May, R., Tilli, M., Newman, J., Clark, P., Collins, R., Cunnigham,D., Ghetie, V., Uhr, W. & Thorpe, P. E. (1991). Phase I immunotoxin trial in patients with B-cell lymphoma. *Cancer Research*, **51**, 4052–4058.

Zalutsky, M. R., Mosley, R. P., Benjamin, J. C., Colapino, E. V., Fuller, G. N., Coakham, H. P. & Bigner, D. D. (1990). Monoclonal antibody and F(ab')₂ fragment delivery to tumour in patients with glioma: comparison of intracarotid and intravenous administration. *Cancer Research*, **50**, 4105–4110.

Zalutsky, M. R., Noska, M. A., Colapinto, E. V., Garg, K. & Bigner, D. (1989). Enhanced tumour localisation and *in-vivo* stability of a monoclonal antibody radioiodinated using N-succinimidyl 3-(tri-n-butylstannyl) benzoate. *Cancer Research*, **49**, 5543–5549.

11A

Monoclonal antibodies in infectious disease: diagnosis

T. G. WREGHITT and J. J. GRAY

11A.1 Introduction

Increasing use is being made of monoclonal antibodies (mab) in the diagnosis of infectious diseases. In this chapter we summarize briefly their use in the diagnosis of bacterial, viral, fungal, mycoplasmal, chlamydial and some other infections.

11A.2 Respiratory infections

Viruses, bacteria, mycoplasmas and chlamydias are associated with human respiratory tract infection. Most infections have a seasonal distribution (Figure 11A.1). Some, such as respiratory syncytial virus (RSV) are associated with

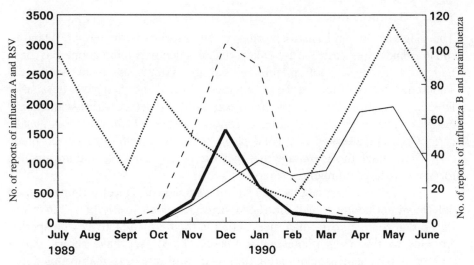

Figure 11A.1. Seasonal distribution of reports by date of specimen for influenza A (—) and B (—) parainfluenza (· · · ·) and respiratory syncytial virus (RSV; – – –). England and Wales, July 1989 to June 1990. Source: Laboratory reports to Communicable Disease Surveillance Centre.

annual epidemics whereas others such as *Mycoplasma pneumoniae* occur in epidemics every 4 years.

Many viral respiratory pathogens can be grown in cell culture. Direct and indirect immunofluorescence tests employing mab are available for detecting influenza A, influenza B, adenovirus, RSV and parainfluenza viruses 1–3 in nasopharyngeal aspirates and inoculated cell cultures (Schmidt *et al.*, 1982; Bell *et al.*, 1983; Kim *et al.*, 1983; Routledge *et al.*, 1985; Mills *et al.*, 1989; Stout *et al.*, 1989). Time-resolved fluoroimmunoassay employing mab has also been used for this purpose (Hierholzer *et al.*, 1989).

Mab against *M. pneumoniae* are being evaluated for use in antigen detection and a fluorescein-labelled antibody against *Chlamydia pneumoniae* is commercially available. The existence of many different strains of *Chlamydia psittaci* preclude the use of mab in antigen detection assays.

Most viral, chlamydial and *M. pneumoniae* respiratory tract infections are diagnosed serologically and mab are not widely used for this purpose but mab have been used on the solid phase in some red cell assays to detect *M. pneumoniae* IgM (Coombs *et al.*, 1988).

Most bacterial respiratory tract infections are detected by isolating the causative organism and mab are not widely used in routine diagnosis. Mab have been produced against several of these organisms. For example, there is a commercially-available fluorescein isothiocyanate (FITC)-conjugated species-specific mab for detecting *Legionella pneumophila* and mab are employed in an enzyme-linked immunosorbent assay (ELISA) to detect *L. pneumophila* serogroup 1 in urine (Birtles *et al.*, 1990).

11A.3 Gastroenteritis

The diagnosis of viral gastroenteritis, often associated with either rotavirus, small round virus, astrovirus, calicivirus or adenovirus infection, has been hampered by the lack of suitable cell culture systems. As these viruses can sometimes be detected in large numbers during the first few days after infection, electron microscopy has been used to detect viruses in clinical samples. There are a few antigen capture assays which use virus-specific antibody either attached to a solid phase or coupled with latex or red blood cells. These have the advantage that they are readily available and are suitable for handling large numbers of samples.

Assays to detect rotavirus antigen in samples of faeces originally used polyclonal antibodies to calf diarrhoea virus (Kapikian *et al.*, 1974) but it was shown that some human rotaviruses varied in their cross-reactivity with specific antibody to this virus (Sanekata & Okada, 1983). We have shown that a reverse passive haemagglutination test with anti-rotavirus mab-coupled red cells used to detect rotavirus antigen in samples of faeces has a sensitivity of 96.0% and a specificity of 98.5% when compared with electron microscopy (Gray *et al.*, 1990). This mab, designated A3M4, is directed against a group-specific epitope of the virion inner capsid (Beards *et al.*, 1984). Monoclonal anti-rotavirus antibodies have also been developed which have specificity for subgroup epitopes (Greenberg *et al.*, 1983). Taniguchi *et al.* (1984) have employed mab which have subgroup specificities in an ELISA for subgrouping human rotavirus isolates.

Mab to astroviruses and enteric adenoviruses, both important causes of gastroenteritis in young children, have also been used in ELISAs to detect virus antigen in samples of faeces (Herrmann *et al.*, 1991).

In bacterial gastroenteritis, culture is relatively easy and the large number of bacterial strains, such as in the salmonellae (1800 or more), make direct immunological assays inappropriate. Mab have been used to identify isolates (Lim & Fok, 1987), differentiate toxin from non-toxin-producing strains or determine the toxins present in a clinical isolate (Padhye *et al.*, 1989). Mab against *Clostridium difficile* toxins have also been produced but they are not as yet used in routine diagnosis. Mab used to diagnose infections caused by Enterobacteriaceae should be well characterized and screened for cross-reactivity with other members of the same family. Husson *et al.* (1989) describe an enzyme immunocapture assay to detect non-diarrhoeal *Escherichia coli*. This assay, using a mab directed against *E. coli* alkaline phosphatase, was able to detect *E. coli* in urine after 2 h incubation or in blood culture but was inappropriate for use with other clinical samples as a cross-reaction between *E. coli* and *Shigella* spp. alkaline phosphatase was observed.

Immunological methods can be used to detect and identify microorganisms in food associated with food-poisoning outbreaks. The Bio-Enzabead Screen Kit (Organon Teknika Ltd, Cambridge) is an ELISA which uses two mab directed against the flagellar antigens of *Salmonella* to detect *Salmonella* spp. in foods after a pre-enrichment procedure.

11A.4 Hepatitis

Hepatitis is associated with a number of viruses and bacteria, including hepatitis viruses A, B, C, D and E, Epstein–Barr virus (EBV), cytomegalovirus (CMV) and *Leptospira* spp.

Hepatitis A virus (HAV) is a picornavirus which is spread by the faecal–oral route, mainly through contaminated food and water. As the virus is difficult to grow in cell culture, infection is usually diagnosed by means of specific antibody tests, such as mu-capture ELISA or radioimmunoassay (RIA) for detecting HAV-specific IgM. MacGregor *et al.* (1983) reported the production of three mab to HAV which were subsequently employed in solid phase RIA and ELISAs to detect HAV antigen and antibodies (Coulepis *et al.*, 1985). HAV antigen detection is only available in reference laboratories.

Hepatitis B virus (HBV) infection, associated with blood-borne transmission, is usually detected by means of assays for hepatitis B surface antigen (HBsAg). Many different kinds of assays are available to detect this virus antigen but

most laboratories currently employ ELISA, RIA or enhanced chemiluminescence for this purpose, many of them incorporating mab directed against
various epitopes of HBsAg. Many of these tests are sensitive and specific but
false positive reactions may be encountered (Ratnam *et al.*, 1989). Mab may
also be included in assays to detect other HBV markers such as anti-hepatitis B
core (anti-HBc) and surface (anti-HBs) antibodies and hepatitis Be antigen
(HBeAg) and anti-hepatitis Be antigen (anti-HBe).

Assays for the detection of hepatitis C virus (HCV) markers are still
evolving. HCV is the major blood-borne non-A, non-B, hepatitis virus. Infection is usually diagnosed by the detection of HCV antibody (by ELISA) or
HCV RNA (by polymerase chain reaction (PCR)). At present, mab are not
employed in assays to detect anti-HCV but it is likely that they will be in the
future.

Hepatitis D virus (HDV), also known as the Delta agent, is a defective virus
that requires active infection with HBV for its replication. Mab have been
developed which recognize the major polypeptides of this virus. These have
been used in assays to detect HDV in human liver samples (Pohl *et al.*, 1987).

As yet, there are no widely available assays for the diagnosis of hepatitis E
virus infection. Mab have been developed in some specialized laboratories to
study leptospira but these are not used widely. Mab are not employed in tests
to diagnose EBV infection. The diagnosis of CMV infection is discussed later
(11A.9).

11A.5 Neurological/congenital infections

Neurological infections can be caused by a wide range of microorganisms
(Table 11A.1). Effective treatment is available for many of these infections;
rapid and accurate identification of the causative agent is essential.

11A.6 Meningitis

Meningitis may be an acute disease caused by a viral (aseptic) or bacterial
(purulent) infection or a chronic condition normally associated with tuberculo-
sis, brucellosis or fungal disease. The need to institute prompt and appropriate
antibiotic therapy in bacterial meningitis may be hampered by the relative
insensitivity of Gram's stain when used to detect bacteria in the cerebrospinal
fluid (CSF). The availability of mab has led to the development of rapid
immunological assays to detect small quantities of some of the more common
bacterial antigens in the CSF. Group B streptococci are one of the leading
causes of meningitis in neonates. Ruch & Smith (1982) described a mab,
designated A9, which reacts with Group B carbohydrate antigen. This antibody, when coupled with latex, was able to detect group B antigen in urine and
CSF samples collected from patients with proven group B streptococcal infec-

Table 11A.1. *Some of the most important microorganisms associated with neurological infections*

Acute bacterial meningitis	Chronic meningitis
Neisseria meningitidis	Tuberculosis
Haemophilus influenzae	Brucellosis
Streptococcus pneumoniae	Cryptococcosis
Listeria monocytogenes	Candidiasis
Group B streptococcus	Coccidioidomycosis
Escherichia coli	Histoplasmosis
Acute viral meningitis	**Encephalitis**
Enterovirus	Arbovirus
Poliovirus	HSV
Coxsackie virus	Varicella-zoster virus (VZV)
Echovirus	EBV
Mumps	CMV
Epstein–Barr virus (EBV)	HIV
Lymphocytic choriomeningitis (LCM) virus	Measles
Human immunodeficiency virus (HIV)	*Chlamydia psittaci*
Herpes simplex virus (HSV)	*Borrelia burgdorferi*
Arboviruses	*Rickettsia rickettsiae*
	Congenital rubella
	Congenital toxoplasmosis
	Congenital CMV
	Congenital syphilis
	Rabies
	Cerebral malaria

tion. A mab directed against VP1 antigen of enteroviruses has been developed for detecting a broad range of enteroviruses growing in cell culture (Yousef *et al.*, 1987).

11A.7 Encephalitis

The identification of a microorganism causing acute encephalitis may rely on detecting antigen *ante mortem* in brain biopsy material or *post mortem* in necropsy tissue. Mab have been used to detect herpes simplex virus (HSV) in smears of brain biopsy material (Rossier *et al.*, 1989) and *Listeria monocytogenes* in necropsy tissue (McLauchlin *et al.*, 1988). In rabies, highly specific mab can be used in epidemiological studies to differentiate specific variants of the street rabies virus (Wiktor *et al.*, 1980) and for diagnosis on brain biopsy and other clinical specimens.

Brain biopsies are not performed in many centres; therefore alternative methods of diagnosis, such as detecting specific IgM in the patient's serum with a sensitive and specific immunological assay, can be employed. In congenitally-acquired neurological infections with rubella, CMV or *Toxoplasma gondii*, specific IgM may be detected in the serum of the infected infant for at least 6 months. Indirect immunoassays with fluorescent, radio or enzyme labels can be used to detect specific IgM in serum but these techniques suffer from interference from specific IgG and rheumatoid factor. IgM capture immunoassays which may use anti-human IgM mab to capture IgM from patient's serum and labelled virus-specific antibodies to detect antigen bound to the patient's IgM, or both, eliminate the need to fractionate and pre-absorb serum (Figure 11A.2).

11A.8   Sexually transmitted disease

The reported incidence of sexually transmitted disease, particularly infection with *Chlamydia trachomatis* and HSV, has increased dramatically over the last 30 years. A dual policy of education to modify behaviour and rapid and accurate diagnosis, leading to effective treatment, has been pursued in an attempt to halt or reverse this trend. The widespread use of mab in immunological assays to detect either *C. trachomatis* antigens or cells infected with HSV in clinical samples has clearly contributed to the increased reporting of such infections (see Figure 11A.3) and has enabled laboratories, with no facilities for culturing these agents, to process large numbers of samples.

Direct immunofluorescence with species-specific mab (which react with *C. trachomatis* elementary bodies) or genus-specific mab (which react with both elementary bodies and the group-specific lipopolysaccharide) has been shown to be highly specific and sensitive when compared with the isolation of *C. trachomatis* in cell culture (Alexander *et al.*, 1985, Thomas *et al.*, 1984) but cannot distinguish between living and dead organisms. Pugh *et al.* (1985) showed that an amplified solid phase ELISA, with a monoclonal antibody directed against genus-specific lipopolysaccharide *C. trachomatis* antigen, had the advantage of detecting low numbers of organisms, which may be undetect-

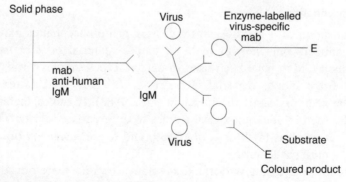

Figure 11A.2. IgM antibody-capture ELISA.

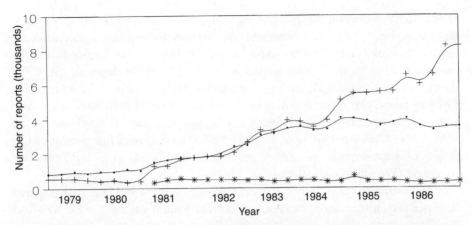

Figure 11A.3. Sexually transmitted diseases. Quarterly Communicable Disease Reports 1979–86. (■) Herpes simplex, (+) *C. trachomatis*, (∗) *N. gonorrhoeae*.

able by direct immunofluorescence, and was suitable for screening large numbers of samples.

The laboratory diagnosis of genital HSV infection again utilizes mab in both direct immunofluorescence assays (Pouletty *et al.*, 1987) and ELISAs (Clayton *et al.*, 1985). Useful epidemiological data can be collected if type-specific mab are used to differentiate HSV type 1 from HSV type 2 (Botcherby *et al.*, 1987).

Although laboratory reports of gonorrhoea caused by *Neisseria gonorrhoeae* have not shown the same dramatic increase as those of *C. trachomatis* and HSV, it is still a major cause of sexually-transmitted disease. Detecting *N. gonorrhoeae* involves the isolation of the organism, then its identification either biochemically (Kellogg & Turner, 1973) or immunologically with polyclonal antibody (Menek, 1976) or mab (Welch & Cartwright, 1988). A single mab directed against an epitope of *N. gonorrhoeae* may not identify all isolates because of the many serotypes of the gonococcus. By pooling mab prepared against different epitopes of the outer membrane protein I of *N. gonorrhoeae*, however, an antibody can be constructed that reacts with serovars containing outer membrane proteins IA and IB (Laughton *et al.*, 1987).

Mab have not found general acceptance in the diagnosis of syphilis. The diagnosis of this disease, caused by infection with *Treponema pallidum*, in the early infectious phase relies on demonstrating treponemes by dark-field microscopy in fluid collected from lesions. In cases of latent or late syphilis, serology is the only practical method of laboratory diagnosis.

11A.9   Infection in the immunocompromised host

Patients who are immunocompromised because of disease (i.e. lymphoma or AIDS) or because of treatment (i.e. organ transplants) are more susceptible to certain infectious agents such as herpesviruses, *Aspergillus* spp., *Pseudomonas* spp., *Pneumocystis carinii*, *Candida* spp. and *Toxoplasma gondii*.

The most important herpesvirus is CMV which produces life-threatening disease in heart–lung and bone marrow transplant recipients in particular. Serious disease may also be experienced by other solid organ transplant recipients, particularly if the infection is acquired from the donor organ. CMV infection is associated with increased morbidity and mortality in AIDS patients. CMV infection can be detected either by means of serological tests or by virus culture or antigen detection. Primary CMV infection may be diagnosed by the detection of CMV-specific IgM. In most clinical laboratories this is achieved by means of a mu-capture ELISA employing a monoclonal anti-CMV antibody conjugate (Wreghitt *et al.*, 1986).

CMV is amenable to antiviral (ganciclovir) treatment but, because it grows slowly in cell culture, more rapid diagnostic techniques such as the DEAFF test (Griffiths *et al.*, 1984) have been developed. In this test, specimens are inoculated on to fibroblast cells. At 24–48 h later, mab directed against early (EA) or immediately early (IEA) CMV antigen are used to identify CMV. This is a rapid technique but it is not as sensitive as culture and to maximize the detection of CMV, conventional culture techiques should also be employed in parallel, particularly with respiratory tract specimens such as bronchoalveolar lavage and lung biopsy. Samples collected from respiratory sites may also contain HSV, which has been associated with fatal pneumonia (Smyth *et al.*, 1990). Mab directed against the IE of CMV may also be used to detect CMV in tissue sections (Hackman *et al.*, 1985) and in peripheral blood (Schirm *et al.*, 1987). Mab directed against a 65 kD matrix protein of CMV have been used to detect CMV antigen in peripheral blood leucocytes (Revello *et al.*, 1992).

HSV infection is frequently encountered by immunocompromised patients, usually manifesting as cold sores or genital herpes, but it may also be associated with mucositis. Isolation in cell culture is the usual method of diagnosis and is usually achieved in 24–48 h. The differentiation between HSV types 1 and 2 is performed by means of indirect immunofluorescence tests employing HSV 1 and 2 type-specific mab (Pereira *et al.*, 1982). ELISAs, employing monoclonal anti-HSV antibodies for the detection of HSV (Clayton *et al.*, 1985) and fluorescein-conjugated mab are also used to detect HSV in clinical samples (Botcherby *et al.*, 1987).

Varicella zoster virus (VZV) primary infection (chickenpox) is usually serious and may be fatal in immunocompromised patients; reactivation of VZV (shingles) is experienced frequently by this group of patients. VZV grows slowly in cell culture and cannot be differentiated from HSV by electron microscopy. Infection is amenable to acyclovir treatment and so rapid, specific, diagnostic techniques are beneficial to patient care. It may be difficult to distinguish clinically between HSV and VZV infection, particularly in patients with shingles. An indirect immunofluorescence test employing mab has been used to detect VZV in vesicle smears (Weigle & Grose, 1984).

Infection with the human immunodeficiency virus (HIV), which in itself is immunosuppressive, may lead to opportunistic infections. Mab have been used in commercial diagnostic tests for detecting HIV antibody and p24 antigen (Kontio, 1991).

Primary *T. gondii* infection may be fatal in organ transplant recipients, particularly if infection is acquired from the donor organ (Wreghitt *et al.*, 1989). In patients with AIDS, space-occupying, ring-enhanced brain lesions are associated with *T. gondii* reactivation. Cerebral toxoplasmosis may also be fatal unless appropriate therapy is given. In transplant recipients, infection is detected serologically. *T. gondii*-specific IgM, found particularly in primary infection, is usually detected by means of a mu-capture ELISA employing a monoclonal antibody (Balfour *et al.*, 1987). AIDS patients may not produce an antibody response and in the absence of brain biopsy material a definitive diagnosis may be difficult.

Pneumonitis associated with *Pneumocystis carinii* infection is found frequently in immunocompromised individuals being particularly prevalent in AIDS and transplant patients. Infection is usually diagnosed by the detection of *P. carinii* antigen in lung biopsy or sputum samples. Mab have been used successfully in indirect (Kovacs *et al.*, 1988) and direct immunofluorescence (Ng *et al.*, 1990) tests with these samples. Cregan *et al.* (1990) have shown that direct and indirect immunofluorescence tests employing mab are more sensitive for the detection of infection than modified Giemsa stain and quick silver stain.

Immunocompromised individuals infected with *Cryptosporidium parvum* experience severe diarrhoea which may be life-threatening. Diagnosis of infection relies on the detection of faecal oocysts. Fluorescein-labelled mab have been used to detect the organism in water (Smith *et al.*, 1989) and an antigen-capture ELISA employing a mab has been developed to detect *C. parvum* in bovine faeces (Krzysztof *et al.*, 1990). This technique should be adaptable for use with human faecal samples. Similarly, ELISAs have been developed for detecting *Giardia lamblia* in faeces (Stibbs, 1989; Rosoff *et al.*, 1989).

Mab are employed in tests to diagnose mycological infections. A liposomal immunoassay (Directigen 1–2–3) for the diagnosis of disseminated candidosis (Walsh *et al.*, 1991) is available from Becton Dickinson and the Diagnostics Pasteur latex agglutination test (Pastorex *Aspergillus*) may be used for the diagnosis of invasive aspergillosis. A similar test (Pastorex *Candida*) uses a mab against *Candida albicans* mannan to diagnose invasive candidosis. Launch Diagnostics market a mab-based ELISA for detecting *Cryptococcus neoformans* antigen in serum and CSF.

11A.10 References

Alexander, I., Paul, I. D. & Caul, E. O. (1985). Evaluation of a genus-reactive monoclonal antibody for the rapid diagnosis of *Chlamydia trachomatis* by direct immunofluorescence. *Genitourinary Medicine*, **61**, 252–254.

Balfour, A. H., Harford, J. P. & Goodall, M. (1987). Use of monoclonal antibodies in an ELISA to detect IgM class antibodies specific for *Toxoplasma gondii*. *Journal of Clinical Pathology*, **40**, 853–857.

Beards, G. M., Campbell, A. D., Cottrell, N. R., Peris, J. S. M., Rees, N., Sanders, R. C., Shirley, J. A., Wood, H. C. & Flewett, T. H. (1984). Enzyme-linked immunosorbent assays based on polyclonal and monoclonal antibodies for rotavirus detection. *Journal of Clinical Microbiology*, **19**, 248–254.

Bell, D. M., Walsh, E. E., Hruska, J. F., Schnabel, K. C. & Hall, C. B. (1983). Rapid detection of respiratory syncitial virus with a monoclonal antibody. *Journal of Clinical Microbiology*, **17**, 1099–1101.

Birtles, R. J., Harrison, T. G., Samuel, D. & Taylor, A. G. (1990). Evaluation of urinary antigen ELISA for diagnosing *Legionella pneumophila* serogroup 1 infection. *Journal of Clinical Pathology*, **43**, 685–690.

Botcherby, M., Gilchrist, C., Bremner, J., Byrne, M. A., Harris, J. R. W. & Taylor-Robinson, D. (1987). Rapid diagnosis of genital herpes by detecting cells infected with virus in smears with fluorescent monoclonal antibodies. *Journal of Clinical Pathology*, **40**, 687–695.

Clayton, A.-L., Beckford, U., Roberts, C., Sutherland, S., Druce, A., Best, J. & Chantler, S. (1985). Factors influencing the sensitivity of herpes simplex virus detection in clinical specimens in a simultaneous enzyme-linked immunosorbent assay using monoclonal antibodies. *Journal of Medical Virology*, **17**, 275–282.

Coombs, R. A., Easter, G., Matejtschuk, P. & Wreghitt, T. G. (1988). Red cell IgM antibody capture assay for the detection of *Mycoplasma pneumoniae*-specific IgM. *Epidemiology and Infection*, **100**, 101–109.

Coulepis, A. G., Veale, M. F., MacGregor, A., Kornitschuk, M. & Gust, I. D. (1985). Detection of hepatitis A virus and antibody by solid-phase radioimmunoassay and enzyme-linked immunosorbent assay with monoclonal antibodies. *Journal of Clinical Microbiology*, **22**, 119–124.

Cregan, P., Yamamoto, A., Lum, A., van der Heide, T., MacDonald, M. & Pulliam, L. (1990). Comparison of four methods for rapid detection of *Pneumocystis carinii* in respiratory specimens. *Journal of Clinical Microbiology*, **28**, 2432–2436.

Gray, J. J., Vasquez, A. M., Kewley, D. R. & Coombs, R. R. A. (1990). Reverse passive haemagglutination with freeze-dried stabilized antibody-coupled red cells for detecting rotavirus in faecal samples. *Serodiagnosis and Immunotherapy in Infectious Diseases*, **4**, 143–149.

Greenberg, H., McAuliffe, V., Valdesuso, J., Wyatt, R., Flores, J., Kalica, A., Hoshino, Y. & Singh, N. (1983). Serological analysis of the subgroup protein of rotavirus using monoclonal antibodies. *Infection and Immunity*, **39**, 91–99.

Griffiths, P. D., Panjwani, D. D., Stirk, P. R., Ball, M. G., Janczakowski, H., Blacklock, H. A. & Prentice, H. G. (1984). Rapid diagnosis of cytomegalovirus infection in immunocompromised patients by detection of early antigen fluorescent foci. *Lancet*, **2**, 1242–1245.

Hackman, R. C., Myerson, D., Meyers, J. D., Shulman, H. M., Sale, G. E., Goldstein, L. C., Rastetter, M., Flournoy, N. & Thomas, E. D. (1985). Rapid diagnosis of cytomegalovirus pneumonia by tissue immunofluorescence with a murine monoclonal antibody. *Journal of Infectious Diseases*, **151**, 325–329.

Herrmann, J. E., Taylor, D. N., Echeverria, P. & Blacklow, N. R. (1991). Astroviruses as a cause of gastroenteritis in children. *New England Journal of Medicine*, **324**, 1757–1760.

Hierholzer, J. G., Bingham, P. G., Coombs, R. A., Johanssohn, K. H., Anderson, L. J. & Halonen, P. E. (1989). Comparison of monoclonal antibody time-resolved fluoroimmunoassay with monoclonal antibody capture-biotinylated detector enzyme immunoassay for respiratory syncitial virus and parainfluenza virus antigen detection. *Journal of Clinical Microbiology*, **27**, 1243–1249.

Husson, M. O., Mielcarek, C., Izard, D. & Leclerc, H. (1989). Alkaline phosphate capture test for the rapid identification of *Escherichia coli* and *Shigella* species based on a specific monoclonal antibody. *Journal of Clinical Microbiology*, **27**, 1518–1521.

Kapikian, A. Z., Kim, H. W., Wyatt, R. G., Rodriguez, W. J., Ross, S., Cline, W. L., Parrott, R. H. & Chanock, R. M. (1974). Reovirus-like agent in stools: association with infantile diarrhea and development of serologic tests. *Science*, **185**, 1049–1053.

Kellogg, D. S. & Turner, E. M. (1973). Rapid fermentation confirmation of *Neisseria gonorrhoeae*. *Applied Microbiology*, **5**, 550–552.

Kim, H. W., Wyatt, R. G., Fernie, B. F., Brandt, C. D., Arrobio, J. O., Jeffries, B. C. & Parrott, R. H. (1983). Respiratory syncitial virus detection by immunofluorescence in nasal secretions with monoclonal antibodies against selected surface and internal proteins. *Journal of Clinical Microbiology*, **18**, 1399–1404.

Kontio, S. (1991). Sensitive one-step enzyme immunoassay for HIV-1 p24 antigen in human blood specimens and cell culture supernatants. *Journal of Immunological Methods*, **139**, 257–263.

Kovaks, J. A., Ng, V. L., Masur, H., Leoung, G., Hadley, W. K., Evans, G., Lane, H. C., Ognibene, F. P., Shelhamer, J., Parrillo, J. E. & Gill, V. J. (1988). Diagnosis of *Pneumocystis carinii* pneumonia: improved detection in sputum with use of monoclonal antibodies. *New England Journal of Medicine*, **318**, 589–593.

Krzysztof, Z. A., Mason, P. H., Riggs, M. W. & Perryman, L. E. (1990). Detection of *Cryptosporidium parvum* oocysts in bovine feces by monoclonal antibody capture enzyme-linked immunosorbent assay. *Journal of Clinical Microbiology*, **28**, 2770–2774.

Laughton, B. E., Ehret, J. M., Tanino, T. T., van der Pol, B., Handsfield, H. H., Jones, R. B., Judson, F. N. & Hook, E. W. (1987). Fluorescent monoclonal antibody for confirmation of *Neisseria gonorrhoea* cultures. *Journal of Clinical Microbiology*, **25**, 2388–2390.

Lim, P.-L. & Fok, Y.-P. (1987). Detection of grouped Salmonellae in blood culture broth and of soluble antigen by tube agglutination using an 0–9 monoclonal antibody latex conjugate. *Journal of Clinical Microbiology*, **25**, 1165–1168.

MacGregor, A., Kornitschuk, M., Hurrell, J. G. R., Lehmann, N. I., Coulepis, A. G., Locarnini, S. A. & Gust, I. D. (1983). Monoclonal antibodies against hepatitis A virus. *Journal of Clinical Microbiology*, **18**, 1237–1243.

McLauchlin, J., Black, A., Green, H. T., Nash, J. Q. & Taylor, A. G. (1988). Monoclonal antibodies show *Listeria monocytogenes* in necropsy tissue samples. *Journal of Clinical Pathology*, **41**, 983–988.

Menek, H. (1976). Identification of *Neisseria gonorrhoeae* in cultures from tonsillo-pharyngeal specimens by means of a slide co-agglutination test (Phadebact gonococcus test). *Acta Pathologica Microbiologica Scandinavica, Section B*, **84**, 139–144.

Mills, R. D., Cain, K. J. & Woods, G. L. (1989). Detection of influenza virus by centrifugal inoculation of MDCK cells and staining with monoclonal antibodies. *Journal of Clinical Microbiology*, **27**, 2505–2508.

Ng, V. L., Virani, N. A., Chaisson, R. E., Yajko, D. M., Sphar, H. T., Cabrian, K., Rollins, N., Charache, P., Krieger, M., Hadley, W. K. & Hopewell, P. C. (1990). Rapid detection of *Pneumocystis carinii* using a direct fluorescent monoclonal antibody stain. *Journal of Clinical Microbiology*, **28**, 2228–2233.

Padhye, V. V., Zhao, T. & Doyle, M. P. (1989). Production and characterization of monoclonal antibodies to verotoxins 1 and 2 from *Escherichia coli* of serotype O157:H7. *Journal of Medical Microbiology*, **30**, 219–226.

Pereira, L., Dondero, D. V., Gallo, D., Devlin, V. & Woodie, J. D. (1982). Serological analysis of herpes simplex virus types 1 and 2 with monoclonal antibodies. *Infection and Immunity*, **35**, 363–367.

Pohl, C., Baroudy, B. M., Bergmann, K. F., Cote, P. J., Purcell, R. H., Hoofnagle, J. & Gerin, J. L. (1987). A human monoclonal antibody that recognizes viral polypeptides and *in vitro* translation products of the genome of hepatitis D virus. *Journal of Infectious Diseases*, **156**, 622–629.

Pouletty, P., Chomel, J. J., Thouvenot, D., Catalan, F., Rabillon, V. & Kadouche, J. (1987). Detection of herpes simplex virus in direct specimens by immunofluorescence assay using a monoclonal antibody. *Journal of Clinical Microbiology*, **25**, 958–959.

Pugh, S. F., Slack, R. C. B., Caul, E. O., Paul, I. D., Appleton, P. N. & Gatley, S. (1985). Enzyme-amplified immunoassay: a novel technique applied to direct detection of *Chlamydia trachomatis* in clinical specimens. *Journal of Clinical Pathology*, **38**, 1139–1141.

Ratnam, S., Stead, F. & Head, C. B. (1989). False-positive results with third-generation monoclonal hepatitis B surface antigen enzyme immunoassay. *Journal of Clinical Microbiology*, **27**, 2102–2104.

Revello, G. M., Percivalle, E., Matteo, A. D., Morini, F. & Gerna, G. (1992). Nuclear expression of the lower matrix protein of human cytomegalovirus in peripheral blood leucocytes of immunocompromised viraemic patients. *Journal of General Virology*, **73**, 437–442.

Rosoff, J. D., Sanders, C. A., Sonnad, S. S., de Lay, P. R., Hadley, W. K., Vincenzi, F. F., Yajko, D. M. & O'Hanley, P. D. (1989). Stool diagnosis of giardiasis using a commercially-available enzyme immunoassay to detect *Giardia*-specific antigen 65 (GSA 65). *Journal of Clinical Microbiology*, **27**, 1997–2002.

Routledge, E. G., McQuillan, J., Samson, A. C. R. & Toms, G. L. (1985). The development of monoclonal antibodies to respiratory syncitial virus and their use in diagnosis by indirect immunofluorescence. *Journal of Medical Virology*, **15**, 305–320.

Ruch, F. E. & Smith, L. (1982). Monoclonal antibody to streptococcal group B carbohydrate: applications in latex agglutination and immunoprecipitin assays. *Journal of Clinical Microbiology*, **16**, 145–152.

Sanekata, T. & Okada, H. (1983). Human rotavirus detection by agglutination of antibody-coated erythrocytes. *Journal of Clinical Microbiology*, **17**, 1141–1147.

Schirm, J., Timmerije, W., van der Bij, W., The, T. H., Wilterdink, J. B., Tegzess, A. M., van Son, W. J. & Schröder, F. P. (1987). Rapid detection of infectious cytomegalovirus in blood with the aid of monoclonal antibodies. *Journal of Medical Virology*, **23**, 31–40.

Schmidt, N. J., Ota, M., Gallo, D. & Fox, V. L. (1982). Monoclonal antibodies for rapid, strain-specific identification of influenza virus isolates. *Journal of Clinical Microbiology*, **16**, 763–765.

Smith, H. V., McDiarmid, A., Smith, A. L., Hinson, A. R. & Gilmour, R. A. (1989). An analysis of staining methods for the detection of *Cryptosporidium* spp. oocysts in water-related samples. *Parasitology*, **99**, 323–327.

Smyth, R. L., Higenbottam, T. W., Scott, J. P., Wreghitt, T. G., Stewart, S., Clelland, C. A., McGoldrick, J. P. & Wallwork, J. (1990). Herpes simples virus infection in heart–lung transplant recipients. *Transplantation*, **49**, 735–739.

Stibbs, H. H. (1989). Monoclonal antibody-based enzyme immunoassay for *Giardia lamblia* antigen in human stool. *Journal of Clinical Microbiology*, **27**, 2582–2588.

Stout, C., Murphy, M. D., Lawrence, S. & Julian, S. (1989). Evaluation of a
   monoclonal antibody pool for rapid diagnosis of respiratory viral infections. *Journal
   of Clinical Microbiology*, **27**, 448–452.
Taniguchi, K., Urasawa, T., Urasawa, S. & Yasuhara, T. (1984). Production of
   subgroup-specific monoclonal antibodies against human rotaviruses and their
   application to an enzyme-linked immunosorbent assay for subgroup determination.
   Journal of Medical Virology, **14**, 115–125.
Thomas, B. J., Evans, R. T., Hawkins, D. A. & Taylor-Robinson, D. (1984).
   Sensitivity of detecting *Chlamydia trachomatis* elementary bodies in smears by use
   of a fluorescein-labelled monoclonal antibody: comparison with conventional
   chlamydial isolation. *Journal of Clinical Pathology*, **37**, 812–816.
Walsh, T. J., Hathorn, J. W., Sobel, J. D., Merz, W. G., Sanchez, V., Maret, S. M.,
   Buckley, H. R. Pfaller, M. A., Schaufele, R., Sliva, C., Navarro, E., Lecciones, J.,
   Chandrasdkar, P., Lee, J. & Pizzo, P. A. (1991). Detection of circulating candida
   enolase by immunoassay in patients with cancer and invasive candidiasis. *New
   England Journal of Medicine*, **324**, 1026–1031.
Weigle, K. A. & Grose, C. (1984). Varicella pneumonitis: immunodiagnosis with a
   monoclonal antibody. *Journal of Pediatrics*, **105**, 265–269.
Welch, W. D. & Cartwright, G. (1988). Fluorescent monoclonal antibody compared
   with carbohydrate utilization for rapid identification of *Neisseria gonorrhoeae*.
   Journal of Clinical Microbiology, **26**, 293–296.
Wiktor, T. J., Flamand, A. & Koprowski, H. (1980). Use of monoclonal antibodies in
   diagnosis of rabies virus infection and differentiation of rabies and rabies-related
   viruses. *Journal of Virological Methods*, **1**, 1–10.
Wreghitt, T. G., Gray, J. J. & Chandler, C. (1986). Prognostic value of cytomegalovirus
   IgM antibody in transplant recipients. *Lancet*, **1**, 1157–1158.
Wreghitt, T. G., Hakim, M., Gray, J. J., Balfour, A. H., Stovin, P. G. I., Stewart, S.,
   Scott, J., English, T. A. H. & Wallwork, J. (1989). Toxoplasmosis in heart and
   heart and lung transplant recipients. *Journal of Clinical Pathology*, **42**, 194–199.
Yousef, G. E., Brown, I. N. & Mowbray, J. F. (1987). Derivation and biochemical
   characterization of an enterovirus group-specific monoclonal antibody.
   International Virology, **28**, 163–170.

11B

Monoclonal antibodies in infectious disease: prophylaxis and therapy

J. COHEN

11B.1 Introduction

Following the introduction of the sulphonamides efforts to improve the treatment of infection focused almost entirely on the development of new and 'better' antimicrobial drugs. There is no doubt that the penicillins, cephalosporins, aminoglycosides, and recent arrivals such as the quinolones, have all had an enormous impact on the treatment of infection; antimicrobials remain the cornerstone of management. That said, it has become apparent in recent years that there are certain instances in which antibiotics alone seem to have reached the limits of their ability, in which case, for one reason or another, some other approach is needed.

The role of specific antibody as part of the host defences against infection has been widely studied and clearly documented. Indeed, historically, antiserum to pneumococcal capsular polysaccharide antedated the use of penicillin in the treatment of lobar pneumonia and the ability to develop protective antibody has been the basis of the successful introduction of vaccines for many important bacterial and viral infections. Passive immunotherapy (the administration of antibody for the prophylaxis and/or therapy of infection) is used in a variety of clinical settings, the most obvious examples being as replacement therapy in individuals with primary immunodeficiency syndromes and as treatment for diseases caused by exotoxins, such as tetanus, diphtheria and botulism. When the technology necessary to produce monoclonal antibodies (mab) became available, the question arose as to whether any of these indications, or others, might benefit from this approach.

In fact, mab have been raised against very many microbial antigens but the clinical applications have been rather limited, at least so far (Larrick, 1989). In part this is probably due to commercial constraints: it is very expensive to develop, test and produce these reagents to a point where they can obtain regulatory approval and in the case of diphtheria, say, the exercise would be uneconomic. In this chapter, I will concentrate on those few areas in which mab have or may soon have clinical use.

11B.2   Bacterial infections

11B.2.1 *Gram-negative sepsis and septic shock*

11B.2.1.1 *Antibody to lipid A and endotoxin core*

Bacteraemia with organisms such as *Escherichia coli*, *Proteus*, *Klebsiella* and *Pseudomonas aeruginosa* has a mortality rate of about 20% but in about 20–25% of all cases the condition is complicated by the development of septic shock when the mortality rises to 75% or more (Ispahani *et al.* 1987). This high mortality has remained virtually unchanged despite the use of modern antibiotics and sophisticated intensive care procedures and has prompted the search for alternative approaches.

Shock is a disorder characterized by hypotension, coagulation abnormalities and multiorgan failure involving the lungs, liver, kidneys and brain. A considerable body of evidence has accumulated indicating that the systemic features of the disease are largely attributable to endotoxin, the lipopolysaccharide (LPS) component of the cell wall of Gram-negative bacteria (Bayston & Cohen, 1990).

In the mid-1960s it was learnt that the lipopolysaccharides of most common Gram-negative bacteria shared a striking degree of common structure (Figure 11B.1). There are three regions. The first, or innermost part, is termed Lipid A and is the most conserved part of the LPS molecule. It consists of a beta-1.6 linked D-glucosamine disaccharide which carries two phosphoryl groups and four ester- or amide-linked 3-hydroxyl fatty acids. The second, or core region, consists of a hetero-oligosaccharide composed of two unusual sugars: heptose and 3-deoxy-D-manno-octulosonic acid (also called keto-deoxyoctonate or KDO) and in the outer core the more common sugars D-glucose, D-galactose

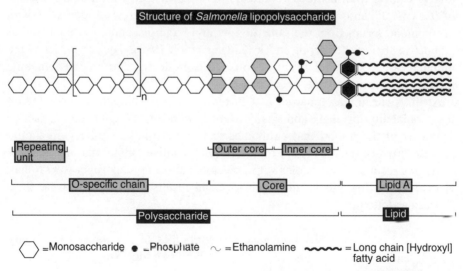

Figure 11B.1. Diagram of the biochemical structure of lipopolysaccharide.

and N-acetyl-D-glucosamine. The third and outermost part of the LPS molecule is made up of a chain of varying length of oligosaccharides and it is the particular configuration of this 'O-specific' side chain that confers serotypic specificity on a particular Gram-negative organism. Thus, while there are more than one hundred 'O' serotypes of *E. coli*, there are only six minor variations in the core and the Lipid A is essentially identical (Rietschel *et al.*, 1982). This understanding of the biochemistry of endotoxin became particularly important when it was appreciated that most of the toxicity of the molecule resided in the Lipid A, raising the possibility of generating antibodies to the core and/or Lipid A which would have broad cross-reactivity to the LPS of most common Gram-negative bacteria and hence be true 'anti-endotoxins'.

The availability of so-called 'rough mutant' strains of Gram-negative bacteria provided the opportunity to produce these antibodies. These strains were deficient in the 'O' chain and varying amounts of the core. Two strains in particular were used: *E. coli* J5 and the 'deep rough' R595 strain of *Salmonella minnesota*. The initial strategy involved the generation of polyclonal antibodies which were tested in a variety of animal models of Gram-negative sepsis. The results were very encouraging: the antibodies seemed able to prevent classical LPS-mediated phenomena, such as the Shwartzman reaction, and could prevent lethality even in models involving challenge with live bacteria. Not all investigators, however, were able to reproduce these findings and it was impossible to exclude the possibility that antibodies (or other components of the antiserum) not directly related to the anti-core activity were responsible for the protection that was seen. A detailed analysis of the literature on polyclonal anti-endotoxins is beyond the scope of this chapter but it has recently been reviewed (Appelmelk & Cohen, 1992). Despite the reservations noted above, the success of at least some of the animal experiments provided the impetus for a large clinical trial in which volunteers were immunized with a boiled vaccine of *E. coli* J5 and then donated immune serum. This was compared with pre-immune serum from the same donors in a large placebo controlled trial as adjunctive therapy for septic shock (Ziegler *et al.*, 1982). The recipients of the immune serum were significantly protected from death, thereby strengthening the case for the use of 'anti-endotoxins'.

At this point it was apparent that further clinical development depended on the availability of mab and many were produced. Despite the attractive simplicity of the notion that antibodies to Lipid A or the core region should provide cross-protection against most Gram-negative organisms and the encouraging results of the studies with polyclonal antisera, experiments with mab yielded conflicting and at times controversial results. The issues can be summarized as follows:

1 It has been difficult to generate antibodies of the desired specificity and to show unequivocally that they bind to endotoxin.

2 It has not been possible to demonstrate that conventional *in-vitro*

assays of antigen–antibody binding predict efficacy in *in-vivo* studies of protection.

3 Animal experiments have produced variable results, even when the same antibody has been used.

4 Very little is known of the mechanism by which some antibodies afford protection in animals.

Let us consider some of these points in more detail.

Ideally, 'anti-endotoxin' mab should react with 'smooth' LPS (i.e. the entire molecule) of the commonest Gram-negative bacteria: *E. coli*, *Klebsiella* and *Pseudomonas*. Nevertheless, it has been a consistent finding that these clones failed to bind to purified smooth LPS. In fact, even binding to LPS from rough mutants is very restricted. Detailed immunochemical analysis of the specificities of many of the anti-core mab has revealed that they are incapable of binding internal residues but that they require both KDO plus part of the Lipid A for binding (Appelmelk & Cohen, 1992). The pattern of reactivity, furthermore, was found to be considerably more restricted than was anticipated; for instance, antibodies raised against the *Salmonella* R595 strain were found to bind only to the homologous deep rough LPS (Pollack *et al.* 1989). Even when these antibodies did seem able to bind LPS *in vitro* it was not clear that it was specific; binding was often equally avid to completely unrelated lipid molecules such as cardiolipin (J. D. Baumgartner & M. P. Glauser, personal communication). Equally curious was the inability to predict efficacy *in vivo* on the basis of screening *in vitro*. We examined a panel of R595 antibodies and ranked them on the basis of their ELISA-binding titres and their ability to neutralize endotoxin in the Limulus assay. We then compared these results with their protective capacity in a mouse protection assay and found no correlation (McConnell *et al.*, 1990).

Animal studies of anti-core antibodies have produced variable results. Some investigators have demonstrated striking protection whereas others have failed. In some cases apparent protection might be explained by experimental arte-facts but in others the observation seems reproducible (reviewed in Appelmelk & Cohen, 1992). It is apparent that the ability to show protection may be highly dependent on the model system used. Teng *et al.* reported that the antibody HA-1A protected neutropenic rabbits from *E. coli* sepsis (Teng *et al.*, 1985) but others could show no effect when the same antibody was tested in mice (Baumgartner *et al.*, 1990).

It is also unclear how these antibodies might work. Antibodies to the outer 'O' side chain are powerfully opsonic but this does not seem to be the case for anti-core antibodies (Mehta *et al.*, 1988). Interestingly, pre-treatment of bacteria with antibiotics enhances the ability of the antibodies to bind to the bacteria and indeed most 'successful' animal models of infection have employed antibiotics. It has been assumed that the effect of the antibiotic is to expose hidden epitopes, thereby allowing the antibody to bind to the LPS and then be cleared, although the evidence for this is controversial (Overbeek *et al.*, 1989*a*, *b*). Curiously, there are no published *in-vivo* data showing that administration of these antibodies is associated with disappearance of LPS from the circulation. Much evidence points to the fact that endotoxin acts by activating cytokines, particularly tumour necrosis factor (TNF) and hence it would be expected that administration of these anti-core antibodies would be reflected in lower TNF levels in protected animals. When we gave a protective anti-core antibody to mice, however, we found no effect on TNF levels (Silva *et al.*, 1990*a*). Recently it has been proposed that the antibody HA-1A might act by binding to LPS and forming a complex with C3b; this complex could then bind to the CR1 receptor and be cleared from the circulation (Krieger *et al.*, 1993).

Despite these unanswered questions, the potential benefits of an effective anti-endotoxin antibody led to the development of two reagents for clinical trial. One, an antibody called E5, is a mouse IgM mab raised against Lipid A. In the first large study to be carried out, 486 patients with suspected Gram-negative sepsis received placebo or two doses of E5 24 h apart (Greenman *et al.*, 1991). Among 316 patients with documented Gram-negative infection, there was no difference in outcome between the placebo and E5 treated groups. When a subgroup of 137 patients not in shock were examined, however, the E5 recipients had a significantly lower 30-day mortality ($p = 0.03$) and significant improvement in the resolution of 'major morbidities' (i.e. complications of shock such as acute renal failure). This trial suggested that E5 was effective in a subgroup of patients, who were defined retrospectively, and so a second trial was carried out to try and verify this finding. Unfortunately, the preliminary results failed to confirm the initial observation, although a meta-analysis of the two studies did indicate some effect (R. Wenzel, data presented at the 31st ICAAC, Chicago, 1991).

The second antibody to be studied was a human IgM to core glycolipid, called HA-1A. In a study similar in design to that carried out with E5, 543 patients received placebo or a single dose of antibody (Ziegler *et al.*, 1991). Once again, the intention-to-treat analysis of all treated patients failed to show any effect but in a subgroup of 200 patients with Gram-negative rod bacteraemia, identified prospectively, antibody recipients benefited from a reduction in mortality from 49% to 30% ($p = 0.014$). In contrast to the results with E5, HA-1A was effective in shocked patients; the placebo mortality rate was 57% compared with 33% in the antibody-treated patients. These encouraging results have led to regulatory approval for this antibody in a number of countries, although many questions remain unanswered (Gazmuri *et al.*, 1991; Tanio & Feldman, 1991; Baumgartner *et al.*, 1991). We still do not know how this antibody works or how to choose those patients who may benefit from it. Unfortunately, a second controlled trial of HA-1A was stopped when an interim safety analysis revealed an increased mortality in mab recipients who did not have Gram-negative bacteraemia.

11B.2.1.2 Antibody to TNF and other cytokines

Much of the toxicity of endotoxin is attributable to its ability to activate a series of mediator cacades (reviewed in Glauser *et al.*, 1991). Central among these is TNF. The evidence implicating TNF as a mediator of endotoxin-induced injury can be summarized as follows:

1 Injection of animals (Mathison *et al.*, 1988) or humans (Michie *et al.*, 1988) with LPS induces a rise in serum TNF levels which coincides with the physiological changes that occur.
2 In animals, injection of TNF can reproduce most of the pathological features of shock (Le & Vilcek, 1987).
3 Clinical studies in sepsis have shown that serum TNF levels on admission correlate with outcome (Girardin *et al.*, 1988) and that persistently high levels reflect a poorer prognosis (Calandra *et al.*, 1990).

Perhaps the most persuasive evidence is that obtained from experiments in which antibody to TNF has been shown to protect animals from Gram-negative sepsis. Beutler first reported that a rabbit polyclonal antibody could protect mice from LPS challenge (Beutler *et al.*, 1985) and the first successful study with mab was carried out (using Fab'$_2$ fragments) in baboons challenged with live *E. coli* 1–2 h after the antibody was given (Tracey *et al.*, 1987). Later we showed in mice that antibody was also effective if given therapeutically after the bacterial challenge, albeit with a rather narrow window of activity (Silva *et al.*, 1990*b*).

The enthusiasm engendered by these early results has been tempered by more recent data which cast doubt on the potential clinical application of anti-TNF antibodies. It appears that while anti-TNF antibodies are highly effective in controlling intravascular infections, they are less active in the setting of focal disease. For example, Bagby *et al.* (1991) showed that anti-TNF IgG was highly effective at protecting rats from intravenous LPS but that it failed to protect them from lethal *E. coli* peritonitis, despite the fact that both models elicited significant serum TNF responses. Another source of concern is that, paradoxically, TNF plays an important role in host defences against infection and hence anti-TNF might be harmful. In mouse models of listeriosis, for example, TNF is protective and anti-TNF enhances lethality (Nakane *et al.*, 1988; Desiderio *et al.*, 1989). Indeed recently, administration of recombinant TNF was shown to protect rodents from Gram-negative infection (Nakano *et al.*, 1990).

Despite these concerns, sufficient evidence has accumulated to warrant clinical evaluation of monoclonal anti-TNF antibodies. A phase II trial has already been reported (Fisher *et al.*, 1993) and large scale trials of efficacy are now in progress.

TNF has been the subject of greatest interest although mab have also been raised against a number of other potential targets. For example, antibodies to interleukin-6 (IL-6) (Starnes *et al.*, 1990) and interferon-gamma (Heinzel, 1990; Silva & Cohen, 1992) have both been shown to be protective in animal models of infection. Other strategies include antibodies to the LPS receptor (Morrison *et al.*, 1990), tissue factor (Colman, 1989), and ingeniously, an anti-idiotype antibody to a mab to Lipid A (Kato *et al.*, 1990). None of these has yet reached clinical trial but they illustrate the wide range of possible therapeutic approaches that are being explored.

11B.2.2 Other bacterial infections

Group B streptococci (*Streptococcus agalactiae*) are an important cause of neonatal sepsis. The organisms are generally susceptible to penicillin but infants lack opsonic activity to the infecting strain. Hill and his colleagues have raised mab to the organism, some of which demonstrate protection in animal models of the infection (Shigeoka *et al.*, 1984; Hill *et al.*, 1991).

Pseudomonas aeruginosa causes nosocomial pneumonia and septicaema, both of which have a high mortality. Theoretically, *Pseudomonas* infections might benefit from the anti-endotoxin monoclonals (the organism shares essentially the same Lipid A structure with the Enterobacteriacae) or indeed anti-TNF but the more limited number of 'O' serotypes has prompted several investigators to raise specific anti-*Pseudomonas* monoclonals (Terashima *et al.*, 1991; Sawada *et al.*, 1984; Zweerink *et al.*, 1988). Rather than rely on just one such monoclonal, the strategy will be to use a pool of reagents which together 'cover' most of the common serotypes. A phase I trial of this approach has been reported recently (Saravolatz *et al.*, 1991).

11B.3 Viral and chlamydial infections

The relative paucity of effective antiviral drugs has been a stimulus to the development of mab for treating serious viral diseases. Many monoclonals have been made although only a few have so far seen clinical application.

11B.3.1 Cytomegalovirus

Cytomegalovirus (CMV) is a major cause of morbidity and mortality, especially in immunosuppressed patients such as bone marrow transplant recipients. During the past 10 years, a number of investigators reported that intravenous immunoglobulin (IVIG) seemed able to modify the course of CMV pneumonitis and this led to trials of hyperimmune CMV globulin in prophylaxis (Emanuel *et al.*, 1987) and, combined with ganciclovir, in the treatment of serious CMV disease (Reed, 1991). Comparison of the functional virus neutralizing properties of IVIG with the hyperimmune preparations, however, failed to show any correlation with the enzyme-linked immunosorbent assay (ELISA) titre, raising questions about the mechanism of any protection seen (Emanuel,

Table 11B.1. *Examples of virus infections for which monoclonal antibodies have been shown to be effective in* in vivo *models*

Virus	Reference
Coxsackie B3	Kishimoto & Abelmann (1989)
Encephalomyocarditis	Sriram *et al.* (1989)
Herpes simplex	Metcalf *et al.* (1988)
Varicella zoster	Foung *et al.* (1985)
Rubella	Van Meel *et al.* (1985)
Measles	Croce *et al.* (1980)
Chlamydia	Rosen *et al.* (1983)
Sendai virus	Carthew *et al.* (1989)

1991). In an attempt to try and address these questions, several investigators have generated mab to CMV, including some human antibodies (Emanuel *et al.*, 1984; Foung *et al.*, 1989) and early clinical trials with these reagents have now begun (Aulitzky *et al.*, 1991). Strains of CMV demonstrate significant antigenic diversity and among one panel of mab to CMV, each of seven antibodies was unable to bind to approximately 20% of a group of 116 clinical isolates of the virus (Emanuel, 1991). Thus eventually it is likely that it will be necessary to use pools of antibodies to provide the range of activity needed.

Other immunotherapeutic approaches to CMV include the use of antibody-targeted antiviral drugs and/or toxins and antireceptor antibodies directed at the CMV receptor.

11B.3.2 Hepatitis virus

Hepatitis B virus (HBV) is a major cause of ill health on a worldwide basis. An effective vaccine exists but passive immunotherapy still plays an important part in the management of the disease, hence the interest in developing mab.

Several such antibodies exist (van Meel *et al.*, 1985; Stricker *et al.*, 1985). The only clinical application to date has been in two patients with hypogamma-globulinaemia who were chronic carriers. An antibody against the viral coat protein was used repeatedly over several months with some success to clear the infection (Lever *et al.*, 1990). Interestingly, in this case a mouse antibody could be used as the patients lacked the ability to make a human anti-mouse response; for more general use a human monoclonal would be necessary.

11B.3.3 Other virus infections

Table 11B.1 lists other viral infections in which the therapeutic use of mab has been demonstrated. In some cases the antibodies might replace an existing

Table 11B.2. *Use of monoclonal antibodies in the treatment of experimental parasitic infection*

Parasite	Reference
Cryptosporidiosis	Bjorneby *et al*. (1991)
	Tilley *et al*. (1991)
Leishmaniasis	Sadick *et al*. (1990)
	Blackwell & Roberts (1987)
Malaria	Peeters *et al*. (1989)
	Schmidt-Ullrich *et al* (1986)
Toxoplasmosis	Israelski *et al*. (1989)
Giardiasis	Butscher & Faubert (1988)
Naegleria fowleri	Lalinger *et al*. (1987)
Schistosomiasis	Sidner *et al*. (1987)

hyperimmune preparation (e.g. varicella zoster), in others monoclonals have been shown to be active in animal models but there is little apparent need for further clinical development (e.g. herpes simplex virus).

11B.4 Additional applications of monoclonal antibodies

So far we have considered mainly mab directed against some component of the organism itself or toxins produced by the organism. In some cases, however, antibodies have been used to modify the immune response to infection or to improve the therapeutic index of antimicrobial agents.

One example is malaria in mice, in which chloroquine-containing liposomes have been directed to the red cells by linking them to an antibody to the erythrocyte membrane (Peeters *et al.*, 1989). In another case, an antibody to the yeast *Cryptococcus neoformans* was shown to enhance the effect of the antifungal drug amphotericin B (Dromer & Charreire, 1991).

Modulation of the immune response has been studied in particular in parasitic infections. For example, antibodies to CD4 and to the mouse major histocompatibility complex (MHC) have both been shown to alter the course of experimental leishmaniasis (Sadick *et al.*, 1990; Blackwell & Roberts, 1987) and anti-CD4 antibodies are also effective in reducing inflammation in toxoplasmic encephalitis (Israelski *et al.*, 1989). The same approach has been considered in AIDS (Dhiver *et al.*, 1991).

Table 11B.2 lists those parasitic infections in which the possible therapeutic use of mabs has been studied.

11B.5 Conclusions

Many hundreds of mab have been generated against a wide range of microorganisms but few have yet found clinical application. In part this is due to practical and commercial constraints; however, it is already apparent that in a growing number of infections, conventional antimicrobial agents have reached the limit of their efficacy. As more is learnt of the underlying mechanisms of host defence to infection, and how it may be modified, the number of clinical uses of mab is set to increase.

11B.6 References

Appelmelk, B. J. & Cohen, J. (1992). The protective role of antibodies to the lipopolysaccharide core region. In *Bacterial Endotoxic Lipopolysaccharides*, ed. D. C. Morrison & J. L. Ryan, New York, CRC Press.

Aulitzky, W. E., Schulz, T. F., Tilg, H. *et al*. (1991). Human monoclonal antibodies neutralising cytomegalovirus (CMV) for prophylaxis of CMV disease: report of a phase I trial in bone marrow transplant recipients. *Journal of Infectious Diseases*, **163**, 1344–1347.

Bagby, G. J., Plessala, K. J., Wilson, L. A., Thompson, J. J. & Nelson, S. (1991). Divergent efficacy of antibody to tumor necrosis factor alpha in intravascular and peritonitis models of sepsis. *Journal of Infectious Diseases*, **163**, 83–88.

Baumgartner, J.-D., Heumann, D., Gerain, J., Weinbreck, P., Grau, G. E. & Glauser, M. P. (1990). Association between protective efficacy of anti-lipopolysaccharide (LPS) antibodies and suppression of LPS-induced tumor necrosis factor alpha and interleukin 6. Comparison of O side chain-specific antibodies and core LPS antibodies. *Journal of Experimental Medicine*, **171**, 889–896.

Baumgartner, J.-D., Heumann, D. & Glauser, M. P. (1991). The HA-1A monoclonal antibody for Gram-negative sepsis. *New England Journal of Medicine*, **324**, 281–282.

Bayston, K. F. & Cohen, J. (1990). Bacterial endotoxin and current concepts in the diagnosis and treatment of endotoxaemia. *Journal of Medical Microbiology*, **31**, 73–83.

Beutler, B., Milsark, I. W. & Cerami, A. (1985). Passive immunization against cachectin/tumor necrosis factor protects mice from lethal effect of endotoxin. *Science*, **229**, 869–871.

Bjorneby, J. M., Hunsaker, B. D., Riggs, M. W. & Perryman, L. E. (1991). Monoclonal antibody immunotherapy in nude mice persistently infected with *Cryptosporidium parvum*. *Infection and Immunity*, **59**, 1172–1176.

Blackwell, J. M. & Roberts, M. B. (1987). Immunomodulation of murine visceral leishmaniasis by administration of monoclonal anti-Ia antibodies; differential effects of anti-Ia vs anti-Ie antibodies. *European Journal of Immunology*, **17**, 1669–1672.

Butscher, W. G. & Faubert, G. M. (1988). The therapeutic action of monoclonal antibodies against a surface glycoprotein of *Giardia muris*. *Immunology*, **64**, 175–180.

Calandra, T., Baumgartner, J.-D., Grau, G. E., Wu, M.-M., Lambert, P.-H., Schellekens, J. F., Verhoef, J., Glauser, M. P. & Swiss-Dutch J5 immunoglobulin study group. (1990). Prognostic values of tumor necrosis factor/cachectin, interleukin-1, interferon-alpha and interferon-gamma in the serum of patients with septic shock. *Journal of Infectious Diseases*, **161**, 982–987.

Carthew, P., Riley, J. & Dinsdale, D. (1989). Amelioration of established Sendai virus pneumonia in the nude mouse using a monoclonal antibody to the virus fusion protein. *British Journal of Experimental Pathology*, **70**, 727–735.

Colman, R. W. (1989). The role of plasma proteases in septic shock. *New England Journal of Medicine*, **320**, 1207–1209.

Croce, C. M., Linnenbach, A., Hall, W., Steplewski, Z. & Koprowski, H. (1980). Production of human hybridomas secreting antibodies to measles virus. *Nature*, **288**, 488–489.

Desiderio, J. V., Kiener, P. A., Lin, P.-F. & Warr, G. A. (1989). Protection of mice against *Listeria monocytogenes* infection by recombinant human tumor necrosis factor alpha. *Infection and Immunity*, **57**, 1615–1617.

Dhiver, C., Oliver, D., Rousseau, S., Tamalet, C., Lopez, M., Galindo, J. R., Mourens, M., Hirn, M., Gastaut, J. A. & Mawas, C. (1991). Pilot phase I study using zidovudine in association with a 10-day course of anti-CD4 monoclonal antibody in seven AIDS patients. *AIDS*, **3**, 835–842.

Dromer, F. & Charreire, J. (1991). Improved amphotericin B activity by a monoclonal anti-*Cryptococcus neoformans* antibody: study during murine cryptococcosis and mechanisms of action. *Journal of Infectious Diseases*, **163**, 1114–1120.

Emanuel, D. (1991). Uses of immunotherapy for control of human cytomegalovirus-associated diseases. *Transplantation Proceedings*, **23** (Suppl. 3), 144–146.

Emanuel, D., Gold, J., Colacino, J., Lopez, C. & Hammerling, U. (1984). A human monoclonal antibody to cytomegalovirus (CMV). *Journal of Immunology*, **133**, 2202–2205.

Emanuel, D., Peppard, J., Chehimi, J., Hammerling, U. & O'Reilly, R. (1987). The diagnostic, prophylactic and therapeutic uses of monoclonal antibodies to human cytomegalovirus. *Transplantation Proceedings*, **19** (Suppl. 7), 132–137.

Fisher, C. J., Opal, S. M., Dhainhaut, J. F. *et al*. (1993). Influence of an anti-tumor necrosis factor monoclonal antibody on cytokine levels in patients with sepsis. *Critical Care Medicine*, **21**, 318–327.

Foung, S. K., Perkins, S., Bradshaw, P., Rowe, J., Rabin, L. B., Reyes, G. R. & Lennette, E. T. (1989). Human monoclonal antibodies to human cytomegalovirus. *Journal of Infectious Diseases*, **159**, 436–443.

Foung, S. K., Perkins, S., Koropchak, C., Fishwild, D. M., Wittek, A. E., Engleman, E. G., Grumet, F. C. & Arvin, A. M. (1985). Human monoclonal antibodies neutralising Varicella-zoster virus. *Journal of Infectious Diseases*, **152**, 280–285.

Gazmuri, R. J., Mecher, C. & Weil, M. H. (1991). The HA-1A monoclonal antibody for Gram-negative sepsis. *New England Journal of Medicine*, **325**, 279–280.

Girardin, E., Grau, G. E., Dayer, J.-M., Roux-Lombard, P. & Lambert, P.-H. (1988). Tumor necrosis factor and interleukin-1 in the serum of children with severe infectious purpura. *New England Journal of Medicine*, **319**, 397–400.

Glauser, M. P., Zanetti, G., Baumgartner, J.-D. & Cohen, J. (1991). Septic shock: pathogenesis. *Lancet*, **338**, 732–736.

Greenman, R. L., Schein, R. M., Martin, M. A., Wenzel, R. P., Macintyre, N. R., Emmanuel, G., Chmel, H., Kohler, R. B., McCarthy, M., Plouffe, J., Russell, J. A. & Xoma Sepsis Study Group. (1991). A controlled clinical trial of E5 murine monoclonal IgM antibody to endotoxin in the treatment of Gram-negative sepsis. *Journal of American Medicine Association*, **266**, 1097–1102.

Heinzel, F. P. (1990). The role of IFN-gamma in the pathology of experimental endotoxemia. *Journal of Immunology*, **145**, 2920–2924.

Hill, H. R., Gonzales, L. A., Knappe, W. A., Fischer, G. W., Kelsey, D. K. & Raff, H. V. (1991). Comparative protective activity of human monoclonal and hyperimmune polyclonal antibody against group B streptococci. *Journal of Infectious Diseases*, **163**, 792–798.

Ispahani, P., Pearson, N. J. & Greenwood, D. (1987). An analysis of community and hospital-acquired bacteraemia in a large teaching hospital in the United Kingdom.

Quarterly Journal of Medicine, **63**, 427–440.

Israelski, D. M., Araujo, F. G., Conley, F. K., Suzuki, Y., Sharma, S. & Remington, J. S. (1989). Treatment with anti-L3T4 (CD4) monoclonal antibody reduces the inflammatory response in toxoplasmic encephalitis. *Journal of Immunology*, **142**, 954–958.

Kato, T., Takazoe, I. & Okuda, K. (1990). Protection of mice against the lethal toxicity of a lipopolysaccharide (LPS) by immunization with anti-idiotype antibody to a monoclonal antibody to Lipid A from *Eikenella corrodens* LPS. *Infection and Immunity*, **58**, 416–420.

Kishimoto, C. & Abelmann, W. H. (1989). Monoclonal antibody therapy for prevention of acute coxsackie B3 myocarditis in mice. *Circulation*, **79**, 1300–1308.

Krieger, J. I., Fletcher, R. C., Siegel, S. A., Fearon, D. T., Neblock, D. S., Boutin, R. H., Taylor, R. P. & Daddona, P. E. (1993). Human anti-endotoxin antibody HA-1A mediates complement-dependent binding of *Escherichia coli* lipopolysaccharide to complement receptor type 1 of human erythrocytes to neutrophils. *Journal of Infectious Diseases*, **167**, 865–875.

Lalinger, G. J., Reiner, S. L., Cooke, D. W., Toffaletti, D. L., Perfect, J. R., Granger, D. L. & Durack, D. T. (1987). Efficacy of immune therapy in early experimental *Naegleria fowleri* meningitis. *Infection and Immunity*, **55**, 1289–1293.

Larrick, J. W. (1989). Potential of monoclonal antibodies as pharmacological agents. *Pharmacological Reviews*, **41**, 539–557.

Le, J. & Vilcek, J. (1987). Tumor necrosis factor and interleukin 1: cytokines with multiple overlapping biological activities. *Laboratory Investigation*, **56**, 234–248.

Lever, A. M., Waters, J., Brook, M. G., Karayiannis, P. & Thomas, H. C. (1990). Monoclonal antibody to HBsAg for chronic hepatitis B virus infection with hypogammaglobulinaemia. *Lancet*, **335**, 1529.

McConnell, J. S., Appelmelk, B. J. & Cohen, J. (1990). Dissociation between Limulus neutralisation and *in-vivo* protection in monoclonal antibodies directed against endotoxin core structures. *Microbial Pathogenesis*, **9**, 55–59.

Mathison, J. C., Wolfson, E. & Ulevitch, R. J. (1988). Participation of tumor necrosis factor in the mediation of Gram-negative bacterial lipopolysaccharide-induced injury in rabbits. *Journal of Clinical Investigation*, **81**, 1925–1937.

Mehta, N. D., Wilson, B. M., Rapson, N. T. & Easmon, C. S. F. (1988). Comparison of the opsonic activity of polyclonal and monoclonal antibodies raised against *Salmonella minnesota* strain R595. *Journal of Medical Microbiology*, **25**, 85–93.

Metcalf, J. F., Chatterjee, S., Koga, J. & Whitley, R. J. (1988). Protection against herpetic ocular disease by immunotherapy with monoclonal antibodies to herpes simplex virus glycoproteins. *Intervirology*, **29**, 39–49.

Michie, H. R., Manogue, K. R., Spriggs, D. R., Revhaug, A., O'Dwyer, S., Dinarello, C. A., Cerami, A., Wolff, S. M. & Wilmore, D. W. (1988). Detection of circulating tumor necrosis factor after endotoxin administration. *New England Journal of Medicine*, **318**, 1481–1486.

Morrison, D. C., Silverstein, R., Bright, S. W., Chen, T.-Y., Flebbe, L. M. & Lei, M.-G. (1990). Monoclonal antibody to mouse lipopolysaccharide receptor protects mice against the lethal effects of endotoxin. *Journal of Infectious Diseases*, **162**, 1063–1068.

Nakane, A., Minagawa, T. & Kato, K. (1988). Endogenous tumor necrosis factor (cachectin) is essential to host resistance against *Listeria monocytogenes* infection. *Infection and Immunity*, **56**, 2563–2569.

Nakano, Y., Onozuka, K., Terada, Y., Shinomiya, H. & Nakano, M. (1990). Protective effect of recombinant tumor necrosis factor-alpha in murine salmonellosis. *Journal of Immunology*, **144**, 1935–1941.

Overbeek, B. P., Machiel de Vos, N., Keller, N., Raponi, G., Rozenberg-Arska, M. & Verhoef, J. (1989*a*). Enhanced binding of murine monoclonal antibodies to lipopolysaccharide structures of Enterobacteriaceae after treatment with antibiotics. *Serodiagnosis and Immunotherapy*, **3**, 167–173.

Overbeek, B. P., Machiel de Vos, N., Schellekens, J. F., Rozenberg-Arska, M. & Verhoef, J. (1989*b*). Beta-lactam antibiotics enhance the binding of antibodies to outer membrane, non-LPS antigenic structures in Enterobacteriaceae. *Serodiagnosis and Immunotherapy*, **3**, 175–183.

Peeters, P. A., Brunink, B. G., Eling, W. M. & Crommelin, D. J. (1989). Therapeutic effect of chloroquine(CQ)-containing immunoliposomes in rats infected with *Plasmodium berghei* parasitised mouse red blood cells: comparison with combinations of antibodies and CQ or liposomal CQ. *Biochimica et Biophysica Acta*, **981**, 269–276.

Pollack, M., Chia, J. K., Koles, N. L., Miller, M. & Guelde, G. (1989). Specificity and cross-reactivity of monoclonal antibodies reactive with the core and lipid A regions of bacterial lipopolysaccharide. *Journal of Infectious Diseases*, **159**, 168–188.

Reed, E. C. (1991). Treatment of cytomegalovirus pneumonia in transplant patients. *Transplantation Proceedings*, **23** (Suppl. 1), 8–12.

Rietschel, E. Th., Schade, U., Jensen, M., Wollenweber, H.-W., Luderitz, O. & Greisman, S. G. (1982). Bacterial endotoxins: chemical structure, biological activity and role in septicaemia. *Scandinavian Journal of Infectious Diseases*, **31**, 8–21.

Rosen, A., Persson, K. & Klein, G. (1983). Human monoclonal antibodies to a genus-specific chlamydial antigen, produced by EBV-transformed B cells. *Journal of Immunology*, **130**, 2899–2902.

Sadick, M. D., Heinzel, F. P., Holaday, B. J., Pu, R. T., Dawkins, R. S. & Locksley, R. M. (1990). Cure of murine leishmaniasis with anti-interleukin-4 monoclonal antibody. *Journal of Experimental Medicine*, **171**, 115–127.

Saravolatz, L. D., Markowitz, N., Collins, M. S., Bogdanoff, D. & Pennington, J. E. (1991). Safety, pharmacokinetics and functional activity of human anti-*Pseudomonas aeruginosa* monoclonal antibodies in septic and non-septic patients. *Journal of Infectious Diseases*, **164**, 803–806.

Sawada, S., Suzuki, M., Kawamura, T., Fujinaga, S., Masuho, Y. & Tomibe, K. (1984). Protection against infection with *Pseudomonas aeruginosa* by passive transfer of monoclonal antibodies to lipopolysaccharides and outer membrane proteins. *Journal of Infectious Diseases*, **150**, 570–576.

Schmidt-Ullrich, R., Brown, J., Whittle, H. & Lin, P.-S. (1986). Human–human hybridomas secreting monoclonal antibodies to the M_r 195 000 *Plasmodium falciparum* blood stage antigen. *Journal of Experimental Medicine*, **163**, 179–188.

Shigeoka, A. O., Pincus, S. H., Rote, N. S. & Hill, H. R. (1984). Protective efficacy of hybridoma type-specific antibody against experimental infection with group B streptococcus. *Journal of Infectious Diseases*, **149**, 363–372.

Sidner, R. A., Carter, C. E. & Colley, D. G. (1987). Modulation of *Schistosoma japonicum* pulmonary egg granulomas with monoclonal antibodies. *American Journal of Tropical Medicine and Hygiene*, **36**, 361–370.

Silva, A. T., Appelmelk, B. J., Buurman, W. A., Bayston, K. F. & Cohen, J. (1990*a*). Monoclonal antibody to endotoxin core protects mice from *Escherichia coli* sepsis by a mechanism independent of tumor necrosis factor and interleukin-6. *Journal of Infectious Diseases*, **162**, 454–459.

Silva, A. T., Bayston, K. F. & Cohen, J. (1990*b*). Prophylactic and therapeutic effects of a monoclonal antibody to tumor necrosis factor-alpha in experimental Gram-negative shock. *Journal of Infectious Diseases*, **162**, 421–427.

Silva, A. T. & Cohen, J. (1992). Role of interferon gamma in experimental

Gram-negative sepsis. *Journal of Infectious Diseases*, **166**, 331–335.

Sriram, S., Topham, D. J., Huang, S. K. & Rodriguez, M. (1989). Treatment of encephalomyocarditis virus-induced central nervous system demyelination with monoclonal anti-T-cell antibodies. *Journal of Virology*, **63**, 4242–4248.

Starnes Jr., H. F., Pearce, M. K., Tewari, A., Yim, J. H., Zou, J.-C. & Abrams, J. S. (1990). Anti-IL-6 monoclonal antibodies protect against lethal *Escherichia coli* infection and lethal tumor necrosis factor-alpha challenge in mice. *Journal of Immunology*, **145**, 4185–4191.

Stricker, E. A., Tiebout, R. F., Lelie, P. N. & Zeijlemaker, W. P. (1985). A human monolonal IgG1 anti-hepatitis B surface antibody. *Scandinavian Journal of Immunology*, **22**, 337–343.

Tanio, C. P. & Feldman, H. I. (1991). The HA-1A monoclonal antibody for Gram-negative sepsis. *New England Journal of Medicine*, **324**, 280.

Teng, N. N., Kaplan, H. S., Hebert, J. M., Moore, C., Douglas, H., Wunderlich, A. & Braude, A. I. (1985). Protection against Gram-negative bacteremia and endotoxemia with human monoclonal IgM antibodies. *Proceedings of the National Academy of Sciences* U.S.A., **82**, 1790–1794.

Terashima, M., Uezumi, I., Tomio, T., Kato, M., Irie, K., Okuda, T., Yokota, S.-I. & Noguchi, H. (1991). A protective human monoclonal antibody directed to the outer core region of *Pseudomonas aeruginosa* lipopolysaccharide. *Infection and Immunity*, **59**, 1–6.

Tilley, M., Upton, S. J., Fayer, R., Barta, J. R., Chrisp, C. E., Freed, P. S., Blagburn, B. L., Anderson, B. C. & Barnard, S. M. (1991). Identification of a 15-kilodalton surface glycoprotein on sporozoites of *Cryptosporidium parvum*. *Infection and Immunity*, **59**, 1002–1007.

Tracey, K. J., Fong, Y., Hesse, D. G., Manogue, K. R., Lee, A. T., Kuo, G. C., Lowry, S. F. & Cerami, A. (1987). Anti-cachectin/TNF monoclonal antibodies prevent septic shock during lethal bacteraemia. *Nature*, **330**, 662–664.

Van Meel, F. C., Steenbakkers, P. G. & Oomen, J. C. (1985). Human and chimpanzee monoclonal antibodies. *Journal of Immunological Methods*, **80**, 267–276.

Ziegler, E. J., Fisher Jr., C. J., Sprung, C., Straube, R. C., Sadoff, J. C., Foulke, G. E., Wortel, C. H., Fink, M. P., Dellinger, R. P., Teng, N. N., Allen, I. E., Berger, H. J., Knatterud, G. L., LoBuglio, A. F., Smith, C. R. & HA-1A Sepsis Study Group. (1991). Treatment of Gram-negative bacteremia and septic shock with HA-1A human monoclonal antibody against endotoxin. A randomized, double-blind, placebo-controlled trial. *New England Journal of Medicine*, **324**, 429–436.

Ziegler, E. J., McCutchan, J. A., Fierer, J., Glauser, M. P., Sadoff, J. C., Douglas, H. & Braude, A. I. (1982). Treatment of Gram-negative bacteremia and shock with human antiserum to a mutant *Escherichia coli*. *New England Journal of Medicine*, **307**, 1225–1230.

Zweerink, H. J., Gammon, M., Hutchison, C. F., Jackson, J., Lombardo, D., Miner, K. M., Puckett, J. M., Sewell, T. J. & Sigal, N. H. (1988). Human monoclonal antibodies that protect mice against challenge with *Pseudomonas aeruginosa*. *Infection and Immunity*, **56**, 1873–1879.

12A

Monoclonal antibodies in transplantation: immunohistology

M. L. ROSE

12A.1 Introduction

Immunohistochemical analysis of events within the graft have been very useful both to help define the nature of cell interactions which take place and to assist the clinical diagnosis of rejection. Although useful in experimental studies, this review must restrict itself to immunohistological analysis of normal human and clinical material. A large number of monoclonal antibodies (mab) reactive with antigens on human tissues are available for investigation of cryostat sections, a much more limited selection can be used on paraffin sections. In the field of solid organ transplantation, mab have been used to define the nature of the infiltrate, expression of Major Histocompatibility Complex (MHC) antigens, expression of adhesion molecules and more recently the presence of cytokines within grafts. In addition, mab against viral or other antigens can be used to diagnose infection within an allografted organ.

12A.2 Nature of the infiltrate

12A.2.1 Kidney

Immunoperoxidase and immunofluorescence methods have been used. Most commonly, mab have been used to identify the common leukocyte antigen, T cells and T cell subsets, monocytes and macrophages, B cells and NK cells (Table 12A.1). In a large study of 279 renal allograft biopsies, McWhinnie *et al*. (1986) used a morphometric analysis and point counting technique to assess the area of graft occupied by various cell types. They demonstrated the level of leukocytes to be 1.7% in day 0 control biopsies and this value increased after transplantation to 11–12%, even in grafts showing stable function. The level was increased further during rejection of leukocytes occupying 21% of the graft. T cells (total CD3) were 15% of the total leukocytes in the control biopsies and increased to 36% during rejection. Although CD8 T cells always exceeded CD4 at every time point, there was no significant difference between

Table 12A.1. *Monoclonal antibodies commonly used to investigate the nature of infiltrates*

Mab	CD (specificity)	Reference/source
Leu 4	CD3 (all T cells)	Becton Dickinson
OKT3	CD3 (all T cells)	Ortho Diagnostics
Leu 3a/3b	CD4 (class II restricted T cells)	Becton Dickinson
OKT4	CD4 (class II restricted T cells)	Ortho Diagnostics
Leu 8	CD8 (class I restricted T cells)	Becton Dickinson
OKT8	CD8 (class I restricted T cells)	Ortho Diagnostics
Leu 7	CD57 (NK cell subset)	Becton Dickinson
Leu 11	CD16 (NK cells and neutrophils)	Becton Dickinson
OKM1	CD11b (monocytes, granulocytes)	Ortho Diagnostics
F10-89-4	CD45 (Leucocyte Common Antigen)	Dalchau *et al.* (1980)
IL-2R	CD25 (activated T cells)	Becton Dickinson

them. These results are in contrast to earlier studies (Platt *et al.*, 1982; Hancock *et al.* 1983, 1985) which had reported a large predominance of CD8 T cells during mild and moderate rejection. Thus although Hancock *et al.* (1983) also reported T cells as being about 30% of the infiltrate during rejection, they found 90% of the T cells were CD8. Other authors have reported CD4 as predominating during rejection (Tufveson *et al.*, 1983; van Es *et al.*, 1984; Hall *et al.*, 1984*a*). Whereas McWhinnie *et al.* (1986) found no significant differences in macrophages correlating either with time after transplantation or clinical status, Hancock *et al.* report increasing numbers with severity of rejection. NK cells were not found in significant numbers at any time by McWhinnie *et al.* (1986) but an early transient increase in the 2–3 days following transplantation was observed by Hancock and colleagues (1985).

It is difficult to reconcile the different results reported from different centres. Many of the centres used the same commercial antibodies (against T cells). All the patients would be receiving different immunosuppressive regimens but a single centre comparison between patients on steroids and azathioprine and those taking cyclosporine (CsA) (McWhinnie *et al.*, 1986) revealed that the patients taking cyclosporine had smaller infiltrates although there was no difference in the composition of the infiltrate. It was acknowledged that mab against CD4 are less than satisfactory because they also bind to macrophages but mab against CD8 give excellent results on tissue sections. Methods of quantifying and expression of results vary between papers. Expressing results as numbers of cells per unit area will underestimate cell number during rejection when there is oedema and tissue expansion. Results from biopsies are subject to sampling error as the biopsy may not be representative of the whole organ.

12A.2.2 Heart

More consistent results have been reported about the nature of the infiltrate in endomyocardial biopsies following cardiac transplantation (perhaps because there have been fewer studies). Rose *et al*. (1984), in an immunoperoxidase study of 17 biopsies from patients receiving azathioprine and steroids, reported a tenfold increase in numbers of CD3 cells in biopsies showing histological signs of rejection compared with control biopsies taken from donor heart prior to transplantation. Approximately 85% of the T cells were of the CD8 subset. Hoshinaga *et al*. (1984) reported a similar magnitude of influx of T cells into the biopsy during rejection and found two to three times as many CD8 cells as CD4 cells. These authors also demonstrated macrophages within the infiltrate (using OKM1), increasing in number with the severity of rejection. Using the mab RFD7 it has been confirmed that macrophages can be a large component of the infiltrate during rejection (Rose *et al*., 1990).

The clinical use of monitoring T cells in endomyocardial biopsies was addressed in a longitudinal study of 111 biopsies from eight patients followed for the first 2 years (de Lourdes Higuchi *et al*., 1991). They concluded that counting numbers of CD8 cells/unit area was a useful adjunct to diagnosis of rejection and anything above three cells/field (using 400 × magnification) was acute rejection. They emphasize the importance of identifying T cells using mab and immunoperoxidase and of not relying on morphological discrimination by eye. The introduction of CsA as the major immunosuppressive reagent produced a curious endocardial infiltrate, or large puddles of cells within the myocardium, called the 'Quilty' effect (Imakita *et al*., 1988, Figure 12A.1a). In the absence of myocytolysis, this infiltrate is not diagnostic of rejection. Immunocytochemical staining has shown the infiltrate to consist of T cells (Figure 12A.1b) as well as macrophages and endothelial cells (unpublished data). The cause of an endocardial cushion of cells and its possible role in rejection is unresolved.

12A.2.3 Liver

In liver transplantation the presence of CD4 cells alone or a mixture of CD4 and CD8 cells in the portal tracts has been associated with rejection (Perkins *et al*., 1987). The same pattern of infiltration, however, was also associated with CMV hepatitis and so immunohistological labelling as an indicator of rejection cannot be used unless CMV hepatitis is excluded.

12A.3   Major histocompatibility complex antigens

MHC antigens are highly polymorphic glycoproteins coded for by chromosome 6 in humans (Jongsma *et al*., 1973). They are the major target of the immune response following allograft rejection. Expression of MHC antigens is not a

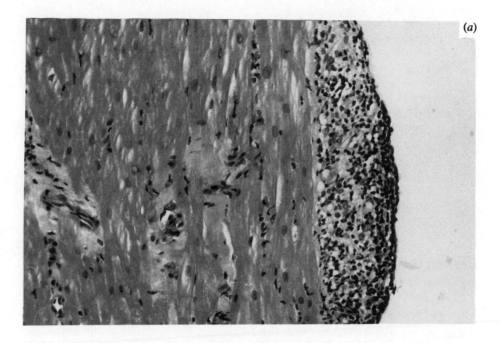

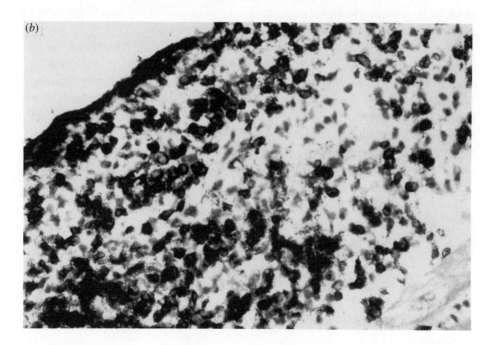

Figure 12A.1. (a) Photomicrograph of endomyocardial biopsy showing a large endocardial cushion of cells. Paraffin section stained with haematoxylin and eosin. (200 X). (b) Cryostat section (6 μm) of endomyocardial biopsy stained with Leu 4 and immunoperoxidase showing the presence of T cells within the endocardial infiltrate. Counterstained with Harris's haematoxylin. (400 X).

Table 12A.2. *Monoclonal antibodies commonly used to detect MHC antigens*

Mab	Specificity	Reference/source
W6/32	Monomorphic class I	Barnstable *et al.* (1978)
PA 2.6	Monomorphic class I	Brodsky *et al.* (1979)
NFK1	Monomorphic class II	Fuggle *et al.* (1983)
L243	DR determinant of class II	Becton Dickinson
B7.21	DP determinant of class II	Becton Dickinson
Leu 10	DQ determinant of class II	Becton Dickinson

MHC, major histocompatibility complex.

constant phenotype: expression can be upregulated or downregulated by cytokines and other factors (reviewed by Halloran *et al.*, 1986). Quantitative differences in MHC expression can affect the magnitude of an immune response. It follows, therefore, that the precise distribution of MHC antigens in donor organs will determine both the target and the strength of the anti-allograft immune response. A brief review follows of the distribution of MHC antigens in normal kidneys, heart, lung and liver and the changes that occur after transplantation and during rejection.

The use of mab on frozen sections has revolutionized our knowledge about the normal distribution of MHC antigens in different tissues. It has revealed patterns of distribution that are quite different to what was previously thought. The idea that HLA class I (HLA-A, B, C) antigens were ubiquitous is now known to be incorrect. They are constitutively present on many nucleated cells but are only weakly expressed or absent on endocrine cells, hepatocytes, smooth muscle (Fleming *et al.*, 1981; Daar *et al.*, 1984*a*; Natali *et al.*, 1984), normal skeletal (Appleyard *et al.*, 1985) and cardiac muscle (Rose *et al.*, 1986). Class II (HLA-DR, DP and DQ) antigens, originally thought to be restricted to macrophages, dendritic cells, monocytes and activated T cells have also been described on human endothelial and epithelial cells (Natali *et al.*, 1981; Daar *et al.*, 1984*b*). The mab commonly used to detect MHC antigens are shown in Table 12A.2

12A.3.1 Kidney transplantation

12A.3.1.1 Normal kidney

MHC class I antigens are detected on all structures in the normal human kidney. The glomeruli, intertubular structures and endothelium of the larger vessels are strongly stained whereas the renal tubules express a much lower level of class I antigen (Fleming *et al.*, 1981; Daar *et al.*, 1984*a*). Using mab against the DR determinant of class II, class II antigens are consistently found on glomerular endothelium, mesangium and intertubular structures (Fuggle *et al.*, 1983). The intertubular structures consist of endothelial and dendritic cells. Expression of class II in the proximal renal tubules is variable, a single study of 46 normal kidneys (Fuggle *et al.*, 1983) found class II in the proximal tubules in 77% of kidneys. The distal tubules are always negative. Variation in expression of class II between individuals and between studies is not surprising in view of the inducibility of class I antigens by different cytokines (see below).

12A.3.1.2 Transplanted kidney

Upregulation of MHC class I antigens in human renal allografts following transplantation has been extensively described (Hall *et al.*, 1984*b*; Fuggle *et al.*, 1986). The most dramatic finding is of intense cytoplasmic and membrane staining of all the renal tubules (Fuggle *et al.*, 1986). There is also induction of class II on the normally negative endothelial cells of the large vessels. Analysis of the induced molecules with polymorphic and locus-specific antibodies (Fuggle *et al.*, 1987) showed it was of donor origin and had HLA-DR, DQ and DP components. It has been well documented that gamma-interferon causes upregulation of class II on many different cell types *in vitro* (reviewed by Halloran *et al.*, 1986) including cultured renal tubule cells (Bishop *et al.*, 1986). It is highly likely that upregulation is caused by local release of cytokines from the inflammatory infiltrate. Indeed, focal upregulation is often located around a focal infiltrate (Milton *et al.*, 1986) and Häyry and von Willebrand observed upregulation of class II only when there was a blastogenic component to the infiltrate (Hayry & von Willebrand, 1986). The question arises whether induction is correlated with episodes of clinical rejection. In general there is a correlation (Hall *et al.*, 1984*b*; Fuggle *et al.*, 1986) but it is not absolute. Thus induced class II are not always detected in biopsies during allograft rejection and induced class II may be found during stable graft function (Fuggle, 1989). It has been suggested that induced class II would be helpful in distinguishing between renal dysfunction caused by rejection and CsA nephrotoxicity (Barrett *et al.*, 1987) but the lack of complete correlation between class II and rejection (Fuggle, 1990) means class II is not reliable as a differential marker.

Class I is also induced during rejection episodes (Barrett *et al.*, 1987), there being increased intensity on the renal epithelial cells. Unlike cardiac transplantation (see below), however, far less attention has been paid to class I induction in renal transplantation. This is partly because all cells constitutively express class I in the kidneys and increased expression is not as obvious as *de novo* expression. Class I induction is not specific to rejection; thus experimental studies have shown transient induction in grafted syngeneic kidneys, presumably due to ischaemic time (Milton *et al.*, 1986).

12A.3.2 Cardiac transplantation

12A.3.2.1 The normal heart

Immunocytochemical staining of normal heart taken prior to transplantation demonstrates that all the interstitial structures are class I positive and the large majority are also class II positive (Figure 12A.2). In contrast, the myocardium plasma membrane is negative for MHC antigens (Rose *et al.*, 1986). Some studies have reported faint staining of the intercalated discs for class I in normal heart (Daar *et al.*, 1984*a*). The interstitial structures in normal heart have been identified as being mostly endothelial cells with a small minority being cells of the monocyte/macrophage/dendritic series (Rose *et al.*, 1990). Thus mab that bind to endothelial cells (EN4 or mab against the CD31 antigen, PECAM) show a pattern of staining (Figure 12A.3) identical to that found with mab against common determinant or DR class II. In contrast, identification of cells of bone marrow origin (with FIO-89-4 or Hel-1) showed sparse numbers of cells (Rose *et al.*, 1990). Quantification of cells binding EN4 and comparison with class II-positive cells showed that 85% of class II positive cells are endothelial (Rose *et al.*, 1990). This is in contrast to rat heart where endothelial cells do not constitutively express class II and the majority of class II-positive cells are dendritic cells (Hart & Fabre, 1981). It has been reported that the endothelial cells in normal human heart are not normally class II-positive (Carforio *et al.*, 1990); however, these authors used vWF to identify endothelial cells. Our studies have shown only about 30% of endothelial cells are vWF-positive in the heart (Hengstenberg *et al.*, 1990) and moreover, it is the larger vessels which are more likely to be vWF-positive and these larger vessels tend to be class II-negative (Page *et al.*, 1992). Fuggle *et al.* (1983) also reported that endothelial cells in the larger vessels tend to be negative for class II antigens whereas the small capillaries are positive.

12A.3.2.2 Transplanted heart

After transplantation, there is a dramatic upregulation of MHC class I on the myocardial plasma membrane and intercalating discs (Figure 12A.4a; Rose *et al.*, 1986; Suitters *et al.*, 1987; Ahmed-Ansari *et al.*, 1988; Steinhoff *et al.*, 1989). This is almost always accompanied by an infiltrate, most of which is also class II positive (Figure 12A.4b). The close apposition of the normally class II positive endothelial cells and class II positive infiltrating cells makes it difficult to determine whether there is upregulation of class II on the endothelial cells. Studies using fluorescent antibody against vWF to identify the larger endothelial cells, have reported more of these cells becoming class II positive after transplantation (Carforio *et al.*, 1990). Our own studies have shown that the normally negative endocardium becomes class II positive following transplantation (P. M. Taylor *et al.*, unpublished data). One study reported upregulation of class II on the myocardium after transplantation (Ahmed-Ansari *et al.*,

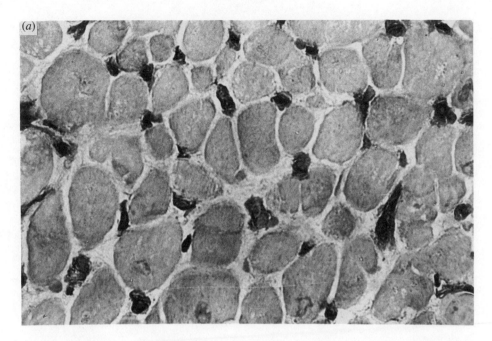

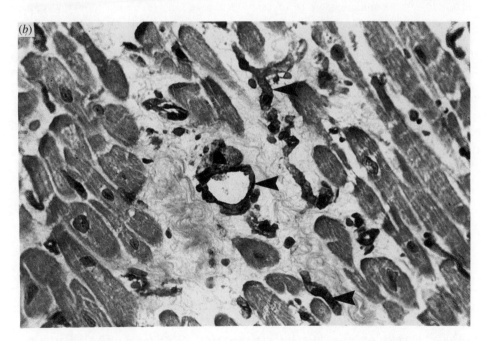

Figure 12A.2. Photomicrograph of cryostat section (6 μm) of normal donor atrium prior to transplantation, stained with W6/32 against monomorphic determinants of MHC class I antigens (a) or L243 against DR determinants of MHC class II antigens (b) and immunoperoxidase. Arrows point to venules which are DR-positive. The myocardium is normally negative for MHC antigen expression. Counterstained with Harris's haematoxylin. (400 X).

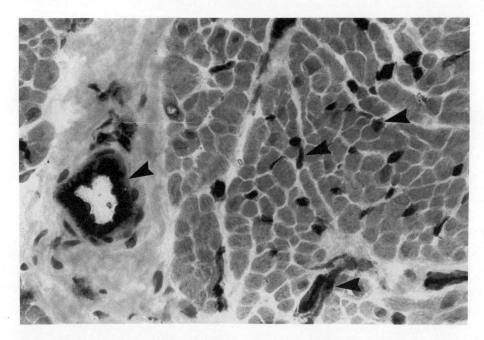

Figure 12A.3. Photomicrograph of cryostat section (6 μm) of normal donor atrium, prior to transplantation, stained with BBIG-P1 against PECAM (CD31) and immuno-peroxidase. Arrows point to an arteriole which is positive and to some of the smaller interstitial structures, the majority of which are CD31-positive. Counterstained with Harris's haematoxylin. (400 X).

1988) but this is something we have never observed and it has not been confirmed by other studies (Steinhoff *et al.*, 1989; Carforio *et al.*, 1990).

Upregulation of class I is easily observed because the cardiac plasma membrane is normally class I negative. Upregulation of donor specific class II antigens on the endothelium may occur, as has been shown in experimental studies in rats (Milton & Fabre, 1985) but because it requires a double-labelling technique to be demonstrated in human tissue the phenomenon has not been extensively studied. Class I is not induced on the myocardium of donor hearts during the 4 h (maximum) ischaemic time prior to transplantation. A sequential study of 114 biopsies from 11 patients showed that upregulation of class I on the myocardium was associated with rejection episodes, diagnosed by histological assessment of endomyocardial biopsy (Suitters *et al.*, 1987). The upregulation is focal and is always in close proximity to an infiltrate which may include T cells or may just be macrophages (Suitters *et al.*, 1987). The assumption is therefore that lymphokines released from the local infiltrate caused upregulation of these antigens. There is no direct evidence for this as yet, as immunocytochemical techniques have not been successful in detecting interferons in tissue sections (see below). As described for induction of MHC antigens during clinical rejection of renal grafts (Fuggle *et al.*, 1986), the

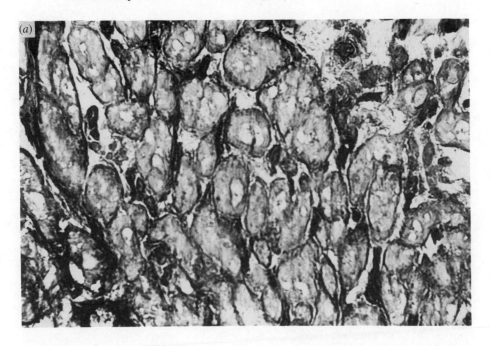

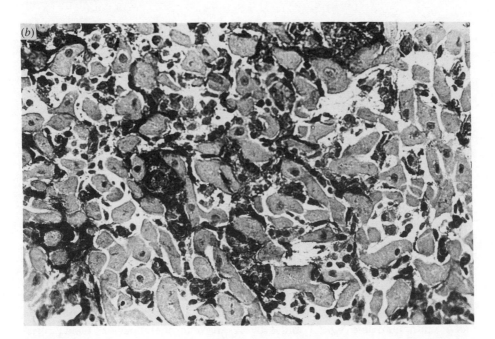

Figure 12A.4. Photomicrograph of cryostat section (6 μm) of endomyocardial biopsy showing histological signs of rejection stained with (a) W6/32 against monomorphic determinants of MHC class I and (b) CA22 against monomorphic determinants of class II. There is *de-novo* expression of class I on the myocardial plasma membrane (a) and the majority of infiltrating cells are class II-positive (b). Sections counterstained with Harris's haematoxylin. (400 X).

correlation between induction of MHC class I on the heart and clinical rejection is not absolute (Suitters et al., 1987; Ahmed-Ansari et al., 1988; Steinhoff et al., 1989). One hundred per cent of first rejection episodes (7 of 7 biopsies) and 79% (11 of 14) of subsequent rejection episodes coincided with class I expression (Suitters et al., 1987). Steinhoff reported that 57 of 78 rejection episodes were characterized by induction of class I on the normally negative myocardium (Steinhoff et al., 1989).

The observation that once induced class I induction takes 3–4 weeks to disappear following treatment (Suitters et al., 1987) explains why, after the first rejection episode, only 31% of biopsies with induced class I are diagnosed as rejection.

Comparison of the effects of immunosuppressive regimens with MHC induction showed that patients taking CsA in conjunction with azathioprine and steroids had significantly less class I induction than patients on CsA and azathioprine or patients taking azathioprine and steroids (Suitters et al., 1987). Not surprisingly, this was associated with fewer rejection episodes in the patients taking triple therapy. Renal transplant patients receiving triple therapy also show less class II induction on their grafts during both rejection and stable periods of graft function (Fuggle, 1990).

12A.3.3 Lung transplantation

Experimental studies in rats have shown induction of class II antigens on the endothelium and epithelium during acute rejection (Romaniuk et al., 1987). It should be remembered, however, that rat endothelial cells, unlike human, do not constitutively express class II antigens. Human lungs 'normally' show a strong and extensive distribution of MHC antigens. Class II antigens are present on all alveolar macrophages and tracheal epithelium but are variably expressed on endothelial cells, tracheal and bronchiolar epithelium (Taylor et al., 1989; Glanville et al., 1989; Yousem et al., 1990). DR and DP antigens are more heavily expressed than DQ in normal lung (Taylor et al., 1989; Yousem et al., 1990). All the above structures were invariably class I positive as well. The strong expression of these antigens in lungs prior to transplantation make any increase difficult to discern. Nevertheless, Taylor and colleagues (1989), in a study of nine lungs removed from heart–lung recipients because of the development of obliterative bronchiolitis, reported enhanced and consistent expression of class II determinants on all endothelial cells and also on bronchiolar epithelium and type I and type II alveolar pneumocytes. Using serial dilutions of mab against class DR, DP and DQ determinants, Yousem et al. (1990) also observed increased expression of DR and DP on all cells within transbro ͏ ͏al biopsies of patients after lung transplantation. Taylor et al. (1989) also found increased expression of DQ in the lung after transplantation.

It is far less easy to know whether the immunocytochemical changes observed in the lungs following transplantation are due to rejection than it is after heart or renal transplantation. The majority of lung transplant patients experience bacterial and cytomegalovirus infections, which directly affect the transplanted organ. A differential diagnosis of rejection and infection is difficult to achieve in the transplanted lungs. The changes described above almost certainly reflect a variety of immunological and infectious stimuli.

12A.3.4 Liver transplantation

In normal liver MHC class I antigens are invariably expressed on the bile duct epithelium, endothelium cells, cells lining sinusoids (including Kupffer cells) and interstitial leukocytes. In contrast, hepatocytes have been described as negative (Gouw *et al.*, 1987; So *et al.*, 1987) or very weakly stained (Daar *et al.*, 1984a; Steinhoff *et al.*, 1988). Class II has been found to be absent or weakly expressed by bile duct epithelium and to be present on all or most of the endothelial cells but absent on hepatocytes (Steinhoff *et al.*, 1988; Gouw *et al.*, 1987; So *et al.*, 1987). There is strong induction of class I antigens on hepatocytes during liver allograft rejection (Steinhoff *et al.*, 1988; So *et al.*, 1987; Gouw *et al.*, 1987). Moreover, using mab against beta$_2$-microglobulin which can be used on paraffin embedded tissue, induction of beta$_2$-microglobulin on hepatocytes has been reported (Nagafuchi *et al.*, 1985). Most studies have not reported induction of class II on hepatocytes but on biliary epithelial cells. Steinhoff and his colleagues (1988) reported two patterns of induction, either class II on biliary epithelium alone associated with weak class I on hepatocytes or class II on both epithelium and hepatocytes associated with strong expression of class I on the hepatocytes.

12A.4 Adhesion molecules

Recently immunocytochemical methods have been employed to investigate expression of adhesion and accessory molecules in allografted organs. Of particular interest in transplantation is the interaction between leukocytes and vascular endothelial cells which control adhesion and extravasation into the tissues. Modulation of leukocyte vessel wall adhesion is mediated by constitutive or cytokine upregulated expression of some or all of the following endothelial molecules: endothelial leukocyte adhesion molecule-1 (ELAM-1), a ligand for neutrophils; vascular adhesion molecule (VCAM), a ligand for monocytes and lymphocytes (Osborn *et al.*, 1989); intercellular adhesion molecule (ICAM-1 or CD54), a ligand involved in adhesion and transmigration of all leukocytes (Van-Epps *et al.*, 1990); and platelet endothelial cell adhesion molecule (PECAM or CD31), found on all endothelial cells and platelets (Parums *et al.*, 1990). We have found ICAM-1 to be constitutively expressed

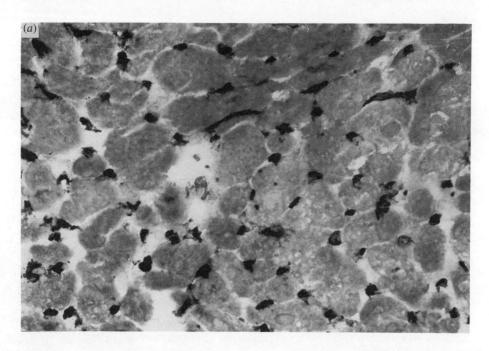

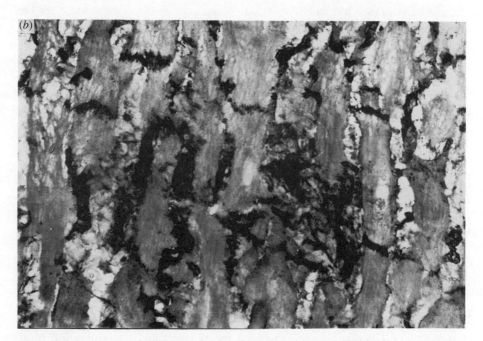

Figure 12A.5. Photomicrograph of cryostat section (6 μm) of normal heart taken before transplantation (a) and endomyocardial biopsy showing histological signs of rejection (b). Sections stained with BBIG-1$_2$ against ICAM-1 (CD54) and immunoperoxidase. Counterstained with Harris's haematoxylin. (400 X).

on the tiny capillary endothelial cells within the normal heart (Figure 12A.5a) and the myocardium and intercalating discs to be normally negative (Rose *et al.*, 1990). During rejection there is dramatic induction of ICAM-1 on the intercalating discs which is closely associated with a focal infiltrate (Figure 12A.5b; Rose *et al.*, 1990). Much of the infiltrate is also strongly ICAM-1 positive. A sequential study, comparing upregulation of class I and ICAM-1 on the myocardium following cardiac transplantation, has shown induction of ICAM-1 to be less common and more specific to rejection than class I (unpublished data). It is also more restricted to areas of myocardium where there is an infiltrate. PECAM was found to stain virtually all interstitial structures (Figure 12A.3) whereas VCAM and ELAM were only minimally expressed in normal heart (Taylor *et al.*, 1992). During rejection episodes, we have found focal induction of VCAM on capillaries associated with an infiltrate (Taylor *et al.*, 1992) confirming recent results (Briscoe *et al.*, 1991). Induction of VCAM and ICAM, both restricted in area and associated with an infiltrate, appear to be important early events preceding mononuclear cell extravasation. Induction of VCAM may be essential for cell migration across the endothelial cells and induction of ICAM-1 on the intercalating discs could be an event preceding damage by LFA-1-positive T cells.

ICAM-1 is constitutively expressed on sinusoidal endothelial and Kupffer cells of the normal liver and it is not detected on hepatocytes and bile ducts (Behrend *et al.*, 1991; Steinhoff *et al.*, 1990). During rejection or infection, however, there was *de novo* induction of ICAM-1 on hepatocyte membranes, with a focal relation to LFA-1 infiltrating lymphocytes (Adams *et al.*, 1989; Steinhoff *et al.*, 1990). On bile duct epithelia that were strongly induced to express class I and HLA-DR antigens during infection and rejection, there was only weak *de novo* expression of ICAM-1 at the apical membranes (Steinhoff *et al.*, 1990). There was also increased expression of ICAM-1 on endothelial cells. Similar to our results in the heart, Steinhoff found the area of induced ICAM-1 on hepatocytes to be more restricted than class I.

12A.5 Cytokines

There is intense interest in identifying cytokines in transplanted tissue in order to understand those that are important in causing the local changes which have been described. To date, the only cytokines which have been identified immunocytochemically are tumour necrosis factor and interleukin-1 beta found in liver biopsies from liver transplant recipients undergoing rejection (Hoffmann *et al.*, 1991). Messenger RNA for interleukin-2 has been identified in allografted experimental kidneys (Dallman *et al.*, 1991) but not the protein. Immunocytochemical identification of other important cytokines of interest (IL-1, IL-4, IL-5, alpha, beta and gamma-interferon) will have to await further developments in immunocytochemistry to improve sensitivity.

12A.6   References

Adams, D. H., Hubscher, S. G., Shaw, J., Rothlein, S. G. & Neuberger, J. M. (1989). Intercellular adhesion molecule 1 on liver allografts during rejection. *Lancet*, **1**, 1122–1125.

Ahmed-Ansari, A., Tadros, T. S., Knopf, W. D., Murphy, D. A., Hertzler, G., Feighan, J., Leatherby, A. & Sell, K. W. (1988). Histocompatibility complex class I and class II expression by myocytes in cardiac biopsies posttransplantation. *Transplantation*, **45**, 972–978.

Appleyard, S. T., Dunn, M. J., Rose, M. L. & Dubowitz, V. (1985). Increased expression of HLA ABC class I antigens by muscle fibres in Duchenne dystrophy, inflammatory myopathy and other neuromuscular disorders. *Lancet*, **1**, 361–363.

Barnstable, C. J., Bodmer, W. F., Brown, G., Galfre, G., Milstein, C., Williams, A. F. & Zieglar, A. (1978). Production of monoclonal antibodies to group A erythryocytes, HLA and other human cell surface antigens – new tools for genetic analysis. *Cell*, **14**, 9–16.

Barrett, M., Milton, A. D., Barrett, J., Taube, D., Bewick, M., Parsons, V. P. & Fabre, J. W. (1987). Needle biopsy evaluation of class II major histocompatibility complex antigen expression for the differential diagnosis of cyclosporine nephrotoxicity from kidney graft rejection. *Transplantation*, **44**, 223–226.

Behrend, M., Steinhoff, G., Wonigeit, K. & Pichlmayr, R. (1991). Patterns of adhesion molecule expression in human liver allografts. *Transplantation Proceedings*, **23**, 1419–1420.

Bishop, G. A., Hall, B. M., Suranyi, M. G., Tiller, D. J., Horvath, J. C. & Duggin, G. G. (1986). Expression of HLA antigens on renal tubular cells in culture. I. Evidence that mixed lymphocyte culture supernatants and gamma interferon increase both class I and class II HLA antigens. *Transplantation*, **42**, 671–679.

Briscoe, D. M., Schoen, F. J., Rice, G. E., Bevilacqua, M. P., Ganz, P. & Pober, J. S. (1991). Induced expression of endothelial-leukocyte adhesion molecules in human cardiac allografts. *Transplantation*, **51**, 537–539.

Brodsky, F. M., Parham, P., Barnstaple, C. J., Crumpton, M. J. & Bodmer, W. F. (1979). Monoclonal antibodies for analysis of the HLA system. *Immunological Reviews*, **47**, 3–33.

Carforio, A. L. P., Botazzo, G. F., Counihan, P. J., Burke, M., Poloniecki, J., Davies, M. J. & Pepper, J. R. (1990). Class II major histocompatibility complex antigens on cardiac endothelium: an early marker of rejection in the transplanted human heart. *Transplantation Proceedings*, **22**, 1830–1833.

Daar, A. S., Fuggle, S. V., Fabre, J. W., Ting, A. & Morris, P. J. (1984a). The detailed distribution of HLA-A, B, C antigens in normal human organs. *Transplantation*, **38**, 287–292.

Daar, A. S., Fuggle, S. V., Fabre, J. W., Ting, A. & Morris, P. J. (1984b). The detailed distribution of MHC class II antigens in normal human organs. *Transplantation*, **38**, 292–297.

Dalchau, R., Kirkley, J. & Fabre, J. W. (1980). Monoclonal antibody to a human leukocyte-specific membrane glycoprotein probably homologous to the leukocyte-common (L-C) antigen of the rat. *European Journal of Immunology*, **10**, 737–744.

Dallman, M. J., Shiho, O., Page, T. H., Wood, K. J. & Morris, P. J. (1991). Peripheral tolerance to alloantigen results from altered regulation of the interleukin-2 pathway. *Journal of Experimental Medicine*, **173**, 79–87.

DeLourdes Higuchi, M., Campas de Assis, R. V., Sambiase, N. V., Reis, M. M., Kalil, J., Bocchi, E., Fiorelli, A., Stolf, N., Bellotti, G., Pileggi, F. & Jatene, A. (1991).

Usefulness of T cell phenotype characteristics in endomyocardial biopsy fragments from human cardiac allografts. *Journal of Heart and Lung Transplantation*, **10**, 235–242.

Fleming, K. A., McMichael, A., Morton, J. A., Woods, J. & McGee, J. (1981). Distribution of HLA class I antigens in normal human tissue and in mammary cancer. *Journal of Clinical Pathology*, **34**, 779–784.

Fuggle, S. V. (1989). MHC antigen expression in vascularised organ allografts: clinical correlations and significance. *Transplantation Reviews*, **3**, 81–103.

Fuggle, S. V., Errasti, P., Daar, A. S., Fabre, J. W., Ting, A. & Morris, P. J. (1983). Localisation of major histocompatibility complex antigens (HLA-ABC and DR) in 46 kidneys. *Transplantation*, **35**, 385–390.

Fuggle, S. V., McWhinnie, D. L., Chapman, J. R., Taylor, H. M. & Morris, P. J. (1986). Sequential analysis of HLA class II antigen expression in human renal allografts. Induction of tubular class II and correlation with clinical parameters. *Transplantation*, **42**, 144–149.

Fuggle, S. V., McWhinnie, D. L. & Morris, P. J. (1987). Precise specificity of induced tubular class II antigens in renal allografts. *Transplantation*, **44**, 214–220.

Fuggle, S. V., McWhinnie, D. L. & Morris, P. J. (1989). Immunohistological analysis of renal allograft biopsies from cyclosporin-treated patients. Induced HLA-class II antigen expression does not exclude a diagnosis of cyclosporin nephrotoxicity. *Transplantation International*, **2**, 123–128.

Glanville, A. R., Tazelaar, H. D. , Theodore, J., Imoto, E., Rouse, R. V., Baldwin, J. C. & Robin, E. D. (1989). The distribution of MHC class I and II antigens on bronchial epithelium. *American Reviews of Respiratory Diseases*, **139**, 330–334.

Gouw, A. S. H., Houthoff, H. J., Huitema, S., Beelen, J. M., Gips, C. H. & Poppema, S. (1987). Expression of major histocompatibility antigens on hepatocytes in rejecting human liver allografts. *Transplantation*, **43**, 291–296.

Hall, B. M., Bishop, G. A., Farnsworth, A., Duggin, G. G., Horvath, J. S., Shiel, A. G. R. & Tiller, D. J. (1984*a*). Identification of the cellular subpopulations infiltrating rejecting cadavar renal allografts. *Transplantation*, **37**, 564–570.

Hall, B., Duggin, G. G., Philips, J., Bishop, G. A., Horvath, J. S. & Tiller, D. J. (1984*b*). Increased expression of HLA-DR antigen on renal tubular cells in renal transplants: relevance to the rejection process. *Lancet*, **2**, 247–249.

Halloran, P. F., Wadgymar, A. & Autenreid, P. (1986). The regulation of the expression of major histocompatibility complex products. *Transplantation*, **4**, 413–420.

Hancock, W. W., Gee, D., de Moerloose, P., Rickles, F. R., Ewan, V. A. & Atkins, R. C. (1985). Immunohistological analysis of serial biopsies taken during human renal allograft rejection. *Transplantation*, **39**, 430–438.

Hancock, W. W., Thomson, N. M. & Atkins, R. C. (1983). Composition of interstitial cellular infiltrate identified by monoclonal antibodies in renal biopsies of rejecting human renal allografts. *Transplantation*, **35**, 458–463.

Hart, D. N. J. & Fabre, J. W. (1981). Demonstration and characterisation of Ia-positive dendritic cells in the interstitial connective tissues of rat heart and other tissues but not brain. *Journal of Experimental Medicine*, **153**, 347–361.

Häyry, P. & von Willebrand, E. (1986). The influence of the pattern of inflammation and administration of steroids on class II MHC antigen expression in renal transplants. *Transplantation*, **42**, 358–363.

Hengstenberg, C., Rose, M. L., Page, C., Taylor, P. M. & Yacoub, M. H. (1990). Immunocytochemical changes suggestive of damage to endothelial cells during rejection of human cardiac allografts. *Transplantation*, **49**, 895–899.

Hoffmann, K., Wonigeit, K., Steinhoff, G., Behrend, M., Herzbeck, H., Flad, H.-D. &

Pilchmayr, R. (1991). Tumour necrosis factor alpha and interleukin-1 beta in rejection human liver allografts. *Transplantation Proceedings*, **23**, 1421–1423.

Hoshinaga, K., Mohanakumar, T., Goldman, M. H., Wolfgang, T. C., Szenrpetry, S., Lee, H. M. & Lower, R. R. (1984). Clinical significance of *in situ* detection of T lymphocyte subsets and monocyte/macrophage lineages in heart allografts. *Transplantation*, **38**, 634–637.

Imakita, M., Cohnert, T. R. & Billingham, M. E. (1988). Endocardial infiltrates: the 'Quilty' effect. *Journal of Heart Transplantation*, **7**, 57–61.

Jongsma, A., van Someven, H., Westerwald, A. Hagemeijer, A. & Pearson, P. (1973). Localisation of human chromosomes by studies of human-Chinese somatic cell hybrids. *Humangenetik*, **20**, 195–202.

McWhinnie, D. L., Thompson, J. F., Taylor, H. M., Chapman, J. R., Bolton, E. M., Carter, N. P., Wood, R. F. M. & Morris, P. J. (1986). Morphometric analysis of cellular infiltration assessed by monoclonal antibody labelling in sequential human renal allograft biopsies. *Transplantation*, **42**, 352–358.

Milton, A. D. & Fabre, J. W. (1985). Massive induction of donor type class I and class II major histocompatibility complex antigens during heart allograft rejection in the rat. *Journal of Experimental Medicine*, **161**, 98–112.

Milton, A. D., Spencer, S. C. & Fabre, J. W. (1986). Detailed analysis and demonstration of differences in the kinetics and induction of class I and class II major histocompatibility complex antigens in rejecting cardiac and kidney allografts in the rat. *Transplantation*, **41**, 499–508.

Nagafuchi, Y., Thomas, H. C., Hobbs, K. E. F. & Scheuer, P. F. (1985). Expression of beta-2 microglobulin on hepatocytes after liver transplantation. *Lancet*, **1**, 552–554.

Natali, P. G., Bigotti, A., Nicotra, M. R., Viora, M., Manfredi, D. & Ferrone, S. (1984). Distribution of human class I (HLA-A, B, C) histocompatibility antigens in normal and malignant tissues of non-lymphoid origin. *Cancer Research*, **44**, 4679–4687.

Natali, P. G., De-Martino, C., Quaranta, V., Nicotra, M. R., Frezza, F., Pellegrino, M. Λ. & Ferrone, S. (1981). Expression of La-like antigens in normal human non-lymphoid tissues. *Transplantation*, **31**, 75–78.

Osborn, L., Hession, R., Tizard, R., Vassallo, C., Lukowsky, S., Chi-Rosso, G. & Lobb, R. (1989). Direct expression cloning of vascular adhesion molecule 1, a cytokine-induced endothelial protein that binds lymphocytes. *Cell*, **59**, 1203–1211.

Page, C., Rose, M. L., Yacoub, M. H., Pigott, R. (1992). Antigenic heterogeneity of vascular endothelium. *American Journal of Pathology*, **141**, 673–683.

Parums, D. V., Cordell, J. L., Micklem, K., Heryet, A. R., Gatter, K. C. & Mason, D. Y. (1990). JC70: a new monoclonal antibody that detects vascular endothelium associated antigen on routinely processed tissue sections. *Journal of Clinical Pathology*, **43**, 752–754.

Perkins, J. D., Weisner, R. H., Banks, P. M., LaRusso, N. F., Ludwig, J. & Krom, R. A. F. (1987). Immunohistologic labelling as an indicator of liver allograft rejection. *Transplantation*, **43**, 105–108.

Platt, J. L., Le Bien, T. W. & Michael, A. F. (1982). Interstitial mononuclear cell populations in renal graft rejection. Identification by monoclonal antibodies in tissue sections. *Journal of Experimental Medicine*, **155**, 17–30.

Romaniuk, A., Prop, J., Petersen, A. H., Wildevuur, C. R. H. & Nieuwenhuis, P. (1987). Expression of class II major histocompatibility complex antigens by bronchial epithelium in rat lung allografts. *Transplantation*, **44**, 209–214.

Rose, M. L., Coles, M. I., Griffin, R. J., Pomerance, A. & Yacoub, M. H. (1986). Expression of class I and class II major histocompatibility antigens in normal and transplanted human heart. *Transplantation*, **41**, 776–780.

Rose, M. L., Gracie, J. A., Fraser, A., Chisholm, P. & Yacoub, M. H. (1984). Use of monoclonal antibodies to quantitate T lymphocyte subpopulations in human cardiac allografts. *Transplantation*, **38**, 230–234.

Rose, M. L., Page, C., Hengstenberg, C. & Yacoub, M. H. (1990). Identification of antigen presenting cells in normal and transplanted human heart: importance of endothelial cells. *Human Immunology*, **28**, 179–185.

Rose, M., Page, C., Hengstenberg, C. & Yacoub, M. (1991). Immunocytochemical markers of activation in cardiac transplant rejection. *European Heart Journal*, **12** (Suppl. D), 147–150.

So, S. K., Platt, J. L., Ascher, N. L. & Snover, D. C. (1987). Increased expression of class I major histocompatibility complex antigens on hepatocytes in rejecting human liver allografts. *Transplantation*, **43**, 79–85.

Steinhoff, G., Behrend, M. & Wonigeit, K. (1990). Expression of adhesion molecules on lymphocyte/monocytes and hepatocytes in human liver grafts. *Human Immunology*, **28**, 123–127.

Steinhoff, G., Wonigeit, K. & Pilchmayer, R. (1988). Analysis of sequential changes in major histocompatibility complex expression in human liver grafts after transplantation. *Transplantation*, **45**, 394–401.

Steinhoff, G., Wonigeit, K., Schafers, H. J. & Haverich, A. (1989). Sequential analysis of monomorphic and polymorphic major histocompatibility complex antigen expression in human heart allograft biopsy specimens. *Journal of Heart Transplantation*, **8**, 360–367.

Suitters, A. J., Rose, M. L., Higgins, A. & Yacoub, M. H. (1987). MHC antigen expression in sequential biopsies from cardiac transplant patients – correlation with rejection. *Clinical and Experimental Immunology*, **69**, 575–583.

Taylor, P. M., Rose, M. L. & Yacoub, M. H. (1989). Expression of MHC antigens in normal lungs and transplanted lungs with obliterative bronchiolitis. *Transplantation*, **48**, 506–510.

Taylor, P. M., Rose, M. L., Yacoub, M. H. & Pigott, R. (1992). Induction of vascular adhesion molecules during rejection of human cardiac allografts. *Transplantation*, **54**, 451–457.

Tufveson, G., Forsum, U., Claesson, K., Klareskog, L., Larsson, E, Karlsson-Parra, A. & Frodin, L. (1983). T lymphocyte subsets and HLA-DR expressing cells in rejected human kidney grafts. *Scandinavian Journal of Immunology*, **18**, 37–40.

Van-Epps, D. E., Potter, J., Vachula, M., Smith, C. W. & Anderson, D. C. (1989). Suppression of human lymphocyte chemotaxis and transendothelial migration by anti-LFA-1 antibody. *Journal of Immunology*, **143**, 3207–3210.

Van Es, A., Meyer, C. J. L. M., Olijans, P. J., Tanke, H. H. & Van Es, L. A. (1984). Mononuclear cells in renal allografts. *Transplantation*, **37**, 134–139.

Yousem, S. A., Curley, J. M., Dauber, J., Paradis, I., Rabinowich, H., Zeevi, A., Duquesnoy, R., Dowling, R., Zenati, M., Hardesty, R. & Griffiths, B. (1990). HLA-class II antigen expression in human heart-lung allografts. *Transplantation*, **49**, 991–995.

12B

Experimental studies on *in-vivo* immunosuppression

N. M. PARISH and A. COOKE

12B.1 Introduction

Monoclonal antibody (mab) technology has had revolutionary effects on diverse areas of biology. In recent years the development of such specific reagents has permitted investigations examining the feasibility of treating diseases and conditions such as autoimmunity and graft rejection. For the purposes of this review, the subject area to be covered will be restricted to literature concerning *in-vivo* treatment of animal models of autoimmune diseases using mab.

In recent years most of the existing animal models of autoimmunity have been shown to have, as central to their disease mechanisms, inappropriately activated T cells. Furthermore, inheritance of certain major histocompatibility complex (MHC) haplotypes can have profound effects on the subsequent incidence of disease. This indicates that an understanding of antigen presentation to autoantigen-specific T cells may be important in devising strategies for intervening in the disease process. The central interaction between the auto-specific T cell and the antigen presenting cell (APC) has a number of direct and indirect effects in that T cell products (cytokines) can upregulate adhesion and homing molecules thereby inducing the infiltration of other cells, e.g. macrophages and neutrophils which may themselves be destructive.

With this in mind we have chosen to structure the following review under sections covering mab treatments directed towards T cell products, antigen-presenting cell markers, cytokines and adhesion molecules representing the key areas currently recognized as showing potential for therapeutic intervention.

Table 12B.1. *Antibodies to pan-T cell markers*

Disease	SLE			Diabetes			EAN	
	MRL	BXSB	F$_1$ (NZB × NZW)	BB rat	NOD (spontaneous)	STZ-induced	Rat	
Effect on disease	↓	→	→	↓	↓	↓	↓	↓↑
Antibody Name	30-H12	30-H12	30-H12	0x 19	–	YTS 154.7	W3/13	0x 19
Isotype	γ2b	γ2b	γ2b	γ1	–	γ2b	γ1	γ1
Specifity	Thy 1.2	Thy 1.2	Thy 1.2	Pan-T cell marker	Thy 1.2	Thy 1.2	Pan-T cell marker	Pan-T cell marker
Side-effects	–	+ (anaphylaxis)	–	–	–	–	–	+ (Exacerbation if given too late)
Reference	Seaman et al. (1983) Wofsy et al. (1985)	Wofsy et al. (1985)	Wofsy et al. (1985)	Like et al. (1986)	Harada & Makino (1986)	Kantwerk et al. (1987)	Strigård et al. (1988)	Strigård et al. (1988)

→, no effect; ⇊, substantially reduced disease incidence/severity; ↓, partially reduced disease incidence/severity; ↑, disease aggravation; EAN, experimental autoimmune neuritis; SLE, systemic lupus erythematosus; STZ, streptozotocin

12B.2   Monoclonal antibody treatments directed towards T cell surface markers

12B.2.1 Pan T cell markers

Table 12B.1 summarizes the major findings of studies using monoclonal antibodies to 'pan T' cell markers.

Animal models of systemic lupus erythematosus (SLE), diabetes and experimental autoimmune neuritis (EAN) have been investigated using antibodies recognizing markers present on the total T cell population of the host animal. There were generally favourable effects in most models studied. In two of the lupus models, however, no improvement of disease manifestations was demonstrated and in fact a fatal anaphylaxis developed in the case of BXSB mice. The preventive effects could not be totally attributed to target cell depletion as in some cases; effective treatment was achieved with non-depleting antibodies.

The studies cited showed that anti-T cell mab could be successful in preventing diverse autoimmune diseases. They also served to show that the disease process is dynamic and evolving and that treatment with any particular antibody may have different effects depending on the stage at which it is given.

12B.2.2 Anti-CD4 treatment

The most-studied antibody therapies have utilized antibodies to the CD4 molecule. Early studies with anti-Thy1 demonstrated that different strains of mice could show a greater or lesser susceptibility to developing anaphylaxis in response to antibody therapy. Furthermore, in some cases the efficacy of the antibody treatment was curtailed by the development of anti-rat immunoglobulin (Ig) antibodies. At an early stage of investigating rat anti-murine CD4 antibodies it was demonstrated that anti-CD4 treatment could induce tolerance to itself, other rat antibodies and to concomitantly administered antigens. This property made such antibodies far more attractive as potential therapeutic agents.

Most of the major animal models of autoimmunity have been studied for possible therapeutic effects of anti-CD4 mab treatment (Table 12B.2). Anti-CD4 antibodies have been effective in some models of lupus, all models of insulin-dependent diabetes mellitus (IDDM), experimental allergic encephalomyelitis (EAE), experimental autoimmune thyroiditis (EAT), EAN, experimental autoimmune myasthenia gravis (EAMG) and rheumatoid arthritis (RA). Depletion of CD4 cells was not always necessary as in some cases $F(ab)_2$ or non-depleting antibody isotypes were effective. Exceptions to the efficacy shown by the variety of anti-CD4 antibodies studied include the MRL mouse in which, although disease amelioration was achieved, this was not sustained on cessation of therapy and the antibody was itself associated with morbidity. A further, less successful anti-CD4 treatment was shown with streptozotocin (STZ)-induced diabetes; this may, however, reflect the possibility that this form of diabetes is not mediated fundamentally by autoimmune mechanisms. The observation that vasculitis induced in BN rats with $HgCl_2$ was completely unaffected by anti-CD4 treatment might suggest that pathology resulting from the activity of Th-2 cells is more refractory to anti-CD4 treatment.

12B.2.3 Anti-CD8 treatments

In diverse cases the infiltration of organs in organ-specific autoimmune models has been shown to involve $CD8^+$ T cells, thereby offering potential for antibody intervention. Table 12B.3 provides a reference for the consideration of these studies.

Anti-CD8 therapy has been used in the treatment of several autoimmune animal models. These include diabetes, EAT, EAN, EAE and SLE. These antibodies appear to achieve more variable results than anti-CD4 treatment. SLE and EAE in macaques were unaffected by anti-CD8 therapy and EAT in the Buffalo rat was exacerbated by such treatment. Diabetes was, however, reduced in most studies by anti-CD8 treatment as was murine EAT and rat EAN. Again, conflicting results have been demonstrated in STZ diabetes, providing further evidence that this disease model may involve a directly toxic element in its development and not just be wholly attributable to an auto-immune aetiology.

The above-cited literature covering antibody treatment targeted to the accessory molecules, CD4 and CD8, shows that such relatively non-specific treatments can be successful, possibly because final effector cell populations are likely to contain multiple specificities in the inflammatory infiltrates that characterize autoimmune diseases. The greater success achieved with anti-CD4 treatments may be due to the role of $CD4^+$ T cells in the induction of further immune effector cells including $CD8^+$ T cells. Thus treatment with anti-CD4 prevents disease progression by, in effect, intervening at an earlier stage in the process. Anti-CD8 therapy, however, can be effective, particularly in the case of the organ-targeted autoimmune diseases (e.g. diabetes, EAT) as opposed to diseases with more diffuse target autoantigens (e.g. SLE).

Anti-CD4 is the more interesting due to its observed effect of not merely preventing CD4 function by depletion or by CD4 blockade but also by inducing long-term protection after treatment has stopped. This seems to be connected with the ability of these antibodies to induce tolerance to both themselves and to antigens/autoantigens present when the antibody is administered.

The above data show that the animal models, even of the same disease, are not consistent with regard to efficacy of therapy. In fact, opposing effects of anti-CD4 and anti-CD8 antibodies have been demonstrated. It has been

Table 12B.2. Antibodies to CD4

Disease	SLE			Diabetes			EAE		
	MRL	B/W F₁	BXSB	NOD	BB rat	STZ-induced	Mouse	Lewis rat	Primates
Effect on disease									
Antibody	→↗ GK1.5	→ GK1.5	→ GK1.5	→ GK1.5/ YTS191.1 YTS177	→ W3/25	↓→ YTS191.1/ GK1.5	→ GK1.5	→ W3/25	→ OKT4+ OKT4a
Isoform	γ2b	Rat γ2b Whole ab and (F(ab)2)	γ2b	γ2b γ2b γ2a	γ1	γ2b γ2b	γ1, γ2a γ2b, γ3 Rat-mouse chimeric antibodies	γ1, γ2a, γ2b Switch variants	γ2b γ1
Reference	Santoro et al. (1988) Jabs et al. (1992)	Ermak et al. (1989) Wofsy et al. (1988) Carteron et al. (1989) Wofsy & Seaman (1985) Connolly et al. (1992)	Wofsy (1986)	Wang et al. (1991) Matsuo et al. (1990) Mandel & Koulmanda (1990) Koike et al. (1987) Shizuru et al. (1988) Charlton & Mandel (1988)	Markmann et al. (1989)	Kantwerk et al. (1987) Dayer-Métroz et al. (1988)	Sriram & Roberts (1986) Alters et al. (1990) Sriram et al. (1988)	Waldor et al. (1987)	van Lambalgen & Jonker (1987)
Side-effects	+ antibody associated deaths	–	–	–	–	–	–	–	–

→, no effect; ↓, substantially reduced disease incidence/severity; ↘, partially reduced disease incidence/severity; ↑, disease aggravation; EAE, experimental allergic encephalomyelitis; EAT, experimental autoimmune thyroiditis; EAN, experimental allergic neuritis; EAMG, experimental autoimmune myasthenia gravis

Disease	EAT	EAN	EAMG	Arthritis	Arthritis Streptococcal cell wall induced (rat)	Pristane induced	Autoimmune nephritis BN rat	HgCl₂ induced vasculitis (BN rat)
Effect on disease Antibody	↓ YTS191.1 YTS177	↓ W3/25	↓ GK1.5	↓ GK1.5	↓ W3/25	↓ L3T4	↓ W3/25	↓ W3/25
Isoform	γ2b γ2a	γ1	γ2b	γ2b	γ1	?	γ1	γ1
Reference	Stull et al. (1988) Kong et al. (1989) Flynn et al. (1989) Hutchings et al. (1993)	Strigård et al. (1988)	Christadoss & Dauphinee (1986)	Ranges et al. (1985)	Van den Broek et al. (1992)	Levitt et al. (1992)	Reynolds & Pusey (1994)	Mathieson et al. (1993)
Side-effects	–	–	–	–	–	–	–	–

Table 12B.3. *Antibodies to CD8*

Disease	Mouse diabetes				Rat diabetes
	Streptozotocin	Adult transfer	Cyclophos-phamide	Islet grafts	Spontaneous
Effect on disease	→ ↓	↓ ↓	↓	→ →	↓
Antibody	H35-17.2 YTS 169.4	YTS 169.4	53–6.7	3.155/ 116–13.1	Ox 8
Isoform	γ γ2b	γ2b	γ2a	μ γ2a	γ_1
Reference	Dayer-Métroz *et al.* (1988) Kantwerk *et al.* (1987)	Hutchings *et al.* (1991)	Charlton *et al.* (1988)	Matsuo *et al* (1990) Wang *et al.* (1991)	Like *et al.* (1986)

⟶, no effect; ↓, substantially reduced disease incidence/severity; ↑, disease aggravation; ↓ , partially reduced disease incidence/severity; EAT, experimental autoimmune thyroiditis; EAE, experimental allergic encephalomyelitis; EAN, experimental allergic neuritis; SLE, systemic lupus erythematosus

Table 12B.4. *Antibodies to T cell receptor*

	Antibody specificity: Anti $\alpha\beta$ T cell receptor				
Disease:	Diabetes			Arthritis	
Form:	Spontaneous	Cyclo-phosphamide	Adult transfer	Collagen	OVA-CFA induced (rat)
Effect on disease	↓	↓	↓	↓	↓ ⟶ Chronic Acute
Antibody	H57-597	H57-597	H57-597	R73	R73
Specificity	$\alpha\beta$ Tcr	$\alpha\beta$ Tcr	$\alpha\beta$ Tcr	$\alpha\beta$ Tcr	
Isoform	Hamster γ	Hamster γ	Hamster γ	Rat γ_1	γ_1
References	Sempé *et al.* (1991)	Sempé *et al.* (1991)	Sempé *et al.* (1991)	Goldschmidt & Holmdahl (1991)	Yoshino & Yoshino (1992)

⟶, no effect; ↓, substantially reduced disease incidence/severity; ↑, disease aggravation; ↓ , partially reduced disease incidence/severity; EAE, experimental allergic encephalomyelitis

Islet grafts	EAT		EAE	EAN	SLE
	Mouse	Buffalo rat	Macaques	Rat	B/W F_1
↓	↓	↑	⟶	↓ ⟶	⟶
Ox 8	YTS 169.4	YTS169.4 YTS156.7 (synergistic pair)	Leu 2a +	Ox8	53–6.7
γ_1	γ_{2b}	γ_{2b}	γ_1	γ_1	γ_{2a}
Markmann et al. (1989)	Kong et al. (1989) Flynn et al. (1989)	Cohen et al. (1990)	Rose et al. (1987)	Strigård et al. (1988)	Wofsy (1988)

	Anti-Vβ				Anti-clonotype	
	Diabetes		EAE (mouse)		EAE	EAT
Adjuvant	Cyclo-phosphamide	Adult transfer	PLJ/SJL	BIO.PL	Lewis rat	Mouse
↓	↓	⟶	↓	↓	↓	↓
R73	F23.1	F23.1	F23.1 MR 12	F23.2 +	10.18	AG7
$\alpha\beta$ Tcr	Vβ 8_{1-3}	Vβ 8_{1-3}	Vβ 8_{1-3}	Vβ 8_2 + Vβ 13	Tcr	
Rat γ_1	Mouse γ_{2a}	Mouse γ_{2a}	Mouse γ_{2a} Mouse γ_1	Mouse γ_1 +		?
Yoshino et al. (1990)	Bacelj et al. (1989)	O'Reilly et al. (1990)	Acha-Orbea et al. (1988)	Zaller et al. (1990)	Owhashi & Heber-Katz (1988)	Texier et al. (1992)

shown, furthermore, that anti-CD4 treatment in humans does not result in tolerance to the therapeutic antibody, possibly as different epitopes are recognized (Pankewicz *et al.*, 1989).

12B.2.4 Anti-CD3 antibody treatment

Most antibody treatments targeted at T cells have concentrated on the CD4 molecule; however, recently anti-CD3 mab have proven efficacious particularly in models of IDDM.

Chatenoud *et al.* (1992, 1994) have shown that a short treatment period with anti-CD3 ε chain (1452C11) prevents cyclophosphamide-induced IDDM in NOD mice. Furthermore, and more dramatically, recent onset full-blown spontaneous IDDM in female NOD mice could be reversed by anti-CD3 treatment in 64–80% of mice (compared with 6% in controls). This remission lasted longer than 4 months.

Remaining with models of diabetes, Vallera *et al.* (1992) prevented low-dose STZ/γ interferon induced autoimmune diabetes in the mouse using an anti-CD3-immunotoxin, in which antibody to the CD3 ε chain was cross-linked to ricin toxin A chain. Protection was complete and long-lived.

12B.2.5 Anti-T cell receptor antibody treatment

Studies of monoclonal anti-T cell receptor (Tcr) antibodies have involved relatively non-specific anti-α/β Tcr therapies which target the monomorphic region of the receptor and also, and more specifically, anti-Vβ antibody treatments which target T cell receptors using particular β chain variable regions (Table 12B.4).

Anti-α/β Tcr antibody has prevented and partially reversed several forms of diabetes and also of arthritis.

Anti-Vβ8 antibody has been shown to protect against cyclophosphamide-induced IDDM in NOD mice but not to prevent transferred diabetes (although in the case of the cyclophosphamide-induced disease animals were only followed for 14 days after the final dose of drug).

Recent evidence seems to demonstrate that no particular Vβ chain shows notable prominence in diabetes. The successful treatment of cyclophosphamide-induced disease by F23.1 (anti-Vβ8.1, 2, 3) may therefore be explained by the fact that a large percentage of T cells in most mouse strains (including the NOD) express Vβ8, so it would not be surprising that in functionally deleting such a large proportion of T cells the disease would be ameliorated.

In contrast to diabetes, EAE has been successfully treated by anti-Vβ reagents in all cases reported here. Anti-Vβ8 and to a lesser extent anti-Vβ13 antibodies were the effective antibodies.

An interesting development of the anti-Vβ therapy approach has been reported in the study of EAE in Lewis rats (Hashim *et al.*, 1990). A synthetic

Table 12B.5. *Antibodies to T cell activation markers*

	Anti-IL-2 receptor							Other activation markers	
Antibody specificity:	Diabetes			SLE	Arthritis	EAE	Autoimmune nephritis	EAE	Arthritis
Disease:	BB rat (spontaneous)	NOD (spontaneous insulitis)	Streptozotocin	B/W F_1	Mouse DBA/1J	Lewis rat	HgCl$_2$-induced (rat)	Lewis rat	Lewis rat (adjuvant)
Effect on disease	↓	↓	↓	↓	↓	↓↑	↓	↓	↓
Antibody	ART18	M7/20	PC61	M7/20	7D4	ART18	NDS61	pta-3	pta-3
Isoform	Mouse γ_1	μ	Rat γ_1	μ	Rat	Mouse γ_1	Mouse ?	Mouse γ_3	Mouse γ_3
Treatment with CsA	+	–	–	–	–	+ –	–	–	–
References	Hahn et al. (1987)	Kelley et al. (1988)	Hatamori et al. (1990)	Kelley et al. (1988)	Banerjee et al. (1988)	Engelhardt et al. (1989)	Dubey et al. (1993)	Schluesener et al. (1986)	Schluesener et al. (1986)

→, no effect; ↓, substantially reduced disease incidence/severity; ↓, partially reduced disease incidence/severity; CsA, cyclosporin A; EAE, experimental allergic encephalomyelitis; NOD, non-obese diabetic; SLE, systemic lupus erythematosus

Table 12B.6. *Antibodies to MHC class II products*

	Disease: Diabetes						EAE
	Form:		NOD Spontaneous	NOD Neonatal transfer	NOD Adult transfer	Streptozotocin	SJL × BALB F_1
	BB rat	BB rat					
Effect on disease	↓	⟶	↓↓	↓	⟶	↓	↓
Antibody	GY15/195	GY15/361	10.2.16	10.2.16	10.2.16	H116-32-RS 13/4/R5	10.3.6
Specificity	I-E	I-A	I-A	I-A	I-A	$I\text{-}A^k$ + $I\text{-}E^k$	$I\text{-}A^s$ β chain
Isoform	γ_{2a}	γ_{2a}	γ_{2a}	γ_{2a}	γ_{2a}	?	γ_{2a}
Side-effects?	+	+	–	–	–	–	–
References	Boitard et al. (1985)	Boitard et al. (1985)	Boitard et al. (1988) Singh et al. (1990)	Boitard et al. (1988)	Boitard et al. (1988)	Kiesel et al. (1989)	Sriram et al. (1987)

⟶, no effect; ↓, substantially reduced disease incidence/severity; ↑, disease aggravation; ↓, partially reduced disease incidence/severity; EAE, experimental allergic encephalomyelitis; EAT, experimental allergic thyroiditis, EAU, experimental allergic uveitis. 1, Monomorphic determinant on RH Class II. 2, Polymorphic determinant on RH LA-DQW.

peptide of the Vβ8 Tcr was prepared (TCR-Vβ8-39-59) as encephalitogenic cell lines show preferential usage of Vβ8 chains. Immunization with this peptide induced peptide-specific antibodies which were protective against EAE induced by either of two distinct myelin basic protein (MBP) encephalitogenic epitopes.

An encephalitogenic T cell hybridoma (5.10) has been used to generate an anti-clonotypic antibody (10.18). This antibody was shown able to abrogate EAE in MBP-primed Lewis rats. EAT in CBA/J mice was also prevented using a mab specific for a T cell hybridoma (HTC2) specific for thyroglobulin and MHC class I (AG7).

The above therapeutic strategies offer attractive possible means for intervention. The more specific methods represented by the anti-Vβ antibodies, however, have the disadvantage that a particular Vβ must be shown to be used preferentially by T cells mediating or initiating the disease in question. In animal models of EAE this has been shown to be true; in other autoimmune disease models, notably diabetes, no single Vβ chain appears to be represented on T cells involved in the disease process. A further alternative has been to target activation markers on T cells, for the obvious reason that in an ongoing aggressive autoimmune response most active T cells would express such markers.

			SLE		EAT	EAU
SJL × BALB F$_1$	Rhesus monkey	Mouse	B/W F$_1$	BALB/c (neonatal CBA/Ca × BALB.Igh^b cells)	AKR mice	Lewis rat
↓	↓	↓	↓	↓ $\longrightarrow$ Tolerance Lupus	↓	↓ ↓
MKD6	GM1 + FN16 Ge−nox 3.53	B.18.7	H10.3.6	10–2.16 (TIB93)	10.3.6 0 × 17	0 × 6
I-A^d β chain	1 and 2^a See footnote	I-A^s + MBP Complex	I-A^z	Ia^k	I-A^k I-E	I-A
γ2a	γ2a + γ1 γ1 + γ2a	Mouse μ	γ2a	Mouse γ2b	γ2a	Mouse γ1 Mouse γ1
−	−	−	−	−	−	
Sriram *et al.* (1987)	Jonker *et al.* (1988)	Aharoni *et al.* (1991)	Adelman *et al.* (1983)	Kramar *et al.* (1993)	Vladutin & Steinman (1987)	Rao *et al.* (1989)

12B.2.6 Anti-T cell activation markers

Some success has been achieved in a variety of autoimmune models with antibodies directed towards the interleukin 2 (IL-2) receptor (IL-2R) and other activation markers (Table 12B.5).

Schluesener *et al.* (1986) describe a mab (pta-3) which recognizes a T cell activation marker and that was able to reduce the inflammatory response in both EAE and adjuvant-induced arthritis in the mouse and rat, respectively.

Most work in this area has been performed using anti-IL-2R antibodies. In most cases reduction in disease severity has been achieved although the effects have often been partial and transient. In some examples combined treatment with subtherapeutic doses of cyclosporin A (CsA) has proven more successful. This may point to a role for such antibodies not so much as single therapeutic agents but as a means of reducing doses of highly toxic immunosuppressive drugs; or the possibility that artificial constructs of antibody and toxins (immunotoxins) could be employed (Strom *et al.*, 1990).

The other major area where mab intervention has been investigated is in preventing the association of T cells with autoantigen presented in association with MHC products by treating with antibodies directed towards antigen-presenting cells. The main antibodies used in this category recognize MHC class II products.

12B.3 Monoclonal antibody therapies targeted at antigen-presenting cells

12B.3.1 Antibodies recognizing MHC class II products

Various models of diabetes, EAE, SLE, EAT and experimental allergic uveitis (EAU) have been studied for the effects of anti-MHC class II antibody (Table 12B.6). Treatment with anti-MHC class II antibodies has been successful in many situations although in a minority of cases anaphylactic reactions have occurred. Such treatment was, however, unsuccessful in preventing spleen cells from diabetic NOD mice passively transferring IDDM to naive recipients. It should be noted that although anti-IA failed to prevent the spontaneous occurrence of IDDM in BB rats, anti-IE antibodies were successful.

Antibodies recognizing the complex of MBP and IA^s have been shown to inhibit EAE in H-2^s mice, demonstrating a more specific refinement in this area.

BALB/c mice injected neonatally with (CBA/Ca × BALB.Igh^b) cells are tolerized to the allogeneic class I. They also show a transient lupus-like autoimmune syndrome. Antibody to I-A^k was able to prevent the lupus while leaving the tolerance unaffected (Kramar et al., 1993).

Table 12B.7. *Antibodies to macrophage markers*

Disease:	Diabetes	Autoimmune nephritis	EAU	EAE
Form:	NOD Adult transfer	Rat	C3H/HeN mice	Lewis rat
Effect on disease	↓	↓	↓	↓
Antibody	5C6	Ox42	Mac1 / LFA-1	ED7/ED8 Ox 42
Isoform	Rat γ_{2b}	Mouse γ_{2a}	Rat γ	Mouse γ_1/γ_1 Mouse γ_{2a}
Specificity	CR3b	CR3	CR3 / CD18	CR3
Reference	Hutchings et al. (1990)	Wu et al. (1993)	Whitcup et al. (1993)	Huitinga et al. (1993)

⟶, no effect; ↓, substantially reduced disease incidence/severity; ↑, disease aggravation; ↓, partially reduced disease incidence/severity.

12B.3.2 Antibody to macrophage surface molecules

Hutchings *et al.* (1990) reported the successful prevention of transferred diabetes in NOD mice using continual treatment with 5C6, a mab to the CR3 receptor on mouse macrophages and neutrophils. This antibody prevents homing of macrophages to inflammatory sites but does not stop antigen presentation or cytokine production. Thus, once macrophages had already infiltrated the pancreas the antibody proved ineffective. This work, in addition to demonstrating a therapeutic possibility, confirmed that the macrophage plays an important role in this model of diabetes (Table 12B.7).

More recently models of EAU, EAE and autoimmune nephritis have all been shown to be ameliorated by treatment with anti-CR3 antibodies. EAE could be prevented by ED7 and ED8 antibodies if given early in the effector phase. Interestingly, Ox42, which also recognizes CR3, had no effect, possibly demonstrating the importance of the isotype in function (i.e. γ_1 versus γ_{2a}). In autoimmune nephritis Ox42 given 16 h prior to disease induction could reduce proteinuria and neutrophil numbers, but not macrophage numbers, in the glomerulus.

12B.4 Monoclonal antibody therapies targeting cytokines

Recent studies using mab directed at cytokines have been particularly success-ful (Table 12B.8). In the case of anti-TNF, success in animal models of arthritis has translated into successful treatment of human disease (Elliott *et al.*, 1993). Antibodies to γ-interferon have successfully ameliorated models of EAT and cyclophosphamide-induced IDDM in NOD mice. The effects on models of SLE are variable. B/W mice treated from age 4 to 7 months with anti-γ interferon, showed improved survival at 11 months; however, MRL-Mp lpr/lpr mice treated from 12 to 20 weeks with DB1 showed no difference in the incidence and severity of lupus nephritis. This may reflect the importance of precise timing in beginning therapy and differences between the two strains of mice in the rate of disease progression.

In collagen-induced arthritis, anti-TNF was effective at ameliorating disease manifestations whether given before or after disease onset. When combined with anti-CD4 therapy a synergistic effect was demonstrated which may in part be due to the prevention of an anti-hamster Ig response curtailing anti-TNF efficacy.

In a model of rat EAU, mab to S-antigen (in S antigen-induced uveitis) prevented disease. The epitope recognized by the antibody displayed homology with a sequence of human TNFα, suggesting the possibility of a role for TNF in the disease process.

BALB/c mice given neonatal (C57Bl/6 × BALB/c)F_1 cells develop tolerance to H-2^b alloantigens but also develop an autoimmune lupus-like disease.

Relatively low levels of anti-IL-4 antibody can prevent the lupus-like syn-

Table 12B.8. *Antibodies to cytokines*

Disease	SLE			EAU	Arthritis		EAT	Diabetes
Form	MRL-Mp-lpr/lpr	(B/W) F1	BALB/c (neonatal BALB × B6 cells)	S-antigen induced (rat)	Collagen induced (mouse)	Collagen induced (mouse)		NOD cyclophosphamide induced
Effect on disease	↓	↓	↓	↓	↓	↓	↓	↓
Antibody	DB1	DB1	11B11	S2D2	TN3-19.12	TN3-19.12 YTS 3.1/ YTS 191.1	AN18	RA642
Isoform	Mouse γ_1	Mouse γ_1	Rat γ_1	–	Hamster γ_1	Hamster γ_1 Rat γ_{2b} Rat γ_{2b}	Rat γ_{2a}	Rat
Specificity	γIfn	γIfn	IL-4	S-antigen (hTNFα)	TNFα/β	TNFα/β CD4/CD4	γIfn	γIfn
Comments	–	–	–	–	Effective if given before or after onset	Synergistic effect of combined therapy	–	–
References	Nicoletti et al. (1992)	Jacob et al. (1987)	Schuurmans et al. (1990)	de Kozak et al. (1992)	Williams et al. (1992)	Williams et al. (1994)	Tang et al. (1993)	Campbell et al. (1991)

⟶, no effect; ↓, substantially reduced disease incidence/severity; ↑, disease aggravation; ↓, partially reduced disease incidence/severity.

Table 12B.9. *Antibodies to adhesion molecules*

Disease	Diabetes		EAE		Autoimmune nephritis	EAU
Form	Adult transfer	Streptozotocin (insulitis)	Lewis rat	SJL/J mouse	CBA/Ca kdkd congenic mice	B10.A mice
Effect on disease	↓	↓	↓	↓	↓	↓
Antibody	R1-2 PS/2	?	1A29 whole and $F(ab)_2$	?	MALA-2	?
Isoform	Rat γ_{2b}	Rat γ_{2b} Rat γ_{2a}	—	?	?	Rat γ
Specificity	VLA-4	ICAM-1 LFA-1	ICAM-1	LFA-1	ICAM-1	ICAM-1 LFA-1
Side effects	—	—	—	Anti-LFA-1 caused adverse effects in one group of mice	—	—
Reference	Burkly et al. (1994)	Hayashi et al. (1994)	Archelos et al. (1993)	Cannella et al. (1993)	Harning et al. (1992)	Whitcup et al. (1993)

→, no effect; ↓, substantially reduced disease incidence/severity; ↑, disease aggravation; ↓, partially reduced disease incidence/severity.

drome without interfering with tolerance induction. Whether such treatments have any relevance to the other lupus models or indeed to human SLE remains to be seen.

12B.5 Monoclonal antibody therapies targeting adhesion molecules

Adhesion molecules may represent potential targets for the prevention of leucocyte adhesion or trafficking into sites of autoimmune destruction (Table 12B.9).

Mab to ICAM-1 and LFA-1 have been shown to be effective in models of diabetic insulitis, EAE in the Lewis rat, EAU and autoimmune glomerulonephritis. EAE induced in SJL mice was unaffected by treatment with mab to either ICAM-1 or LFA-1. Diabetes induced by transfer of diabetic spleen cells into irradiated adult NOD recipients was prevented by anti-VLA-4 therapy. Insulitis was completely inhibited during treatment but progressed once treatment was suspended.

These results serve to demonstrate a key role for adhesion molecules in the cellular interactions characterizing a range of autoimmune diseases.

Table 12B.10. *Antibodies to miscellaneous cell markers*

Disease	SLE			Diabetes	EAE
Form	MRL/lpr lymphadenopathy	MRL/lpr lymphadenopathy	BXSB	Spontaneous and transferred (BB/Wor rat)	Lewis rat
Effect of disease	↓	↓	↓	↓	↓
Antibody	RA3.6B2	MEL 14	104.2	Ox34; Ox53; Ox54; Ox55	Ox19
Isoform	μ	γ2a	γ2a	γ2a; γ1 / γ1; γ1	γ1
Specificity	B220	Gp90. Mel 14	Ly5.2	CD2	CD5
Reference	Mountz *et al.* (1988)	Mountz *et al.* (1988)	Yakura *et al.* (1989)	Barlow & Like (1992)	Sun *et al.* (1992)

⟶, no effect; ↓, substantially reduced disease incidence/severity; ↑, disease aggravation; ↓, partially reduced disease incidence/severity.

12B.6 Monoclonal antibodies directed towards miscellaneous cell markers

Most of the therapeutic strategies employed in animal models so far using mab have been covered above. There are, however, several other reports of mab therapies that do not readily fit into the two main areas addressed above (Table 12B.10).

The anti-homing receptor antibody Mel14 and 6B2 (anti-B220) have been shown to reduce certain disease manifestations in MRL mice.

Reduced mortality due to SLE has been achieved in the BXSB mouse using an anti-Ly5 antibody (Ly5 is distributed on all haematopoietic cells).

The mechanism of action of this antibody is unknown but it may be that autoreactive B cells show increased expression of this marker and so are more sensitive to the antibody. CD5 mab were shown to be capable of preventing both induced and adoptively transferred EAE in Lewis rats.

Both spontaneous and transferred diabetes in the BB/Wor rat have been reduced by a range of different mab recognizing the CD2 molecule. CD2 is an antigen/signalling molecule present on thymocytes, mature T cells and NK cells. In most cases CD4$^+$T cells were depleted by the treatments which may be the means by which anti-CD2 treatment operates or by interfering with the CD2/ligand interaction between effector and target cells such that tolerance develops.

Mab therapy, therefore, has been investigated from a diversity of different standpoints and the literature demonstrates the potential such therapies could represent either alone or in combination. Moreover, understanding the underlying mechanisms involved in the major autoimmune diseases, or at least the animal models of these diseases, has been broadened by such studies.

In terms of extending such antibody treatment to human disease several problems remain, not least the relative non-specificity of for example anti-CD4 and anti-MHC treatments, and the side-effects observed with some therapies (e.g. anaphylaxis). There is also the question of tolerance induction to the therapeutic antibody which has been a fortuitous feature of rodent models of autoimmune disease but so far has not been demonstrated in humans treated with such antibodies.

On the face of it, it would seem to be preferable to have more specific strategies such as antibodies targeting the T cell receptor or antibodies to the IA/autoantigen complex. These are attractive possibilities but the autoantigen in autoimmune diseases is not always known. Even if it were, particular T cell receptors would have to be identified which were involved in the disease process in all or most cases presenting with the disease in question; this may not prove to be true in human disease.

There are formidable problems still to be overcome before many of the above methods can be applied to the human situation; the innovative approaches adopted so far make this field a fast developing and fascinating area in which to be involved.

12B.7   References

Acha-Orbea, H., Mitchell, D. J., Timmermann, L., Wraith, D. C., Tausch,
    G. S., Waldor, M. K., Zamvil, S. S., McDevitt, H. O. & Steinman, L. (1988).
    Limited heterogeneity of T cell receptors from lymphocytes mediating autoimmune
    encephalomyelitis allows specific immune intervention. *Cell*, **54**, 263–273.
Adelman, N. E., Watling, D. L. & McDevitt, H. O. (1983). Treatment of
    (NZB × NZW)F$_1$ disease with anti-IA monoclonal antibodies. *Journal of
    Experimental Medicine*, **158**, 1350–1355.
Aharoni, N. E., Teitelbaum, D., Arnon, R. & Puri, J. (1991). Immunomodulation of
    experimental allergic encephalomyelitis by antibodies to the antigen-IA complex.
    Nature, **351**, 147–150.
Alters, S. E., Sakai, K., Steinman, L. & Oi, V. T. (1990). Mechanisms of
    anti-CD4-mediated depletion and immunotherapy. A study using a set of chimeric
    anti-CD4 antibodies. *Journal of Immunology*, **144**, 4587–4592.
Archelos, J. J., Jung, S., Maurer, M., Schmied, M., Lassmann, H., Tamatani, T.,
    Miyasaka, M., Toyka, K. V. & Hartung, H. P. (1993). Inhibition of autoimmune
    encephalomyelitis by an antibody to the intercellular adhesion molecule ICAM-1.
    Annals of Neurology, **34**, 145–154.
Bacelj, A., Charlton, B. & Mandel, T. E. (1989). Prevention of cyclophosphamide
    induced diabetes by anti-Vβ8 T lymphocyte receptor monoclonal antibody therapy
    in NOD/Wehi mice. *Diabetes*, **38**, 1492–1495.
Banerjee, S., Wei, B.-Y., Hillman, K., Luthra, H. S. & David, C. S. (1988).
    Immunosuppression of collagen-induced arthritis in mice with an anti-IL2 receptor
    antibody. *Journal of Immunology*, **141**, 1150–1154.
Barlow, A. K. & Like, A. A. (1992). Anti-CD2 monoclonal antibodies prevent
    spontaneous and adoptive transfer of diabetes in the BB/Wor rat. *American
    Journal of Pathology*, **141**, 1043–1051.
Boitard, C., Bendelac, A., Richard, M. F., Carnaud, C. & Bach, J.-F. (1988).
    Prevention of diabetes in nonobese diabetic mice by anti-IA monoclonal antibodies:
    Transfer of protection by splenic T cells. *Proceedings of the National Academy of
    Sciences of the U.S.A.*, **85**, 9719–9723.
Boitard, C., Minchie, S., Serrurier, P., Butcher, G. W., Larkins, A. P. & McDevitt, H.
    O. (1985). *In-vivo* prevention of thyroid and pancreatic autoimmunity in the BB rat
    by antibody to class II MHC gene products. *Proceedings of the National Academy
    of Sciences of the U.S.A.*, **82**, 6627–1631.
Burkly, L. C., Jakubowski, A. & Hattori, M. (1994). Protection against adoptive
    transfer of autoimmune diabetes mediated through very late antigen-4 integrin.
    Diabetes, **43**, 529–533.
Campbell, I. L., Kay, T. W. H., Oxbrow, L. & Harrison, L. C. (1991). Essential role
    for γ-interferon and interleukin-6 in autoimmune insulin-dependent diabetes in
    NOD/Wehi mice. *Journal of Clinical Investigation*, **87**, 739–742.
Cannela, B., Cross, A. H. & Raine, C. S. (1993). Anti-adhesion molecule therapy in
    experimental autoimmune encephalomyelitis. *Journal of Neuroimmunology*, **46**,
    43–55.
Carteron, N. L., Schimenti, C. L. & Wofsy, D. (1989). Treatment of murine lupus with
    F(ab')$_2$ fragments of monoclonal antibody to L3T4. Suppression of autoimmunity
    does not depend on T helper cell depletion. *Journal of Immunology*, **142**,
    1470–1475.
Charlton, B., Bacelj, A. & Mandel, T. E. (1988). Administration of silica particles or
    anti-Lyt2 antibody prevents β cell destruction in NOD mice given
    cyclophosphamide. *Diabetes*, **37**, 930–935.

Charlton, B. & Mandel, T. E. (1988). Progression from insulitis to β cell destruction in NOD mice requires L3T4$^+$ T lymphocytes. *Diabetes*, **37**, 1108–1112.

Chatenoud, L., Thervet, E., Primo, J. & Bach, J.-F. (1992). Remission de la maladie etablie chez la souris NOD diabetique par l'anticorps monoclonal anti-CD3. *Complete Rende Academie Sciences III*, **315**, 225–228 (English abstract).

Chatenoud, L., Thervet, E., Primo, J. & Bach, J.-F. (1994). Anti-CD3 antibody induces long-term remission of overt autoimmunity in nonobese diabetic mice. *Proceedings of the National Academy of Sciences of the U.S.A.*, **91**, 123–127.

Christadoss, P. & Dauphinee, M. J. (1986). Immunotherapy for myasthenia gravis: a murine model. *Journal of Immunology*, **136**, 2437–2440.

Cohen, S. B., Diamantstein, T. & Weetman, A. P. (1990). The effect of T cell subset depletion on autoimmune thyroiditis in the Buffalo strain rat. *Immunology Letters*, **23**, 263–268.

Connolly, K., Roubinian, J. R. & Wofsy, D. (1992). Development of murine lupus in CD4-depleted NZB/NZW mice. Sustained inhibition of residual CD4$^+$ T cells is required to suppress autoimmunity. *Journal of Immunology*, **149**, 3083–3088.

Dayer-Métroz, M.-D., Kimoto, M., Izui, S., Vassalli, P. & Renold, A. E. (1988). Effect of helper and/or cytotoxic T lymphocyte depletion on low-dose streptozotocin-induced diabetes in C57BL/6J mice. *Diabetes*, **37**, 1082–1089.

Dubey, D., Kuhn, J., Vial, M. C., Druet, P. & Bellon, B. (1993). Anti-interleukin-2 receptor monoclonal antibody therapy supports a role for Th-1-like cells in HgCl$_2$-induced autoimmunity in rats. *Scandinavian Journal of Immunology*, **37**, 406–412.

Elliott, M. J., Maini, R. N., Feldmann, M. *et al*. (1993). Treatment of rheumatoid arthritis with chimeric monoclonal antibodies to tumor necrosis factor-α. *Arthritis and Rheumatism*, **36**, 1681–1690.

Engelhardt, B., Diamantstein, T. & Wekerle, H. (1989). Immunotherapy of experimental autoimmune encephalomyelitis (EAE): differential effect of anti-IL2 receptor antibody therapy on actively induced and T cell line mediated EAE of the Lewis rat. *Journal of Autoimmunity*, **2**, 61–73.

Ermak, T. H., Steger, H. J. & Wofsy, D. (1989). Treatment of murine lupus with monoclonal antibody to L3T4. II. Effects on immunohistopathology of thymus, spleen and lymph node. *Laboratory Investigation*, **61**, 447–456.

Flynn, J. C., Conaway, D. H., Cobbold, S., Waldmann, H. & Kong, Y. M. (1989). Depletion of L3T4+ and Lyt2+ T cells by rat monoclonal antibodies alters the development of adoptively transferred experimental autoimmune thyroiditis. *Cellular Immunology*, **122**, 377–390.

Goldschmidt, T. J. & Holmdahl, R. (1991). Anti-T cell receptor antibody treatment of rats with established autologous collagen-induced arthritis: suppression of arthritis without reduction of anti-type II collagen autoantibody levels. *European Journal of Immunology*, **21**, 1327–1330.

Hahn, H. J., Lucke, S., Klöting, I., Volk, H. D., Baehr, R. V. & Diamantstein, T. (1987). Curing BB rats of freshly manifested diabetes by short-term treatment with a combination of a monoclonal anti-interleukin 2 receptor antibody and a subtherapeutic dose of cyclosporin A. *European Journal of Immunology*, **17**, 1075–1078.

Harada, M. & Makino, S. (1986). Immunological modulation of diabetes prodution in NOD mice. *Experimental Animal (Tokyo)*, **35**, 501–504.

Harning, R., Pelletier, J., Van, G., Takei, F. & Merluzzi, V. J. (1992). Monoclonal antibody to MALA-2 (ICAM-1) reduces acute autoimmune nephritis in kdkd mice. *Clinical Immunology and Immunopathology*, **64**, 129–134.

Hashim, G. A., Vandenbark, A. A., Galang, A. B., Diamanduros, T., Carvalho, E.,

Srinivasan, J., Jones, R., Vainiene, M., Morrison, W. J. & Offner, H. (1990). Antibodies specific for Vβ8 receptor peptide suppress experimental autoimmune encephalomyelitis. *Journal of Immunology*, **144**, 4621–4627.

Hatamori, N., Yokono, K., Hayakawa, M., Taki, T., Ogawa, M., Nagata, M., Hari, J., Shii, K., Taniguchi, H. & Baba, S. (1990). Anti-interleukin-2 receptor antibody attenuates low-dose streptozotocin induced diabetes in mice. *Diabetologia*, **33**, 266–271.

Hayashi, T., Hashimoto, S. & Kameyama, Y. (1994). Reduced steptozotocin-induced insulitis in CD-1 mice by treatment with anti-cellular adhesion molecule-1 and anti-lymphocyte function associated antigen-1 monoclonal antibodies together with lactic dehydrogenase virus infection. *International Journal of Experimental Pathology*, **75**, 117–121.

Huitinga, I., Damoiseaux, J. G., Dopp, E. A. & Dijkstra, C. D. (1993). Treatment with anti-CR3 antibodies ED7 and ED8 suppresses experimental allergic encephalomyelitis in Lewis rats. *European Journal of Immunology*, **23**, 709–715.

Hutchings, P., Rosen, H., O'Reilly, L., Simpson, E., Gordon, S. & Cooke, A. (1990). Transfer of diabetes in mice prevented by blockade of adhesion-promoting receptor in macrophages. *Nature*, **348**, 639–642.

Hutchings, P. R., Simpson, E., O'Reilly, L. A., Lund, T., Waldmann, H. & Cooke, A. (1991). The involvement of Lyt2+ cells in β cell destruction. *Journal of Autoimmunity*, **3**, 101–109.

Hutchings, P. R., Cooke, A., Dawe, K., Waldmann, H. & Roitt, I. M. (1993). Active suppression induced by anti-CD4. *European Journal of Immunology*, **23**, 965–968.

Jabs, D. A., Burek, C. L., Hu, Q., Kuppers, R. C., Lee, B. & Prendergast, R. A. (1992). Anti-CD4 monoclonal antibody therapy suppresses autoimmune disease in MRL/Mp-lpr/lpr mice. *Cellular Immunology*, **141**, 496–507.

Jacob, C. O., van der Meide, P. H. & McDevitt, H. O. (1987). *In vivo* treatment of (NZB × NZW)F$_1$ lupus-like nephritis with monoclonal antibodies to γ interferon. *Journal of Experimental Medicine*, **166**, 798–803.

Jonker, M., van Lambalgen, R., Mitchell, D. J., Durham, S. K. & Steinman, L. (1988). Successful treatment of EAE in Rhesus monkeys with MHC class II-specific monoclonal antibodies. *Journal of Autoimmunity*, **1**, 399–414.

Kantwerk, G., Cobbold, S., Waldmann, H. & Kolb, H. (1987). L3T4+ and Lyt2+ T cells are both involved in the generation of low-dose streptozotocin-induced diabetes in mice. *Clinical Experimental Immunology*, **70**, 585–592.

Kelley, V. E., Gaulton, G. N., Hattori, M., Ikegami, H., Eisenbarth, G. & Strom, T. B. (1988). Anti-interleukin 2 receptor antibody suppresses murine diabetic insulitis and lupus nephritis. *Journal of Immunology*, **140**, 59–61.

Kiesel, U., Oschilewski, M., Taniguchi, M. & Kolb, H. (1989). Modulation of low-dose streptozotocin-induced diabetes in mice by administration of antibodies to I-A, I-E and I-J determinants. *Diabetologia*, **32**, 173–176.

Koike, T., Itoh, Y., Ishii, I., Takabayashi, K., Maruyama, N., Tomioka, H. & Yoshida, S. (1987). Preventive effect of monoclonal anti-L3T4 antibody on development of diabetes in NOD mice. *Diabetes*, **36**, 539–541.

Kong, Y. M., Waldmann, H., Cobbold, S., Giraldo, A. A., Fuller, B. E. & Simon, L. L. (1989). Pathogenic mechanisms in murine autoimmune thyroiditis: short- and long-term effects of *in vivo* depletion of CD4+ and CD8+ cells. *Clinical Experimental Immunology*, **77**, 428–433.

DeKozak, Y., Stiemer, R. H., Mirshahi, M., Frank, R. W., de Smet, M. & Faure, J. P. (1992). Humoral response against the S-antigen/TNF alpha common epitope in rat EAU suppressed by the monoclonal antibody S2D2. *Current Eye Research*, **11** (Suppl.), 119–127.

Kramar, G., Schurmans, S., Aguado, T., Izui, S., Del-Guidice, G. & Lambert, P. H. (1993). Anti-Ia treatment prevents lupus-like autoimmune syndrome in mice neonatally tolerised to alloantigens. *Journal of Autoimmunity*, **6**, 27–37.

Levitt, N. G., Fernandez-Madrid, F. & Wooley, P. H. (1992). Pristane induced arthritis in mice. IV. Immunotherapy with monoclonal antibodies directed against lymphocyte subsets. *Journal of Rheumatology*, **19**, 1342–1347.

Like, A. A., Biron, C. A., Weringer, E. J., Byman, K., Sroczynski, E. & Guberski, D. L. (1986). Prevention of diabetes in Biobreeding/Worcester rats with monoclonal antibodies that recognise T lymphocytes or natural killer cells. *Journal of Experimental Medicine*, **164**, 1145–1159.

Mandel, T. E. & Koulmanda, M. (1990). The effect of continuous anti-CD4 monoclonal antibody therapy on fetal pig pancreas xenografts in nonobese diabetic mice. *Transplantation Proceedings*, **22**, 2093–2094.

Markmann, J. F., Jacobson, J. D., Brayman, K. L., Kimura, H., Barker, C. F. & Naji, A. (1989). Prevention of recurrent diabetes in BB rats after islet transplantation by monoclonal antibody therapy. *Diabetes*, **38**, (Suppl. 1), 165–167.

Mathieson, P. W., Qasim, F. J., Esnault, V. L. & Oliveira, D. B. (1993). Animal models of vasculitis. *Journal of Autoimmunity*, **6**, 251–264.

Matsuo, S., Mullen, Y., Wicker, L. S., Peterson, L. B., Nagata, M., Tsunoda, T. & Clare-Salzier, M. (1990). Prolongation of islet isograft survival in diabetic NOD mice by anti-L3T4 and anti-Lyt2 monoclonal antibodies. *Transplantation Proceedings*, **22**, 880–881.

Mountz, J. D., Gause, W. C., Finkelman, F. D. & Steinberg, A. D. (1988). Prevention of lymphadenopathy in MRL-lpr/lpr mice by blocking peripheral lymph node homing with Mel-14 *in vivo*. *Journal of Immunology*, **140**, 2943–2949.

Nicoletti, F., Meroni, P., DiMarco, R., Barcellini, W., Borghi, M. O., Gariglio, M., Mattina, A., Grasso, S. & Landolfo, S. (1992). *In vivo* treatment with a monoclonal antibody to interferon-gamma neither affects the survival nor the incidence of lupus-nephritis in the MRL/lpr-lpr mouse. *Immunopharmacology*, **24**, 11–16.

O'Reilly, L. A., Hutchings, P. R., Parish, N., Simpson, E., Tomonari, K., Lund, T., Crocker, P. & Cooke, A. (1990). Factors affecting diabetes in rodent models of insulin dependent diabetes mellitus. In *The Molecular Biology of Autoimmune Disease*, ed. H. G. Demaine. NATO ASI Series H38 p. 302.

Owhashi, M. & Heber-Katz, E. (1988). Protection from experimental allergic encephalomyelitis conferred by a monoclonal antibody directed against a shared idiotype on rat T cell receptors specific for myelin basic protein. *Journal of Experimental Medicine*, **168**, 2153–2164.

Pankewicz, O., Strom, T. B. & Kelley, V. E. (1989). Therapeutic strategies using monoclonal antibodies in autoimmune disease. *Current Opinion in Immunology*, **1**, 757–763.

Ranges, G. E., Sriram, S. & Cooper, S. M. (1985). Prevention of type II collagen induced arthritis by *in vivo* treatment with anti-L3T4. *Journal of Experimental Medicine*, **162**, 1105–1110.

Rao, N. A., Atalla, L., Linker-Israeli, M., Chen, F. Y., George, F. W., Martin, W. J. & Steinman, L. (1989). Suppression of experimental uveitis in rats by anti-IA antibodies. *Investigative and Ophthalmological and Visual Sciences*, **30**, 2348–2355.

Reynolds, J. & Pusey, C. D. (1994). *In vivo* treatment with a monoclonal antibody to T helper cells in experimental autoimmune glomerulonephritis in the BN rat. *Clinical and Experimental Immunology*, **95**, 122–127.

Rose, L. M., Alvord, E. C., Hruby, S., Jackevicius, S., Petersen, R., Warner, N. & Clark, E. A. (1987). *In vivo* administration of anti-CD4 monoclonal antibody prolongs survival in long-tailed macaques with experimental allergic encephalomyelitis. *Clinical Immunology and Immunopathology*, **45**, 405–423.

Santoro, T. J., Portanova, J. P. & Kotzin, B. L. (1988). The contribution of L3T4+ T cells to lymphoproliferation and autoantibody production in MRL-lpr/lpr mice. *Journal of Experimental Medicine*, **167**, 1713–1718.

Schluesener, H., Brunner, C., Vass, K. & Lassmann, H. (1986). Therapy of rat autoimmune disease by a monoclonal antibody specific for T lymphoblasts. *Journal of Immunology*, **137**, 3814–3820.

Schurmans, S., Heusser, C. H., Qin, H.-Y., Merino, J., Brighouse, G. T. & Lambert, P.-H. (1990). *In vivo* effects of anti-IL4 monoclonal antibody on neonatal induction of tolerance and on an associated autoimmune syndrome. *Journal of Immunology*, **145**, 2465–2473.

Seaman, W. E., Wofsy, D., Greenspan, J. S. & Ledbetter, J. A. (1983). Treatment of autoimmune MRL/lpr mice with monoclonal antibody to Thy1.2: a single injection has sustained effects on lymphoproliferation and renal disease. *Journal of Immunology*, **130**, 1713–1718.

Sempé, P., Bédossa, P., Richard, M.-F., Villà, M.-C., Bach, J.-F. & Boitard, C. (1991). Anti-α/β T cell receptor monoclonal antibody provides an efficient therapy for autoimmune diabetes in nonobese diabetic (NOD) mice. *European Journal of Immunology*, **21**, 1163–1169.

Shizuru, J. A., Taylor-Edwards, C., Banks, B. A., Gregory, A. K. & Fathman, C. G. (1988). Immunotherapy of the nonobese diabetic mouse: treatment with an antibody to T-helper lymphocytes. *Science*, **240**, 659–662.

Singh, B., Dillon, T., Fraga, E. & Lauzon, J. (1990). Role of the first external domain of IA beta chain in immune responses and diabetes in nonobese diabetic (NOD) mice. *Journal of Autoimmunity*, **3**, 507–521.

Sriram, S., Carroll, L., Fortin, S., Cooper, S. & Ranges, G. (1988). *In vivo* immunomodulation by monoclonal anti-CD4 antibody. II. Effect on T cell response to myelin basic protein and experimental allergic encephalomyelitis. *Journal of Immunology*, **141**, 464–468.

Sriram, S. & Roberts, C. A. (1986). Treatment of chronic relapsing experimental allergic encephalomyelitis in SJL/J mice with anti-L3T4 antibodies. *Journal of Immunology*, **136**, 4464–4469.

Sriram, S., Topham, D. J. & Carroll, L. (1987). Haplotype suppression of experimental allergic encephalomyelitis with anti-IA antibodies. *Journal of Immunology*, **139**, 1485–1489.

Strigård, K., Olsson, T., Larsson, P., Holmdahl, R. & Klareskog, L. (1988). Modulation of experimental allergic neuritis in rats by *in vivo* treatment with monoclonal anti-T cell antibodies. *Journal of Neurological Science*, **83**, 283–291.

Strom, T. B., Anderson, P. L., Rubin-Kelley, V. E., Williams, D. P., Kiyokawa, T. & Murphy, J. R. (1990). Immunotoxins and cytokine toxin fusion proteins. *Seminars in Immunology*, **2**, 467–479.

Stull, S. J., Kyriakos, M., Sharp, G. C. & Braley-Mullen, H. (1988). Prevention and reversal of experimental autoimmune thyroiditis (EAT) in mice by administration of anti-L3T4 monoclonal antibody at different stages of disease development. *Cellular Immunology*, **117**, 188–.

Sun, D., Branum, K. & Sun, Q. (1992). Prevention of experimental autoimmune encephalomyelitis in Lewis rats by treatment with an anti-rat CD5 antibody (OX19). *Cellular Immunology*, **145**, 263–271.

Tang, H., Mignon-Godefroy, K., Meroni, P. L., Garotta, G., Charreire, J. & Nicoletti, F. (1993). The effects of a monoclonal antibody to interferon-gamma on experimental autoimmune thyroiditis (EAT): prevention of disease and decrease of

EAT-specific cells. *European Journal of Immunology*, **23**, 275–278.

Texier, B., Bedin, C., Roubaty, C., Brezin, C. & Charreire, J. (1992). Protection from experimental autoimmune thyroiditis conferred by a monoclonal antibody to T cell receptor from a cytotoxic hybridoma specific for thyroglobulin. *Journal of Immunology*, **148**, 439–444.

Vallera, D. A., Carroll, S. F., Brief, S. & Blazar, B. R. (1992). Anti-CD3 immunotoxin prevents low-dose STZ/interferon-induced autoimmune diabetes in mouse. *Diabetes*, **41**, 457–464.

Van Lambalgen, R. & Jonker, M. (1987). Experimental allergic encephalomyelitis in rhesus monkeys: II. Treatment of EAE with anti-T lymphocyte subset monoclonal antibodies. *Clinical Experimental Immunology*, **68**, 305–312.

Vladutiu, A. O. & Steinman, L. (1987). Inhibition of experimental autoimmune thyroiditis in mice by anti-IA antibodies. *Cellular Immunology*, **109**, 169–180.

Waldor, M. K., Mitchell, D., Kipps, T. J., Herzenberg, L. A. & Steinman, L. (1987). Importance of immunoglobulin isotype in therapy of experimental autoimmune encephalomyelitis with monoclonal anti-CD4 antibody. *Journal of Immunology*, **139**, 3660–3664.

Wang, Y., Pontesilli, O., Gill, R. G., LaRosa, F. G. & Lafferty, K. J. (1991). The role of CD4+ and CD8+ T cells in the destruction of islet grafts by spontaneously diabetic mice. *Proceedings of the National Academy of Sciences of the U.S.A.*, **88**, 527–531.

Whitcup, S. M., DeBarge, L. R., Caspi, R. R., Harning, R., Nussenblatt, R. B. & Chan, C. C. (1993). Monoclonal antibodies against ICAM-1 (CD54) and LFA-1 (CD11a/CD18) inhibit experimental autoimmune uveitis. *Clinical Immunology and Immunopathology*, **67**, 143–150.

Whitcup, S. M., DeBarge, L. R., Rosen, H., Nussenblatt, R. B. & Chan, C. C. (1993). Monoclonal antibody against CD11b/CD18 inhibits endotoxin-induced uveitis. *Investigations in Ophthalmology and Visual Science*, **34**, 673–681.

Williams, R. O., Feldmann, M. & Maini, R. N. (1992). Anti-tumor necrosis factor ameliorates joint disease in murine collagen-induced arthritis. *Proceedings of the National Academy of Sciences of the U.S.A.*, **89**, 9784–9788.

Williams, R. O., Mason, L. J., Feldmann, M. & Maini, R. N. (1994). Synergy between anti-CD4 and anti-TNF in the amelioration of established collagen-induced arthritis. *Proceedings of the National Academy of Sciences of the U.S.A.*, **91**, 2762–2766.

Wofsy, D. (1986). Administration of monoclonal anti-T cell antibodies retards murine lupus in BXSB mice. *Journal of Immunology*, **136**, 4554–4560.

Wofsy, D. (1988). The role of Lyt2+ T cells in the regulation of autoimmunity in murine lupus. *Journal of Autoimmunity*, **1**, 207–217.

Wofsy, D., Chiang, N. Y., Greenspan, J. S. & Ermak, T. H. (1988). Treatment of murine lupus with monoclonal antibody to L3T4.I. Effects on the distribution and function of lymphocyte subsets and on the histopathology of autoimmune disease. *Journal of Autoimmunity*, **1**, 415–431.

Wofsy, D., Ledbetter, J. A., Hendler, P. L. & Seaman, W. E. (1985). Treatment of murine lupus with monoclonal anti-T cell antibody. *Journal of Immunology*, **134**, 852–857.

Wofsy, D. & Seaman, W. E. (1985). Successful treatment of autoimmunity in NZB/NZW F_1 mice with monoclonal antibody to L3T4. *Journal of Experimental Medicine*, **161**, 378–391.

Wu, X., Pippin, J. & Lefkowith, J. B. (1993). Attenuation of immune-mediated glomerulonephritis with an anti-CD11b monoclonal antibody. *American Journal of Physiology*, **264**, F715–F721.

Yakura, H., Ashida, I., Kawabata, I. & Katagiri, M. (1989). Alleviation of
  autoimmunity in BXSB mice by monoclonal antibody to Ly5 (CD45). *European
  Journal of Immunology*, **19**, 1505–1508.
Yoshino, S., Schlipköter, E., Kinne, R., Hünig, T. & Emmrich, F. (1990). Suppression
  and prevention of adjuvant arthritis in rats by a monoclonal antibody to the α/β T
  cell receptor. *European Journal of Immunology*, **20**, 2805–2808.
Yoshino, S. & Yoshino, J. (1992). Suppression of chronic antigen-induced arthritis in
  rats by a monoclonal antibody against the T cell receptor $\alpha\beta$. *Cellular Immunology*,
  144, 382–391.
Zaller, D. M., Osman, G., Kanagawa, O. & Hood, L. (1990). Prevention and treatment
  of murine experimental allergic encephalomyelitis with T cell receptor Vβ-specific
  antibodies. *Journal of Experimental Medicine*, **171**, 1943–1955.

12C

Monoclonal antibodies in transplantation: prophylaxis and treatment of graft-versus-host disease after bone marrow transplantation

L. BOSTRÖM and O. RINGDEN

12C.1 Introduction

12C.1.1 Indications for bone marrow transplantation (BMT)

By 1993, more than 40 000 allogeneic transplants had been carried out. The most common diagnoses for BMT are acute myeloid leukaemia (AML), acute lymphoblastic leukaemia (ALL), chronic myeloid leukaemia (CML), severe aplastic anaemia (SAA), advanced Hodgkin's disease, lymphomas and myeloma. Severe combined immunodeficiency (SCID), thalassemia major and various metabolic disorders are also successfully treated.

12C.1.2 Results after bone marrow transplantation

For AML and ALL in first complete remission, most BMT teams and registers report a 5-year leukaemia-free survival of 35–60% in patients, including children and adults (Blume *et al.*, 1980; Champlin, 1987; Ringden *et al.*, 1987*a*; Gale *et al.*, 1989; Sullivan *et al.*, 1989). Patients with acute leukaemia beyond first complete remission have a 5-year leukaemia-free survival of about 25–30%. In patients with CML in first chronic phase long-term survival varies between 49 and 70% compared with between 14 and 29% in patients in second chronic phase, accelerated phase or blast crisis (Zwaan *et al.*, 1985; Ringden *et al.*, 1987*a*; Thomas, 1987; Grathwohl *et al.*, 1988; Sullivan *et al.*, 1989). From different studies it is reported that long-term survival in patients with SAA varies between 52 and 82% when the donor is HLA-identical and between 15 and 50% for non-HLA-identical donors (Bacigalupo *et al.*, 1988; Sullivan *et al.*, 1989; Locasciulli *et al.*, 1990).

12C.1.3 Acute graft-versus-host disease

Following bone marrow transplantation between HLA-identical siblings 10–60% of the patients develop clinically significant acute graft-versus-host disease (GVHD) (Prentice *et al.*, 1984; Santos *et al.*, 1985; Storb & Deeg, 1986). The incidence depends in part on the method of prophylaxis against GVHD (Storb & Deeb, 1986; Prentice *et al.*, 1984). Donor T lymphocytes reacting against host histocompatibility antigens are thought to be responsible for GVHD (Grebe & Streilein, 1976).

The classically recognized target organs of acute GVHD in humans are skin, gastrointestinal tract and liver. The disorder may appear from 1 week up to 2 months after BMT. Acute GVHD is graded on a scale from 0–IV (Glucksberg *et al.*, 1974; Thomas *et al.*, 1975). Severe immunological deficiency accompanies acute GVHD (Paulin *et al.*, 1987; Gale *et al.*, 1978; Noel *et al.*, 1978) and the treatment of acute GVHD by anti-thymocyte globulin and steroids may induce further immunosuppression (Witherspoon *et al.*, 1981).

12C.1.4 Chronic graft-versus-host disease

Among long-term survivors following BMT one major complication is chronic GVHD with an incidence of 25–50% (Sullivan *et al.*, 1981; Storb *et al.*, 1983; Ringden *et al.*, 1985). Acute GVHD often precedes chronic GVHD (Ringdén *et al.*, 1985). The major clinical manifestations are skin disease, keratoconjuctivitis, generalized sicca syndrome, oral mucositis and liver disease. In more advanced disease, oesophageal and vaginal strictures, malabsorption, wasting and pulmonary insufficiency may also appear (Saurat *et al.*, 1975; Hood *et al.*, 1977; Siimes *et al.*, 1977; Sullivan *et al.*, 1981). Chronic GVHD is not only a negative complication, it also may have an antileukaemic effect (Weiden *et al.*, 1981).

12C.1.5 Rejection

Graft failure owing to rejection and other causes remains an important, life-threatening complication following allogeneic BMT in humans. Two immune-mediated aetiologies of graft failures have been proposed from animal experiments. In the first case, prior sensitization to donor antigens occurs; lethally irradiated dogs or mice, previously sensitized to MHC-matched or mismatched allogeneic donors through infusions of whole blood or marrow cells, reject marrow grafts by what is presumed to be a classic immune response (Storb *et al.*, 1970, 1971; Dennert *et al.*, 1985; Storb & Deeg, 1986). In the second proposed mechanism, unsensitized, lethally irradiated recipient mice are able to reject marrow from either H-2 non-identical (allogeneic) or H-2 compatible first generation (F_1) parental strain marrow donors (Cudkowicz & Bennet, 1971*a*, *b*; Bonmassar *et al.*, 1975). It is believed that this form of resistance is mediated by natural killer (NK) cells (Bortin & Saltzstein 1969; Kiessling *et al.*, 1977). In patients transplanted for leukaemia the rejection rate was increased among patients with haploidentical donors (5%) compared with patients with HLA genotypically identical siblings (0.1%) (Beatty *et al.*, 1985).

The rejection rate increases with increased HLA disparity between donor and recipient (Ash *et al.*, 1991).

12C.1.6 *Prevention of graft-versus-host disease*

Methotrexate (MTX) was found to be effective in preventing GVHD in dogs (Storb *et al.*, 1970) and was used in humans by the group from Seattle. When cyclosporin A (CsA) was introduced (Powles *et al.*, 1980) this was not more effective than MTX according to five randomized trials (Ringdén *et al.*, 1986). More recently, CsA has been combined with the first four doses of MTX, a combination shown to decrease the incidence of acute GVHD in HLA-identical and HLA-mismatched recipients and also to improve patient survival (Storb *et al.*, 1986*a*, *b*; Tollemar *et al.*, 1989). The ability to prevent GVHD by removing T cells from donor marrow has been demonstrated in numerous experimental models. In clinical studies there was approximately a 10% incidence of clinically significant acute GVHD among durably engrafted patients transplanted with HLA-identical T cell-depleted marrow even when no post-transplant immunosuppression was administered (Lowenberg *et al.*, 1986; Gale, 1987; Hale *et al.*, 1988). This is in contrast to a GVHD incidence of at least 80% when post-transplant immunosuppression is omitted in patients given unmodified marrow (Sullivan *et al.*, 1986). In patients given MTX or CsA as monotherapy the incidence of acute GVHD in patients with HLA-identical donors varies between 30 and 60% (Ringdén *et al.*, 1986).

12C.1.7 *Treatment of graft-versus-host disease*

Several immunosuppressive agents have been used to treat established acute GVHD, including high doses of prednisolone, methylprednisolone, antithymocyte globulin (ATG), various types of mab against T cells, CsA, psoralen treatment and ultraviolet light (PUVA), interleukin 2 (IL-2) and thalidomide (Weiden *et al.*, 1978; Groth *et al.*, 1979; Prentice *et al.*, 1980; Gratama *et al.*, 1984; Deeg *et al.*, 1985; Hymes *et al.*, 1985; Hervé *et al.*, 1988; Vogelsang *et al.*, 1988; Pico *et al.*, 1989). In a randomized study comparing CsA and ATG with or without additional methylprednisolone, patients with methylprednisolone had a worse outcome (Deeg *et al.*, 1985). In general, treatment of moderate to severe acute GVHD has been unsatisfactory. Chronic GVHD is treated with prednisolone and/or CsA (Sullivan *et al.*, 1988*a*, *b*).

12C.2. Prevention of GVHD with *in-vitro* use of monoclonal antibodies

Monoclonal antibodies (Mab) have great potential in the field of bone marrow transplantation both for *in-vivo* use and for *ex-vivo* use in marrow purging. The use of mab in allogeneic transplantation has primarily been for the removal of T cells from the donor marrow in an effort to overcome GVHD

Table 12C.1. *Monoclonal antibodies used for T cell depletion of donor bone marrow to prevent GVHD*

Author	Anti-human T cell antibodies against	With or without complement
Filipovich *et al.* (1982)	CD3	—
Prentice *et al.* (1982)	CD3	ALS
Hayward *et al.* (1982)	CD3	C′
Reinherz *et al.* (1982)	T12	C′
Martin *et al.* (1983)	CD3, CD11, CD4, CD8	—
Prentice *et al.* (1984)	CD3/CD6 + CD8	C′
Waldman *et al.* (1984)	Campath I	C′
Hervé *et al.* (1985)	CD2 + CD3	C′
Trigg *et al.* (1985)	CT-2	C′
Martin *et al.* (1985)	CD2-CD6, CD8	—
Kohler *et al* (1986)	CT-2	C′
Mitsuyasu *et al.* (1986)	CT-2	C′
Hervé *et al.* (1987)	CD2 + CD3, CD2 + CD5 + CD7	C′
Maraninchi *et al.* (1987)	CD4 + CD5 + CD8, CD2 + CD5 + CD7	C′
Filipovich *et al.* (1987)	CD3 + CD5 + CD11a	IT
Siena *et al.* (1987)	CD5	IT
Vartdal *et al.* (1987*a*)	CD2 + CD3	MB
Maraninchi *et al.* (1988)	CD8	C′
Fauser *et al.* (1988)	CD5	IT
Antin *et al.* (1990)	CD5	IT
Champlin *et al.* (1990)	CD8	C′
Henslee *et al.* (1989)	CD5	RTA
Filipovich *et al.* (1990)	CD5	IT

C′, complement; CD, clusters of differentiation; IT, immunotoxin; RTA, ricin A chain (Hemitoxin); ALS, anti-lymphocyte sera; MB, magnetic beads.

(Table 12C.1). A number of groups has performed evaluations with a variety of anti-human T cell antibodies. In many of the reports a mixture of mab is used. Experimental studies have shown that various mab are additive or synergistic when used in combination (Vallera *et al.*, 1983; Stong *et al.*, 1985). T cell depletion, although effective in GVHD prevention, has been associated with graft failure and an increased incidence of leukaemic relapse (Apperley *et al.*, 1986; Mitsuyasu *et al.*, 1986; Maraninchi *et al.*, 1987; Ringdén *et al.*, 1987*a*; Hale *et al.*, 1988; Martin *et al.*, 1988*b*)).

Both antibody-based and physical methods have been used for depletion of T cells in human donor marrow. Anti-T cell antibodies have been employed alone (Filipovich *et al.*, 1982; Prentice *et al.*, 1982; Martin *et al.*, 1984*a*), together with homologous or heterologous complement (Prentice *et al.*, 1984; Waldmann *et al.*, 1984; Hervé *et al.*, 1985; Martin *et al.*, 1985; Sondel *et al.*,

1985; Mitsuyasu *et al.*, 1986; Reinherz *et al.*, 1982; Trigg *et al.*, 1985), conjugated to immunotoxins (Filipovich *et al.*, 1987; Martin *et al.*, 1988*b*) or combined with immunomagnetic beads (Vartdal *et al.*, 1987*a*, *b*) (Table 12C.1). Most antibody-based methods are capable of a T cell depletion of at least two orders of magnitude.

Different methods of physical separation of lymphocytes from marrow progenitors have been used: discontinuous albumin gradients, cell elutriation, soybean agglutination and sheep erythrocyte rosetting and the combination of mab with physical separation procedures. Mab can also be used to destroy or disable T cells directly.

Methods using mab together with rabbit or human complement (C′) to achieve *in-vitro* cytolysis have also been described. Another method described is immunopharmacological depletion using mab toxin conjugates, such as ricin (Brenner *et al.*, 1986).

12C.2.1 Monoclonal antibodies with or without complement

12C.2.1.1 Experimental models

In an experimental model it was shown that treatment of donor grafts with a standardized mab anti-Thy-1.2 plus C′ protects recipients (mice) in a system that favours the development of lethal GVHD (Vallera *et al.*, 1981). The same group also showed that donor bone marrow treated with the mab anti-Lyt-1.2 plus C′ protected recipients from lethal GVHD but did not have any effect on the stem cell activity (Vallera *et al.*, 1982). Treatment with mab anti-Lyt-2.2 plus C′ did not prevent GVHD.

In a study by Thierfelder *et al.* (1985) 11 mab of rat or mouse origin directed against the mouse pan T antigen Thy-1 were compared for their ability to reduce mortality of GVHD when incubated with donor bone marrow. Two of two rat IgG2b anti-Thy-1 mab suppressed acute GVHD without the need for complement. All mab were complement-fixing, seven with specificity for Thy-1 and two with specificity for Thy-1.2.

Cobbold *et al.* (1986) showed that removal of mature T cells from the marrow by the use of mab can reduce GVHD and rejection of the marrow in mouse models. The mab were specific for L3/T4$^+$ (CD4$^+$) and Lyt-2$^+$ (CD8$^+$) cells.

12C.2.1.2 Campath-I

The most extensive experience worldwide has been with the rat IgM mab Campath-I (Hale *et al.*, 1983), which recognizes a heterogeneous 23–30 kDa glycoprotein expressed on all lymphocytes and monocytes (Cobbold *et al.*, 1987). Campath-I gave very effective cell lysis with human complement: more than 99% of lymphocytes were killed and viable T cells could no longer be detected. In the clinical situation Prentice *et al.* (1984) showed that T cell depletion with Campath-I minimized acute GVHD in 14 matched transplants. Other reports have confirmed that T cell depletion with Campath-I significantly reduces the incidence of acute GVHD but increases the incidence of graft-rejection and leukaemic relapse in HLA-identical transplants (Apperley *et al.*, 1986; Heit *et al.*, 1986). In 282 patients with leukaemia receiving marrow depleted of T cells with Campath-I and autologous complement, the incidence of grade II–IV acute GVHD was only 12% but the maximum incidence of graft failure was 15% (Hale *et al.*, 1988). In this patient series no significant increase in relapse was detected in patients with acute leukaemia but the relapse incidence in CML patients was substantially above that reported before T cell depletion. In a study from the International Bone Marrow Transplantation Registry (IBMTR) it was also found that T cell depletion dramatically increased the risk of relapse in patients with CML and to a smaller degree in patients with acute leukaemia compared with pharmacological immunosuppression (Horowitz *et al.*, 1990).

12C.2.1.3 Various monoclonal antibodies

Pure muromonab CD3, not the preparation used for *in-vivo* treatment which contains polysorbate 80, has been used for the *ex-vivo* pretreatment of donor bone marrow to deplete residual T lymphocytes. Several preliminary and pilot studies involving small numbers of patients have been published (Filipovich *et al.*, 1982; Prentice *et al.*, 1982; Gilmore *et al.*, 1983; Zepp *et al.*, 1984; Hervé *et al.*, 1985). Prentice *et al.* (1982) used *ex-vivo* T cell opsonization with pure muromonab CD3 in conjunction with prophylactic MTX in 17 patients undergoing allogeneic BMT. During 60 days observation three patients developed grade II–IV acute GVHD (18%), compared with 79% in 14 patients treated with the same dose of MTX alone. The death rate of acute GVHD was also lower in the group treated with muromonab CD3 (12% versus 29%). Filipovich *et al.* (1982) used almost the same technique in 10 patients. Five developed grade II–IV acute GVHD, which was not different when compared with their past experience with MTX.

In 1985 Hervé and co-workers combined muromonab CD2 (anti-T11), with muromonab CD3 in 10 patients to effect more complete T cell depletion in allogeneic bone marrow *ex vivo*. MTX was also given. Of the 10 patients so treated none developed acute GVHD during 90 days follow-up.

Kohler *et al.* (1986) treated the marrow from 23 consecutive donors with CT-2 (anti-T cell mab) and complement *in vitro*. This resulted in 99% T cell depletion measured as E-rosette, OKT3 and OKT11 positive cells. Prompt engraftment with minimal GVHD, despite no post-transplant GVHD prophylaxis, was seen in seven of eight HLA-matched patients. Among 15 non-HLA-identical patients, failure of engraftment occurred in 11 patients. Grades III–IV acute GVHD were seen in two of the four patients who engrafted.

A number of mab have been utilized in preclinical and clinical studies of T cell depletion of human marrow (Table 12C.1). These mab define cell surface antigens expressed mainly on T lymphocytes. Antibodies against CD2, CD3, CD5, CD7 and against other pan-T specificities have frequently been used. Using mab without complement seems less effective in preventing acute GVHD compared with mab together with complement (Filipovich *et al.*, 1982; Martin *et al.*, 1983; Mitsuyasu *et al.*, 1986).

Patients with congenital T lymphocyte deficiency disorders received transplants with parental bone marrow depleted of mature T cells by the use of an anti-T cell mab (CT-2) and complement (Moen *et al.*, 1987). All 16 patients (20 transplants) showed engraftment. No patient received prophylaxis against GVHD and only one patient developed grade II–IV or greater acute GVHD.

Racadot *et al.* (1987) evaluated T cell depletion in 62 consecutive patients (nine BMT centers) with poor prognosis leukaemia or haematosarcoma and HLA-identical donors. A combination of three pan-T cell mab (CD2 'D66', CD5 'A50', CD7 '121') with a single incubation of rabbit complement was used. Twenty-six patients received additional immunosuppression. Only one case of significant acute GVHD was observed but the graft failure rate was 19% in this multicentre study.

Selective depletion of $CD8^+$ cells from donor bone marrow was assessed in 36 leukaemic patients with HLA-identical siblings (Champlin *et al.*, 1990). Anti-Leu-2 mab and complement was used as *ex-vivo* treatment. CsA was given for 6 months post-transplant. The actuarial incidence of grade II–IV acute GVHD was $28 \pm 18\%$, 33 of 36 patients engrafted and the actuarial relapse rate was $11 \pm 10\%$.

12C.2.2 Monoclonal antibodies and immunotoxins (IT)

Henslee *et al.* (1989) describe in a case report the use of XomaZyme-H65 following a partially T cell depleted, histoincompatible marrow graft utilizing a single murine IgM mab, T10B9, activated with rabbit serum complement. The patient developed grade II acute and limited chronic GVHD, which responded to immunosuppressive therapy. XomaZyme-H65 was safely infused in the early post-marrow grafting period.

Immunotoxins have an advantage because they are stable, in contrast to complement which is labile. The toxins covalently bound to antibody are ricin, pokeweed antiviral protein, saponin and gelonin. Ricin is very effective as a cytotoxic agent when directed to a cell by a mab (Vallera *et al.*, 1983; Stong *et al.*, 1985; Ramsay & Kersey, 1988). Vallera *et al.* (1982) demonstrated that *ex-vivo* treatment with T cell antibodies linked to ricin will eliminate T cells and prevent lethal GVHD in a mismatched marrow transplantation model in the mouse.

Uckun *et al.* (1986) showed the inhibitory effect of two immunotoxins synthesized by linking two different anti-CD2 (T, p50) murine mab to intact ricin (R). Pretreatment with 1000 ng/ml 35.1-R or OKT11$_a$-R inhibited PHA-induced T cell proliferation by 93% and 86%, respectively. At this immuno-toxin concentration both 35.1-R and OKT11$_a$-R inhibited the generation of alloreactive cytotoxic T cells by more than 99% and were minimally toxic to NK effectors and pluripotent bone marrow progenitor cells.

In 1987 Filipovich and coworkers presented a study including 17 transplanted patients with HLA-identical marrow that had been depleted of T lymphocytes by *ex-vivo* immunotoxin treatment. A mixture of three anti-T cell mab conjug-ated to ricin were used in this study: TA-1, UCHT-1 (anti-CD3) and T101 (anti-CD5). No other GVHD prophylaxis was used. Twelve patients had high risk acute leukaemia, and five had CML. Four patients developed grade II skin GVHD, 13 had relapse of leukaemia.

In a study from Italy (Siena *et al.*, 1987) optimal conditions for *ex-vivo* elimination of mature T cells from human marrow by T101 immunotoxin were studied. The method used induced T cell depletion of two orders of magnitude. If the same T101-IT treatment in addition was preceded by fractionation with soybean lectin, T cell depletion of three orders of magnitude was accom-plished.

In two clinical studies the effectiveness in decreasing the severity of acute GVHD by treating the donor bone marrow with an immunotoxin, which couples A chain of ricin with a monoclonal anti-T cell antibody T101 (anti-CD5), was studied (Fauser *et al.*, 1988; Filipovich *et al.*, 1990). There were less than 5% T cells left after treatment of the marrow. In the first study 10 patients were included and two patients developed grade II acute GVHD. In the second study 29 patients were included and a statistically significant reduction in acute GVHD was achieved for patients receiving marrow pre-treated with 1000 ng of immunotoxin compared with recipients treated with 300 ng.

12C.2.3 Monoclonal antibodies and immunomagnetic beads

A relatively new technique for depletion of T cells from bone marrow is the use of magnetic monosized polymer microspheres coated with T lympho-cyte-specific mab. Bone marrow cells are rosetted with magnetic beads coated with mab specific for T cell CD2 and CD3 antigens. Rosetted T cells are subsequently removed from non-T cells with the aid of a magnet. The separa-tion procedure is carried out in less than 40 min and less than 0.02% T cells were detected by a T cell limiting dilution assay (Vartdal *et al.*, 1987*a, b*).

12C.3 Randomized clinical studies comparing pharmacological GVHD prophylaxis with T cell depletion

In two independent studies patients receiving T cell-depleted allogeneic bone marrow treated with mab had a lower incidence of acute GVHD compared with patients receiving non-manipulated bone marrow and CsA or MTX (controls) (Maraninchi *et al.*, 1987; Mitsuyasu *et al.*, 1986). On the other hand graft failure and relapse of leukaemia were increased in the patients receiving T cell-depleted marrow. This was also confirmed in a non-randomized study by MacDonald *et al.* (1988).

In a study from Huddinge hospital including adult leukaemic marrow recipients of HLA-identical sibling marrow, 23 patients were randomized to T cell depletion and 25 received combination therapy of MTX and CsA to prevent GVHD (Ringden *et al.*, 1991). Anti-CD8 and anti-CD6 antibodies plus complement depleted $95.3 \pm 5.8\%$ CD3 cells. The incidence of grade II–III acute GVHD was 23% following T cell depletion and 12% for those receiving CsA + MTX. Recipients of T cell-depleted marrow who developed grade I–III acute GVHD received more T cells compared with those without acute GVHD ($p = 0.02$). The cumulative relapse incidence at 4 years was 39% in the recipients of T cell-depleted marrow and 54% in the CsA + MTX group. The 3-year actuarial leukaemia-free survival was 42% and 44% in the two groups, respectively.

12C.4 Monoclonal antibodies *in vivo* for prevention of GVHD

12C.4.1 Anti-CD3 monoclonal antibodies (OKT3)

Prophylactic use of muromonab CD3 for 14 days (20 patients) or antithymocyte globulin (ATG) (19 patients) was compared in a randomized study where the drugs were adminstered soon after transplantation in patients receiving concomitant MTX and steroids (Filipovich *et al.*, 1985). Acute GVHD was diagnosed in 14 of 20 patients who received OKT3-pred-MTX and in eight of 19 patients who received ATG-pred-MTX ($p = 0.06$). One-year actuarial patient survival was 65% in the OKT-3 group and 44% in the ATG group.

12C.4.2 Anti-IL-2 receptor monoclonal antibodies

In mice, the prophylactic use of mab against the IL-2 receptor significantly decreased the incidence and severity of GVHD with a success rate intermediate between that attained by T cell depletion and the rate in untreated controls (Ferrara *et al.*, 1987).

In 18 patients, all received short-term MTX and CsA as GVHD prophylaxis combined with an anti-IL-2 receptor mab (33 B3.1 rat IgG2). All patients engrafted; GVHD did not occur during anti-IL-2R therapy (30 days). GVHD was observed after 35 days in three of eight patients (Blaise *et al.*, 1989).

In a prospective randomized multicentre study 108 patients with standard risk leukaemias were included. Fifty-three patients received an anti-IL-2 receptor (CD25) mab (33B3.11) together with MTX + CsA and 55 patients received

MTX + CsA alone as GVHD prophylaxis. In the first study group severe GVHD was significantly delayed; however, the overall incidence of acute and chronic GVHD was the same in the two groups (Blaise *et al.*, 1991).

12C.4.3 Anti-LFA-1 monoclonal antibodies

In a European multicentre study 46 children with immunodeficiency disorders, malignant osteopetroses or Fanconi's anaemia were transplanted with T cell-depleted bone marrow from HLA-identical siblings (Fischer *et al.*, 1991). To prevent graft failure, a mouse mab specific for the CD11a-lymphocyte function-associated antigen 1 (LFA-1) molecule was infused into the patients. The overall sustained engraftment rate was 72% instead of 26% in a retrospective control group of 24 patients similarly treated except for the infusion of the anti-LFA-1 antibody. No late rejections occurred. Acute GVHD of grade II or more occurred in 35% of the patients and the rate of chronic GVHD was 13%. Epstein–Barr virus-induced B cell proliferative syndrome was observed in seven patients (six with Wiskott–Aldrich syndrome).

12C.5 Treatment of GVHD with monoclonal antibodies

12C.5.1 Anti-CD3 monoclonal antibodies (OKT3)

Gratama *et al.* (1984) administered muromonab CD3 for 14 days to eight patients with grade II–IV acute GVHD, five of them were resistant to steroid treatment. The patients received MTX as GVHD prophylaxis. Four patients experienced a complete response, two a partial response and two no response. The response to muromonab CD3 (OKT3) was rapid, within 48 h. All patients, however, died within 19–398 days after the introduction of OKT3 treatment, most from infectious complications related to profound immunosuppression.

In a second study of 10 patients with grades III–IV acute GVHD resistant to treatment with CsA and steroids, mab (OKT3) induced a complete response in five and a partial response in four patients within 1–4 days of treatment (Gluckman *et al.*, 1984). Acute GVHD frequently recurred, however, and all four surviving patients developed chronic GVHD. One patient in addition developed a monoclonal B cell lymphoma.

In a case report, Faure *et al.* (1986) described the occurrence of an immunoblastic lymphoma after BMT in a patient with severe steroid-resistant acute GVHD and treated with OKT3.

Two patients with severe GVHD were treated with an anti-CD3 mab (64.1; IgG2a) (Martin *et al.*, 1984*b*). The GVHD responded but both patients developed a fatal polyclonal lymphoproliferative disorder arising in donor-derived B cells. Hybridization studies showed Epstein–Barr virus in both tumours. The same IgG2a anti-CD3 mab was given to treat acute GVHD in 24

BMT recipients in a dose-escalation trial. Although skin disease responded at doses of 0.15 mg/kg per day, gastrointestinal tract or liver disease only responded at higher doses. Four of 24 patients developed Epstein–Barr virus-associated lymphoproliferative disorders (Martin *et al.*, 1988*a*).

12C.5.2 *Other monoclonal antibodies for treatment of GVHD*

Four different murine mab against T cells were administered to 15 patients with severe steroid-resistant GVHD. The four mab were: 9.6 (CD2), 35.1 (CD2), 10.2 and 12.1. The patients received in total 151 infusions (range 1–20 mg/day). Six of ten patients receiving 5–20 mg had partial improvement in GVHD in at least one involved organ system (Remlinger *et al.*, 1984).

12C.5.3 *Anti-IL-2 monoclonal antibodies*

Hervé *et al.* (1988) treated 13 patients with acute GVHD that was refractory to corticosteroids with B-B10, a mouse mab of IgG kappa isotype, with an inhibitory activity against IL-2-induced T cell proliferation. GVHD was eliminated in eight cases, improved in three cases and no response was seen in two cases. In a subsequent study the same group reported results from 32 patients with steroid-resistant grade II–IV acute GVHD (Hervé *et al.*, 1990). The same anti-IL-2 receptor mab B-B10 (anti-CD25), was given. Overall, 84% of the patients responded (65% completely and 19% partially). The group included recipients of marrow from HLA-identical siblings, non-HLA-identical siblings and unrelated donors. After discontinuation of therapy GVHD recurred in 38% of patients. In a multicentre study, 58 patients with steroid-resistant acute GVHD were treated with anti-IL-2 mab (B-B10) (Hervé *et al.*, 1991*a*). A complete response was achieved in 29 patients (50%) and 17 showed no response (30%). In the same patient series, ten patients with GVHD resistant to steroids and anti-IL-2R antibody were given an anti-TNF-alpha mab (clone B-C7, IgG1 isotype). GVHD was eliminated in three patients, improved in six and no response was seen in one patient.

From the Seattle group a study was reported that included 10 patients with grade II–IV acute GVHD treated with a murine IgG1 antibody specific for the IL-2 receptor beta chain (CD25). Among seven patients treated within 40 days after BMT, one had a complete response and three had a partial response. No responses were achieved with liver disease or in patients treated for more than 40 days after BMT (Anasetti *et al.*, 1990).

In a single centre pilot study 31 patients with acute GVHD following allogeneic BMT were treated with a mab B-B10, directed at the IL-2 receptor. All received CsA as GVHD prophylaxis. All patients received both B-B10 and high-dose methylprednisolone intravenously (i.v.) at diagnosis of significant GVHD. In 17 of 31 (55%) patients the GVHD responded completely, a partial response was obtained in six (20%) and eight patients failed to respond. In those who had previously responded (completely or partially), GVHD recurred in 12 patients (52%) at a median of 10 days after completion of the B-B10 therapy (Anasetti *et al.*, 1991).

12C.5.4 Anti-CD5 immunotoxin (ricin A chain)

Mab immunotoxin conjugates have been constructed for use both *in vitro* and *in vivo* to ensure destruction of the target cell. In 34 patients with steroid-resistant grade II–IV acute GVHD, a ricin A chain conjugated mab, Xoma-Zyme-H65 (IgG; anti-CD5) was given for 14 days (Byers *et al.*, 1990). Of 32 evaluable patients, 72% responded in at least one organ and another 16% had stable disease; however, recurrence of GVHD was frequent.

12C.5.5 Anti TNFα monoclonal antibody

In mice it has been shown that antibodies to TNFα prevented GVHD (Piguet *et al.*, 1987). This finding formed the basis for subsequent clinical trials. In 18 patients suffering from acute GVHD grade III–IV, uncontrolled with both steroids and anti-IL-2 receptor mab (B-B10), a murine mab specific for TNFα (clone B-C7) was administered and was well tolerated (Hervé *et al.*, 1991b). In 21% of patients there was a complete response and 61% improved; however, among the 14 evaluable responders, active GVHD reappeared rapidly in eight patients (57%). Only 22% of the patients have survived; the main causes of death were GVHD and infectious complications.

12C.6 Monoclonal antibodies in the diagnosis of GVHD

Mab have been used to determine lymphocyte subpopulations in blood after BMT. After BMT CD8+ cells generally increase compared with CD4+ cells which decrease (De Bruin *et al.*, 1981; Forman *et al.*, 1982). The CD4/CD8 ratio is increased in patients with acute GVHD, chronic GVHD and during CMV infection (Persson *et al.*, 1987). This is due to a reduced absolute number of CD4+ cells during acute GVHD and a significantly increased number of CD8+ cells during CMV infection.

Mab have also been used *in situ* in affected tissue of patients with GVHD. In particular, CD8 antigen-bearing lymphocytes have been found in skin biopsies from patients with acute GVHD (Lampert *et al.*, 1981). CD8+ lymphocytes have also been found in biopsies from patients with oral lichenoid-like lesions in patients with chronic GVHD (Fujii *et al.*, 1988).

In a study by Muller (1983) immunohistological analysis of GVHD-mediated lesions was performed with selected mab against differentiation antigens in 31 BMT patients. Cutaneous acute or chronic GVHD reactivity was associated with infiltrates of activated mature CD4+ and CD8+ lymphocytes within the dermis and epithelium, as well as with HLA class II antigen expression on keratinocytes.

Expression of HLA class II antigen on keratinocytes has been advocated as a diagnostic marker of acute GVHD. Synovec *et al*. (1990) analysed LN-3 staining pattern (LN-3 is a murine mab marking an HLA class II antigen that survives formalin fixation and paraffin embedding) on 56 skin biopsies from patients treated with BMT or peripheral stem cell transplantation, non-transplantation, non-transplant patients receiving conventional chemotherapy and/ or radiation therapy as controls. The most predictive parameter for GVHD was labelling of endothelial cells by LN-3 which was present in 12 of 16 (75%) biopsies from patients with GVHD. Endothelial staining was found in a total of 19 biopsies of which 12 (63%) had GVHD.

12C.7 Outlook

Acute GVHD remains a major complication in allogeneic BMT. T cell depletion raised the hope that it might be possible to obtain a substantial decrease in GVHD incidence. However, the incidence of graft failure and leukaemic relapse increased and the overall survival has not improved compared with pharmacological immunosuppression.

The graft-versus-leukaemia (GVL) effect is probably associated with GVHD; perhaps the T cells from the donor react with remaining tumour cells in the recipient, as well as with normal cells in association with MHC.

With the use of biological response-modifying agents and new approaches for T cell depletion, a better control of GVHD in high-risk patients may be achieved. A major task would be to abrogate the loss of the GVL effect. For GVHD prevention this would involve depletion only of alloreactive T cells. This would require a more accurate understanding of the phenotype of the T cells responsible for GVHD.

The addition of mab or other biological effectors to conditioning regimens will give better eradication of disseminated tumours. The use of mab in the treatment of alloreactivity events is still at its early stage.

In the future it may be possible to modify the mab with class switch technology, antibody isotope conjugates, bispecific antibodies, reshaped human antibodies and construction of A + B chain conjugates (which lack lectin activity yet retain the capacity to facilitate A chain entry). It is concluded that mab will be increasingly used for the diagnosis, prevention and treatment of various immunological events in BMT.

12C.8 References

Anasetti, C., Martin, P. J., Hansen, J. A., Appelbaum, F. R., Beatty, P. G., Doney, K., Harkonen, S., Jackson, A., Reichert, T., Stewart, P., Storb, R., Sullivan, K. M., Thomas, E. D., Warner, N. & Witherspoon, R. P. (1990). A phase I–II study evaluating the murine anti-IL-2 receptor antibody 2A3 for treatment of acute graft-versus-host disease. *Transplantation*, **50**, 49–54.

Anasetti, C., Martin, P. J., Storb, F. R., Appelbaum, F. R., Beatty, P. G., Calori, E., Davis, J., Doney, K., Reichert, T., Stewart, P., Sullivan, K. M., Thomas, E. D., Witherspoon, R. P. & Hansen, J. A. (1991). Prophylaxis of graft-versus-host disease by administration of the murine anti-IL-2 receptor antibody 2A3. *Bone Marrow Transplantation*, **7**, 375–381.

Antin, J. H., Bierer, B. E., & Smith, B. R. (1990). Depletion of bone marrow T-lymphocytes with an anti-CD5 monoclonal immunotoxin (ST-1 immunotoxin): effective prophylaxis for graft-versus-host disease. In *Bone Marrow Purging and Processing*, New York, Alan R Liss, pp. 207–215.

Apperley, J. F., Jones, L., Hale, G., Waldmann, H., Hows, J., Rombos, Y., Tsatalas, C., Marcus, R. E., Goolden, A. W. G., Gordon-Smith, E. C., Catovsky, D., Galton, D. A. G. & Goldman, J. M. (1986). Bone marrow transplantation for patients with chronic myeloid leukaemia: T-cell depletion with Campath-I reduces the incidence of graft-versus-host disease but may increase the risk of leukaemic relapse. *Bone Marrow Transplantation*, **1**, 53–66.

Ash, R. C., Horowitz, M. M., Gale, R. P., van Bekkum, D. W., Casper, J. T., Gordon-Smith, E. C., Henslee, P. J., Kolb, H. J., Lowenberg, B., Masaoka, T., McGlave, P. B., Rimm, A. A., Ringden, O., van Rood, J. J., Sondel, P. M., Vowels, M. R. & Bortin, M. M. (1991). Bone marrow transplantation from related donors other than HLA-identical siblings: effect of T cell depletion Registry analysis. *Bone Marrow Transplantation*, **7**, 443–452.

Bacigalupo, A., Hows, J., Gluckman, E., Nissen, C., Marsh, J., van Lint, M. T., Congiu, M., De Planque, M. M., Ernst, P., McCann, S., Ragavashar, A., Frickhufen, N., Wursch, A., Marmont, A. M. & Gordon-Smith, E. C. (1988). Bone marrow transplantation (BMT) versus immunosuppression for the treatment of severe aplastic anemia (SAA): a report of the EBMT SAA Working Party. *British Journal of Hematology*, **70**, 177–182.

Beatty, P. G., Clift, R. A., Mickelson, E. M., Nisperos, B. B., Flournoy, N., Martin, P. J., Sanders, J. E., Stewart, P., Buckner, C. D., Storb, R., Thomas, E. D. & Hansen, J. A. (1985). Marrow transplantation from related donors other than HLA-identical siblings. *New England Journal of Medicine*, **313**, 765–771.

Blaise, D., Guyotat, D., Reiffers, J., Olive, D., Michallet, M., Bellanger, C., Vernaut, J. P., Ifrah, N., Attal, M. & Vilmer, E. (1991). Prospective randomized study of GVHD prevention using an anti IL2 receptor (CD25) MoAb after allogeneic bone marrow transplantation (BMT). *Bone Marrow Transplantation*, **7**(Suppl. 2), 150.

Blaise, D., Maraninchi, D., Mawas, C., Stoppa, A. M., Hirn, M., Guyotat, D., Attal, M. and Reiffers, J. (1989). Prevention of graft-versus-host disease by monoclonal antibody to interleukin-2 receptor. *Lancet*, **1**, 1333–1334.

Blume, K. G., Beutler, E., Bross, K. J., Chillar, R. K., Ellington, O. B., Fahey, J. L., Farbstein, M. J., Forman, S. J., Schmidt, G. M., Scott, E. P., Spruce, W. E., Turner, M. A. & Wolf, J. L. (1980). Bone marrow ablation and allogeneic marrow transplantation in acute leukemia. *New England Journal of Medicine*, **302**, 1041–1046.

Bonmasser, E., Campanile, F., Houchens, D., Crino, L. & Goldwin, A. (1975). Impaired growth of a radiation induced lymphoma in intact or lethally irradiated allogeneic athymic (nude) mice. *Transplantation*, **20**, 343–346.

Bortin, M. M. & Saltzstein, E. C. (1969). Graft versus host inhibition: fetal liver and thymus cells minimize secondary disease. *Science*, **164**, 316–318.

Brenner, M. K., Grob, J.-P. & Prentice, H. G. (1986). The use of monoclonal antibodies in graft versus host disease prevention. *Haematologia*, **19**, 167–176.

Byers, V., Henslee, P. J., Kernan, N. A., Blazar, B. R., Gingrich, R., Phillips, G. L., LeMaistre, C. F., Gilliland, G., Antin, J. H., Martin, P., Tutscha, P. J., Trown, P., Ackerman, S. K., O'Reilly, R. J. & Scannon, P. J. (1990). Use of an anti-Pan-T-lymphocyte ricin A chain immunotoxin in steroid-resistant acute graft-versus-host disease. *Blood*, **75**, 1426–1432.

Champlin, R. E. (1987). For the Advisory Committee for the IBMTR. Bone marrow transplantation for acute leukemia: a preliminary report from the International Bone Marrow Transplant Registry. *Transplantation Proceedings*, **19**, 2626–2628.

Champlin, R., Ho, W., Gajewski, J., Feig, S., Burnison, M., Holley, G., Greenberg, P., Lee, K., Schmid, I., Giorgi, J., Yam, P., Petz, L., Winston, D., Warner, N. & Reichert, T. (1990). Selective depletion of CD8$^+$ T lymphocytes for prevention of graft-versus-host disease after allogeneic bone marrow transplantation. *Blood*, **76**, 418–423.

Cobbold, S., Hale, G. & Waldmann, H. (1987). Non-lineage, LFA-1 family and leukocyte common antigens: new and previously defined clusters. In *Leucocyte Typing III, White Cell Differentiation Antigens*, ed. A. J. McMichael, pp. 788–803. Oxford, Oxford University Press.

Cobbold, S., Martin, G. & Waldmann, H. (1986). Monoclonal antibodies for the prevention of graft-versus-host disease and marrow graft rejection. *Transplantation*, **42**, 239–247.

Cudkowicz, G. & Bennet, M. (1971*a*). Peculiar immunobiology of bone marrow allografts. I. Graft rejection by irradiated responder mice. *Journal of Experimental Medicine*, **134**, 83–102.

Cudkowicz, G. & Bennet, M. (1971*b*). Peculiar immunobiology of bone marrow allografts. II. Rejection of parental grafts by resistance F$_1$ hybrid mice. *Journal of Experimental Medicine*, **134**, 1513–1529.

De Bruin, H. G., Astaldi, A., Leupers, T., Van de Griend, R., Dooren, L. J., Schellekens, P. T. A., Tanke, H. J., Roos, M. & Vossen, J. M. (1981). T lymphocyte characteristics in bone marrow-transplanted patients. II. Analysis with monoclonal antibodies. *Journal of Immunology*, **127**, 244–251.

Deeg, H. J., Loughran, Jr., T. P., Storb, R., Kennedy, M. S., Sullivan, K. M., Doney, K., Appelbaum, F. R. & Thomas, E. D. (1985). Treatment of human acute graft-versus-host disease with antithymocyte globulin and cyclosporine with or without methylprednisolone. *Transplantation*, **40**, 162–166.

Dennert, G., Anderson, C. G., & Warner, J. (1985). T killer cells play a role in allogeneic bone marrow graft rejection but not in hybrid resistance. *Journal of Immunology*, **135**, 3729–3734.

Faure, P., d'Agay, M. F. & Tricot, G. (1986). Lymphome immunoblastique apres greffe de moelle osseuse. *Annales de Pathologie*, **6**, 137–143.

Fauser, A. A., Shustik, C., Langleben, A., Laurent, G., Kanz, L., Spurll, G. M., Price, G., Ahlgren, P. D. & Cooper, B. A. (1988). T cell depletion with ricin A-chain T101 in allogeneic bone marrow transplantation to prevent severe graft-versus-host disease. *Clinical and Investigative Medicine*, **11**, 40–46.

Ferrara, J., Marion, A., Murphy, G. & Burakoff, S. (1987). Acute graft-versus-host disease: pathogenesis and prevention with a monoclonal antibody *in vitro*. *Transplantation Proceedings*, **19**, 2662–2663.

Filipovich, A. H., Krawczak, C. L., Kersey, J. H., McGlave, P., Ramsay, N. K. C., Goldman, A. & Goldstein, G. (1985). Graft-versus-host disease prophylaxis with anti-T-cell monoclonal antibody OKT3, prednisone and methotrexate in allogeneic bone marrow transplantation. *British Journal of Haematology*, **60**, 143–152.

Filipovich, A. H., McGlave, P. B., Ramsay, N. K. C., Goldstein, G., Warkentin, P. I. & Kersey, J. H. (1982). Pretreatment of donor bone marrow with monoclonal antibody OKT3 for prevention of acute graft-versus-host disease in allogeneic histocompatible bone-marrow transplantation. *Lancet*, **1**, 1266–1269.

Filipovich, A. H., Vallera, D., McGlave, P., Polich, D., Gajl-Peczalska, K., Haake, R., Lasky, L., Blazar, B., Ramsay, N. K. C., Kersey, J. & Weisdorf, D. (1990). T cell depletion with anti-CD5 immunotoxin in histocompatible bone marrow transplantation. *Transplantation*, **50**, 410–415.

Filipovich, A. H., Vallera, D. A., Youle, R. J., Haake, R., Blazar, B. R., Arthur, D., Neville, D. M. Jr., Ramsay, N. K. C., McGlave, P. & Kersey, J. H. (1987). Graft-versus-host disease prevention in allogeneic bone marrow transplantation from histocompatible siblings. *Transplantation*, **44**, 62–69.

Fischer, A., Friedrich, W., Fasth, A., Blanche, S., Le Deist, F., Girault, D., Veber, F., Vossen, J., Lopez, M., Griscelli, C. & Hirn, M. (1991). Reduction of graft failure by a monoclonal antibody (anti-LFA-1 CD11a) after HLA nonidentical bone marrow transplantation in children with immunodeficiencies, osteopetrosis and Fanconi's anemia: a European Group for Immunodeficiency/European group for Bone Marrow Transplantation report. *Blood*, **77**, 249–256.

Forman, S. J., Nöcker, P., Gallagher, M., Zaia, J., Wright, C., Bolen, J., Mills, B. & Hecht, T. (1982). Pattern of T cell reconstitution following allogeneic bone marrow transplantation for acute hematological malignancy. *Transplantation*, **34**, 96–98.

Fujii, H., Ohashi, M. & Nagura, H. (1988). Immunohistochemical analysis of oral-lichen-planus-like eruptions in graft-versus-host disease after allogeneic bone marrow transplantation. *American Journal of Clinical Pathology*, **89**, 177–186.

Gale, R. P., (1987). T cells bone marrow transplantation and immunotherapy: use of monoclonal antibodies. In *Immune Interventions in Disease*, (moderator). J. L. Fahey, *Annals of Internal Medicine*, **106**, 257–274.

Gale, R. P., Horowitz, M. M., Biggs, J. C., Herzig, R. H., Kersey, J. H., Marmont, A. M., Masaoka, T., Rimm, A. A., Speck, B., Weiner, R. S., Zwaan, F. E. & Bortin, M. M. (1989). Transplant or chemotherapy in acute myelogenous leukaemia. *Lancet*, **1**, 1119–1122.

Gale, R. P., Opelz, G., Mickey, M. R., Graze, P. R. & Saxon, A. for the UCLA Bone Marrow Transplant Team (1978). Immunodeficiency following allogeneic bone marrow transplantation. *Transplantation Proceedings*, **10**, 223–227.

Gilmore, M. J. M. L., Prentice, H. G., Price Jones, E., Blacklock, H. A., Tidman, N., Schey, S., Goldstein, G., Janossy, G. & Hoffbrand, A. V. (1983). Allogeneic bone marrow transplantation: the monitoring of granulocyte macrophage colonies following the collection of bone marrow mononuclear cells and after the subsequent *in vitro* cytolysis of OKT3 positive lymphocytes. *British Journal of Haematology*, **55**, 587–593.

Gluckman, E., Devergie, A., Varin, F., Rabian, C., D'Agay, M. F. D. & Benbunan, M. (1984). Treatment of steroid resistant severe acute graft versus host disease with monoclonal PAN T OKT3 antibody. *Experimental Hematology*, **12** (Suppl. 15), 66–67.

Glucksberg, H., Storb, R. & Fefer, A. (1974). Clinical manifestations of graft-versus-host disease in human recipients of marrow from HLA-matched sibling donors. *Transplantation*, **18**, 295–304.

Gratama, J. W., Jansen, J., Lipovich, R. A., Tanke, H. J., Goldstein, G. & Zwaan, F. E. (1984). Treatment of acute graft-versus-host disease with monoclonal antibody OKT3. Clinical results and effect on circulating T lymphocytes. *Transplantation*, **38**, 469–474.

Grathwohl, A., Hermans, J., Barrett, A. J., Ernst, P., Frassoni, F., Gahrton, E., Granena, A., Kolb, H. J., Marmont, H., Prentice, G., Speck, B., Vernant, J. P. & Zwaan, F. J. (1988). Allogeneic bone marrow transplantation for leukaemia in

Europe. *Lancet*, **1**, 1379–1382.

Grebe, S. C. & Streilein, J. W. (1976). Graft-versus-host reactions: a review. *Advances in Immunology*, **22**, 119–221.

Groth, C-G., Gahrton, G., Lundgren, G., Möller, E., Pihlstredt, P., Ringdén, O. & Sundelin, P. (1979). Successful treatment with prednisolone of graft-versus-host disease in an allogeneic bone marrow transplant recipient. *Scandinavian Journal of Hematology*, **22**, 333–338.

Hale, G., Bright, S., Chumbley, G., Hoang, T., Metcalf, D., Munro, A. J. & Waldmann, H. (1983). Removal of T cells from bone marrow for transplantation: a monoclonal antilymphocyte antibody that fixes human complement. *Blood*, **62**, 873–882.

Hale, G., Cobbold, S. & Waldmann, H. (1988). T-cell depletion with Campath-1 in allogeneic bone marrow transplantation. *Transplantation*, **45**, 753–759.

Hayward, A., Murphy, S., Githens, J., Troup, G. and Ambruso, D. (1982). Failure of a pan-reactive anti-T cell antibody, OKT3, to prevent graft-versus-host disease in severe combined immunodeficiency. *Journal of Pediatrics*, **100**, 665–668.

Heit, W., Bunjes, D., Wiesneth, M. Schmeiser, T., Arnold, R., Hale, G., Waldmann, H. and Heimpel, H. (1986). *Ex-vivo* T-cell depletion with the monoclonal antibody Campath-1 plus human complement effectively prevents acute graft-versus-host disease in allogeneic bone marrow transplantation. *British Journal of Haematology*, **64**, 479–486.

Henslee, P. J., Byers, V. S. & Jennings, C. D. (1989). A new approach to the prevention of graft-versus-host disease using XomaZyme-H65 following histo-incompatible partially T-depleted marrow grafts. *Transplantation Proceedings*, **21**, 3004–3007.

Hervé, P., Bordigoni, P. & Cahn, J. Y. (1991*a*). Use of monoclonal antibodies *in vivo* as a therapeutic strategy for acute GVHD in matched and mismatched bone marrow transplantation. *Transplantation Proceedings*, **23**, 1692–1694.

Hervé, P., Cahn, J. Y. & Flesch, M. (1987). Successful graft versus host disease prevention without graft failure in 32 HLA identical allogeneic bone marrow transplantations with marrow depleted of T cells by monoclonal antibodies and complement. *Blood*, **69**, 388–393.

Hervé, P., Racadot, E. & Wijdenes, J. (1991*b*). Monoclonal anti TNF alpha antibody in the treatment of acute GVHD refractory both to corticosteroids and anti IL-2 R antibody. *Bone Marrow Transplantation*, **7** (Suppl. 2), 149.

Hervé, P., Flesch, M., Cahn, J. Y., Racadot, E., Plouvier, E., Lamy, B., Rozenbaum, A., Noir, A., D'es Floris, R. L. and Peters, A. (1985). Removal of marrow T cells with OKT3-OKT11 monoclonal antibodies and complement to prevent acute graft-versus-host disease. *Transplantation*, **39**, 138–143.

Hervé, P., Wijdenes, J. & Bergerat, J. P. (1990). Treatment of corticosteroid resistant acute graft-versus-host disease by *in vivo* administration of anti-interleukin-2 receptor monoclonal antibody (B-B10). *Blood*, **75**, 1017–1023.

Hervé, P., Wijdenes, J., Bergerat, J. P., Milpied, N., Gaud, C. & Bordigoni, P. (1988). Treatment of acute graft versus host disease with monoclonal antibody to IL2 receptor. *Lancet*, **2**, 1072–1073.

Hood, A. F., Soter, N. A., Rappeport, J. & Gigli, I. (1977). Graft-versus-host reaction: cutaneous manifestations following bone marrow transplantation. *Archives of Dermatology*, **113**, 1087–1091.

Horowitz, M. M., Gale, R. P., Sondel, P. M., Goldman, J. M., Kersey, J., Kolb, H. J., Rimm, A. A., Ringden, O., Rozman, C., Speck, B., Truitt, R. L., Zwaan, F. E. & Bortin, M. M. (1990). Graft-versus-leukemia reactions after bone marrow transplantation. *Blood*, **75**, 555–562.

Hymes, S. R., Morison, W. L., Farmer, E. R., Walters, L. L., Tutschka, P. J. & Santos, G. W. (1985). Methoxsalen and ultraviolet A radiation in treatment of chronic cutaneous graft-versus-host reaction. *Journal of the American Academy of Dermatology*, **12**, 30–37.

Kiessling, R., Hochman, P. S., Haller, O., Shearer, G. M., Wigzell, H. & Cudkowics, G. (1977). Evidence for a similar or common mechanism for natural killer activity and resistance to hemopoietic grafts. *European Journal of Immunology*, **7**, 665–673.

Kohler, P. C., Erickson, C., Finlay, J. L., Trigg, M. E., Edwards, B., Hong, R., Hank, J. A., Billing, R., Bozdech, M. & Sondel, P. M. (1986). *In vitro* analysis of donor bone marrow following monoclonal antibody treatment for the prevention of acute graft-versus-host disease. *Cancer Research*, **46**, 5413–5418.

Lampert, I. A., Suitters, A. J., Janossy, G., Thomas, J. A., Palmer, S. & Gordon-Smith, E. (1981). Lymphoid infiltrates in skin in graft-versus-host disease. *Lancet*, **2**, 1352 (letter).

Locasciulli, A., van't Veer, L., Bacigalupo, A., Hows, J., Van Lint, M. T., Gluckman, E., Nissen, C., McCann, S., Vossen, J., Schrezenmeier, A., Hinterberger, W. & Marin, A. (1990). Treatment with marrow transplantation or immunosuppression of childhood acquired severe aplastic anemia: a report from the EBMT SAA Working Party. *Bone Marrow Transplantation*, **6**, 211–217.

Lowenberg, B., Wagemaker, E. & van Bekkum, D. W. (1986). Graft-versus-host disease following transplantation of 'one log' versus 'two log' T-lymphocyte depleted bone marrow from HLA-identical donors. *Bone Marrow Transplantation*, **1**, 133–140.

MacDonald, D., Poynton, C. H. & McCarthy, D. (1988). T depletion versus cyclosporin as GVHD prophylaxis in leukaemia recipients of matched marrow allografts. *Bone Marrow Transplantation*, **3** (Suppl. 1), 229.

Maraninchi, D., Gluckman, E., Blaise, D., Guyotat, D., Rio, B., Pico, J. L., Leblond, V., Michallet, M., Dreyfus, F. & Ifrah, N. (1987). Impact of T-cell depletion on outcome of allogeneic bone-marrow transplantation for standard-risk leukaemias. *Lancet*, **2**, 175–178.

Maraninchi, D., Mawas, C. & Guyotat, D. (1988). Selective depletion of marrow-T cytotoxic lymphocytes (CD8) in the prevention of graft-versus-host disease after allogeneic bone-marrow transplantation. *Transplant International*, **1**, 91–94.

Martin, P. J., Hansen, J. A. & Anasetti, C. (1988a). Treatment of acute graft-versus-host disease anti-CD3 monoclonal antibodies. *American Journal of Kidney Diseases*, **XI**, 149–152.

Martin, P. J., Hansen, J. A., Buckner, C. D., Sanders, J. E., Deeg, J., Stewart, P., Appelbaum, F. R., Clift, R., Fefer, A., Witherspoon, R. P., Kennedy, M. S., Sullivan, K. M., Flournoy, N., Storb, R. & Thomas, E. D. (1985). Effects of *in vitro* depletion of T cells in HLA-identical allogeneic marrow grafts. *Blood*, **66**, 664–672.

Martin, P. J., Hansen, J. A. & Remlinger, K. (1983). Murine monoclonal antihuman T cell antibodies for the prevention and treatment of graft-versus-host disease. In *Recent Advances in Bone Marrow Transplantation*, ed. R. P. Gale, New York, pp. 313–329. Alan R. Liss.

Martin, P. J., Hansen, J. A. & Thomas, E. D. (1984a). Preincubation of donor marrow cells with a combination of murine monoclonal anti-T-cell antibodies without complement does not prevent graft-versus-host disease after allogeneic marrow transplantation. *Journal of Clinical Immunology*, **4**, 18–22.

Martin, P. J., Hansen, J. A., Torok-Storb, B., Durnam, D., Przepiorka, D., O'Quigley, J., Sanders, J., Sullivan, K. M., Witherspoon, R. P., Deeg, J. J.,

Appelbaum, F. R., Stewart, P. & Weiden, P. (1988b). Graft failure in patients receiving T cell depleted HLA-identical allogeneic marrow transplants. *Bone Marrow Transplantation*, 3, 445–456.

Martin, P. J., Shulman, H. M., Schubach, W. H., Hansen, J. A., Fefer, A., Miller, E. & Thomas, E. D. (1984b). Fatal Epstein–Barr-virus-associated proliferation of donor B cells after treatment of acute graft-versus-host disease with a murine anti-T-cell antibody. *Annals of Internal Medicine*, 101, 310–315.

Mitsuyasu, R. T., Champlin, R. E., Gale, R. P., Ho, W. G., Lenarsky, C., Winston, D., Selch, M., Elashoff, R., Giorgi, J. V., Wells, J., Terasaki, P., Billing, R. & Feig, S. (1986). Treatment of donor bone marrow with monoclonal anti-T-cell antibody and complement for the prevention of graft-versus-host disease. *Annals of Internal Medicine*, 105, 20–26.

Moen, R. C., Horowitz, S. D., Sondel, P. M. Borcherding, W. R., Trigg, M. E., Billing, R. & Höng, R. (1987). Immunologic reconstitution after haploidentical bone marrow transplantation for immune deficiency disorders: treatment of bone marrow cells with monoclonal antibody CT-2 and complement. *Blood*, 70, 664–669.

Muller, C. (1983). Charakterisierung GvH-bedingter Hautläsionen mit Hilfe monoklonaler Antikörper am Gefrierschnitt. *Verhandlungen der Deutschen Gesellschaft für Pathologie*, 67, 362–366.

Noel, D. R., Witherspoon, R. P., Storb, R., Atkinson, K., Doney, K., Mickelson, E. M., Ochs, H. D., Warren, R. P., Weiden, P. L. & Thomas, E. D. (1978). Does graft-versus-host disease influence the tempo of immunologic recovery after allogeneic human marrow transplantation? An observation on 56 long-term survivors. *Blood*, 51, 1087–1104.

Paulin, T., Ringdén, O. & Nilsson, B. (1987). Immunological recovery after bone marrow transplantation: role of age, graft-versus-host disease, prednisolone treatment and infections. *Bone Marrow Transplantation*, 1, 317–328.

Persson, U., Myrenfors, P., Ringdén, O., Sundberg, B., Larsson, P. & Johansson, S. G. O. (1987). T lymphocyte subpopulations in bone-marrow-transplanted patients in relation to graft-versus-host disease and cytomegalovirus-induced infection. *Transplantation*, 43, 663–668.

Pico, J. L., Kuentz, M., Hervé, P., Morizet, J., Beaujean, F., Racadot, E., Vernant, J. P., Flesch, M., Baume, D., Hayat, M. & Bernard, A. (1989). Efficacy of monoclonal antibodies (mAb) CD5+CD8 for the treatment of steroid resistant graft versus host disease (GvHD). *Bone Marrow Transplantation*, 4 (Suppl. 2), 68.

Piguet, P.-F., Grau, G. E., Allet, B. & Vassalli, P. (1987). Tumor necrosis factor/cachetin is an effector of skin and gut lesions of the acute phase of graft-versus-host disease. *Journal of Experimental Medicine*, 166, 1280–1289.

Powles, R. L., Clink, H. M., Spence, D., Morgenstern, E., Watson, J. G., Selby, P. J., Woods, M., Barrett, A., Jameson, B., Sloane, J., Lawler, S. D., Kay, H. E. M., Lawson, D., McElwain, T. J. & Alexander, P. (1980). Cyclosporin A to prevent graft-versus-host disease in man after allogeneic bone marrow transplantation. *Lancet*, 1, 327–329.

Prentice, H. G., Bateman, S. M., Bradstock, K. F. & Hoffbrand, A. V. (1980). High dose methyl prednisolone therapy in established acute graft-versus-host disease. *Blut*, 41, 175–177.

Prentice, H. G., Blacklock, H. A., Janossy, G., Bradstock, K. F., Skeggs, D., Goldstein, G. & Hoffbrand, A. V. (1982). Use of anti-T cell monoclonal antibody OKT3 to prevent acute graft-versus-host disease in allogeneic bone-marrow transplantation for acute leukemia. *Lancet*, 1, 700–703.

Prentice, H. G., Blacklock, H. A., Janossy, G., Gilmore, M. J. M. L, Price-Jones, L.,

Tidman, N., Trejdosiewicz, L. K., Skeggs, D. B. L., Panjwani, D., Ball, S., Graphakos, S., Patterson, J., Ivory, K. & Hoffbrand, A. V. (1984). Depletion of T lymphocytes in donor marrow prevents significant graft versus host disease in matched allogeneic leukaemic marrow transplant recipients. *Lancet*, **1**, 472–475.

Racadot, E., Hervé, P., Beaujean, F., Vernant, J-P., Flesch, M., Plouvier, E., Andreu, G., Rio, B., Phillipe, N., Souillet, G., Pico, J., Bordigoni, P., Ifrah, N., Paitre, M-L., Lutz, P., Morizet, J. and Bernard, A. (1987). Prevention of graft-versus-host disease in HLA-matched bone marrow transplantation for malignant diseases: a multicentric study of 62 patients using 3-Pan-T monoclonal antibodies and rabbit complement. *Journal of Clinical Oncology*, **5**, 426–435.

Ramsay, N. K. C. & Kersey, J. H. (1988). Bone marrow purging using monoclonal antibodies. *Journal of Clinical Immunology*, **8**, 81–88.

Reinherz, E. L., Geha, R., Rappeport, J. M., Wilson, M., Penta, A. C., Hussey, R. E., Fitzgerald, K. A., Daley, J. F., Levine, H., Rosen, F. S. & Schlossman, S. F. (1982). Reconstitution after transplantation with T-lymphocyte-depleted HLA haplotype-mismatched bone marrow for severe combined immunodeficiency. *Proceedings of the National Academy of Sciences of the U.S.A.*, **79**, 6047–6051.

Remlinger, K., Martin, P. J. & Hansen, J. A. (1984). Murine monoclonal anti-T cell antibodies for treatment of steroid-resistant acute graft-versus-host disease. *Human Immunology*, **9**, 21–35.

Ringdén, O., Bäckman, L. & Lönnqvist, B. (1986). A randomized trial comparing the use of cyclosporin and methotrexate for graft-versus-host disease prophylaxis in bone marrow transplant recipients with haematologic malignancies. *Bone Marrow Transplantation*, **1**, 41–51.

Ringdén, O., Deeg, H. J., Beschorner, W. & Slavin, S. (1987*b*). Effector cells of graft-versus-host disease, host resistance and the graft-versus-leukemia effect: summary of a workshop on bone marrow transplantation. *Transplantation Proceedings*, **19**, 2758–2761.

Ringdén, O., Paulin, T., Lönnqvist, B. & Nilsson, B. (1985). An analysis of factors predisposing for chronic graft-versus-host disease. *Experimental Hematology*, **13**, 1062–1067.

Ringden, O., Pihlstedt, P., Markling, L., Aschan, J., Baryd, I., Ljungman, P., Lönnqvist, B., Tollemar, J., Janossy, G. & Sundberg, B. (1991). Prevention of graft-versus-host disease with T cell depletion or cyclosporin and methotrexate. A randomized trial in adult leukemic marrow recipients. *Bone Marrow Transplantation*, **7**, 221–226.

Ringdén, O., Zwaan, F. E., Hermans, J. & Gratwohl, A. for the Leukemia Working Party of the European Group for Bone Marrow Transplantation (1987*a*): European experience of bone marrow transplantation for leukemia. *Transplantation Proceedings*, **19**, 2600–2604.

Santos, G. W., Hess, A. D. & Vogelsang, G. B. (1985). Graft-versus-host reaction and disease. In *Immunological Reviews*, ed. G. Moller, **88**, 169–192.

Saurat, J. H., Didier-Jean, L., Gluckman, E. & Bussel, A. (1975). Graft versus host reaction and Lichen planus-like eruption in man. *British Journal of Dermatology*, **92**, 591–592.

Siena, S., Villa, S., Bonadonna, G., Bregni, M. & Gianni, A. M. (1987). Specific *ex-vivo* depletion of human bone marrow T lymphocytes by an anti-pan-T cell (CD5) ricin A-chain immunotoxin. *Transplantation*, **43**, 421–426.

Siimes, M. A., Johansson, E. & Rapola, J. (1977). Scleroderma-like graft-versus-host disease as late consequence of bone-marrow trafting. *Lancet*, **2**, 831–832.

Sondel, P.M., Bozdech, M. J., Trigg, M. E., Hong, R., Finlay, J. L., Kohler, P. C., Longo, W., Hank, J. A., Billing, R., Steeves, R. & Flynn, B. (1985). Additional immunosuppression allows engraftment following HLA-mismatched T cell-depleted bone marrow transplantation for leukemia. *Transplantation Proceedings*, **17**, 460–461.

Stong, R. C., Uckun, F., Youle, R. J., Kersey, J. H. & Vallera, D. A. (1985). Use of multiple T-cell directed intact ricin immunotoxins for autologous bone marrow transplantation. *Blood*, **66**, 627–635.

Storb, R. & Deeg, H. J. (1986). Failure of allogeneic canine marrow grafts after total body irradiation: allogeneic 'resistance' versus transfusion-induced sensitization. *Transplantation*, **42**, 571–580.

Storb, R., Deeg, H. J., Farewell, V., Doney, K., Appelbaum, F., Beatty, P., Bensinger, W., Buckner, C. D., Clift, R., Hansen, J., Hill, R., Longton, G., Lum, L., Martin, P., McGuffin, R., Sanders, J., Singer, J., Stewart, P., Sullivan, K., Witherspoon, R. and Thomas, E. D. (1986*b*). Marrow transplantation for severe aplastic anemia: methotrexate alone compared with a combination of methotrexate and cyclosporine for prevention of acute graft-versus-host disease. *Blood*, **68**, 119–125.

Storb, R., Deeg, H. J., Whitehead, J., Appelbaum, F., Beatty, P., Bensinger, W., Buckner, C. D., Clift, R., Doney, K., Farewell, V., Hansen, J., Hill, R., Lum, L., Martin, P., McGuffin, R., Sanders, J., Stewart, P., Sullivan, K., Witherspoon, R., Pharm, G. Y. & Thomas, E. D. (1986*a*). Methotrexate and cyclosporine compared with cyclosporine alone for prophylaxis of acute graft versus host disease after marrow transplantation for leukemia. *New England Journal of Medicine*, **314**, 729–735.

Storb, R., Epstein, R. B., Graham, T. C. & Thomas, E. D. (1970). Methotrexate regimens for control of graft-versus-host disease in dogs with allogeneic marrow grafts. *Transplantation*, **9**, 240–246.

Storb, R., Prentice, R. L., Thomas, E. D., Appelbaum, F. R., Deeg, H. J., Doney, K., Fefer, A., Goodell, B. W., Mickelson, E., Stewart, P., Sullivan, K. M. & Witherspoon, R. P. (1983). Factors associated with graft rejection after HLA-identical marrow transplantation for aplastic anemia. *British Journal of Haematology*, **55**, 573–585.

Storb, R., Rudolph, R. H., Graham, T. C. & Thomas, E. D. (1971). The influence of transfusions from unrelated donors upon marrow grafts between histocompatible canine siblings. *Journal of Immunology*, **107**, 409–413.

Sullivan, K. M., Deeg, H. J., Sanders, J. Klosterman, A., Amos, D., Schulman, H., Sale, G., Martin, P., Witherspoon, R., Appelbaum, F., Doney, K., Stewart, P., Meyers, J., McDonald, G. B., Weiden, P., Fefer, A., Buckner, C. D., Storb, R. & Thomas, E. D. (1986). Hyperacute graft-versus-host disease in patients not given immunosuppression after allogeneic marrow transplantation. *Blood*, **67**, 1172–1175.

Sullivan, K. M., Schulman, H. M., Storb, R., Weiden, P. L., Witherspoon, R. P., McDonald, G. B., Schubert, M. M., Atkinson, K. and Thomas, E. D. (1981). Chronic graft-versus-host disease in 52 patients: adverse natural course and successful treatment with combination immunosuppression. *Blood*, **57**, 267–276.

Sullivan, K. M., Witherspoon, R. P., Storb, R., Buckner, C. D., Sanders, J. & Thomas, E. D. (1989). Long-term results of allogeneic bone marrow transplantation. *Transplantation Proceedings*, **21**, 2926–2928.

Sullivan, K. M., Witherspoon, R. P., Storb, R., Deeg, H. J., Dahlberg, S., Sanders, J. E., Appelbaum, F. R., Doney, C., Weiden, P., Anasetti, C., Loughran, T. P., Hill, R., Shields, A., Yee, G., Schulman, H., Nims, J., Strom, S. & Thomas, E. D. (1988*b*). Alternating-day cyclosporine and prednisolone for treatment of high-risk chronic graft-v-host disease. *Blood*, **72**, 555–561.

Sullivan, K. M., Witherspoon, R. P., Storb, R., Weiden, P., Flournoy, N., Dahlberg, S., Deeg, H. J., Sanders, J. E., Doney, K. C., Applebaum, F. R., McGuffin, R., McDonald, G. B., Meyers, J., Schubert, M. M., Gaureau, J., Shulman, H. M., Sale, G. E., Anasetti, C., Loughran, T. P., Strom, S., Nims, J. & Thomas, E. D. (1988a). Prednisolone and azathioprine compared with prednisolone and placebo for treatment of chronic graft-v-host disease: prognostic influence of prolonged thrombocytopenia after allogeneic marrow transplantation. *Blood*, **72**, 546–554.

Synovec, M. S., Braddock, S. W. & Jones, J. (1990). LN-3: diagnostic adjunct in cutaneous graft-versus-host disease. *Modern Pathology*, **3**, 643–647.

Thierfelder, S., Cobbold, S. & Kummer, U. (1985). Antilymphocytic antibodies and marrow transplantation. VII. Two of nine monoclonal anti-Thy-1 antibodies used for pretreatment of donor marrow suppressed graft-versus-host reactions without added complement. *International Society for Experimental Hematology*, **13**, 948–955.

Thomas, E. D., Storb, R. & Clift, R. A. (1975). Bone-marrow transplantation I and II. *New England Journal of Medicine*, **292**, 832–843, 895–902.

Thomas, E. D. (1987). Marrow transplantation for malignant disease. *American Journal of the Medical Sciences*, **294**, 75–79.

Tiley, C., Powles, R. & Teo, C. P. (1991). Treatment of acute graft versus host disease with a murine monoclonal antibody to the IL-2 receptor. *Bone Marrow Transplantation*, **7** (Suppl. 2), 151.

Tollemar, J., Ringdén, O., Bäckman, L., Janossy, G., Lönnqvist, B., Markling, L., Philstedt, P. & Sundberg, B. (1989). Results of four different protocols for prophylaxis against graft-versus-host disease. *Transplantation Proceedings*, **21**, 3008–3010.

Trigg, M. E., Billing, R. & Sondel, P. M. (1985). Clinical trial depleting T lymphocytes from donor marrow for matched and mismatched allogeneic bone marrow transplants. *Cancer Treatment Reports*, **69**, 377–386.

Uckun, F. M., Azemove, S. M., Myers, D. E. & Vallera, D. A. (1986). Anti-CD2 (T, p50) intact ricin immunotoxins for GVHD-prophylaxis in allogeneic bone marrow transplantation. *Leukemia Research*, **10**, 145–153.

Vallera, D. A., Ash, R. C., Zanjani, E. D., Kersey, J. H., Le Bien, T. W., Beverley, P. C., Neville, D. M. Jr. & Youle, R. J. (1983). Anti-T-cell reagents for human bone marrow transplantation: Ricin linked to three monoclonal antibodies. *Science*, **222**, 512–515.

Vallera, D. A., Soderling, C. C., Carlson, G. J. & Kersey, J. H. (1981). Bone marrow transplantation across major histocompatibility barriers in mice. Effect of elimination of T cells from donor grafts by treatment with monoclonal Thy-1.2 plus complement or antibody alone. *Transplantation*, **31**, 218–222.

Vallera, D. A., Soderling, C. C. B. & Kersey, J. H. (1982). Bone marrow transplantation across major histocompatiblity barriers in mice. *Journal of Immunology*, **128**, 871–875.

Vartdal, F., Albrechtsen, D. & Ringden, O. (1987b). Immunomagnetic treatment of bone marrow allografts. *Bone Marrow Transplantation*, **2** (Suppl. 2), 94–98.

Vartdal, F., Kvalheim, G., Lea, T. E., Bosnes, V., Gaudernack, G., Ugelstad, J. & Albrechtsen, D. (1987a). Depletion of T lymphocytes from human bone marrow. *Transplantation*, **43**, 366–371.

Vogelsang, G. B., Santos, G. W., Colvin, O. M. & Chen, T. (1988). Thalidomide for graft-versus-host disease. *Lancet*, **1**, 827.

Waldmann, H., Polliak, A. & Hale, G. (1984). Elimination of graft-versus-host disease by *in vitro* depletion of alloreactive lymphocytes with a monoclonal rat anti-human lymphocyte antibody (Campath-I). *Lancet*, **2**, 483–486.

Weiden, P. L., Doney, K., Storb, R. & Thomas, E. D. (1978). Anti-human thymocyte globulin (ATG) for prophylaxis and treatment of graft-versus-host disease in recipients of allogeneic marrow grafts. *Transplantation Proceedings*, **10**, 213–6.

Weiden, P. L., Sullivan, K. M., Flournoy, N., Storb, R. & Thomas, E. D. and the Seattle Marrow Transplant Team (1981). Antileukemic effect of chronic graft-versus-host disease. Contribution to improved survival after allogeneic marrow transplantation. *New England Journal of Medicine*, **304**, 1529–1533.

Witherspoon, R. P., Storb, R., Ochs, H. D., Flournoy, N., Kopecky, K. J., Sullivan, K. M., Deeg, H. J., Sosa, R., Noel, D. R., Atkinson, K. & Thomas, E. D. (1981). Recovery of antibody production in human allogeneic marrow graft recipients: Influence of time posttransplantation, the presence or absence of chronic graft-versus-host disease, and antithymocyte globulin treatment. *Blood*, **58**, 360–368.

Zepp, F., Mannhardt, W., Duber, J., Gehler, J., Beetz, R. & Schulte-Wisserman, H. (1984). Successful bone marrow transplantation (BMT) in two patients with severe combined immunodeficiency (SCID) using SBA-lecitin and OKT-3 pretreated non-identical (unrelated) bone marrow (BM). *Experimental Hematology*, **12** (suppl. 15), 89–90.

Zwaan, F. E., Hermans, J. & Lyklema, A. (1985). Bone marrow transplantation for leukemia in Europe: Factors influencing the possibility of long-term leukemia-free survival. *Experimental Hematology*, **13** (Suppl. 17), 3–5.

12D

Monoclonal antibodies in transplantation: use as therapeutic agents in clinical organ transplantation

M. GIRAL, J. DANTAL, D. CANTAROVICH,
M. HOURMANT, R. BAATARD, B. LE MAUFF,
Y. JACQUES and J. P. SOULILLOU

12D.1 Introduction

Antibodies directed to graft recipient lymphocytes used in allograft transplantation were first restricted to rabbit anti-lymphocyte polyclonal gammaglobulins (ALG) (Monaco *et al.*, 1967; Bonneville *et al.*, 1989; Hourmant *et al.*, 1989) but now comprise a growing family of monoclonal antibodies (mab) recognizing targets not restricted to lymphocytes. ALGs are associated with side-effects (fever, serum sickness, etc.) and with a high incidence of severe opportunistic infections and lymphomas when used with other immunosuppressive drugs, particularly at the beginning of the cyclosporin A (CsA) era (Touraine *et al.*, 1985). A better knowledge of the surface membrane molecules involved in the immune response and the capacity to produce mab against a wide range of surface determinants have enabled the design of new specific and 'intelligent' means of immunosuppression.

To 1993, besides rabbit or horse ALG or antithymocyte globulins (ATG), only Ortho pan-T OKT3 (OKT3) (Ortho Multicentre Transplant Study Group, 1985) (a mouse mab directed against the ε component of the CD3 complex) has been used on a large scale in the treatment of human allograft recipients. Many other mabs directed at several different surface membrane molecules involved in immune recognition are under study in pilot or randomized trials. In this chapter, we focus on the mab that have been already used in the treatment of human allograft recipients. We also discuss the new possibilities offered by some of the mab that are still studied in experimental models as well as the new therapeutic tools that have emerged from molecular biology techniques such as chimeric or humanized mab or fusion molecules that comprise parts of the immunoglobulin (Ig) structure involved in opsonization or complement-mediated killing.

340

12D.2   Monoclonal antibodies reacting with all T lymphocytes

12D.2.1 Anti-T12 monoclonal antibody

Anti-T12 is a murine IgM mab that recognizes a 130 kDa glycoprotein (CD6) present on the cell surface membrane of mature T cells. The effect of this mab (which was one of the first studied) has been assessed in 19 acute renal rejection episodes (Kirkman *et al.*, 1983) and in a second multicentre report in 46 recipients (including the 19 previously mentioned episodes) (Milford *et al.*, 1987). The patients were treated for 7–10 days by intravenous (i.v.) infusion of 200–600 μg/kg of the mab; 43% of patients experienced an early response attributed to anti-T12 treatment alone. The graft survival rate at 1 year was the same in both anti-T12 treated patients and in all other grafts treated in these centres. Blood monitoring showed a decrease in $T12^+$ cells followed by their reappearance after 2 or 3 days of treatment, 60% of the patients treated developed an immune response against mouse immunoglobulins. This first study strongly suggested that surface membrane determinants not involved in allorecognition (Gangemi *et al.*, 1989) or effector function may not be suitable in the treatment of allograft recipients and that effort should be directed to mab that interfere with 'functional' target molecules.

12D.2.2 Anti-CD3 monoclonal antibody

OKT3 is a mouse IgG2a antibody directed against the 20 kDa glycoprotein chain of the CD3 complex (ε chain), which flanks the T cell receptor (TCR) (Ortho Multicentre Transplant Study Group, 1985). OKT3 was first used in kidney transplant patients by Cosimi *et al.*, (1981) and marketed in 1986. OKT3 is now widely recognized as a powerful immunosuppressive agent for reversing acute rejection (Vigeral *et al.*, 1986) and has been shown to be as effective as ATG in prophylactic protocols (Benvenisty *et al.*, 1990). In these studies, OKT3 was used i.v. at a daily dose of 5 mg for 10–14 days but lower doses (i.e. 22 mg over 10 days) have been reported to give good results in induction protocols of renal transplantation (Norman *et al.*, 1991). OKT3 reversed 94% of acute kidney rejection (versus 85% with high-dose steroids) (Ortho Multicentre Transplant Study Group, 1985) and was also effective in the rescue of steroid (or ATG)-resistant rejection (Oh *et al.*, 1988*a*). In kidney transplantation, the response to OKT3 occurs within 20 days after the onset of the treatment but more delayed responses were reported in cases of steroid or ATG-resistant rejection episodes (Oh *et al.*, 1988*a*). Recurrent rejection episodes were observed, however, in 66% (without CsA) (Ortho Multicentre Transplant Study Group, 1985) to 33% (with CsA) (Hricik, *et al.*, 1989) of the OKT3 treated patients.

In prophylactic protocols, cardiac transplant recipients treated with OKT3 experienced fewer acute rejection episodes during the first 3 months post-transplantation than those treated with ATG (1.5 ± 0.2 versus 2.2 ± 0.2 rejection episodes per patient) and required less chronic maintenance immunosuppression (Renlund *et al.*, 1989). A recent randomized, prospective trial in kidney transplantation showed that OKT3 and ATG produced similar results (Frey *et al.*, 1991).

OKT3 mab that recognizes the CD3-TCR complex and targets all mature T-lymphocytes, including resting T cells, is therefore more specific than ALG which also binds to monocytes, natural killer (NK) and B cells. *In vitro*, OKT3 inhibits the generation of functional effector T cells and the activity of mature cytotoxic effector lymphocytes (Chang *et al.*, 1981). Peripheral blood lymphocyte counts drop dramatically after OKT3 administration and the reappearing T lymphocytes fail to express CD3 whereas other T cell antigens are normally expressed (Chatenoud *et al.*, 1982). This modulation is reversible after the OKT3 interruption but, during the treatment, T lymphocytes cannot respond to the antigen carried by the transplant. The monitoring of CD3 treatment is based therefore on the decrease of circulating $CD3^+$ cells and, to a lesser extent, on the measurement of the OKT3 plasma levels (levels of approximately 900 ng/ml correspond to a concentration that blocks cytotoxic T cell function *in vitro*). In acute kidney rejection, there is not always a complete elimination of $CD3^+$ cells in the graft at usual OKT3 doses (Kerr & Atkins, 1989; Caillat-Zucman *et al.*, 1990), and some reports describe changes in the local T lymphocyte populations with a shift toward an increase in $CD8^+$ and $2H4^+$ cells (Chauhan *et al.*, 1990).

The major problems associated with the use of OKT3 are the severe adverse side-effects present in a majority of patients which start 45–60 min after the first two or three injections of OKT3 and last for several hours. They include high grade fever (96%), chills (57%), tremor (10%), gastrointestinal symptoms (vomiting 11%, diarrhoea 13%), pseudomeningitis and increased vascular permeability (Thistlethwaite *et al.*, 1987). OKT3 nephrotoxicity was also reported (Goldman *et al.*, 1990) with an average increase of 31% in blood creatinine levels before improvement. Pulmonary oedema is rarely seen and only in patients with previous fluid overload (Ortho Multicentre Transplant Study Group, 1985; Cosimi *et al.*, 1981); therefore, care must be taken to prepare adequately the patients prior to the first injection. It has been shown that these side-effects are related to the massive (although transient) release of cytokines such as tumour necrosis factor (TNF), interferon (IFN) gamma and interleukins (IL-2, IL-3, IL-6) (Chatenoud *et al.*, 1990) before CD3 modulation (Chatenoud *et al.*, 1988). Three main, but not mutually exclusive, mechanisms could explain this. (1) The opsonization, trapping and lympholysis of OKT3-coated T cells by macrophages with a subsequent release of cytokines; however, other anti-T cell mab do not provoke this phenomenon (anti-CD2, anti-CD4). (2) The capacity of OKT3 to induce T cell activation *in vitro* and *in vivo*. (3) The lymphokines released could, in turn, activate macrophages or

OKT3 could bridge T lymphocytes and macrophage/monocytes (via Fc receptors) resulting also in activation (Wong *et al.*, 1990). The side-effects are reduced by the administration of high-dose steroids (0.5–1 g i.v.) bolus 1 h before injection (Chatenoud *et al.*, 1991) which inhibits the transcription of the specific cytokine mRNAs. The recommended steroid dosage is 8 mg/kg 1 h before the first OKT3 injection (Goldman *et al.*, 1989). Anti-TNF mab have been shown to decrease OKT3 side-effects in mice and in humans, confirming the major involvement of TNF in this syndrome (Ferran *et al.*, 1991).

No serum sickness is observed but the xenosensitization may result in total abrogation of the mab effectiveness. Recipient anti-OKT3 (IgM and IgG) of both anti-isotype and anti-idiotype specificities are usually produced. Neutralizing antibodies are anti-idiotypic (Chatenoud *et al.*, 1986). Anti-OKT3 decreases with an increase in associated immunosuppressive treatment: 70–100% immunization was reported when OKT3 was used alone (Ortho Multicentre Transplant Study Group, 1985) compared with 25% when OKT3 was given in association with low-dose steroids and azathioprine (AZA) (Schroeder *et al.*, 1990) and 15% when a quadruple therapy was administered with CsA given at 50% of its usual maintenance dose (Hricik *et al.*, 1989). In animal studies, the concomitant use of anti-CD4 and anti-CD3 mab suppresses not only the antibody responses to the anti-CD4 mab but also that to the anti-CD3 mab (Hirsch *et al.*, 1989).

A comparison of available data concerning OKT3 and ATG shows no differences in infectious disease incidence (Frey *et al.*, 1991) while this incidence was significantly increased in OKT3 treatment compared with conventional treatment (Oh, 1988*b*). Finally, one report (Swinnen *et al.*, 1990) shows that prolonged use (or re-use) of OKT3 is associated with a dramatic increase in the incidence of lymphoproliferative disorders in cardiac transplantation (35.7% in patients who received more than 75 mg versus 6.2% of patients who received less than 75 mg). This was confirmed by other cardiac transplantation groups (Emery & Lake, 1991).

Several other mab directed also against CD3 or against TCR monomorphic epitopes have been recently tested in human kidney transplantation. While other anti-CD3 did not reduce cytokine release (Frenken *et al.*, 1991), results with mab against the TCR were promising (Waid *et al.*, 1991), showing a reversal of acute kidney rejection episodes with fewer severe side-effects than expected. This was probably related to the absence of a mitogenic effect of this mab although it does modulate the CD3-TCR complex at the T lymphocyte surface. Another anti-β TCR mab (BMA 031, a murine IgG2b) was also studied in prophylaxis but was poorly effective at the dose used (Land *et al.*, 1988). An alternative approach may be the use of F(ab')$_2$ fragments. In mice, 145 2C11 (a murine equivalent of OKT3) F(ab')$_2$ caused neither T cell activation nor an increase in animal morbidity/mortality whereas the survival of skin allografts was prolonged (Hirsch *et al.*, 1990). Moreover, recent *in-vitro* data confirm that OKT3 F(ab')$_2$ fragments cause markedly less potent T cell

activation than whole mab (Springer, 1990). Thus, these mab or the corresponding F(ab')$_2$ fragments may represent an alternative to ALG or OKT3.
The available data are so far too preliminary to draw firm conclusions.

12D.2.3 Anti-LFA1 and ICAM1 monoclonal antibodies

Cell–cell interactions that operate through a variety of molecules expressed on
the surface membrane of immunoreactive cells and their targets are necessary
for obtaining an optimal immune response. Among these, the molecules of the
integrin family are involved in the early adhesion process. They all have a
structure composed of two non-covalently linked polypeptide chains ($\alpha + \beta$)
(for review see Springer, 1990). Different subfamilies are defined by different
β chains. The $\beta 2$ chain, or CD18, can associate with one of three different α
chains (CD11 a, b or c) to constitute the LFA1, Mac 1/CR3 and p150/95
molecules, respectively. These three molecules are mainly expressed on leucocytes whereas their ligands (e.g. ICAM1 and ICAM2 for LFA1) are widely
distributed. LFA1 molecules are present on vascular endothelial cells, macrophages, monocytes and activated B lymphocytes. They are upregulated by
TNFα, IL-2 and IFN-gamma and can also be induced on fibroblasts, keratinocytes and epithelial cells. LFA1 was first defined by anti-CD11a mab which
inhibited cell–cell adhesion and several effector functions *in vitro*: CTL and
NK lysis, T-B cell cooperation leading to antibody production and T monocytes
and T vascular endothelial cell interactions. The cellular adhesion in which
LFA1 is involved enhances TCR/Ag recognition and provides auxiliary signals
for T cell activation. T cell activation leads also to an increase in cell
'adhesiveness' through conformational changes of the LFA1 molecule.

In humans, all but one study have been conducted in bone marrow transplantation (Heagy *et al.*, 1984). Fischer and colleagues have, for the first time,
successfully used a rat anti-CD11a (mab 25-3; IgG1) in children with inherited
disease to prevent rejection in HLA-mismatched bone marrow transplantation
(Fischer *et al.*, 1986). Unfortunately, this was not reproducible in leukaemic
adults receiving a T cell-depleted bone marrow transplant, with either the same
mab (Maraninchi *et al.*, 1989) or with an anti-CD18 mab (β chain) in another
pilot study (Baume, 1989). Anti-LFA1 mab 25-3 (Le Mauff *et al.*, 1991) has
recently been used in our centre in the curative treatment of initial acute
rejection episodes in seven recipients of a first kidney transplant with concurrent CsA and AZA. This anti-CD11a mab has few side-effects, except for a
transient fever after the first injection, but was not effective in six of the seven
patients treated for an ongoing acute rejection, although 25-3 circulating levels
were high. These concentrations were 3–12-fold higher than the mab dissociation constant ($K_d = 5$ nM) suggesting that this lack of effectiveness was not a
consequence of low drug concentration. Interestingly, only one patient of the
seven developed (low level) anti-25-3 IgG at day 17. This may be related to the
property of anti-CD11a to interfere in cell–cell interactions leading to antibody

production. It is possible that this antibody production is more sensitive to 25-3 than the immunological events involved in acute cellular rejection. If confirmed in further studies in humans, this property of anti-LFA1 mab, which was also observed in animals (Benjamin *et al.*, 1986), may offer a new possibility of decreasing or delaying the recipient immune response against other admin- istered mab. Although attempts to treat acute cellular rejection episodes with this anti-CD11a mab in kidney transplantation were unsuccessful, the results obtained in recipients suggest that further studies may be interesting, particu- larly in prophylaxis protocols. The combination of an anti-CD2 mab and an anti-CD11a mab is also under evaluation in bone marrow transplantation. Eight of nine patients are without rejection at 1.5–5 months and these preliminary results are encouraging (A. Fischer, personal communication).

R6.5, an anti-ICAM1 mouse IgG2 has recently been tested in cynomolgus monkey kidney and heart transplantation, in which it has been able to delay and reverse acute cellular rejection (Cosimi *et al.*, 1990). Two points were particularly interesting: (i) Anti-ICAM1 mab triggered an immune response in the primate, and (ii) although the kidney endothelial cells were covered by mab in treated animals the function of graft was unimpaired and histological examination showed no vasculitis. This mab is currently being studied in humans (B. Cosimi, personal communication).

12D.2.4 Anti-CD7 monoclonal antibody

Anti-CD7 mab recognize a 40 kDa antigen (CD7) present on T cells and preferentially on T cell blasts (Morishima *et al.*, 1982). RFT2, a mouse anti-CD7 IgG2a, has been used (Raftery *et al.*, 1985) in a prophylactic regimen in renal allograft recipients. Five milligrams per day (2–12 days) were given i.v. to five recipients, associated with conventional CsA and prednisolone immuno- suppression. No adverse effects were reported but two acute rejection episodes were noted. Lymphocyte counts decrease gradually with the presence of $CD3^+CD4^+CD8^+$, $RFT2^-$ lymphocytes and revert to pretreatment levels by day 7. Recipient anti-mouse IgG antibodies were present from approximately day 14. Additional data are expected from a multicentre trial using a chimeric anti-CD7 mab derived from the RFT2 hybridoma (Heinrich *et al.*, 1989).

12D.2.5 CBL1 monoclonal antibody

CBL1 mab (a mouse IgM) directed against a determinant present on human lymphoblast cells was used (5 mg/day for 9 days) in acute steroid-resistant rejection episodes. A beneficial effect was reported in 27 of the 30 episodes treated (Takahashi, 1983) or 50% of responsive treatment (Oei *et al.*, 1985). Despite this promising initial study, results concerning the prophylactic utiliza- tion of CBL1 mab in recipients of living, related kidney allografts were inconclusive (Takahashi *et al.*, 1985). No adverse effect was described although CBL1 mab reacted with other normal tissues (Terasaki *et al.*, 1985).

12D.2.6 Campath-I

Campath-I is a rat monoclonal IgM antibody that recognizes more than 95% of human peripheral mononuclear cells, binds human complement (Hale *et al.*, 1983) and has been shown to be effective in purging bone marrow from T cells through human complement-mediated cytotoxicity (Gazitt *et al.*, 1987; Theobald *et al.*, 1990). One pilot study (Hale *et al.*, 1986) has detailed its effect in steroid-resistant acute rejection.

Campath-I has also been administered prophylactically to 11 combined kidney/pancreas and 36 liver recipients without conclusive reduction of the rejection rate episodes (Hale *et al.*, 1986). In another randomized trial (Friend *et al.*, 1987, 1989), Campath-I has been evaluated in 52 kidney allografts. The protocol compares Campath-I (25 mg/day for 10 days) and CsA at high doses (17 mg/kg) versus CsA at high doses alone. The incidence of rejection episodes at 6 months was identical within the two groups but the incidence of major infection episodes was increased after mab treatment. No other adverse reactions were observed, although anti-rat Ig antibodies were detectable on day 10 and further increased during the next 7 days.

12D.2.7 Chal 1

Chal 1, an IgM mab (anti-T cell, anti-B cell and anti-monocyte), was given at 12–24 mg daily for 9 days in 28 renal allograft recipients during acute cortico-steroid-resistant rejection episodes (4 living related grafts, 18 first and 6 second cadaveric grafts). Fourteen cadaver recipients received CsA and prednisolone, the others received prednisolone and AZA. The reversal rate was higher among CsA-treated patients than among AZA-treated patients (81% versus 50%) (Oei *et al.*, 1985) but in this preliminary report 33% of the patients treated with Chal 1 had rejection recurrence.

12D.3   Antibodies that react against a subset of T lymphocytes

12D.3.1 Anti-CD4 monoclonal antibody

During antigen recognition by TCR, CD4 molecules on T cells bind major histocompatibility complex (MHC) class II molecules on antigen presenting cells, increasing cell–cell interactions. CD4 is also intimately involved in T cell activation or inactivation (CD4 is associated with the $p56^{lck}$, a tyrosine protein kinase) (Parnes, 1989) and may represent an original target for manipulation of the immune response. Several CD4 mab are available in various species and encouraging results have emerged from experimental organ transplantation in rodents and primates. Post-graft treatment by anti-CD4 mab in rhesus monkeys has been shown to prolong kidney graft survival (Jonker *et al.*, 1985, 1987; Cosimi *et al.*, 1991). In rodents, anti-CD4 mab were used for induction of donor-specific unresponsiveness. Survival of a second graft from the same donor strain was prolonged compared with acute rejection of a third party organ (Herbert & Roser, 1988; Shizuru *et al.*, 1990; Alters *et al.*, 1991). The mechanisms responsible for the tolerance induced by anti-CD4 mab remain, however, unclear. To date only depleting anti-CD4 mab have been used in experimental organ transplantation (non-depleting mab are under investigation). Induced tolerance may result from the emergence of new T cells that have matured in a new environmental situation (presence of graft antigens) resulting in specific inactivation of T cell clones against alloantigens.

Anti-CD4 mab may be non-immunogenic, inducing self-tolerance (Alters *et al.*, 1991; Benjamin & Waldmann, 1986). It was previously shown that concomitant injection of soluble antigen and anti-CD4 mab (or $F(ab')_2$ fragments) results in a specific, long-lasting, unresponsiveness to subsequent challenge with the same antigen (Benjamin & Waldmann, 1986; Gutstein & Wofsy, 1986). As it has been demonstrated that donor-specific blood transfusion or cells can induce specific unresponsiveness to organ allografts (Peugh *et al.*, 1988), a combined treatment with donor antigen (blood transfusion) and anti-CD4 mab before transplantation in mice has been tested and resulted in an indefinite acceptance of the graft (Wood *et al.*, 1991). The unresponsive state, however, was effective and specific only at optimal blood transfusion volume and mab dosage. In this model, non-depleting CD4 or $F(ab')_2$ fragments were also effective when given at a high dose (tenfold). Recently an anti-CD4 (BL4; IgG2a) has been used immediately after transplantation until days 3–14 in humans. This patient series was too limited to allow any definitive conclusions on the effect of BL4 on the incidence of early rejection (4 episodes in 12 patients) but only one patient developed anti-BL4 antibodies, suggesting that some anti-CD4 antibodies can mimic in humans what was observed in mice (Morel *et al.*, 1990).

12D.4 Monoclonal antibodies against interleukin-2 receptors

The availability of antibodies directed at activation determinants such as mab targeting IL-2R, offer a new possibility for more selective immunosuppression. Resting T cells do not express the functional high-affinity IL-2R. Following antigenic stimulation through the T cell receptor, specific T lymphocytes are activated (Smith, 1980); IL-2 is then secreted and functional IL-2R transiently expressed (Robb *et al.*, 1981; Cantrell & Smith, 1983). This process permits antigen-specific lymphocytes to expand. Three chains constitute the functional IL-2R. The α or Tac chain was the first component to be recognized (Leonard *et al.*, 1984; Robb & Greene, 1983; Cosman *et al.*, 1984; Nikaido *et al.*, 1984; Robb *et al.*, 1984). This 55 kDa glycoprotein is the antigen-inducible structure of the system and after antigenic stimulation its expression increases by at least tenfold (Robb *et al.*, 1981; Cantrell & Smith, 1983). This chain alone has a low affinity for IL-2 (kDa 20 nM) (Robb *et al.*, 1984) and is not able to internalize IL-2 (Weissman *et al.*, 1986). More recently, a second chain has been characterized. This β chain of 75 kDa has an intermediate affinity for IL-2, is able to internalize IL-2 and allows signal transduction. This chain is also present on resting T lymphocytes and NK cells. After antigenic stimulation, 10% of α chains associate with the β chains forming the high-affinity IL-2R (kDa 30 pM) (Sharon *et al.*, 1986; Tsudo *et al.*, 1986; Teshigawara *et al.*, 1987) that is the functional entity (this high-affinity receptor is also expressed on activated B lymphocytes and monocytes). A third component might also be implicated in the IL-2R structure: the γ chain (Edidin *et al.*, 1988; Herrmann & Diamantstein, 1988).

Mab directed at the IL-2 binding site of the α chain are potent inhibitors of IL-2-driven proliferation. Antibodies directed against the IL-2R have been demonstrated to be effective immunosuppressive agents in a variety of animal model systems and in humans. In the mouse, treatment for only 10 days results in indefinite graft survival in over 50% of recipients (Kirkman *et al.*, 1985, 1987). In the rat, anti-IL-2R antibodies have been shown to be effective as single agents and also to be synergistic with CsA (Kupiec-Weglinski *et al.*, 1986, 1988). The anti-Tac itself allows the prolongation of renal allografts in cynomolgus monkeys (Reed *et al.*, 1989).

We have characterized a rat IgG2a mab (33B3.1) which belongs to a cluster of mab that are able to inhibit IL-2 binding on both p55 and high-affinity IL-2R and to block IL-2-driven proliferation (Olive *et al.*, 1986; Le Mauff *et al.*, 1987). We then investigated the effect of this mab on the recipient's immune response to kidney transplantation (Soulillou *et al.*, 1987). In April 1987, a 43-year-old woman received, for induction treatment following cadaveric renal transplantation, the anti-I55 mab 33B3.1. Since this date, 135 recipients of first and second renal and renal/pancreas transplants have been treated with this mab at our institution.

We showed firstly, that 33B3.1 was well tolerated by almost all recipients (Soulillou *et al.*, 1987), secondly, that 5 mg/day were insufficient to obtain 'therapeutic' trough levels (Soulillou *et al.*, 1987) and, finally, that 10 mg/day were as efficient as ATG in the prevention of acute rejection episodes when given immediately after transplantation for 2 weeks in association with corticosteroids and AZA (Cantarovich *et al.*, 1988). As a result of these pilot studies, a prospective randomized controlled trial was conducted (Soulillou *et al.*, 1990).

One hundred consecutive recipients of primary cadaveric renal transplant were allocated to receive either 33B3.1 ($n = 50$) or the rabbit ATG produced by Mérieux Institut ($n = 50$). 33B3.1 was given at 10 mg/day in a saline solution administered i.v. into a peripheral vein for 10 min during the first 2 weeks after surgery (the first injection was immediately following surgery). In association with the mab, 1 mg/kg methylprednisolone and 2 mg/kg AZA were given (corticosteroids and AZA were withdrawn between days 45 and 60). At the end of the mab course (day 14), CsA was started at an oral dose of 8 mg/kg per day and then adjusted according to the trough whole blood CsA level. For rejection episodes that occurred during 33B3.1 treatment, a 7–10 day course of rabbit ATG was given, while the mab was discontinued. After day 14, rejection episodes were treated with daily i.v. infusions of methylprednisolone. The 50 recipients randomly assigned to received ATG were given the same immuno-suppressive regimen. For rejection episodes during or after the ATG course, corticosteroid pulses were given.

Only one patient from the 50 patients treated with 33B3.1 required drug interruption because of major clinical intolerance versus 32% of patients in the ATG group. A similar number of rejection episodes was observed during the first 3 months (15 versus 12 in 33B3.1 and ATG group, respectively). The 33B3.1-treated recipients experienced more rejection episodes during the first 2 weeks (6 versus 1). In both of the two groups, subacute vascular or hyperacute rejection episodes were noted. Only one patient in the 33B3.1 group (and none in the ATG group) had a rebound rejection during the first 3 months. Thereafter, between months 4 and 12, seven patients in the ATG group experienced a total of nine rejection episodes and three patients in the mab group experienced three rejection episodes (difference not significant). After the first year, the incidence of rejection episodes was 5% in both groups of patients.

Fewer episodes of infection were observed in the 33B3.1 group than in the ATG one (47 versus 72). Regarding viral infections, eight of the nine cases of cytomegalovirus (CMV) disease in the mab group were mild whereas half were severe in the ATG group. After the third month, the number of infectious episodes remained statistically lower in patients who received mab compared with those treated with ATG (9 versus 23). As during the first 3 months, the difference was essentially due to the increased incidence of urinary tract infections occurring in patients who received ATG.

Patient survival was 96% in both groups at 1 year and 94 and 96% at 2 years in 33B3.1 and ATG groups, respectively. Graft survival was 85% in both groups at 1 year and 80 and 82% at 2 years in the 33B3.1 and ATG groups, respectively. Graft survival was 85% in both groups at 1 year and 80 and 82% at 2 years in the 33B3.1 and ATG groups, respectively.

Trough levels of 33B3.1 have been determined in pilot and randomized studies. The results clearly demonstrated a different bioavailability between the two doses: with 5 mg/day, trough levels were below 0.5 μg/ml and with 10 mg/day they reached a mean level of 4 μg/ml.

A classical pattern of immunization against the xenogeneic protein was observed: 80% of patients had developed anti-33B3.1 antibodies at day 20. An anti-idiotype response was detected more than 7 days after the end of treatment; however, the trough levels seem to be impaired by the host response, as patients with anti-rat antibodies before the end of mab treatment had significantly lower circulating mab levels.

Similar good results have been obtained following renal retransplantation (M. Hourmant, unpublished data) and simultaneous renal/pancreas transplantation (Cantarovich et al., 1992); both randomized trials are in current study.

Almost all of the second renal transplants were carried out in hypersensitized patients. Compared with ATG immunoprophylaxis (15 recipients in each group), the induction therapy with 33B3.1 for the first 10 post-operative days, in association with corticosteroids and AZA (CsA was started at day 10), achieved similar patient and transplant survival rates: one patient died in each group; 1-year renal survival of 77 and 71% in ATG and 33B3.1 groups, respectively. The incidence of rejection episodes was similar under both regimens (45 and 44%).

Following simultaneous pancreas and renal transplant, excellent results were obtained. All type 1 diabetic uraemic recipients ($n = 35$) received segmental neoprene-occluded pancreatic transplants and were transplanted without regard to tissue matching. 33B3.1 (17 patients) and ATG (18 patients) were given for induction treatment, in association with corticosteroids, AZA and CsA. No differences were seen in the incidence of rejection episodes (58% in 33B3.1-treated patients versus 33% in ATG patients; all were restricted to the kidney and none was during bioreagent treatment), patient survival (83 and 100% in ATG and 33B3.1 groups, respectively) and transplant survival (pancreas 72 and 70%, kidney 78 and 100% in ATG and 33B3.1 groups, respectively).

As a result of the efficacy of the 33B3.1 mab in the prevention of rejection episodes and the capacity to reverse ongoing rejection in animals, we undertook a pilot study to assess the effect of 33B3.1 in the treatment of 10 cellular acute active rejection episodes (Cantarovich et al., 1989). Six episodes were reversed and four required rescue treatment. Several hypotheses can explain this partial failure, principally the fact that the mab was given too late, after effector cells had already proliferated and expanded within the transplant.

Other clinical trials have been performed following renal transplantation with different anti-p55 mab. Recently, Kirkman et al. (1991), reported a randomized trial of anti-Tac, a murine IgG2a mab directed against the p55 chain of the human IL-2R, in human renal transplantation. As in our trial, anti-Tac mab was given for induction therapy but in combination with CsA, steroids and AZA. The results also confirm the ability of anti-Tac to prevent early renal allograft rejection. Another rat IgG2b anti-IL-2R mab (Campath-6) was given with success as a part of a quadruple immunosuppressive therapy after human liver transplantation. The prophylactic use of this mab results in a reduction in the incidence and severity of rejection. Current studies are to test the efficacy of a rat IgG2b mab directed to the human IL-2R 55 kDa chain (LOTAC-1) and a mouse IgG1 mab also directed against the α chain of the human IL-2R (BT563) in renal and liver transplantation. Preliminary data seem to confirm their efficacy in preventing both renal and liver rejection episodes and with reasonably good clinical tolerance.

All these trials, including those in marrow transplantation and type 1 diabetes, confirm the main interest of targeting IL-2R$^+$ cells. Several improvements are necessary, however, to decrease host immunization against the mab (humanized bioreagents). Furthermore, combinations of mab against different clusters might ameliorate clinical results.

12D.5   Engineered monoclonal antibody molecules: chimeric, 'humanized' and fusion proteins

The use of murine mab is severely restricted by their immunogenicity. To avoid this, genetic engineering allows the production of constructs aimed at eliminating foreign sequences of the mab (Rodwell, 1989; Co & Queen, 1991; Chapters 7 and 8). For example, chimeric antibodies were obtained by the fusion of rearranged murine DNA encoding specific VH and VL regions of mab, with DNA encoding human CH and CL regions. The resulting antibody combines the entire variable region (V) binding domain of the foreign (rodent) antibody with the human antibody constant (C) domain. Unfortunately, the V region framework may have residual immunogenicity (Jaffers *et al.*, 1986).

Alternatively, it is now possible to place the six murine complementary regions (CDRs or hypervariable regions) involved in the binding site of the antigen, into the human V region framework. This characterizes the 'humanized' or 'reshaped' antibodies (Rodwell, 1989; Co & Queen, 1991; Winter & Milstein, 1991). Both humanized and chimeric antibodies retain the human effector region (Fc) and are less immunogenic; however, anti-idiotypic immunization is still possible (Riechmann *et al.*, 1988).

Queen *et al.* (1989) have produced chimeric and humanized anti-Tac antibody using computerized modelling to identify several framework amino acids in the rodent mab which they introduced together with the CDRs into the human framework allowing a better conformation for the antigen-binding site. The resulting affinity of this engineered mab for the IL-2 receptor is 3×10^9 M^{-1}, around one-third of the affinity of the original mouse anti-Tac. In animal studies, this chimeric mab prolonged primate cardiac allograft survival and was less immunogenic than the rodent anti-Tac (Brown *et al.*, 1991). A humanized Campath-I has been obtained by Riechman *et al.* (1988). This mab was more efficient in complement-mediated cell lysis (using a B cell leukaemia target) than the original Campath-I. Finally, Heinrich *et al.* (1989) have produced a chimeric CD7 mab (SHEET) which is currently being used in clinical studies (see above).

Genetic engineering can also provide alternative molecules to obtain fully humanized reagents that contain specific constant region components from IgG or IgM (CH2—CH3 or CH2—CH4, respectively). Such human cDNA sequences can be fused to other cDNAs coding for molecules that will target the resulting fusion protein to a membrane receptor; for example human cytokines, such as IL-2 or adhesion molecules, can be used in these fusion proteins. Recently, a fusion molecule between human IL-2 and IgG constant sequences has been shown to interact specifically with IL-2 receptor-bearing cells and to induce complement-mediated killing (Landolfi, 1991). Moreover, the use of the IgM heavy chain can provide multimeric fusion molecules that can activate complement-mediated killing but which may also be able to inhibit internalization of the ligand-receptor complex and its resulting signal (Kumar *et al.*, 1987).

Milstein & Cuello (1983) described the procedure to produce bispecific mab that hybridize immunoglobulins with two different antigen-binding sites. Bispecific antibodies may have, for instance, one Fab arm with an anti-toxin specificity and the other Fab arm with an anti-cell marker specificity. The toxin could then be delivered to the target cells after the mab has bound to the specific target cell. (For further details of bispecific antibodies see Chapter 6 and for details of antibody engineering see Chapters 7 and 8).

12D.6 Comments

ATG has been well recognized as being effective in the prevention or treatment of rejection; however, several disadvantages are associated with the use of polyclonal sera. These include variability between batches, reactivity with antigen unrelated to lymphocytes and serum sickness. Mab therapy should circumvent these problems as they have a single defined specificity, a unique target and are used at low doses (no serum sickness); in addition their effectiveness can be followed using specific monitoring.

The prophylactic use of mab focuses on the prevention of the recipient's immune response during the first days after transplantation. This scheme allows the introduction of CsA in kidney transplantation to be delayed until a stable graft function is obtained. Most mab are targeted at all T lymphocytes (as is ALG), irrespective of the specific allorecognition determined by the TCR. OKT3 is very powerful but its use is limited by a risk of over-immunosuppression when administered to patients without high immunological risk (e.g. first graft in a non-responding patient), with an increased incidence in infectious episodes and lymphoproliferative disorders and important side-effects which cannot be controlled by the use of high doses of steroids (raising the immunosuppression) without consequences. The new generation of anti-TCRβ mab which do not stimulate T cells may help to circumvent these side-effects, if their effectiveness is confirmed.

Another approach discriminates specific anti-donor cells (less than 1% of the total lymphocyte pool as assessed by limiting dilution assay). Under normal conditions, donor tissue antigens are the major stimulus after transplantation. IL-2R (p55) was a good target candidate in this strategy as it is only expressed after antigenic stimulation in the first steps of the clonal expansion of alloreactive cells. In practice, it seems that this 'anti-donor specificity' is operational as shown by the first clinical studies obtained with 33V3.1, a rat IgG2a. It is possible that the graft could have carried over CMV infections with this therapeutic approach. The strategy faces problems of a possibly completely different nature in the indication of ongoing rejection. In this situation, clearly expanding T lymphocytes have accumulated in the rejecting graft and have recruited many non-specific effector cells (lymphocytes/monocytes/macrophages) which represent the majority of graft infiltrating cells. At this stage it is probably insufficient to target donor-specific cells, as shown from the 33B3.1 study. Efficient immunointervention may require interaction with all lymphocytes and with non-lymphoid cells. In keeping only with reagents related to immunoglobulin, other means of immunocompetent cell targeting are also promising. Firstly, a combination of two mab targeting functionally related molecules such as the combination of anti-p55 with anti-p55 (Tsudo *et al.*, 1989) that produced a synergistic effect *in vivo* (Audrain *et al.*, 1991). Such a combination of these two mab may be more effective on high affinity IL-2R$^+$ cells in clinical practice. Other approaches are hybrid dimeric mab, fusion molecules and chimeric or CDR engineered mab such as constructs comprising human IL-2 and the constant part of human Ig.

Other possibilities arise from the observation that certain mab, such as anti-LFA1 or anti-CD4, may prevent the recipient's immune response against the mab itself. If not powerful when used alone, these mab may be of interest in association with other immunosuppressively effective but immunogenic mab.

Finally, although the cost of these new strategies offered by bioreagents is considerable and their efficacy in the clinic not yet fully assessed, they are nevertheless promising and far from being completely explored. Clinical trials are critically needed to define the molecules that will be, in the future, the targets of choice in immunointervention. Ultimately, these new therapeutic molecules (mab, chimeric or 'humanized' mab, fusion proteins) should make 'intelligent' and specific targeting possible in the clinic and may also lead to the development of new bioreagents, such as molecular antagonists.

12D.7 Acknowledgements

We are grateful to Ms Aline Bertho for excellent secretarial assistance.

12D.8 References

Alters, S. E., Shizuru, J. A., Ackerman, J., Grossman, D., Seydel, K. B. & Fathman, C. G. (1991). Anti-CD4 mediates clonal energy during transplantation tolerance induction. *Journal of Experimental Medicine*, **173**, 491–494.

Audrain, M., Boeffard, F., Soulillou, J. P. & Jacques, Y. (1991). Synergistic action of monoclonal antibodies directed at p55 and p75 chains of the human IL-2 receptor. *Journal of Immunology*, **146**, 884–892.

Baume, D., Kuentz, M., Pico, J. L., Beaujean, F., Cordonnier, C., Vernant, J. P., Hayat, M. & Bernard, A. (1989). Failure of a CD18/anti-LFA1 monoclonal antibody infusion to prevent graft rejection in leukemic patients receiving T-depleted allogeneic bone marrow transplantation. *Transplantation*, **47**, 472–474.

Benjamin, R. J., Cobbold, S. P., Clark, M. R. & Waldmann, H. (1986). Tolerance to rat monoclonal antibodies. Implications for serotherapy. *Journal of Experimental Medicine*, **163**, 1539–1552.

Benjamin, R. J. & Waldmann, H. (1986). Induction of tolerance by monoclonal antibody therapy. *Nature*, **320**, 449–451.

Benvenisty, A. I., Cohen, D., Stegall, M. D. & Hardy, M. A. (1990). Improved results using OKT3 as induction immunosuppression in renal allograft recipients with delayed graft function. *Transplantation*, **49**, 321–327.

Bonneville, M., Carcagne, J., Vie, H., Moreau, J. F., Chevalier, S., Latour, M., Carosella, E. & Soulillou, J. P. (1989). Polyclonal rabbit gamma globulins against a human cytotoxic CD4$^+$ T cell clone. I. Clone characteristics and antiblast globulin preparation (published erratum appears in *Transplantation*, 1990, **49**, 664). *Transplantation*, **48**, 253–260.

Brown, P. S., Jr, Parenteau, G. L., Dirbas, F.M., Garsia, R. J., Goldman, C. K., Bukowski, M. A., Junghans, R. P., Queen, C., Hakimi, J., Benjamin, W. R., Clark, R. E. & Waldman, H. (1991). Anti-Tac-H, a humanized antibody to the interleukin 2 receptor, prolongs primate cardiac allograft survival. *Proceedings of the National Academy of Sciences of the U.S.A.*, **88**, 2663–2667.

Caillat-Zucman, S., Blumenfeld, N., Legendre, C., Noel, L. H., Bach, J. F., Kreis, H. & Chatenoud, L. (1990). The OKT3 immunosuppressive effect. *In situ* antigenic modulation of human graft-infiltrating T cells. *Transplantation*, **49**, 156–160.

Cantarovich, D., Le Mauff, B., Hourmant, M., Giral, M., Denis, M., Hirn, M., Jacques, Y. & Soulillou, J. P. (1989). Anti-interleukin 2 receptor monoclonal antibody in the treatment of ongoing acute rejection episodes of human kidney graft: a pilot study. *Transplantation*, **47**, 454–457.

Cantarovich, D., Le Mauff, B., Hourmant, M., Giral, M., Denis, M., Hirn, M., Jacques, Y. & Soulillou, J. P. (1992). Randomized trial of induction immunosuppression with anti-IL-2R monoclonal antibody 33B3.1 and rabbit antithymocyte globulin following simultaneous pancreas and kidney transplantation. *Transplantation Proceedings*, **24**, 911.

Cantarovich, D., Le Mauff, B., Hourmant, M., Peyronnet, P., Jacques, Y., Boeffard, F., Hirn, M. & Soulillou, J. P. (1988). Prophylactic use of a monoclonal antibody (33B3.1) directed against interleukin 2 receptor following human renal transplantation. *American Journal of Kidney Disease*, **11**, 101–106.

Cantrell, D. A. & Smith, K. A. (1983). Transient expression of interleukin 2 receptors. Consequences for T cell growth. *Journal of Experimental Medicine*, **158**, 1895–1911.

Chang, T. W., Kung, P. C., Gingras, S. P. & Goldstein, G. (1981). Does OKT3 monoclonal antibody react with an antigen-recognition structure on human T cells? *Proceedings of the National Academy of Sciences of the U.S.A.*, **78**, 1805–1808.

Chatenoud, L., Baudrihaye, M. F., Kreis, H., Goldstein, G., Schindler, J. & Bach, J. F. (1982). Human *in vivo* antigenic modulation induced by the anti-T cell OKT3 monoclonal antibody. *European Journal of Immunology*, **12**, 979–982.

Chatenoud, L., Ferran, C., Legendre, C., Renter, A., Franchimont, P., Dreis, H. & Bach, J. F. (1988). Clinical use of OKT3: the role of cytokine release and xenosensitization. *Journal of Autoimmunity*, **1**, 631–635.

Chatenoud, L., Ferran, C., Legendre, C., Thouard, I., Merite, S., Reuter, A., Gevaert, Y., Kreis, H., Franchimont, P. & Bach, J. F. (1990). *In vivo* cell activation following OKT3 administration. Systemic cytokine release and modulation by corticosteroids. *Transplantation*, **49**, 697–702.

Chatenoud, L., Jonker, M., Villemain, F., Goldstein, G. & Bach, J. F. (1986). The human immune response to the OKT3 monoclonal antibody is oligoclonal. *Science*, **232**, 1406–1408.

Chatenoud, L., Legendre, C., Ferran, C., Bach, J. F. & Kreis, H. (1991). Cortico-steroid inhibition of the OKT3-induced cytokine-related syndrome: dosage and kinetics prerequisites. *Transplantation*, **51**, 334–338.

Chauhan, B., Mohanakumar, T. & Flye, M. W. (1990). Immunohistological analysis of T lymphocyte subpopulations in needle core biopsies from OKT3-treated renal allograft recipients. *Transplantation*, **50**, 1058–1060.

Co., M. S. & Queen, C. (1991). Humanized antibodies for therapy. *Nature*, **351**, 501–502.

Cosimi, A. B., Burton, R. C., Colvin, R. B., Goldstein, G., Delmonico, F. L., LaQuaglia, M. P., Tolkoff-Rubin, N., Rubin, R. H., Herrin, J. T. & Russell, P. S. (1981). Treatment of acute renal allograft rejection with OKT3 monoclonal anti-body. *Transplantation*, **32**, 535–539.

Cosimi, A. B., Conti, D., Delmonico, F. L., Preffer, F. I., Wee, S. L., Rothlein, R., Faanes, R. & Colvin, R. B. (1990). *In vivo* effects of monoclonal antibody to ICAM-1 (CD54) in nonhuman primates with renal allografts. *Journal of Immuno-logy*, **144**, 4604–4612.

Cosimi, A. B., Delmonico, F. L., Wright, J. K., Wee, S. L., Preffer, F. I., Bedle, M. & Colvin, R. B. (1991). OKT4A monoclonal antibody immunosuppression of cynomologus renal allograft recipients. *Transplantation Proceedings*, **23**, 501–503.

Cosman, D., Cerretti, D. P., Larsen, A., Park, L., March, C., Dower, S., Gillis, S. & Urdal, D. (1984). Cloning, sequence and expression of human interleukin-2 receptor. *Nature*, **312**, 768–771.

Edidin, M., Aszalos, A., Damjanovich, S. & Waldmann, T. A. (1988). Lateral diffusion measurements give evidence for association of the Tac peptide of the IL-2 receptor with the T27 peptide in the plasma membrane of HUT-102-B2 T cells. *Journal of Immunology*, **141**, 1206–1210.

Emery, R. W. & Lake, K. D. (1991). Post-transplantation lymphoproliferative disorder and OKT3. *New England Journal of Medicine*, **324**, 1437–1441.

Ferran, C., Sheehan, K., Schreiber, R., Bach, J. F. & Chatenoud, L. (1991). Anti-TNF abrogates the cytokine-related anti-CD3 induced syndrome. *Transplantation Proceedings*, **23**, 849–850.

Fischer, A., Griscelli, C., Blanche, S., Le Deist, F., Veber, F., Lopez, M., Delaage, M., Olive, D., Mawas, C. & Janossy, G. (1986). Prevention of graft failure by an anti-HLFA-1 monoclonal antibody in HLA-mismatched bone marrow transplant-ation. *Lancet*, **2**, 1058–1061.

Frenken, L. A., Hoitsma, A. J., Tax, W. J. & Koene, R. A. (1991). Prophylactic use of anti-CD3 monoclonal antibody WT32 in kidney transplantation. *Transplantation Proceedings*, **23**, 1072–1073.

Frey, D. J., Matas, A. J., Gillingham, K. J., Canafax, D., Payne, W. D., Dunn, D. L., Sutherland, D. E. & Najarian, J. S. (1991). MALG versus OKT3 following renal transplantation: a randomized prospective trial. *Transplantation Proceedings*, **23**, 1048–1049.

Friend, P. J., Calne, R. Y., Hale, G., Waldmann, H., Evans, D. B., Rolles, K., Thiru, S. & Gore, S. (1987). Prophylactic use of an antilymphocyte monoclonal antibody following renal transplantation: a randomized controlled trial. *Transplantation Proceedings*, **19**, 1898–1900.

Friend, P. J., Hale, G., Waldmann, H., Gore, S., Thiru, S., Joysey, V., Evans, D. B. &

Calne, R. Y. (1989). Campath-IM: prophylactic use after kidney transplantation. A randomized controlled clinical trial. *Transplantation*, **48**, 248–253.

Gangemi, R. M., Swack, J. A., Gaviria, D. M. & Romain, P. L. (1989). Anti-T12, an anti-CD6 monoclonal antibody, can activate human T lymphocytes. *Journal of Immunology*, **143**, 2439–2447.

Gazitt, Y., Or, R., Mumcuoglu, M. & Slavin, S. (1987). Monoclonal rat anti-human lymphocyte antibody Campath-I binds to T and B lymphocytes but effectively lyses only T cells. *Bone Marrow Transplantation*, **2**, 427–433.

Goldman, M., Abramowicz, D., De Pauw, L., Alegre, M. L., Widera, I., Vereer-straeten, P. & Kinnaert, P. (1989). OKT3-induced cytokine release attenuation by high-dose methylprednisolone *Lancet*, **2**, 802–803 (letter).

Goldman, M., van Laethem, J. L., Abramowicz, D., De Pauw, L., Kinnaert, P. & Vereerstraeten, P. (1990). Evolution of renal function during treatment of kidney graft rejection with OKT3 monoclonal antibody. *Transplantation*, **50**, 158–159.

Gutstein, M. L. & Wofsy, D. (1986). Administration of F(ab')$_2$ fragments of monoclonal antibody to L3T4 inhibits humoral immunity in mice without depleting L3T4$^+$ cells. *Journal of Immunology*, **137**, 3414–3419.

Hale, G., Bright, S., Chumbley, G., Hoang, T., Metcalf, D., Munro, A. J. & Waldmann, H. (1983). Removal of T cells from bone marrow for transplantation: a monoclonal antilymphocyte antibody that fixes human complement. *Blood*, **62**, 873–882.

Hale, G., Waldmann, H., Friend, P. & Calne, R. (1986). Pilot study of Campath-I, a rat monoclonal antibody that fixes human complement, as an immunosuppressant in organ transplantation. *Transplantation*, **42**, 308–311.

Heagy, W., Walterbangh, C. & Martz, E. (1984). Potent ability of anti-LFA-1 mono-clonal antibody to prolong allograft survival. *Transplantation*, **37**, 520–523.

Heinrich, G., Gram, H., Kocher, H. P., Schreier, M. H., Ryffel, B., Akbar, A., Amlot, P. L. & Janossy, G. (1989). Characterization of a human T cell-specific chimeric antibody (CD7) with human constant and mouse variable regions. *Journal of Immunology*, **143**, 3589–3597.

Herbert, J. & Roser, B. (1988). Strategies of monoclonal antibody therapy that induce permanent tolerance of organ transplants. *Transplantation*, **46**, 128S–134S.

Herrmann, T. & Diamantstein, T. (1988). The high affinity interleukin 2 receptor: evidence for three distinct polypeptide chains comprising the high affinity inter-leukin 2 receptor. *Molecular Immunology*, **25**, 1201–1207.

Hirsch, R., Bluestone, J. A., DeNenno, L. & Gress, R. E. (1990). Anti-CD3 F(ab')$_2$ fragments are immunosuppressive *in vivo* without evoking either the strong humoral response or morbidity associated with whole mab. *Transplantation*, **49**, 1117–1123.

Hirsch, R., Chatenoud, L., Gress, R. E., Sachs, D. H., Bach, J. F. & Bluestone, J. A. (1989). Suppression of the humoral response to anti-CD3 monoclonal antibody. *Transplantation*, **47**, 853–857.

Hourmant, M., Babinet, F., Cantarovich, D., Latour, M., Carcagne, J., Vie, H., Bonneville, M., Moreau, J. F., Carosella, E., Bignon, J. D., & Soulillou, J. P. (1989). Polyclonal rabbit gamma globulins against a human cytotoxic CD4 T cell clone. II. Use in prevention of rejection in kidney transplantation: a pilot study. *Transplantation*, **48**, 260–263.

Hricik, D. E., Zarconi, J. & Schulak, J. A. (1989) Influence of low-dose cyclosporine on the outcome of treatment with OKT3 for acute renal allograft rejection. *Trans-plantation*, **47**, 272–7.

Jaffers, G. J., Fuller, T. C., Cosimi, A. B., Russell, P. S., Winn, H. J. & Colvin, R. B. (1986). Monoclonal antibody therapy. Anti-idiotypic and non-anti-idiotypic antibodies to OKT3 arising despite intense immunosuppression. *Transplantation*, **41**, 572–578.

Jonker, M., Neuhaus, P., Zurcher, C., Fucello, A. & Goldstein, G. (1985). OKT4 and OKT4A antibody treatment as immunosuppression for kidney transplantation in rhesus monkeys. *Transplantation*, **39**, 247–253.

Jonker, M., Nooij, F. J. & Steinhof, G. (1987) Effects of CD4 and CD8 specific monoclonal antibodies *in vitro* and *in vivo* on T cells and their relation to the allograft response in rhesus monkeys. *Transplantation Proceedings*, **19**, 4308–4314.

Kerr, P. G. & Atkins, R. C. (1989). The effects of OKT3 therapy on infiltrating lymphocytes in rejecting renal allografts. *Transplantation*, **48**, 33–36.

Kirkman, R. L., Araujo, J. L., Busch, G. J., Carpenter, C. B., Milford, E. L., Reinherz, E. L., Schlossman, S. F., Strom, T. B. & Tilney, N. L. (1983) Treatment of acute renal allograft rejection with monoclonal anti-T12 antibody. *Transplantation*, **36**, 620–626.

Kirkman, R. L., Barrett, L. V., Gaulton, G. N., Kelley, V. E., Ythier, A. & Strom, T. B. (1985). Administration of an anti-interleukin 2 receptor monoclonal antibody prolongs cardiac allograft survival in mice. *Journal of Experimental Medicine*, **162**, 358–362.

Kirkman, R. L., Barrett, L. V., Koltun, W. A. & Diamantstein, T. (1987). Prolongation of murine cardiac allograft survival by the anti-interleukin-2 receptor monoclonal antibody AMT-13. *Transplantation Proceedings*, **19**, 618–619.

Kirkman, R. L., Shapiro, M. E., Carpenter, C. B., McKay, D. B., Milford, E. L., Ramos, E. L., Tilney, N. L., Waldmann, T. A., Zimmerman, C. E. & Strom, T. B. (1991). A randomized prospective trial of anti-Tac monoclonal antibody in human renal transplantation. *Transplantation*, **51**, 107–113.

Kumar, A., Moreau, J. L., Gibert, M. & Theze, J. (1987). Internalization of interleukin 2 (IL-2) by high affinity IL-2 receptors is required for the growth of IL-2-dependent T cell lines. *Journal of Immunology*, **139**, 3680–3684.

Kupiec-Weglinski, J. W., Diamantstein, T., Tilney, N. L. & Strom, T. B. (1986). Therapy with monoclonal antibody to interleukin 2 receptor spares suppressor T cells and prevents or reverses acute allograft rejection in rats. *Proceedings of the National Academy of Sciences of the U.S.A.*, **83**, 2624–2627.

Kupiec-Weglinski, J. W., Hahn, H. J., Kirkman, R. L., Volk, H. D., Mouzaki, A., DiStefano, R., Tellides, G., Dallman, M., Morris, P. J. & Strom, T. B. (1988). Cyclosporine potentiates the immunosuppressive effects of anti-interleukin 2 receptor monoclonal antibody therapy. *Transplantation Proceedings*, **20**, 207–216.

Land, W., Hillebrand, G., Illner, W. D., Abendroth, D., Hancke, E., Schleibner, S., Hammer, C. & Racenberg, J. (1988). First clinical experience with a new TCR/CD3-monoclonal antibody (BMA 031) in kidney transplant patients. *Transplant International*, **1**, 116–117 (letter).

Landolfi, N. F. (1991). A chimeric IL-2/Ig molecule possesses the functional activity of both proteins. *Journal of Immunology*, **146**, 915–919.

Le Mauff, B., Hourmant, M., Rougier, J. P., Hirn, M., Dantal, J., Baatard, R., Cantarovich, D., Jacques, Y. & Soulillou, J. P. (1991). Effect of anti-LFA1 (CD11a) monoclonal antibodies in acute rejection in human kidney transplantation. *Transplantation*, **52**, 291–296.

Le Mauff, B., Gascan, H., Olive, D., Moreau, J. F., Mawas, C., Soulillou, J. P. & Jacques, Y. (1987). Parameters of interaction of a novel monoclonal antibody (33B3.1) with the human IL2-receptors: interrelationship between 33B3.1, anti-Tac, and IL2 binding sites. *Human Immunology*, **19**, 53–68.

Leonard, W. J., Depper, J. M., Crabtree, G. R., Rudikoff, S., Pumphrey, J., Robb, R. J., Kronke, M., Svetlik, P. B., Peffer, N. J., Waldmann, T. A. &

Greene, W. C. (1984). Molecular cloning and expression of cDNAs for the human interleukin-2 receptor. *Nature*, **311**, 626–631.

Maraninchi, D., Mawas, C., Stoppa, A. M., Gaspard, M. H., Marit, G., van Ekthoven, A., Reiffers, J., Olive, D., Hirn, M., Delaage, M., Burgues, F. & Laurent, G. (1989). Anti LFA1 monoclonal antibody for the prevention of graft rejection after T cell-depleted HLA-matched bone marrow transplantation for leukemia in adults. *Bone Marrow Transplantation*, **4**, 147–150.

Milford, E. L., Carpenter, C. B., Kirkman, R. L., Tilney, N. L., Mazoujian, G., Strom, T. B., Lazarus, J. M., Schlossman, S. F., Guttman, R. D., Lowry, R., Rocher, L., Campbell, D. A., Salomon, D. R. & Pfaff, W. W. (1987). Anti-T12 monoclonal antibody therapy of acute renal allograft rejection. *Transplantation Proceedings*, **19**, 1910.

Milstein, C. & Cuello, A. C. (1983). Hybrid hybridomas and their use in immunohisto-chemistry. *Nature*, **305**, 537–540.

Monaco, A. P., Wood, M. L. & Russell, P. S. (1967). Some effects of purified hetero-logous antihuman lymphocyte serum in man. *Transplantation*, **5**, 1106–1114.

Morel, P., Vincent, C., Cordier, G., Panaye, G., Carosella, E. & Revillard, J. P. (1990). Anti-CD4 monoclonal antibody administration in renal transplanted patients. *Clinical Immunology and Immunopathology*, **56**, 311–322.

Morishima, Y., Kobayashi, M., Yang, S. Y., Collins, N. H., Hoffmann, M. K. & Dupont, B. (1982). Functionally different T lymphocyte subpopulations determined by their sensitivity to complement-dependent cell lysis with the monoclonal antibody 4A. *Journal of Immunology*, **129**, 1091–1098.

Nikaido, T., Shimizu, A., Ishida, N., Sabe, H., Teshigawara, K., Maeda, M., Uchiyama, T., Yodoi, J. & Honjo, T. (1984). Molecular cloning of cDNA encoding human interleukin-2 receptor. *Nature*, **311**, 631–635.

Norman, D. J., Barry, J. M., Bennett, W. M., Munson, J. L., Meyer, M., Henell, K., Kimball, J. & Hubert, B. (1991). OKT3 for induction immunosuppression in renal transplantation: a comparative study of high versus low doses. *Transplantation Proceedings*, **23**, 1052–1054.

Oei, J., Cicciarelli, J., Terasaki, P., Hardiwidjaja, S. & Mendez, R. (1985). Treatment of kidney graft rejection with CHAL1 and CBL1 monoclonal antibodies. *Transplantation Proceedings*, **17**, 2740–2741.

Oh, C. S., Sollinger, H. W., Stratta, R. J., Kalayoglu, M. & Belzer, F. O. (1988*a*). Delayed response to orthoclone OKT3 treatment for renal allograft rejection resistant to steroid and antilymphocyte globulin. *Transplantation*, **45**, 65–67.

Oh, C. S., Stratta, R. J., Fox, B. C., Sollinger, H. W., Belzer, F. O. & Maki, D. G. (1988*b*). Increased infections associated with the use of OKT3 for treatment of steroid-resistant rejection in renal transplantation. *Transplantation*, **45**, 68–73.

Olive, D., Raymond, J., Dubreuil, P., Charmot, D., Jacques, Y. & Mawas, C. (1986). Anti-interleukin 2 receptor monoclonal antibodies. Respective role of epitope mapping and monoclonal antibody-receptor interactions in their antagonist effects on interleukin 2-dependent T cell growth. *European Journal of Immunology*, **16**, 611–616.

Ortho Multicenter Transplant Study Group. (1985). A randomized clinical trial of OKT3 monoclonal antibody for acute rejection of cadaveric renal transplants. *New England Journal of Medicine*, **313**, 337–342.

Parnes, J. R. (1989). Molecular biology and function of CD4 and CD8. *Advances in Immunology*, **44**, 265–311.

Peugh, W. N., Wood, K. J. & Morris, P. J. (1988). Genetic aspects of the blood trans-fusion effect. *Transplantation*, **46**, 438–443.

Queen, C., Schneider, W. P., Selick, H. E., Payne, P. W., Landolfi, N. F.,

Duncan, J. F., Avdalovic, N. M., Levitt, M., Junghans, R. P. & Waldmann, T. A. (1989). A humanized antibody that binds to the interleukin 2 receptor. *Proceedings of the National Academy of Sciences of the U.S.A.*, **86**, 10029–10033.

Raftery, M. J., Lang, C. J., Ivory, K., Sweny, P., Fernando, O. N., Moorhead, J. F. & Janossy, G. (1985). Use of RFT2 (CD7) monoclonal antibody as prophylaxis against renal allograft refection. *Transplantation Proceedings*, **17**, 2737–2738.

Reed, M. H., Shapiro, M. E., Strom, T. B., Milford, E. L., Carpenter, C. B., Weinberg, D. S., Reimann, K. A., Letvin, N. L., Waldmann, T. A. & Kirkman, R. L. (1989). Prolongation of primate renal allograft survival by anti-Tac, an anti-human IL-2 receptor monoclonal antibody. *Transplantation*, **47**, 55–59.

Renlund, D. G., O'Connell, J. B., Gilbert, E. M., Hammond, M. E., Burton, N. A., Jones, K. W., Karwande, S. V., Doty, D. B., Menlove, R. L., Herrick, C. M., Lee, H. R., Gay, W. A. & Bristow, W. R. (1989). A prospective comparison of murine monoclonal CD-3 (OKT3) antibody-based and equine antithymocyte globulin-based rejection prophylaxis in cardiac transplantation. Decreased rejection and less corticosteroid use with OKT3. *Transplantation*, **47**, 599–605.

Riechmann, L., Clark, M., Waldmann, H. & Winter, G. (1988). Reshaping human antibodies for therapy. *Nature*, **332**, 323–327.

Robb, R. J. & Greene, W. C. (1983). Direct demonstration of the identity of T cell growth factor binding protein and the Tac antigen. *Journal of Experimental Medicine*, **158**, 1332–1337.

Robb, R. J., Greene, W. C. & Rusk, C. M. (1984). Low and high affinity cellular receptors for interleukin 2. Implications for the level of Tac antigen. *Journal of Experimental Medicine*, **160**, 1126–1146.

Robb, R. J., Munck, A. & Smith, K. A. (1981). T cell growth factor receptors. Quantitation, specificity and biological relevance. *Journal of Experimental Medicine*, **154**, 1455–1474.

Rodwell, J. D. (1989). Engineering monoclonal antibodies. *Nature*, **342**, 99–100.

Schroeder, T. J., First, M. R., Mansour, M. E., Hurtubise, P. E., Hariharan, S., Ryckman, F. C., Munda, R., Melvin, D. B., Penn, I., Ballistreri, W. F. & Alexander, J. W. (1990). Antimurine antibody formation following OKT3 therapy. *Transplantation*, **49**, 48–51.

Sharon, M., Klausner, R. D., Cullen, B. R., Chizzonite, R. & Leonard, W. J. (1986). Novel interleukin-2 receptor subunit detected by cross-linking under high-affinity conditions. *Science*, **234**, 859–863.

Shizuru, J. A., Seydel, K. B., Flavin, T. F., Wu, A. P., Kong, C. C., Hoyt, E. G., Fujimoto, N., Billingham, M. E., Starnes, V. A. & Fathman, C. G. (1990). Induction of donor-specific unresponsiveness to cardiac allografts in rats by pretransplant anti-CD4 monoclonal antibody therapy. *Transplantation*, **50**, 366–373.

Smith, K. A. (1980). T-cell growth factor. *Immunological Reviews*, **51**, 337–357.

Soulillou, J. P., Cantarovich, D., Le Mauff, B., Giral, M., Robillard, N., Hourmant, M., Hirn, M. & Jacques, Y. (1990). Randomized controlled trial of a monoclonal antibody against the interleukin-2 receptor (33B3.1) as compared with rabbit antithymocyte globulin for prophylaxis against rejection of renal allografts (see comments). *New England Journal of Medicine*, **322**, 1175–1182.

Soulillou, J. P., Peyronnet, P., Le Mauff, B., Hourmant, M., Olive, D., Mawas, C., Delaage, M., Hirn, M. & Jacques, Y. N. (1987). Prevention of rejection of kidney transplants by monoclonal antibody directed against interleukin 2. *Lancet*, **1**, 1339–1342.

Springer, T. A. (1990). Adhesion receptors of the immune system. *Nature*, **346**, 425–434.

Swinnen, L. J., Costanzo-Nordin, M. R., Fisher, S. G., O'Sullivan, E. J., Johnson, M. R., Heroux, A. L., Dizikes, G. J., Pifarre, R. & Risher, R. I. (1990). Increased incidence of lymphoproliferative disorder after immunosuppression with the monoclonal antibody OKT3 in cardiac-transplant recipients (see comments). *New England Journal of Medicine*, 323, 1723–1728.

Takahashi, H., Okazaki, H., Terasaki, P. I., Iwaki, Y., Kinukawa, T., Miura, K., Oguma, S. & Ishizaki, M. (1985). Follow-up on initial trials of kidney transplant rejection reversal by a monoclonal antiblast antibody. *Transplantation Proceedings*, 17, 69–70.

Takahashi, H., Okazaki, H., Terasaki, P. I., Iwaki, Y., Kinukawa, T., Taguchi, Y., Chia, D., Hardiwidjaja, S., Miura, K., Ishizaki, M. & Billing, R. (1983). Reversal of transplant rejection by monoclonal antiblast antibody. *Lancet*, 2, 1155–1158.

Terasaki, P., Cats, S., Cicciarelli, F., Toyome, A., Iwaki, Y., Kinukawa, T., Wakisaka, A., Takahashi, H., Hardiwidjaja, S. & Mendez, R. (1985). Use of monoclonal antibodies for kidney transplant patients. *Transplantation Proceedings*, 17, 1521–1522.

Teshigawara, K., Wang, H. M., Kato, K. & Smith, K. A. (1987). Interleukin 2 high-affinity receptor expression requires two distinct binding proteins. *Journal of Experimental Medicine*, 165, 223–238.

Theobald, M., Hoffmann, T., Bunjes, D. & Heit, W. (1990). Comparative analysis of *in vivo* T cell depletion with radiotherapy, combination chemotherapy and the monoclonal antibody Campath-IG, using limiting dilution methodology. *Transplantation*, 49, 553–559.

Thistlethwaite, J. R., Jr, Gaber, A. O., Haag, B. W., Aronson, A. J., Broelsch, C. E., Stuart, J. K. & Stuart, F. P. (1987). OKT3 treatment of steroid-resistant renal allograft rejection. *Transplantation*, 43, 176–184.

Touraine, J. L., Bozi, E. & El Yafi, S. (1985). Infectious lymphoproliferative syndrome in transplant patients under immunosuppressive treatment. *Transplantation Proceedings*, 17, 96–97.

Tsudo, M., Kitamura, F. & Miyasaka, M. (1989). Characterization of the interleukin 2 receptor beta chain using three distinct monoclonal antibodies. *Proceedings of the National Academy of Sciences of the U.S.A.*, 86, 1982–1986.

Tsudo, M., Kozak, R. W., Goldman, C. K. & Waldmann, T. A. (1986). Demonstration of a non-Tac peptide that binds interleukin 2: a potential participant in a multichain interleukin 2 receptor complex. *Proceedings of the National Academy of Sciences of the U.S.A.*, 83, 9694–9698.

Vigeral, P., Chkoff, N., Chatenoud, L., Campos, H., Lacombe, M., Droz, D., Goldstein, G., Bach, J. F. & Kreis, H. (1986). Prophylactic use of OKT3 monoclonal antibody in cadaver kidney recipients. Utilization of OKT3 as the sole immunosuppressive agent. *Transplantation*, 41, 730–733.

Waid, T. H., Lucas, B. A., Thompson, J. S., Munch, L. C., Brown, S., Kryscio, R., Prebeck, R., VanHoy, M. A. & Jezek, D. (1991). Treatment of acute rejection with anti-T-cell antigen receptor complex alpha beta (T10B9.1A-31) or anti-CD3 (OKT3) monoclonal antibody: results of a prospective randomized double-blind trial. *Transplantation Proceedings*, 23, 1062–1065.

Weissman, A. M., Harford, J. B., Svetlik, P. B., Leonard, W. L., Depper, J. M., Waldmann, T. A., Greene, W. C. & Klausner, R. D. (1986). Only high-affinity receptors for interleukin 2 mediate internalization of ligand. *Proceedings of the National Academy of Sciences of the U.S.A.*, 83, 1463–1466.

Winter, G. & Milstein, C. (1991). Man-made antibodies. *Nature*, 349, 293–299.

Wong, J. T., Eylath, A. A., Ghobrial, I. & Colvin, R. B. (1990). The mechanism of anti-CD3 monoclonal antibodies. Mediation of cytolysis by inter-T cell bridging. *Transplantation*, 50, 683–689.

Wood, K. J., Pearson, T. S., Darby, C. & Morris, P. J. (1991). CD4: a potential target molecule for immunosuppressive therapy and tolerance induction. *Transplantation Reviews*, **5**, 150–158.

13

Monoclonal antibodies and the skin

A. C. CHU and E. TSELE

13.1 Introduction

Monoclonal antibodies (mab) have been of enormous value in the study of the skin, both in health and disease. Mab against keratins have established the changes in the pattern of keratin production with maturation of the keratinocyte and how this is disrupted in diseases of the epidermis. Antibodies against structural antigens of the basement membrane zone have provided a viable alternative to electron microscopy in the study of this important part of the skin. Antibodies have helped in the identification of different cell types within the skin and the differentiation of different tumours of the skin.

The immunophenotyping of the cellular infiltrate of various dermatoses has given valuable information about cell migration through the skin and the interaction of different cell types within the skin but has not provided the means to accurately diagnose a specific disease. We still have no disease specific mab. In this chapter we review the current literature pertaining to mab and their use in the investigation of the skin and skin diseases.

13.2 Structure of the skin

The skin is conventionally divided into two parts: the superficial epidermis, which is a stratified squamous epithelium composed of keratinocytes and some migrant cell types, and the dermis, which provides the structural support for the epidermis and contains blood vessels, nerves and other mesenchymal elements. These two parts are joined by a basement membrane zone which may be the target for various disease processes. A schematic representation of the skin is given in Figure 13.1.

13.3 The keratinocyte

The keratinocyte is the indigenous cell population of the epidermis. The keratinocyte matures from a dividing basal cell layer through the Malpighian or

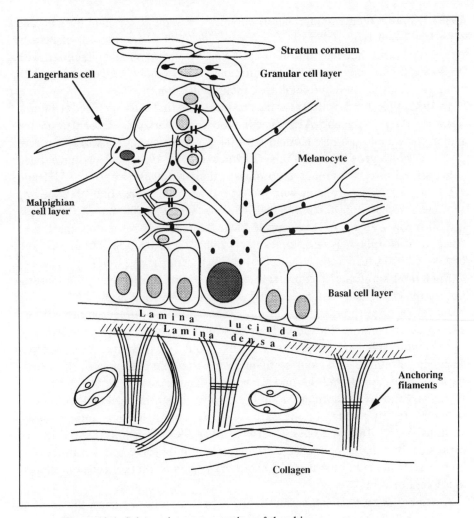

Figure 13.1. Schematic representation of the skin.

prickle cell layers to the granular cell layer and finally, with loss of the nucleus, to the stratum corneum. The major marker of the keratinocyte is a family of water-insoluble proteins, the keratins. The pattern of expression of keratins changes with maturation of the keratinocyte but expression of certain keratins is conserved even after malignant transformation of the cells.

Nineteen keratins have been described with molecular weights of between 40,000 and 70,000 and pH from 5.2 to 7.8 (Moll *et al.*, 1982). Based on the molecular weights and isoelectric focusing, keratins have been identified and numbered 1–19. This avoids the confusion of the variation in the precise molecular weights determined by polyacrylamide gel electrophoresis in the presence of sodium dodecyl sulphate (SDS-PAGE) from one study to another.

There are two gene families of keratins, type I that is relatively basic (keratins 1–8) and type II that is relatively acidic (keratins 9–19) (Fuchs *et al.*,

1987). Keratin filaments are heteropolymers of equimolar quantities of one type I and one type II keratin (Eichner *et al.*, 1986). The pattern of keratin expression varies between different epithelia, within the same epithelium, with anatomical site, degree of differentiation, environment of cellular growth (culture versus *in vivo*) and fetal age (Tseng *et al.*, 1982).

In 1982, Woodcock-Mitchell *et al.* produced the first mab specific for human keratins: AE1, AE2 and AE3. These mab can be used to recognize all the major epidermal keratins. Human keratinocytes express at least nine keratins under various growth conditions (Eichner *et al.*, 1984), which have been subclassified into two groups according to their reactivity with mab AE1 and AE3. Subfamily A correlates with the type II acidic keratins (pH < 5.5) having molecular weights of 40,000, 46,000, 48,000, 50,000/50,000 and 56,000; these are all recognized by AE1 except 46 kDa. Subfamily B represents the type I basic keratins (pH > 6) with molecular weights of 52,000, 56,000, 58,000 and 65,000–67,000 which are recognized by AE3 (Eichner *et al.*, 1984).

Epidermal keratinocyte expression of the keratins changes with the maturation of the cell (Fuchs & Green, 1980; Woodcock-Mitchell *et al.*, 1982). In the basal cell layer of the skin, the keratinocytes synthesize primary keratins 5 and 14. These are retained in the cells as they mature in the suprabasal layer. In the epibasal cells, the secondary keratins 1 and 10 are synthesized. In non-cornifying stratified squamous epithelium, for example oesophagus, the secondary keratins are 4 and 13 and in corneal epithelium they are 3 and 12. Keratins 6 and 16 are normally found in high-turnover mucosal epithelia but in hyperproliferative states in the skin, such as wound healing and psoriasis, keratins 6 and 16 are found (Weiss *et al.*, 1983). Keratins 8 and 18 are expressed by simple epithelial cells and are not observed in keratinocytes; however, in the skin, sweat gland excretory cells and Merkel cells do express these keratins.

A number of monoclonal antibodies have been produced against the keratins and have helped to establish the pattern of keratin production in the development of the skin and in skin disease. LL001 and LL002 (Purkis *et al.*, 1990) were raised against keratin 14 and stain epidermal cells up to the granular cell layer. 2.1.D7 and RaK5 (Purkis *et al.*, 1990) label keratin 5 and stain all basal and parabasal cells. LH6, LH8 (Purkis *et al.*, 1990) and PAb421 (Leigh *et al.*, 1990) recognise epitopes of keratins 5 and 14 specific for basal keratinocytes. LH1, LH2, RKSE60, KK8.60 and RaK1 (Lane *et al.*, 1985) label keratins 1 and 10 and thus all suprabasal keratinocytes. LMM3 (Gardner *et al.*, 1986) and Ks8.12 (de Mare *et al.*, 1989) label keratin 16.

Immunoblot, SDS-PAGE and histochemical studies using mab have clearly shown that the expression of keratins is altered in normal and pathological hyperproliferative conditions and pre-cancerous and cancerous lesions (Moll *et al.*, 1984; Kariniemi & Virtanen, 1989; Shimizu *et al.*, 1989). *In situ* studies have shown that AE1 stains the basal layer of epidermis in specimens from normal skin and skin from ichthyosis vulgaris (Woodcock-Mitchell *et al.*, 1982).

A suprabasal pattern of staining with AE1 is seen in hyperproliferative diseases (psoriasis, seborrhoeic keratosis, actinic keratosis and verruca vulgaris) (Weiss *et al.*, 1983).

Similar findings were shown in other studies using the mab Ks8.12 in frozen sections of psoriatic and stripped skin (de Mare *et al.*, 1989). Ks8.12 recognizes keratins 6 and 16. Recently, Schofield *et al.* (1991) used a panel of mab and showed that keratins 6 and 16, characteristic of hyperproliferative disorders, are expressed in genital and extragenital lichen planus.

The study of keratin expression by cells has given inconclusive and sometimes conflicting results. It is clear, however, that there is no disease-specific keratin and that the alteration in keratin composition is the result of rather than the cause of the diseases. Although the anti-keratin mab are valuable in the study of the pathogenesis of skin disorders, their major application is in the differentiation of epithelial from non-epithelial tumours. CAM 5.2 is a pan-cytokeratin mab which labels keratins 8, 18 and 19 and can be used in formalin-fixed paraffin-embedded sections. It labels all epithelia except stratified squamous epithelium (Makin *et al.*, 1983) and is conserved after malignant transformation.

Another mab, LP 34, labels keratins of high molecular weight which are expressed in stratified squamous epithelium (Cerio & MacDonald, 1988) and can be similarly used in paraffin-embedded specimens to identify malignancies of such epithelia.

Keratinocytes express a variety of surface antigens, both constitutively and following stimulation of the cells by cytokines such as interferon (IFN)-γ. Class II major histocompatibility complex (MHC) molecules (HLA-DR) are expressed by keratinocytes following stimulation by gamma-interferon either *in vivo* or *in vitro* (Lampert *et al.*, 1981; Basham *et al.*, 1985). The functional significance of this remains to be elucidated but HLA-DR expression may help in the migration of leukocytes through the epidermis, as a ligand to CD4, or it may confer some additional immunological properties to the keratinocyte.

MAC 387 recognizes the L1 antigen (Brandtzaeg *et al.*, 1985). L1 antigen is a 36 kDa calcium-binding protein (Dale *et al.*, 1983) expressed by myelomonocytic cells. L1 was found to be expressed by keratinocytes in inflammatory skin diseases (Gabrielson *et al.*, 1986). Expression of MAC 387 in the epidermis overlying inflammatory, bullous and hyperproliferative skin disorders has subsequently been described in two different studies. In one study (Kelly *et al.*, 1989), MAC 387 staining in the epidermis was found to be identical to that of mab CF145 and CF557, which recognize the calgranulins A and B, respectively. Calgranulins are intracellular calcium-binding proteins with inflammatory cytokine activity. It appears that MAC 387 recognizes epitopes on both proteins.

In the other study (Kirkham *et al.*, 1990), MAC 387 was expressed by keratinocytes in association with activated T cells in the dermis but independent of HLA-DR expression. The precise binding site of MAC 387 has not been defined but it seems likely that the antigen consists of two polypeptide chains, α and β, that are linked by disulphide bonds at different points in monocytes and granulocytes.

13.4   Melanocytes

Melanocytes are of neural crest origin and are thus an immigrant population to the epidermis. These cells are responsible for skin pigmentation by the production of melanin. Melanocytes are evenly distributed in the basal cell layer of the epidermis and transfer melanin to keratinocytes via a network of dendrites. Benign tumours of melanocytes generally start in the basal cell layer but with growth and maturation extend down into the dermis to form compound naevae and eventually become wholly dermal. Melanocytic lesions may begin in the dermis (blue naevus, naevus of Ota and Ita) but are less common. Malignancies of melanocytes may occur in pre-existing junctional or compound naevae or may start *de novo* in previously normal looking skin.

Mab may help in differentiating benign from malignant melanocytic lesions and between malignant melanoma and other cutaneous tumours such as epithelioma, sarcoma, carcinoma and lymphoma. So far, the most widely used marker for melanocytic lesions is the S-100 protein. This is a calcium-binding, acidic protein which was originally isolated from brain tissue by Moore in 1965. Since then it has been described in several other tissues; in the skin it labels Langerhans cells, peripheral nerves, some normal melanocytes and interdigitating reticulum cells. Anti-S-100 monoclonal and polyclonal antibodies give a sensitive but non-specific method of identifying cell types and can be used in routinely processed formalin-fixed and paraffin-embedded tissue (Cerio & MacDonald, 1988). In melanocytic lesions, S-100 cannot distinguish between benign and malignant melanocytes but is a very useful marker for the routine detection of primary and secondary melanomas, including amelanotic melanomas (Springall *et al.*, 1983). It has been demonstrated that S-100 immunoreactivity does not correlate with the degree of pleomorphism, level of invasion or thickness of the melanoma (Springall *et al.*, 1983).

Anti-non-specific enolase antibodies have also been used in the differential diagnosis of melanocytic tumours (Dhillon *et al.*, 1982) but this marker is of limited value because of its low sensitivity (Springall *et al.*, 1983) and specificity (MacKie *et al.*, 1983).

NK1 C3 is a mab that was produced by the Netherlands Cancer Institute against an as yet unidentified antigen. It does not discriminate between benign and malignant melanocytes but it does give stronger staining in malignant melanoma lesions than anti-S-100. As with anti-S-100, it can be used in formalin-fixed, paraffin-embedded sections and is very useful in the retrospective evaluation of melanocytic lesions.

Another mouse mab, HMB-45, was raised by Gown *et al.* (1986), and is claimed to be specific and highly sensitive for melanocytic tumours. It defines a cytoplasmic antigen which is not related to the pigment-producing apparatus. Holbrook *et al.* (1989) demonstrated that HMB-45 stained fetal melanocytes at embryonic stages of development before melanosomes were present. HMB-45 can be used in routinely processed sections. It labels primary and secondary melanomas, junctional naevae and fetal, neonatal and atypical melanocytes but not normal adult melanocytes, dermal naevus cells in compound naevae or intradermal naevae. It also labels the cells of blue naevae (Sun *et al.*, 1990), labelling the non-pigmented immature melanocytes in these benign tumours.

HMSA-1 (Akutsu & Jimbow, 1986) and HMSA-2 (Maeda & Jimbow, 1987) recognize epitopes on melanosomes and endoplasmic reticulum. They react with intradermal naevae and the dermal component of compound naevae but not with junctional naevae or normal epidermal melanocytes. In dysplastic naevae, these antibodies label both junctional and dermal naevus cells. They label malignant melanoma, metastatic melanoma and amelanotic melanoma. Both antibodies are of the IgG1, κ-type subclass and can be used in paraffin-embedded sections.

PAL-M1 and PAL-M2 mab (Ruiter *et al.*, 1985) have been used in frozen sections for the differential diagnosis of malignant melanoma from melanocytic naevi. PAL-M1 defines a transferrin receptor (van Muijen *et al.*, 1990) and labels primary and secondary malignant melanomas and some dysplastic naevae but not common melanocytic naevae. The antigen defined by PAL-M2 is yet to be identified but this mab only stains more advanced primary malignant melanomas of Breslow thickness of 0.76 or greater. These mab are non-specific and their prognostic significance has not been established.

Studies of HLA-DR expression in malignant melanoma on frozen sections (anti-HLA-DR) and in paraffin-embedded sections (TAL-1 B9 and LN3 mab) (West *et al.*, 1989) have shown inconsistent results and HLA-DR expression is not regarded as a reliable marker of malignant transformation of melanocytes (MacKie, 1983).

13.5 Langerhans cells

The Langerhans cell (LC) is the antigen-presenting, dendritic cell of the epidermis. It is of bone marrow origin (Katz *et al.*, 1979) and is a mobile cell population, migrating to regional lymph nodes via the lymphatics and being replenished by as yet uncharacterized circulating progenitor cells.

The Langerhans cell belongs to the group of potent antigen-presenting cells, the dendritic cells, and is pivotal in both induction and elicidation phases of contact allergic dermatitis, is the target cell in skin graft rejection and is involved in all cellular immune reactions in the skin (Austyn, 1987). The cell constitutively expresses HLA-DR, DQ and DP and in normal epidermis the LC remains the only cell to be labelled with mab against HLA-DR. Probably the most important marker of LC is the CD1 antigen, different epitopes of which are recognized by the mab OKT6, Leu 6 (Reinherz *et al.*, 1980) and NAI/34 (McMichael *et al.*, 1979). This antigen was first identified as a marker for cortical thymocytes but was later demonstrated to label Langerhans cells (Fithian *et al.*, 1981) and the putative precursor of LC in the epidermis (Chu *et al.*, 1982).

In normal skin, the only cell that expresses CD1 is the LC. CD1 may be observed in various T cell malignancies and is consistently seen in the abnormal proliferating LC in Langerhans cell histiocytosis (Chu *et al.*, 1987). A mab against CD1 that can be used in paraffin-embedded tissue has yet to be produced.

LC have been shown to express ICAM-1, LFA-3, CD11b, CD11c, CD18, CD54, CD58 and CDw32 (Teuissen *et al.*, 1990). In addition, the LC, usually in an activated state, expresses CD4 (Schmidt *et al.*, 1984). S-100 is a sensitive but non-specific marker for LC and the lesional cells of Langerhans cell histiocytosis. It can be used in paraffin-embedded tissue.

Lag is a mouse mab specific for LC. It defines a 40 kDa heterogeneously glycosylated protein with pI 4.7–6.5 which is apparently sited on Birbeck granules (Kashihara *et al.*, 1986) Lag$^+$ cells were found in stratified squamous epithelia of lip, tongue, buccal mucosa, oesophagus, vagina and uterine cervix. These Lag$^+$ cells were found on immunoelectron microscopy to have Birbeck granules. Lag does not react with monocytes, macrophages, follicular dendritic cells or interdigitating reticulum cells. In Letterer–Siwe disease 70% of CD1$^+$ cells in lymph nodes were Lag$^+$ but in skin lesions almost all CD1$^+$ cells were Lag$^+$ (Kashihara-Sawami *et al.*, 1988).

13.6   Basement membrane zone (BMZ)

This zone separates the epidermis from the dermis and maintains cohesion between these two parts of the skin. It is composed of an upper lamina lucida which is derived from the basal keratinocytes and a lower lamina densa, a product of dermal cellular elements. The main marker for the lamina lucida is the so-called bullous pemphigoid antigen which is the target for the autoantibodies produced in this disease. The major marker for the lamina densa is type IV collagen.

Using antibodies directed against the bullous pemphigoid antigen and type IV collagen, the anatomical site of the cleft seen in bullous diseases can be easily identified, i.e. if the cleft is in the epidermis, both type IV collagen and bullous pemphigoid antigen are found in the floor of the blister; if the cleft is through the lamina lucida, the bullous pemphigoid antigen is found in the roof and the floor of the blister and type IV collagen only in the floor; if the cleft is subbasement membrane, both the bullous pemphigoid antigen and type IV collagen can be found in the roof of the blister.

Identification of the site of the cleft is important in differentiating the different subtypes of the acquired or genetic diseases encompassed by the term epidermolysis bullosa. Differentiation of these subtypes is important as each variety carries a different prognosis.

Epidermolysis bullosa (EB) is a term that encompasses a heterogeneous group of disorders, characterized by trauma-induced blisters of skin and mucous membranes. Three main variants have been recognized:

1. EB simplex, the only form with true epidermolysis, in which the cleft occurs through the epidermal basal cells.
2. Junctional EB (JEB), in which the cleft occurs within the lamina lucida.
3. Dystrophic EB (DEB), in which the blisters appear below the basal lamina of which two subtypes are recognized, an autosomal dominant and an autosomal recessive type.

In the inherited forms of EB, the prenatal and post-natal diagnosis has been routinely performed by means of electron microscopy studies of fetal skin, taken with fetoscopy at 18 weeks' gestation (Eady *et al.*, 1985) or post-natally. Preliminary studies have shown that immunohistochemistry using mab against type IV collagen and bullous pemphigoid antigen in newly developed blisters provides us with a rapid and, in some cases, equally reliable method of diagnosis. Other antibodies have also proven to be of value in the diagnosis of the difficult types of EB where no blisters are present at the time of biopsy.

The rabbit polyclonal antibody AA3 was initially used in the diagnosis of recessive or lethal JEB. It was raised against deoxycholate-solubilized human amnion and recognizes an antigen within the BMZ, mainly the lamina lucida (Hsi *et al.*, 1985).

AA3 was superseded by a mab, GB3, which shows similar binding characteristics. It has not been shown whether it shares the same antigenic sites with AA3. GB3 defines a 600 kDa glycoprotein within the lamina lucida (Verrando *et al.*, 1991). In indirect immunofluorescence, GB3 shows markedly reduced or absent binding to BMZ in specimens from patients with lethal JEB. In contrast, it labels intensely the BMZ in skin samples of EB simplex, DEB (dominant and recessive), non-lethal forms of JEB and normal controls (Heagerty *et al.*, 1986*a*). In the indeterminate form of JEB there is faint labelling. Verrando *et al.* (1991) showed that in patients with lethal JEB, GB3 immunoreactivity is absent not only in the skin but in other epithelial basement membranes as well, suggesting a widespread defect in the basement membranes of these patients.

In the diagnosis of recessive DEB, the following mab have been used: KF1 AF1, AF2, LH7:2. KF1 is a murine IgG3 mab which defines a collagenase-resistant primate-specific antigen restricted to the basement membrane of stratified squamous epithelia (Breatnach *et al.*, 1983). It has been characterized as a 72 kDa polypeptide (Bernard, 1986) localized in the lamina densa. KF1 staining is absent in skin samples from recessive DEB patients and can be used in the prenatal diagnosis of recessive DEB in conjunction with electron microscopy. KF1 is also the only available mab for the diagnosis of dominant DEB. Fine *et al.* (1988), however, showed that immunostaining of fetal skin biopsies of dominant DEB, studied in parallel with electron microscopy, gave inconsistent results and cautioned that KF1 should not be used by itself in the prenatal diagnosis of this form of EB.

LH7:2 is a mab which recognizes an antigen in the lamina densa of the basement membrane of stratified squamous epithelia (Leigh & Perkis, 1985) and has been used in the pre and post-natal diagnosis of recessive DEB (Heagerty *et al.*, 1986*b*). LH7:2 immunoreactivity is reduced or absent in normal-appearing skin in patients with severe mutilating recessive DEB and patchily reduced in localized non-mutilating recessive DEB. Skin samples from dominant DEB, JEB, EB simplex and normal skin showed intense labelling (Heagerty *et al.*, 1985).

Two other murine mab, AF1 and AF2, both of IgG1 type, were raised against anchoring fibrils and used in the diagnosis of recessive DEB by Goldsmith & Briggaman (1983). These mab showed somewhat different distribution patterns and it appears they recognize different antigenic epitopes of anchoring fibrils. Both of them showed no immunoreactivity in biopsies from recessive DEB patients whereas they label very intensely the sub-basal area in dominant DEB and normal skin.

An acquired form of EB, EB acquisita, is an autoimmune disease in which antibodies are directed against a normal constituent of the BMZ, the EBA antigen. The EBA antigen consists of two components; a 290 kDa major protein and a 145 kDa minor protein, which may be the breakdown product of the major protein. In immunoelectron microscopic studies using serum from EBA patients, the antigen was identified immediately below the lamina densa (Woodley *et al.*, 1984). EBA antigen is different from collagen I, IV, V, laminin, fibronectin, bullous pemphigoid antigen and elastin. A mouse mab H3a was raised against the EBA antigen by Paller *et al.* (1985). It recognizes both 290 and 145 kDa proteins of the EBA antigen. The distribution of H3a was identical with that of polyclonal sera from patients with EBA (Paller *et al.*, 1985).

13.7   Dermal infiltrates

Mab directed against different leucocyte antigens have provided valuable reagents for the investigation of dermal cellular infiltrates and clues as to the pathogenesis of certain diseases. These reagents are important in defining the originating cell type in various cutaneous malignancies but have failed to provide the means to diagnose accurately benign skin disease. These mab are detailed in their relevant chapters but their use in the investigation of cutaneous T cell lymphoma (CTCL) and benign dermatoses will be briefly outlined.

13.8   Cutaneous T cell lymphoma

The major problem in the study of CTCL is its diagnosis in early stages. Despite the large number of mab used in immunohistochemical studies, no single mab gives unique staining for CTCL. It is now well established that the malignant cells in CTCL are of the helper/inducer phenotype, $CD3^+$, $CD4^+$ (Chu, 1983; Turbitt & MacKie, 1986). Chu *et al.* (1984), in a large study of 91 patients with CTCL, found that there was selective loss of reactivity with mab OKT1 and BE3 and concurrent expression of CD4 and CD8 antigens by some cells in the lesion of CTCL. Another feature, helpful in the diagnosis of CTCL, was the presence of $OKT10^+$ cells (mean 3%) in the dermal infiltrates of CTCL and the absence of $OKT10^+$ cells from benign dermal infiltrates. This was confirmed by Turbitt & MacKie (1986), although they found a smaller proportion of $OKT10^+$ cells (1.4%).

Two other mab have been used in the study of CTCL: Leu 8 and Leu 9 (anti-CD7). Leu 8 recognizes a subset of regulatory T cells of both helper/inducer and suppressor/cytotoxic subpopulations (Gatenby *et al.*, 1982). Leu 9 antigen is expressed by approximately 90% of mature T cells (Link *et al.*, 1983). There is general agreement that lesional cells in CTCL are Leu 8^- (Abel *et al.*, 1985; Turbitt & MacKie, 1986; Wood *et al.*, 1986) and also Leu 9^- (Wood *et al.*, 1986). In addition Wood *et al.* (1986) found that Leu 8^- and Leu 9^- cells are present in early and late stages of CTCL and that the lack of these markers correlated with confidence in the diagnosis. It has been postulated that the Leu 9 antigen (CD7) and the 3A1 antigen (Haynes *et al.*, 1981) represent different epitopes of the same antigen. Haynes *et al.* (1981) reported that circulating Sezary cells in CTCL were $3A1^-$ but cells within the cutaneous infiltrate of CTCL were $3A1^+$.

More recently, the MY7 mab has been used in the study of CTCL (Dreno *et al.*, 1990). This mab labels peripheral granulocytes and monocytes and cross-reacts with epidermal basal cells. CTCL cells were $CD4^+$ $MY7^+$ in the dermis and $MY7^-$ in the epidermis; in contrast, T cells in benign inflammatory lesions were $CD4^+$ $MY7^-$ in the dermis and $MY7^+$ in the epidermis.

13.9   Benign cellular infiltrates

Lupus erythematosus is characterized by a predominance of $CD4^+$ cells with varying numbers of $CD8^+$ cells. Jessner's lymphocytic infiltrate was initially thought to be a prodromal stage of lupus erythematosus and Rijlaarsdam *et al.* (1989) using mab were unable to differentiate between Jessner's lymphocytic infiltrate and lupus erythematosus. Smolle *et al.* (1990), however, used a large panel of mab to study the pseudolymphomas and classified Jessner's lymphocytic infiltrate as nodular T cell pseudolymphoma. This was supported by Cerio *et al.* (1990) who identified perivascular $LN1^+$ cells (follicular centre B cells) in more than half of the Jessner's lymphocytic infiltrate lesions they studied. They proposed that the B cell subtype of Jessner's lymphocytic infiltrate belong to the pseudolymphomas and the T cell subtype to persistent or figurate erythemas.

13.10   Adhesion molecules

Adhesion molecules are a group of cell receptors involved in cell–cell and cell–matrix interactions. They allow the adhesion of leucocytes to other leucocytes, to endothelial cells, to keratinocytes and to extracellular molecules. Three superfamilies have been described: the integrins (Hynes, 1987), the 'ELAM' molecules (Marx, 1989) and the immunoglobulin superfamily (Williams & Barclay, 1988).

Integrins are non-covalently linked heterodimers with a subfamily-specific β chain and a variable α chain. They interact with extracellular ligands which 'contain' the RGD tripeptide. The intracellular portion interacts with the actin filaments, providing a link between the cytoskeleton and the extracellular environment (Hynes, 1987). Integrins consist of four subfamilies, defined by the type of β chain of the $\alpha\beta$ heterodimer.

1. β_1-integrins or VLA (very late antigens) molecules which are primarily involved in cell–matrix interactions (Hemler et al., 1987).
2. β_2-integrins, including LFA-1, MAC-1 and p150,95, which are restricted to leucocytes.
3. β_3-integrins include the vitronectin receptor and the IIb/IIIa platelet complex.
4. β_4-integrins which are found in epithelial tissues (Kajiji et al., 1989).

Studies in normal skin using mab (Konter et al., 1989) have shown that VLA-α_2 expression is restricted to epithelial cells, basal keratinocytes in the epidermis and hair follicles and sweat and sebaceous gland cells. VLA-α_3 is restricted to basal and suprabasal keratinocytes, sweat and sebaceous gland cells and endothelium and VLA-α_6 to basal keratinocytes with more intense labelling on the dermal pole of their membrane (Konter et al., 1989). The latter is in agreement with the studies of Zambruno et al. (1991) and Nazzaro et al. (1990) who also suggested that VLA-α_6 staining could replace the use of the bullous pemphigoid antigen in the study of JEB. Zambruno et al. (1991) also found that LC express VLA-α_4 and VLA-α_6 and melanocytes express VLA-α_3 and VLA-α_6 integrins. VLA-α_1 is not expressed in the epidermis and is the only integrin without a known ligand.

As the VLA molecules mediate cell adhesion with collagen, laminin and fibronectin they are considered to be involved in cell anchorage, cell polarity, differentiation of keratinocytes and stability of basal keratinocytes at the dermoepidermal junction (Konter et al., 1989; Zambruno et al., 1991).

The ELAM (selectin) superfamily consists of the lymph node homing receptor (L-selectin), ELAM-1 (E-selectin) and GMP-140 (P-selectin) molecules. ELAM-1 is a surface glycoprotein found on endothelial cells which selectively binds neutrophils and possibly monocytes (Bevilacqua *et al.*, 1989). In normal human skin, dermal blood vessels show minimal labelling for ELAM-1. This is upregulated in the presence of dermal infiltrates associated with cell-mediated conditions, hyperproliferative disorders such as psoriasis, and malignant and premalignant proliferation of keratinocytes (Groves *et al.*, 1991). Endothelial expression of ELAM-1 has been shown to be upregulated by both UVB exposure and subcutaneous injection with PPD but persists longer after PPD injection (Norris *et al.*, 1991).

The immunoglobulin superfamily includes CD2, LFA-3 and ICAM-1. CD2 is the sheep red blood cell receptor found on T cells and is the ligand for LFA-3. LFA-3 has been shown to be constitutively expressed on both keratinocytes and Langerhans cells (Panfilis *et al.*, 1991) which may be of functional importance in traffiking of T cells through the epidermis. ICAM-1 is expressed by various cells. In normal human skin it has been shown to be expressed by all endothelial cells, especially on the luminal side, and occasionally on keratinocytes, particularly where T cells were present in the epidermis (Konter *et al.*, 1989). The same authors found ICAM-1$^-$ keratinocytes in close apposition with LFA-1$^+$ T cells and therefore suggested that ICAM-1 expression is not a prerequisite for T cell recruitment into the epidermis, although Dustin *et al.* (1988) showed that adhesion of T cells to keratinocytes was mediated by ICAM-1 and regulated by INF-γ. Endothelial cells constitutively express ICAM-1 which is upregulated by IL-1, TNF and to a lesser extent by IFN-γ (Dustin & Springer, 1988). In one study, basal keratinocytes were induced to express ICAM-1 after intracutaneous PPD injection but not UVB exposure (Norris *et al.*, 1991).

ICAM-1 is expressed by melanoma cells and melanoma cell lines. The degree of expression of ICAM-1 on melanoma cells has been correlated with the metastatic potential of the primary tumour. Hansen *et al.* (1991), however, found that ICAM-1 was expressed by both malignant melanoma and benign naevi and that there was no correlation between ICAM-1 expression and the depth of invasion in malignant melanoma. They suggested that ICAM-1 is not of prognostic importance in malignant melanoma.

13.11 References

Abel, E. A., Wood, G. S., Hoppe, R. T. & Warnke, R. A. (1985). Expression of Leu 8 antigen, a majority T-cell marker is uncommon in mycosis fungoides. *Journal of Investigative Dermatology*, **85**, 199–202.

Akutsu, Y. & Jimbow, K. (1986). Development and characterization of a mouse monoclonal antibody. MoAb HMSA-1 against a melanosomal fraction of human malignant melanoma. *Cancer Research*, **46**, 2904–2911.

Austyn, J. M. (1987). Lymphoid dendritic cells. *Immunology*, **62**, 161–170.

Basham, T. Y., Nickoloff, B. J., Merigan, T. C. & Morhenn, V. B. (1985). Recombinant gamma interferon differentially regulates class II antigen expression and biosynthesis on cultured normal keratinocytes. *Journal of Interferon Research*, **5**, 23–32.

Bernard, B. A. (1986). Biochemical characterization of the epithelial basement membrane antigen defined by the monoclonal antibody KF-1. *Journal of Investigative Dermatology*, **87**, 86–88.

Bevilacqua, M. P., Stengelin, S., Gimbrone, M. A. & Seed, B. (1989). Endothelial leucocyte adhesion molecule 1: an inducible receptor for neutrophils related to complement regulatory proteins and lectins. *Science*, **243**, 1160–1164.

Brandtzaeg, P., Jones, D. B., Flavell, D. J. & Fagerhol, M. K. (1985). A monoclonal antibody to human monocytes that reacts with the formalin resistant myelomonocytic L1 antigen. *Journal of Clinical Pathology*, **41**, 963–970.

Breatnach, S. M., Fox, P. A., Neises, G. R., Stanley, J. R. & Katz, S. I. (1983). A unique epithelial basement membrane antigen defined by the monoclonal antibody KF-1. *Journal of Investigative Dermatology*, **80**, 392–395.

Cerio, R. & MacDonald, D. M. (1988). Monoclonal antibodies in diagnostic dermatology. *Advances in Dermatology*, **3**, 123–140.

Cerio, R., Oliver, G. F., Wilson Jones, E. & Winkelmann, R. K. (1990). The heterogenicity of Jessner's lymphocytic infiltration of the skin: immuno-histochemical studies suggesting one form of perivascular lymphocytoma. *Journal of the American Academy of Dermatology*, **23**, 63–67.

Chu, A. C. (1983). The use of monoclonal antibodies in the in situ identification of T-cell subpopulations in cutaneous T-cell lymphoma. *Journal of Cutaneous Pathology*, **10**, 479–498.

Chu, A. C., D'Angio, G. J., Favara, B., Ladisch, S., Nesbit, M. & Pritchard, J. (1987). Histiocytosis syndromes in children. *Lancet*, **1**, 208–209.

Chu, A. C., Eisinger, M., Takezaki, S., Kung, P. C. & Edelson, R. L. (1982). Immunoelectron microscopic identification of Langerhans cells using a new antigenic marker. *Journal of Investigative Dermatology*, **78**, 177–180.

Chu, A. C., Patterson, J., Berger, C., Vonderheid, E. & Edelson, R. (1984). *In situ* study of T-cell subpopulations in cutaneous T-cell lymphoma. *Cancer*, **54**, 2414–2422.

Dale, I., Fagerhol, M. K. & Naesgaard, I. (1983). Purification and partial characterization of a highly immunogenic human leukocyte protein, the L1 antigen. *European Journal of Biochemistry*, **134**, 1–6.

De Mare, S., van Erp, P. E. J. & van de Kerkhof, P. C. M. (1989). Epidermal hyperproliferation assessed by the monoclonal antibody Ks8.12 on frozen sections. *Journal of Investigative Dermatology*, **92**, 130–131.

Dhillon, A. P., Rode, J. & Leatham, A. (1982). Neurone specific enolase. An aid to the diagnosis of melanoma and neuroblastoma. *Histopathology*, **3**, 205–211.

Dreno, B., Bureau, B., Stalder, J.-F. and Litoux, P. (1990). MY7 monoclonal antibody for diagnosis of cutaneous T-cell lymphoma. *Archives of Dermatology*, **126**, 1454–1456.

Dustin, M. L., Singer, K. H., Tuck, D. T. & Springer, T. A. (1988). Adhesion of T lymphoblasts to epidermal keratinocytes is regulated by interferon gamma and is mediated by intercellular adhesion molecule-1 (ICAM-1). *Journal of Experimental Medicine*, **167**, 1323–1340.

Dustin, M. L. & Springer, T. A. (1988). Lymphocyte function-associated antigen-2 (LFA-1) interaction with inter-cellular adhesion molecule-1 (ICAM-1) is one of at least three mechanisms for lymphocyte adhesion to cultured endothelial cells. *Journal of Cell Biology*, **107**, 321–331.

Eady, R. A. J., Gunner, D. B., Tidman, M. J., Heagerty, A. H. M., Nicolaides, K. H. & Rodeck, C. H. (1985). Prenatal diagnosis of genetic skin disease by fetoscopy and electron microscopy: report on 5 years' experience. *British Journal of Dermatology*, (Suppl. 29), 45.

Eichner, R., Bonitz, P. & Sun, T.-T. (1984). Classification of epidermal keratins according to their immunoreactivity, isoelectric point and mode of expression. *Journal of Cell Biology*, **98**, 1388–1396.

Eichner, R., Sun, T.-T. & Aebi, U. (1986). The role of keratin subfamilies and keratin pairs in the formation of human epidermal intermediate filaments. *Journal of Cell Biology*, **102**, 1767–1777.

Fine, J.-D., Eady, R. A. J., Levy, M. L., Hejtmancik, J. F., Courtney, K. B., Carpenter, R., Holbrook, K. A. & Hawkins, H. K. (1988). Prenatal diagnosis of dominant and recessive dystrophic epidermolysis bullosa: application and limitations in the use of KF1 and LH 7:2 monoclonal antibodies and immunofluorescence mapping technique. *Journal of Investigative Dermatology*, **91**, 465–471.

Fithian, E., Kung, P., Goldstein, G., Rubenfeld, M., Fenoglio, C. & Edelson, R. (1981). Reactivity of Langerhans cells with hybridoma antibody. *Proceedings of the National Academy of Sciences of the U.S.A.*, **78**, 2541–2544.

Fuchs, E. & Green, H. (1980). Changes in keratin gene expression during terminal differentiation of the keratinocyte. *Cell*, **9**, 1033–1042.

Fuchs, E., Tyrer, A. L., Giudice, G. J., Marchuk, D., RayChaudhury, A. & Rosenberg, M. (1987). The human keratin genes and their differential expression. *Developmental Biology*, **22**, 5–34.

Gabrielson, T., Dale, I., Brandtzaeg, P., Hoel, P. S., Fagerhol, M. K., Larsen, T. E. & Thune, P. O. (1986). Epidermal and dermal distribution of a myelomonocytic antigen (L12) shared by epithelial cells in various inflammatory skin diseases. *Journal of American Academy of Dermatology*, **15**, 173–199.

Gardner, I. D., Whitehead, R. H. & Burgess, A. W. (1986). Production and characterisation of monoclonal antibodies reactive with subsets of epidermal cells. *Pathology*, **18**, 314–320.

Gatenby, D. A., Kansas, G. S., Xian, C. Y., Evans, R. L. & Engleman, E. G. (1982). Dissections of immunoregulatory subpopulations of T lymphocytes within helper and suppressor sublineages in man. *Journal of Immunology*, **129**, 1295–1303.

Goldsmith, L. A. & Briggaman, R. A. (1983). Monoclonal antibodies to anchoring fibrils for the diagnosis of epidermolysis bullosa. *Journal of Investigative Dermatology*, **81**, 464–466.

Gown, A. M., Vogel, A. M., Hoak, D., Gough, F. & McNutt, M. A. (1986). Monoclonal antibodies specific for melanocytic tumours distinguish subpopulations of melanocytes. *American Journal of Pathology*, **123**, 195–203.

Groves, R. W., Allen, M. H., Barker, J. N. W. N., Haskard, D. O. & MacDonald, D. M. (1991). Endothelial leucocyte adhesion molecule-1 (ELAM-1) expression in cutaneous inflammation. *British Journal of Dermatology*, **124**, 117–123.

Hansen, N. L., Ralfkiaer, E., Hou-Jensen, K., Thomson, K., Drzewiecki, K. T., Rothlein, R. & Vejlsgaard, G. L. (1991). Expression of intercellular adhesion molecule-1 (ICAM-1) in benign nevi and malignant melanomas. *Acta Dermato-Venereologica (Stockholm)*, **71**, 48–51.

Haynes, B. F., Metzger, R. S., Minna, J. D. & Bunn, P. A. (1981). Phenotype characterization of cutaneous T cell lymphoma. Use of monoclonal antibodies to compare with other malignant T cells. *New England Journal of Medicine*, **304**, 1319–1323.

Heagerty, A. H. M., Kennedy, A. R., Eady, R. A. J., Hsi, B.-L., Verrando, P., Yeh, G.-J. & Ortonne, J.-P. (1986a). GB3 monoclonal antibody for diagnosis of junctional epidermolysis bullosa. *Lancet*, **1**, 860.

Heagerty, A. H. M., Kennedy, A. R., Gunner, D. B. & Eady, R. A. J. (1986*b*). Rapid prenatal diagnosis and exclusion of epidermolysis bullosa using novel antibody probes. *Journal of Investigative Dermatology*, **86**, 603–605.

Heagerty, A. H. M., Kennedy, A. R., Leigh, I. M. & Eady, R. A. J. (1985). LH 7:2 monoclonal antibody defines a common dermo-epidermal junction defect in recessive forms of dystrophic epidermolysis bullosa. *Journal of Investigative Dermatology*, **84**, 448 (abstract).

Hemler, M. E., Huang, C. & Schwarz, L. (1987). The VLA protein family. Characterization of five distinct cell surface heterodimers each with a common 130000 molecular weight β submit. *Journal of Biological Chemistry*, **262**, 3300–3309.

Holbrook, K. A., Underwood, R. A., Vogel, A. M., Gown, A. M. & Kimball, H. (1989). The appearance, density and distribution of melanocytes in human embryonic and fetal skin revealed by the anti-melanoma monoclonal antibody HMB-45. *Anatomical Embryology*, **180**, 443–455.

Hsi, B.-L., Yeh, C.-J. & Faulk, P. W. (1985). Characterization of antibodies to antigens of the human amnion. *Placenta*, **5**, 513–522.

Hynes, R. O. (1987). Integrins: a family of surface receptors. *Cell*, **48**, 549–554.

Kajiji, I., Tamura, R. & Quaranta, V. (1989). A novel integrin (alpha-e beta-4) from human epithelial cells suggests a fourth family of integrin adhesion receptors. *EMBO Journal*, **8**, 673–680.

Kariniemi, A.-L. & Virtanen, I. (1989). Altered keratin expression in benign and malignant skin diseases revealed with monoclonal antibodies. *American Journal of Dermatopathology*, **11**, 202–208.

Kashihara, M., Ueda, M., Horiguchi, Y., Furukawa, F., Hanaoka, M. & Imamura, S. (1986). A monoclonal antibody specifically reactive to human Langerhans cells. *Journal of Investigative Dermatology*, **87**, 602–607.

Kashihara-Sawami, M. N., Horiguchi, Y., Ikai, K., Takigawa, M., Ueda, M., Hanaoka, M. & Imamura, S. (1988). Letter–Siwe disease: immunopathological study with a new monoclonal antibody. *Journal of the American Academy of Dermatology*, **18**, 646–654.

Katz, S. I., Tamaki, J. & Sachs, D. H. (1979). Epidermal Langerhans cells are derived from cells originating in the bone marrow. *Nature (London)*, **282**, 324–326.

Kelly, S. E., Jones, D. B. & Fleming, S. (1989). Calgranulin expression in inflammatory dermatoses. *Journal of Pathology*, **159**, 17–21.

Kirkham, N., Peacock, S. J. & Jones, D. B. (1990). Monoclonal antibody MAC 387 recognizes a myelomonocytic antigen shared by epithelial cells in inflammatory skin diseases. *British Journal of Dermatology*, **122**, 61–69.

Konter, U., Kellner, I., Klein, E., Kaufmann, R., Mielke, V. & Sterry, W. (1989). Adhesion molecule mapping of normal human skin. *Archives of Dermatological Research*, **281**, 454–462.

Lampert, I. A., Smitters, A. J. & Chisholm, P. M. (1981). Expression of Ia antigen on epidermal keratinocytes in graft-versus-host disease. *Nature (London)*, **293**, 149.

Lane, E. B., Bartek, J., Purkis, P. E. & Leigh, I. M. (1985). Keratin antigens in differentiating skin. *Annals of the New York Academy of Science*, **455**, 241–258.

Leigh, I. M., Pulford, K. A., Ramaekers, F. C. & Lane, E. B. (1990). Psoriasis: maintenance of an intact monolayer of basal cells in complex epithelial. *Journal of Cell Science*, **97**, 39–50.

Leigh, I. M. & Purkis, P. E. (1985). LH 7:2 a new monoclonal antibody to a lamina densa protein. *Journal of Investigative Dermatology*, **84**, 448 (abstract).

Link, M. P., Roper, M., Dorfman, R. F., Crist, W. M., Cooper, M. D. & Levy, R. (1983). Cutaneous lymphoblastic lymphoma with pre-B markers. *Blood*, **61**,

838–841.

MacKie, R. M., Campbell, I. & Turbitt, M. L. (1983). Use of NK1 C3 monoclonal antibody in the assessment of benign and malignant melanocytic lesions. *Journal of Clinical Pathology*, **37**, 367–372.

McMichael, A. J., Pilch, J. R., Galfre, G., Mason, D. Y., Fabre, J. W. & Milstein, C. (1979). A human thymocyte antigen defined by a hybrid myeloma monoclonal antibody. *European Journal of Immunology*, **9**, 205–210.

Maeda, K. & Jimbow, K. (1987). Development of MoAb HMSA-2 for melanosomes of human melanoma and its application to immunohistopathological diagnosis of neoplastic melanocytes. *Cancer*, **59**, 415–423.

Makin, C. A., Bobrow, L. B. & Bodmer, W. F. (1983). Monoclonal antibody to cytokeratin for use in routine histopathology. *Journal of Clinical Pathology*, **37**, 975–983.

Marx, J. L. (1989). New family of adhesion proteins discovered. *Science*, **243**, 1144.

Moll, R., Franke, W. W., Schiller, D. L., Geiger, B. & Krepler, R. (1982). The catalog of human cytokeratins: patterns of expression in normal epithelia, tumors and culture cells. *Cell*, **31**, 11–24.

Moll, R., Moll, I. & Franke, W. W. (1984). Differences of expression of cytokeratin polypeptides in various epithelial skin tumours. *Archives of Dermatological Research*, **276**, 349–363.

Moore, B. W. (1965). A soluble protein characteristic of the nervous system. *Biophysical Communications*, **19**, 739–744.

Nazzaro, V., Berti, E., Cerri, A., Brosasco, A., Cavalli, R. & Caputo, R. (1990). Expression of integrins in junctional dystrophic epidermolysis bullosa. *Journal of Investigative Dermatology*, **95**, 60–64.

Norris, P., Poston, R. N., Thomas, D. S., Thornhill, M., Hawk, J. & Haskard, D. O. (1991). The expression of endothelial leucocyte adhesion molecule-1 (ELAM-1), intercellular adhesion molecule-1 (ICAM-1), vascular cell adhesion molecule-1 (VCAM-1) in experimental cutaneous inflammation: a comparison of ultraviolet B erythema and delayed hypersensitivity. *Journal of Investigative Dermatology*, **96**, 763–770.

Paller, A. S., Queen, L. L., Woodley, D. T., Gammon, W. R., O'Keefe, E. J & Briggaman, R. A. (1985). A mouse monoclonal antibody against a newly discovered basement membrane component, the epidermolysis bullosa aquisita antigen. *Journal of Investigative Dermatology*, **84**, 215–217.

Panfilis, G. D., Manara, G. C., Ferrari, C. & Torresani, C. (1991). Adhesion molecules on the plasma membrane of epidermal cells. III. Keratinocytes and Langerhans cells constitutively express the lymphocyte function associated antigen 3. *Journal of Investigative Dermatology*, **96**, 512–517.

Purkis, P. E., Steel, J. B., Mackenzie, I. C., Nathrath, W. B. J., Leigh, I. M. & Lane, E. B. (1990). Antibody markers of basal cells in complex epithelia. *Journal of Cell Science*, **97**, 39–50.

Reinherz, E. L., Kung, P. C., Goldstein, G., Levey, R. H. & Schlossman, S. F. (1980). Discrete stages of human intrathymic differentiation. Analysis of normal thymocytes and leukemic lymphoblasts of T cell lineage. *Proceedings of the National Academy of Sciences of the U.S.A.*, **77**, 1588–1592.

Rijlaarsdam, J. U., Nieboer, C., de Vries, E. & Willemze, R. (1989). Characterization of the dermal infiltrates in Jessner's lymphocytic infiltrate of the skin, polymorphous light eruption and cutaneous lupus erythematosus: differential diagnostic and pathogenetic aspects. *Journal of Cutaneous Pathology*, **17**, 2–8.

Ruiter, D. J., Dingjan, G. M., Steijen, P. M., Veveren-Hooyer, M., De Graaf-Reitsma, C. B., Berman, W., van Muigen, G. N. P. & Warnaar, S. O. (1985). Monoclonal antibodies selected to discriminate between malignant melanomas and nevolcellular nevi. *Journal of Investigative Dermatology*, **85**, 4–8.

Schmidt, D., Faure, M., Dambuyant-Dezutter, C. & Thivolet, J. (1984). The semi-quantitative distribution of T4 and T6 surface antigens on human Langerhans cells. *British Journal of Dermatology*, **111**, 655–659.

Schofield, J. K., Neill, S. M., Milligan, A., Graham-Brown, R., Rohloff, W. & Leigh, I. M. (1991). Genital and non-genital, lichen planus: an immunophenotypic study of keratin expression. *British Journal of Dermatology*, **125** (Suppl. 38), 95.

Shimizu, N., Ito, M., Tazawa, T. & Sato, Y. (1989). Immunohistochemical study on keratin expression in certain cutaneous epithelial neoplasms: basal cell carcinoma, pilomatricoma and seborrheic keratosis. *American Journal of Dermapathology*, **11**, 534–540.

Smolle, J., Torne, R., Soyer, H. P. & Kerl, H. (1990). Immunohistochemical classification of cutaneous pseudolymphomas: delineation of distinct patterns. *Journal of Cutaneous Pathology*, **17**, 149–159.

Springall, D. R., Gu, J., Cocchia, D., Michetti, F., Levene, A., Levene, M. M., Marangos, P. J., Bloom, S. R. & Polak, J. M. (1983). The value of S-100 immunostaining as a diagnostic tool in human malignant melanomas. *Virchows Archives (Pathologische und Anatomische)*, **400**, 331–343.

Sun, J., Morton, T. H. & Gown, A. M. (1990). Antibody HMB-45 identifies the cells of blue nevi. *American Journal of Surgical Pathology*, **14**, 748–751.

Teuissen, M. B. M., Wormmeester, J., Krieg, S. R., Peters, P. J., Vogels, I. M. C., Kapsenberg, M. L. & Bos, J. (1990). Human epidermal Langerhans cells undergo profound morphologic and phenotypical changes during *in vitro* culture. *Journal of Investigative Dermatology*, **94**, 166–174.

Tseng, S. C. G., Jarvinen, M. J., Nelson, W. G., Huang, J.-W., Woodcock-Mitchell, J. & Sun, T.-T. (1982). Correlation of specific keratins with different types of epithelial differentiation: monoclonal antibody studies. *Cell*, **30**, 361–372.

Turbitt, M. L. & MacKic, R. M. (1986). An assessment of the diagnostic value of the monoclonal antibodies Leu 8, OKT9, OKT10 and Ki67 in cutaneous lymphocytic infiltrates. *British Journal of Dermatology*, **115**, 151–158.

Van Muijen, G. N. P., Ruiter, D. J., Hoefakker, S. & Johnson, J. P. (1990). Monoclonal antibody PAL-M1 recognizes the transferrin receptor and I a progession marker in melanocytic lesions. *Journal of Investigative Dermatology*, **95**, 65–69.

Verrando, P., Blanchet-Bardon, C., Pisani, A., Thomas, L., Cambazard, F., Eady, R. A. J., Schofield, O. & Ortonne, J.-P. (1991). Monoclonal antibody GB3 defines a widespread defect of several basement membranes and a keratinocyte dysfunction in patients with lethal junctional epidermolysis bullosa. *Laboratory Investigation*, **64**, 85–92.

Weiss, R. A., Eichner, R. & Sun, T.-T. (1984). Monoclonal antibody analysis of keratin expression in epidermal diseases: a 48- and 56-kdalton keratin as molecular markers for hyperproliferative keratinocytes. *Journal of Cell Biology*, **98**, 1397–1406.

Weiss, R. A., Guiollet, G. Y. A., Freedberg, I. M., Farmer, E. R., Small, E. A., Weiss, M. M. & Sun, T.-T. (1983). The use of monoclonal antibody to keratin in human epidermal disease: alterations in immunohistochemical staining pattern. *Journal of Investigative Dermatology*, **81**, 224–230.

West, K. P., Priyakumar, P., Jagjivan, R. & Colloby, P. S. (1989). Can HLA-DR expression help in the routine diagnosis of malignant melanoma. *British Journal of Dermatology*, **121**, 175–178.

Williams, A. F. & Barclay, A. N. (1988). The immunoglobulin superfamily-domains for cell surface recognition. *Annual Review in Immunology*, **6**, 381–405.

Wood, G. S., Abel, E. A., Hoppe, R. T. & Warnke, R. A. (1986). Leu-8 and Leu-9 antigen phenotypes: immunologic criteria for the distinction of mycosis fungoides from cutaneous inflammation. *Journal of the American Academy of Dermatology*, **14**, 1006–1013.

Woodcock-Mitchell, J., Eichner, R., Nelson, W. G. & Sun, T.-T. (1982). Immunolocalization of keratin polypeptides in human epidermis using monoclonal antibodies. *Journal of Cell Biology*, **95**, 580–588.

Woodley, D. T., Briggaman, R. A., O'Keefe, E. J., Inman, A. O., Queen, L. L. & Gammon, W. R. (1984). Identification of the skin basement-membrane autoantigen in epidermolysis bullosa aquisita. *New England Journal of Medicine*, **310**, 1007–1013.

Zambruno, G., Manca, V., Santantonio, M. L., Soligo, D. & Giannetti, A. (1991). VLA protein expression on epidermal cells (keratinocytes, Langerhans cells, melanocytes): a light and electron microscopic immunohistochemical study. *British Journal of Dermatology*, **124**, 135–145.

14

Monoclonal antibodies in endocrinology

E. HILLHOUSE and C. H. SELF

14.1 Introduction

In considering the influence that scientific achievements have had on endocrinology it is important to appreciate the close relationship that exists between clinical endocrinology, physiology, cell biology, genetics, biochemistry and immunology. In recent years advances in these disciplines have helped to modify the concept of a rigid endocrine system in order to encompass an ever-expanding list of chemical messengers. Many of these humoral mediators have similar chemical structures and many organ systems appear to share common secretory products and receptor mechanisms. Thus, it has become increasingly important to develop specific and sensitive techniques for discriminating between these substances. In this chapter we review the impact that monoclonal antibody (mab) technology has had on the development of both basic and clinical endocrinology.

14.2 Assay of hormones

The cornerstone of endocrinology is an ability to measure hormonal activity in biological samples. This is essential both in terms of understanding how endocrine cells work and in assessing endocrine disease states in patients. A variety of techniques are available to measure biologically active molecules (Table 14.1). For many years the standard for determining hormonal activity was the bioassay and this still has a central role to play in basic research today. Bioassays also provide a valuable contribution to clinical endocrinology by helping to discriminate between active and inactive fragments in biological samples, e.g. in the assessment of parathyroid disease. Bioassays are dependent on the ability of hormones to produce measurable biological effects on various target organs. They may use either direct or indirect measures of hormonal activity. Their great advantage over immunoassays is that they measure only the bioactive hormone. Unfortunately bioassays have many problems that limit their usefulness. They are time-consuming and require a source of biological material. Consequently they have a wide intra- and

Table 14.1. *Use of monoclonal antibody immunometric assays in discriminating between clinically important related molecules*

LH and hCG
GH and HPL
Insulin, proinsulin and split proinsulins
Intact PTH and fragments of PTH
PTH-related peptide and PTH
ACTH and precursor molecules

ACTH, adrenocorticotrophic hormone; LH, luteinizing hormone; GH, growth hormone; hCG, human chorionic gonadotrophin; HPL, human placental lactogen; PTH, parathyroid hormone

interassay coefficient of variation along with significant variability between laboratories. All of this makes comparison of data difficult, particularly if good standards and quality control are not available.

While bioassays can occasionally be surprisingly sensitive, as demonstrated by Branch *et al*. (1991) with their report of a specific and reliable bioassay of femtomolar sensitivity for murine tumour necrosis factor, generally speaking, they have very restricted sensitivity when compared with current immunoassays. For example, Fukuda *et al*. (1991) have reported an ELISA for human interleukin 5 which is 10 000 times more sensitive than their corresponding bioassay. It is not at all surprising that there is often a difference found between bioassays and immunoassays as the requirements of analyte to be measured may be quite different between the very different assays. The goal of making a simple immunoassay measure the same as a more complex bioassay can, however, be achieved sometimes, as Adolf and Lamche have recently demonstrated with their mab-based immunoassay for tumour necrosis factor (TNF) beta which was found to give parallel results to bioassay (Adolf & Lamche, 1990).

The question of specificity has been addressed by the application of assays designed to make use of the physical properties of the hormone under investigation, such as its ability to migrate to a certain position on a gel because of its size and charge (electrophoresis). Unfortunately, many hormones of biological interest have similar physical properties and are difficult to separate using such techniques. More sophisticated chromatographic techniques such as high pressure liquid chromatography (HPLC) or gas chromatography are more specific but require expensive equipment, are time consuming and lack the sensitivity required to measure hormones in the minute quantities present in many biological samples. HPLC will separate different molecular forms of hormones and is the method of choice for assay of the catecholamines (Guan & Dluzen, 1991). For most routine applications, however, the technique is time consuming and expensive.

Thus, the challenge in clinical endocrinology has been to develop assays which combine high specificity with high sensitivity and reproducibility. With the advent of radioimmunoassay (RIA) it was thought that these problems had been largely overcome. These assays have a number of advantages compared with bioassay. In particular they allow for discrimination between different hormones with similar biological activities. There are inherent problems in RIAs in that they are dependent on measuring analyte unbound rather than analyte bound sites (as discussed in Chapter 9).

Some of these problems can be overcome by the use of immunometric assays (Chapter 9). The use of a double antibody immunometric technique has the potential to improve both specificity and sensitivity and also enables direct measurements to be made on biological samples. Many antiserum-based assays require the prior affinity purification of the antisera, however, which is time-consuming and may be expensive and high concentrations of labelled detection antibody. This tends to reduce the utility of such assays. Access to mab removes these problems.

14.3   Generation of suitable monoclonal antibodies

The vast majority of mab employed in endocrinology has been prepared by simple immunization regimens followed by conventional screening and clonal expansion. Indeed, the ease with which such antibodies can be obtained against a wide variety of antigens is one of the major reasons for the increasing dominance of this technology. There are, however, situations where such straightforward approaches are not productive of suitable antibodies. As pointed out by Lerner (1982), the immunogenicity of an amino acid sequence in an intact protein may be less than that of the synthetic peptide sequence itself. While the approach is by no means always successful (Lerner, 1984), the fact that such short synthetic sequences can serve to make highly specific antibodies reactive with the intact molecule has been very widely used to solve many problems. Through such approaches it is, for example, possible to raise antibodies against materials that are highly conserved between species. Groome (1991) has recently employed such an approach to raise mab against inhibin-A and activin-A and Ratcliffe et al. (1990) have employed the increased immunogenicity of an N-terminal sequence of parathyroid hormone-related protein (highly homologous with parathyroid hormone) to produce antibodies specific for it. In the case where the intact molecule is toxic or immunosuppressive, this is clearly a route of choice and has been taken by Wakefield et al. (1988) with respect to raising polyclonal antibodies to transforming growth factor. The approach is particularly useful in allowing antibodies to be raised against materials that have not themselves been isolated but for which the gene sequence has been obtained (Amara *et al.*, 1982).

In addition to the nature of the immunogen, the nature of the immune system immunized may be very important. For example, it has long been known that BALB/c mice do not respond well to parathyroid hormone (PTH) immunogens (Nussbaum *et al.*, 1981) whereas in other studies rats have been shown to respond usefully. Clearly, this is an area where methods such as intrasplenic immunization (Spitz *et al.*, 1984), *in-vitro* immunization (van Ness *et al.*, 1984) and genetically-engineered antibodies (Winter & Milstein, 1991) will find increasing use.

14.4   Use of monoclonal antibodies

The increasing availability and application of mab technology has significantly enhanced the assay of hormones using immunometric techniques. When mab technology was first introduced it was thought that mab might have low affinity for biological materials and would not therefore supersede polyclonal antisera as assay tools. It has now become apparent that high-affinity mab can be generated and these can be used to construct highly specific, sensitive and reproducible immunoassays. Crucial to this process is the screening assay, which should be closely linked to the contemplated assay, to enable clones secreting appropriate antibodies to be selected and propagated. Mab provide distinct advantages over polyclonal antisera in immunoassays. Firstly, in sequential immunometric assays the high degree of epitope specificity provided by the mab means that affinity purification is unnecessary. Also, polyclonal antisera may bind to many antigenic sites on the hormones, possibly reducing sensitivity, whereas a mab will bind to a single site and leave other epitopes free to bind to the solid phase. Also, mab are superior owing to the lack of competition between the binding sites of capturing and labelled antibody. Secondly, the higher capacity of the solid phase to bind mab delays the saturation effect seen at extremely high antigen concentrations. Finally, the mab, unlike polyclonal antisera, represent only one subclass of immunoglobulins with a single affinity constant. This ability to produce limitless quantities of antibodies of defined specificity has had a great impact on clinical endocrinology. Using defined reagents many assays can be automated, so reducing their cost and making them more widely available. It also allows for better comparison of results obtained by different laboratories.

14.4.1 Enhancement of binding

Another interesting characteristic of certain mab in immunoassays is that the binding of one mab to a soluble antigen can enhance the binding of a second antibody. In the case of human chorionic gonadotrophin (hCG) some mab produced a ten-fold increase in avidity when used in combination (Erlich &

Moyle, 1983). This effect was observed with $F(ab)_2$ fragments but not with $F(ab)$ fragments suggesting that in this case the phenomenon is a characteristic of bivalent antibodies and not a property of antibody–hCG interactions. Similar increases in avidity can be obtained using single mab under certain experimental conditions. Thus, the inclusion of dithiothreitol in the incubation medium can break disulphide bonds binding the heavy chains together and allow the Fab arms of the molecule greater flexibility to bind antigen molecules (Thompson & Jackson, 1984). This favours formation of large molecular cyclic complexes and increased antibody avidity. Such effects may be usefully applied to the immunoassay of hormones.

14.4.2   Two-site immunometric assays in clinical endocrinology

The availability of mab in large quantities has revolutionized the clinical diagnosis of certain endocrine disorders. A good example of this is thyroid disease where immunometric assays for the detection of thyrotropin (TSH) are now available as kits. The diagnosis of thyroid disease provides the bulk of work for most routine diagnostic endocrine laboratories. The most reliable indicator of abnormal thyroid function is the plasma TSH concentration which may be extremely low in thyrotoxicosis. This provided the impetus to develop ultrasensitive and highly specific immunoassays for TSH. Prior to the development of mab for TSH assay, specificity was a problem because of cross-reactivity of polyclonal antisera with other pituitary and placental glycoprotein hormones, often leading to a spurious diagnosis of thyrotoxicosis, particularly in pregnancy. The introduction of immunoradiometric assays was a great advance and provided specific and sensitive assay of circulating TSH concentrations (Seth et al., 1984). These assays were further improved by the use of non-isotopic techniques such as immunochemoluminescence (Weeks et al., 1983, 1984), time-resolved fluorescence (Ekins & Dakabu, 1985; Paterson et al., 1985) and enzyme amplification (Roddis et al., 1985; Stanley et al., 1985; Blunt et al., 1988). The sensitivity of these assays is dependent on the quality of the mab themselves and not on the quality of the detection system.

Other clinically important hormones which may be measured using similar techniques are adrenocorticotrophin (White et al., 1987; Raff & Findling, 1989), gonadotrophins (Pettersson & Soderholm, 1990, 1991), growth hormone (Smith & Norman, 1990; Rudd, 1991), insulin (Sobey et al., 1989), parathyroid hormone (Addison et al., 1971; Dechaud et al., 1986; Logue et al., 1991a, b) and prolactin (Smith & Norman, 1990). The great advantage of these assays over conventional immunoassays is an increase in both specificity and sensitivity. Thus, the assays have enabled discrimination between chemically closely related molecules (Table 14.1) with subsequent improvement in diagnostic precision. They have also enabled pathologically low circulating concentrations of hormones to be measured with confidence.

Perhaps the area where these type of assays have proved most useful has been in discriminating between circulating intact biologically-active forms and precursor or partially processed forms. The two hormones that have been most investigated have been insulin and adrenocorticotrophic hormone (ACTH). Both hormones are synthesized as larger precursor molecules (proinsulin and pro-opiomelanocortin, respectively) which undergo extensive post-translational modifications to produce the biologically-active molecule. As part of this process a number of important circulating cleavage products are produced. In normal subjects proinsulin-like molecules account for some 10–20% of the plasma insulin-like immunoreactivity. In diabetic patients this proportion is considerably increased (Mako *et al.*, 1977) and may give rise to inappropriate estimates of plasma insulin concentrations. To address this problem Hales and his co-workers developed mab that recognized epitopes contained within the entire proinsulin molecule. By careful selection of the mab they were able to produce immunoradiometric assays capable of distinguishing between insulin, proinsulin, 32–33 split proinsulin and 65–66 split proinsulin (Sobey *et al.*, 1989). These studies have shown that much of the proinsulin-like immunoreactivity in plasma is in fact 32–33 split proinsulin. This may be in part because the 65–66 split molecule has a significantly shorter half-life in plasma. During an oral glucose tolerance test the major proinsulin-like molecule found in the plasma is the 32–33 split molecule (Gray *et al.*, 1984; Sobey *et al.*, 1989). This may cause considerable confusion with regard to the insulin status of patients with non-insulin-dependent diabetes mellitus if conventional immunoassays are used. These assays are finding increasing application both clinically and in research and recent high sensitivity enzyme amplified forms of the assay (Cox *et al.*, 1991; Dhahir *et al.*, 1992) should be useful. They enable for the first time accurate measurement of the insulin status of patients. They will also undoubtedly contribute to our knowledge of insulin synthesis and processing. This technology has now been applied to ACTH and its precursors (White *et al.*, 1986). These assays are proving extremely useful in the analysis of ACTH hypersecretion states. The assays can discriminate between intact ACTH and the 22 kDa precursor molecule which has biological activity similar to ACTH 1–39, potentiates ACTH bioactivity and circulates in patients with ectopic ACTH-secreting tumours.

The field of cytokine analysis has recently become extremely active with respect to mab-based immunoassays. In particular, the interleukins (IL) are well served with many assays such as described by Grassi *et al.* (1989) for IL-1 alpha and IL-1 beta with a sensitivity down to 1 pg/ml. Importantly, it has also been possible to employ specific mab to discriminate between intact recombinant IL-1 and its deaminated derivative (Sunahara *et al.*, 1989).

14.4.3 *Immunocytochemistry*

The technique of immunocytochemistry has found wide application within endocrinology and has helped to formulate modern ideas on the existence of a diffuse endocrine system. Using this technique many hormones and neuropeptides have been shown to have a widespread distribution within the body. A classic example of this is somatostatin which was originally isolated from the sheep hypothalamus but has now been shown to exist in cells throughout the brain, pancreas, gut and placenta (Polak & Bloom, 1986). A major drawback of many immunocytochemical techniques has been the quality of the reagents used which have often been poorly characterized polyclonal antisera and which may still contain contaminating immunoglobulins even after extensive absorption. These will often show cross-reactivity with unrelated peptides and peptide fragments and will almost certainly recognize some precursor forms containing the mature peptide sequence. This can best be illustrated by reference to somatostatin which is synthesized as a large precursor molecule that undergoes extensive post-translational modifications to produce the biologically active form. This process appears to generate at least seven different molecular forms in mammalian brain all displaying varying amounts of cross-reactivity with the different terminally-directed antisera (Benoit *et al.*, 1982). Furthermore, there are often considerable variations in the specificities of antisera obtained from commercial sources or from successive bleeds from the same animal. All this helps to reduce the discriminative power of immunocytochemical techniques.

It is not surprising, therefore, that well characterized mab are finding increasing applications as tools in endocrine diagnosis and research. The advantages are mainly those of specificity, purity and availability in unlimited quantities. It must be borne in mind that mab can still cross-react with epitopes in unrelated tissues and can cause serious diagnostic problems for the histopathologist. Alternatively, inaccurate diagnosis could result if the mab did not recognize a functionally active genetic variant lacking the epitope or if the epitope in question was inaccessible in the tissue section. Immunocytochemistry has proved invaluable in the diagnosis of endocrine tumours, particularly pituitary adenomas. Adjacent sections of tumour tissue can be stained with mab to the different anterior pituitary hormones and this, together with the clinical details and endocrine function testing, can provide an accurate diagnosis. This is essential for both clinical management and research.

14.4.4 Flow cytometry

Flow cytometry is now a well established diagnostic and research tool in the fields of immunology, haematology and oncology (Ryan *et al.*, 1988). It has only recently, however, begun to have an impact on endocrinology. The technique is particularly suitable for the analysis and sorting of cell populations but may also be used for analysing subcellular particles and soluble proteins. A commonly employed technique is to label a cell with a fluorochrome-conjugated mab directed against specific cell surface proteins or receptors. Fluorochromes with different absorption and emission peaks can be combined to allow multitarget analysis of individual cells. The main use of cell sorting is in research, particularly in trying to separate either hormone-producing or hormone-sensitive cells from heterogenous cell populations. It may also be of use clinically to identify a particular cell population of interest in a patient. Clinical applications so far have mainly centred on its use in the diagnosis of endocrine tumours but there are many potential clinical applications, particularly in the field of gynaecological endocrinology. For example, it has been used for the cytometric characterization of cell populations in human pregnant decidua (Vince *et al.*, 1990) and for the detection of antibodies to sperm in infertile men (Sinton *et al.*, 1991). Future studies should see the increasing use of this technology in endocrine research, particularly now that many endocrine cell surface markers and receptors are being characterized. As mab to these membrane-bound proteins become available then it should be possible to isolate the cells by flow cytometry and produce homogenous cell populations. This will allow more precise studies on endocrine cells, including single cell studies utilizing technology such as patch clamping and measurement of intracellular calcium flux.

14.4.5   *Analysis of antigenic epitopes in autoimmune endocrine disease*

Mab have proved particularly useful in the dissection of the structure of antigenic molecules and have proved invaluable in helping to characterize the antigen–antibody interactions involved in autoimmunity. The best example of this is autoimmune thyroid disease (AITD) in which mab provided the first evidence that thyroid peroxidase (TPO) is the microsomal antigen. A mab was found which was able to bind preparations of human thyroid membranes, human TPO, bovine TPO and lactoperoxidase and such binding was strongly inhibited by sera from patients with AITD. The mab was subsequently used to purify human TPO from solubilized thyroid membranes using immunoaffinity chromatography (Czarnocka *et al.*, 1985). It was also shown (by indirect immunofluorescence) to bind to the surface of human thyroid cells in culture. Subsequent studies with mab helped to show that the thyroid microsomal antigen and thyroid peroxidase are identical and consist of two separate polypeptide bands of 101 and 107 kDa (Portmann *et al.*, 1988).

An important step in the understanding of the pathogenesis of Hashimoto's thyroiditis will be definition of the epitopes recognized by anti-thyroid peroxidase antibodies. This approach has been limited by the difficulty in obtaining highly purified hTPO for analysis. The recent cloning of the cDNA for hTPO (Magnusson *et al.*, 1987) has circumvented this difficulty and made the production of recombinant TPO possible. This has led to an interesting approach to define the important pathogenic epitopes on hTPO in which a hTPO library expressing random fragments of the protein has been constructed. None of these fragments was recognized by serum from patients with Hashimoto's thyroiditis but they did cross-react with mab raised against denatured hTPO suggesting that the pathogenic epitopes are highly conformational (Finke *et al.*, 1990). Indeed, so far only one mab has been shown to recognize a linear epitope expressed by the library (Finke *et al.*, 1991). This is further evidence for the importance of discontinuous epitopes in autoimmune disease processes.

14.4.6 *Monoclonal antibodies against cell surface determinants on endocrine cells*

Mab have been generated that display exquisite specificity for cellular differentiation antigens and other important cell surface molecules. These have proved useful reagents for identifying and characterizing cell types. Many apparently diverse cell types share common antigenic determinants which are recognized by specific mab. Typically, such cells share common developmental pathways prior to functional differentiation. Analysis of such cell surface markers with mab have proved useful in the study of human autoimmune endocrine disease as these antigens may serve as autoantigens. In certain endocrine disorders the autoimmune response is predominantly organ-specific (e.g. Hashimoto's thyroiditis); however, in others there is multiple organ involvement. This raises the question as to whether the response in such patients is polyclonal with multiple autoantigens or whether it is more restricted with a limited number of autoantibodies recognizing common antigenic determinants in multiple endocrine organs. From the studies available so far it would appear that human mab (prepared by fusion of lymphocytes from patients with various autoimmune endocrine disorders with either mouse or human myeloma cell lines) cross-react with multiple endocrine organs (Satoh *et al.*, 1983).

14.4.7 *Analysis of neuroendocrine cell function*

It has been demonstrated recently that mab directed against neuropeptides can be taken up specifically by neurones when microinjected into the brains of rats (Burlet *et al.*, 1987). These antibodies are transported to the nerve terminals of neurosecretory neurones where they can interfere with neuroendocrine function. The uptake of antibodies is dependent on the functional activity of the neuroendocrine system. Thus, arginine vasopressin (AVP)-mab uptake into AVP neurones is increased in dehydrated rats. Similarly, treatment of rats with a corticotrophin-releasing factor (CRF)-mab results in inhibition of stress-induced ACTH release (Menzaghi *et al.*, 1991). This technique is proving invaluable as a tool for probing discrete neuroendocrine function.

14.4.8 *Identification of new peptides*

Most hormones are produced as larger precursor molecules from which the active hormone is cleaved by proteolysis. This process generates a number of peptides of uncertain biological significance. These gene products can be sequenced and the biological activity investigated (MacIntyre *et al.*, 1982;

Hillyard *et al.*, 1983). Antibodies can also be raised against synthetic peptides and the tissue distribution and circulating concentrations determined (Amara *et al.*, 1982; Hillyard *et al.*, 1983).

14.4.9 Hormone receptor antibodies

Hormone receptor antibodies may be of three types (inhibitory, stimulatory or without effect) and the clinical picture may vary depending on the ratio of the various autoantibodies within the circulation. In the case of Graves' disease, functional TSH-receptor antibodies may either activate the receptor (TSH-stimulating antibodies) or block the receptor (TSH-blocking antibodies). The discovery of endocrine diseases associated with anti-receptor autoimmune reaction has provided the stimulus to produce anti-receptor antibodies. Such antibodies have emerged as important agents for the analysis of receptor structure and function. Several different types of antibody are recognized all of which have different but important roles in endocrine research and clinical practice. These antibodies can be used to clearly distinguish the hormone-binding domain and characterize other portions of the receptor molecule.

14.4.9.1. Purification and characterization of hormonal receptors

Mab have proved extremely useful in the purification of hormonal receptors by immunoaffinity chromatography. This can be achieved in one of two ways: (i) utilizing mab against the receptor itself, or (ii) utilizing antibodies against the ligand. In the latter case the mab is used to purify the receptor–ligand complex as has been shown for the luteinizing hormone (LH) receptor (Vuhai-Luuthi *et al.*, 1990). Immunoprecipitation with mab can be used to further characterize the receptor. In the case of the insulin-like growth factor (IGF)-1 receptor this technique was used to show that, like the insulin receptor, it is autophosphorylated on tyrosine residues. Furthermore, phorbol esters induce phosphorylation of both receptors at serine and threonine residues (Jacobs & Cuatrecasas, 1986). Mab can also be useful in characterizing different molecular forms of hormonal receptors. They can either be used in conventional Western blotting following size separation by SDS-polyacrylamide gel electrophoresis (SDS-PAGE) or the receptor complex can be immunoprecipitated, subjected to SDS-PAGE and then Western-ligand blotted. These techniques are equally applicable to circulating binding proteins as well as to hormonal receptors. Metabolically-labelled newly synthesized binding proteins can also be immunoprecipitated and separated by SDS-PAGE.

14.4.9.2 Epitope mapping of immunogenic domains on hormonal receptors and ligands

The precise mapping of epitopes recognized by mab is important for the definition of immunogenic and functional domains of hormonal receptors and

Table 14.2. *Monoclonal antibody techniques for epitope mapping of hormonal receptors*

Protein proteolysis followed by identification and sequencing of the peptides recognized by antibodies

Chemical modification of amino acids involved in antigen–antibody reactions

Synthesis of peptides and study of their immunological recognition

In vitro mutagenesis followed by study of immunological recognition

Construction of expression vectors containing fragments of the receptor cDNA and study of immunological recognition

Use of carboxy-terminally truncated protein obtained by transcription-translated or cloned cDNA and study of immunological recognition

ligands and has provided much important information. The various techniques utilized in such studies are listed in Table 14.2 but for fine mapping of the epitope structure competitive inhibition studies utilizing synthetic peptides are required. Each of these techniques is not without problems, particularly with respect to discontinuous epitopes, i.e. epitopes that comprise amino acids localized at a distance in the primary structure of the protein but brought together by formation of the tertiary structure.

An approach to the determination of receptor-binding domains on peptide hormones has involved the generation of mab to epitopes on the native molecule. This can be illustrated best by reference to members of the prolactin and growth hormone (GH) family. These are proteins of about 190–200 amino acids in length which share a number of common biological, immunological and structural features. Human GH (hGH) is capable of binding to GH and prolactin receptors from a wide variety of species (Isaksson *et al.*, 1985). The relationship between the structure of hGH and hormone-receptor interaction has been investigated using as probes mab to hGH of defined epitope specificity. These studies have helped to define the functional domains in the hGH molecule responsible for its somatotrophic and lactogenic activities. The GH receptor-binding activity of hGH may be located on two sites, one at the N-terminus and one close to the C-terminus whereas the prolactin receptor-binding activity of hGH is mainly confined to the N-terminus (Strasburger *et al.*, 1989).

The pioneering work of Kabat has shown that the complementary relationships in the recognition of antigens by antibodies is due to the hypervariable nature of the complementarity-determining regions of the antigen-binding site (Wu & Kabat, 1970; Chen & Kabat, 1985; Kabat *et al.*, 1987). This type of technology has been applied to the determination of antigenic regions on hormones using mab to peptides (Lerner, 1984). This has provided important information on structure–activity relationships of hormones.

14.4.9.3 Functional analysis of hormonal receptors

Mab have been used extensively to characterize the structure–activity relationships of hormonal receptors. This is best illustrated with reference to the human insulin receptor. Most mab against this receptor are directed to the cytoplasmic domain of the receptor β subunit which has four main antigenic regions. Using mab the β_2 region has been shown to be associated with the receptor kinase activity. Mab directed against this region were unique in being able to completely inhibit both receptor autophosphorylation and phosphorylation of an exogenous substrate (Morgan & Roth, 1986). These antibodies were also able to recognize the IGF-1 receptor. In contrast, mab to the α subunit of the insulin receptor can inhibit glucose transport but not receptor kinase activity (Forsayeth *et al.*, 1987). Thus, mab can help to separate functional components of the receptor complex. They can also be used to probe the fate of activated receptors at a cellular level. In the case of the insulin receptor, it has been shown that receptor internalization can be induced by mab which are either agonists or antagonists of receptor activity. Such internalization is followed by recycling of the receptor to the cell surface and does not necessarily lead to enhanced receptor degradation. Such degradation was only induced by either insulin or the mab insulin receptor agonist (Trischitta *et al.*, 1989).

Similar studies have shown that epidermal growth factor (EGF)-mediated responses, such as receptor clustering and internalization, receptor phosphorylation, alterations in membrane transport and changes in cell morphology, may either be mimicked or prevented by mab to the EGF receptor (Schreiber *et al.*, 1983; Gill *et al.*, 1984; Gregoriou & Rees, 1984). Also mab directed against both the α and β subunits of the hLH molecule can inhibit hLH-induced steroidogenesis, suggesting that both subunits are required for expression of biological activity (Alonso-Whipple *et al.*, 1988). Mab can also be used to analyse the biological activity of structurally-related hormones. For example, mab that block IGF-I activity, but not IGF-II or insulin activity, can inhibit the growth of MC-7 cells (a human breast carcinoma cell line) in culture, suggesting that such cells require IGF-I as an autocrine growth factor (Rohlik *et al.*, 1987). Mab can also be used to probe functional aspects of intracellular receptors. In the case of the glucocorticoid receptor, mab have been shown to be able to inhibit both steroid binding to the receptor and DNA binding of the activated steroid–receptor complex (Robertson *et al.*, 1987).

14.4.9.4 Anti-idiotypic antibodies

Anti-idiotypic antibodies may mimic the binding characteristics of the hormone itself and can thus be used as a probe of receptor structure and function. This is based on the theory that an anti-ligand antibody represents a negative molecular image of the ligand (Linthicum *et al.*, 1988). Useful information can be gained by generating anti-idiotypic antibodies against the binding site of hormone antibodies. Anti-idiotypes have been produced which bind to, for example, receptors to insulin (Sege & Peterson, 1978: Scechter *et al.*, 1982), TSH (Hill & Erlanger, 1988), prolactin (Amit *et al.*, 1986), progesterone (Wang *et al.*, 1989), glucocorticoids (Cayanis *et al.*, 1986), GH (Elbashir *et al.*, 1990) and beta-adrenergic ligands (Schreiber *et al.*, 1980). Insulin-like stimulation of glucose uptake and activation of catecholamine-sensitive lipase have confirmed the specificity of the reaction between the mab and the receptors. More detailed studies on structural and functional relationships of receptors will undoubtedly lead to a better understanding of the process of signal transduction.

14.4.9.5 TSH receptor antibodies

In autoimmune thyroid disease there appears to be a spectrum of TSH receptor stimulating and blocking antibodies and the clinical picture is dependent on the prevalence of antibody type. Receptor-blocking antibodies undoubtedly play a role in the development of atrophic thyroiditis (primary myxoedema). Antibodies from such patients have been shown to prevent the production of cAMP by human thyroid cells in response to TSH (Konishi *et al.*, 1983). In contrast, TSH stimulating antibodies are responsible for the pathogenesis of hyperthyroidism in Graves' disease. These antibodies are also capable of crossing the placenta and causing transient neonatal hyperthyroidism (McKenzie, 1964). There is also a subgroup of patients who demonstrate fluctuating thyroidal status, either hyperthyroidism followed by hypothyroidism or *vice versa*. This has now been shown to be due to changes in the TSH-receptor antibody status of such patients (McGregor, 1990). Thus there is little doubt that TSH receptor autoantibodies contribute to the pathogenesis of autoimmune thyroid disease. How and why this happens is totally unknown. Autoanti-idiotypes to the TSH receptor have been generated by immunizing BALB/c mice with a mixture of bovine and human TSH (Hill & Erlanger, 1988). These antibodies shared similar binding characteristics to antibodies secreted by Graves' heterohybridomas, suggesting that idiotypic networks may play a role in the pathogenesis of Graves' disease.

The recent cloning of the TSH receptor (Libert *et al.*, 1989; Nagayami *et al.*, 1989) has generated much excitement in the field. It should now be possible to probe the molecular events underlying autoantibody stimulation. Mab against purified receptor or receptor fragments (either native or recombinant) will undoubtedly play an important role in this process. They will be used to develop sensitive and specific immunoassays and also as specific probes to investigate the nature of the receptor–antibody interaction. Another approach which is currently receiving attention is the preparation of TSH receptor antibodies by fusion of lymphocytes from Graves' patients with suitable human or animal myeloma cell lines.

14.4.10 Immunoaffinity purification

The power of mab as a tool in the purification of hormones is finding increasing application both in research and in industry. In this technique the mab is bound to a solid matrix such as sepharose and packed in a column. The tissue extract or solution of interest can then be applied to the column and any hormone present will bind to the column from which it can be eluted. In this way hormones are isolated from complex mixtures in a single step with high yield and purity. Such immunoaffinity techniques are finding increasing application in the purification of recombinant hormones such as bovine somatotropin. They are simple to implement, rapid and easy to automate compared with conventional procedures such as ion exchange chromatography which often requires multiple purification steps to achieve satisfactory purity. The mab used for such techniques, however, must be carefully selected and, if used to purify hormones for the pharmaceutical industry, must be subjected to stringent, standard procedures for production and purification to ensure that the products do not become contaminated.

14.5 Specific modification

14.5.1 Modification of hormonal activity by monoclonal antibodies

Mab can modify hormonal activity by binding to either the hormone or its receptor. The overall effect may be either inhibitory or stimulatory depending on the specificity of the antibody. It has been known for some time that many patients receiving hormone replacement therapy develop antibodies to the hormone. Thus in diabetes mellitus patients may exhibit circulating insulin antibodies which either increase, decrease or have no effect on insulin requirements. Similarly, refractoriness to hGH treatment in children, following the appearance of antibodies, occurs in about 5% of individuals. These observations can only be understood when it is appreciated that the binding of an antibody to an antigen can result in diverse effects depending on the specificity of the antibody. Additionally, antigen-antibody complexes can manifest markedly different effects in the body depending on which epitope the antibody recognizes.

14.5.1.1 Immunoneutralization of hormonal activity

It is normally expected that the effect of an antibody on a hormone is to neutralize the activity of that hormone. Such hormone neutralization may be brought about either by direct masking of the hormone 'active site' or by conformational changes which inhibit hormone-receptor binding. Such inhibition has been observed with monoclonals to a wide variety of hormones including prolactin (Scammell *et al.*, 1990), hGH (Ivanji, 1982), insulin-like growth factor I (Russel *et al.*, 1984; Morrell *et al.*, 1989) and CRF (Milton *et al.*, 1990*a*, *b*).

The observed effects may not be species-specific because of the ability of many mab to cross-react with hormones from different species. In our own studies we have shown that mab raised to human/rat CRF-41 can cross-react with rabbit and mouse CRF-41 (Milton *et al.*, 1990*a*, *b*). Similarly, mab generated to sheep prolactin have been shown to cross-react with monkey and rat prolactin (Scammell *et al.*, 1990). Interestingly, some antibodies were able to selectively neutralize the lactogenic activity of rat prolactin whereas others were able to neutralize sheep lactogenic activity. This raises an important point with respect to screening of clones secreting antibodies to hormones. The screening assay must take account of the purpose for which the mab are being generated. Thus, if the antibodies are required for the study of a particular biological activity of a hormone then the screening procedure must incorporate some measure of such biological activity. Immunization with a mouse mab against progesterone (DB$_3$) prevents pregnancy in several species (Wright *et al.*, 1982; Phillips *et al.*, 1988). It appears to do so by binding to a progesterone-membrane-binding protein complex on uterine epithelial cells and thus preventing implantation (Wang *et al.*, 1990). A mab to IGF-I has been shown to block the action of IGF-I on cartilage growth and sulphation *in vitro* and the insulin-like activity of IGF-I on adipocytes *in vitro* (Morrell *et al.*, 1989).

Numerous reports of inhibition of cytokines by mab have been made including human IL-4 (Chretien *et al.*, 1989), human IL-5 (Schumacher *et al.*, 1988), human IL-6 (Helle *et al.*, 1991) and TNF-β (Adolf & Lamche, 1990). Similarly, mab against cytokine receptors such as mouse IL-5 receptor (Rolink *et al.*, 1989) and human IL-2 receptor (Ohbo, 1991) have provided important information on signal transduction. It has been possible to raise a mab which distinguishes different forms (high and low affinity) of the IL-2 receptor (Takeshita *et al.*, 1990). D'Andrea *et al.* (1989) employed the power of high affinity mab against human recombinant erythropoietin (EPO) to obtain evidence that a recombinant form of the receptor bound to EPO in the same orientation as from the cells from which it was derived. Taga *et al.* (1989) have used a mab against the IL-6 receptor to suggest that binding of IL-6 to its receptor caused association of the receptor with a possible signal transducer gp130. Antibody reagents are being increasingly used as means of analysing cellular events. A clear example of this, albeit with polyclonal antibodies, was the evidence obtained for an autocrine loop operating in the oncogenesis of human myeloma as a result of the production of B cell stimulating factor (BSF-2) growth factor (Kawano *et al.*, 1988). The inhibitory action of the antibodies stopped the feed-back loop. In contrast, Schreurs *et al.* (1989) have identified a mab with stimulatory action. This antibody has been shown to have IL-3-like activity. It both blocks IL-3 binding and stimulates tyrosine phosphorylation. Clearly the availability of specific mab against cytokines and their receptors will be extremely important in understanding their mode of action.

14.5.2 Enhancement of hormonal activity

Some mab have been shown to prolong hormonal activity of, for example, GH (Bates *et al.*, 1992) and TSH (Holder *et al.*, 1987). Recent studies have provided a molecular basis for such interactions and have gone some way in helping to explain certain clinical phenomena. Perhaps the most commonly proposed mechanism for antibody-mediated enhancement of hormonal activity is that of prolongation of half-life in the circulation. Most hormones have a very short half-life (hGH, 20 min; insulin, 9 min) either as a result of a receptor clearance or degradation by specific enzymes. An antibody may protect a hormone from degradation by virtue of its ability to act as a 'carrier protein' in the circulation. It can then prolong hormonal activity by slowly releasing the active hormone into the circulation or because the antibody–hormone complex is able to bind to the receptor and activate it.

Another mechanism whereby mab might enhance hormone activity is by interfering with hormone-receptor binding either by virtue of bivalency or by inducing conformational changes resulting in a more favourable hormone-receptor interaction. In such a way the hormone may either acquire greater affinity for its receptor or be protected from proteolytic mechanisms. The existence of different receptor specificities for a particular hormone and the ability of mab to interfere with hormone binding to one class of receptor, but not to another, may provide a means of regulating or directing hormonal activity. Whether or not such manipulation of hormone activity could be of clinical use is as yet unclear.

14.5.3 Future prospects

In this chapter we have covered some of the potential applications of mab technology in endocrinology. Undoubtedly, as the technology develops, so will the applied science. The next decade should see considerable progress in immunoassays and one can confidently expect new, monoclonal-based immunoassays to revolutionize analyte measurement, particularly with regard to difficult small molecules such as steroids. Other diagnostic uses will involve improved imaging and histological diagnosis of endocrine tumours. Further progress in recombinant DNA technology and mab should greatly improve our knowledge of normal cell biology and the pathogenesis of various diseases and, in particular, autoimmune endocrine disease. This basic knowledge will enhance the therapeutic potential for endocrine diseases. No doubt mab will be at the forefront here as well. Once the problems of producing genetically-engineered human antibodies have been overcome then we should see the production of mab, or their isolated specific binding sites, for therapeutic purposes. The main targets will be the autoimmune disorders such as thyroid disease and diabetes mellitus; however, other potential targets will be endocrine tumours and ectopic hormone-secreting tumours.

14.6   References

Addison, G., Hales, C., Woodhead, J. & O'Riordan, J. (1971). Immunoradiometric assay of parathyroid hormone. *Journal of Endocrinology*, **49**, 521–530.

Adolf, G. A. & Lamche, H. R. (1990). Highly sensitive enzyme immunoassay for human lymphotoxin (tumor necrosis factor β) in serum. *Journal of Immunological Methods*, **130**, 177–185.

Alonso-Whipple, C., Couet, M., Doss, R., Koziarz, J., Ogunro, E. & Crowley, W. (1988). Epitope mapping of human luteinizing hormone using monoclonal antibodies. *Endocrinology*, **123**, 1854–1860.

Amara, S., Jonas, V., O'Neill, J., Vale, W., Rivier, J., Roos, B., Evans, R. & Rosenfield, M. (1982). Calcitonin COOH-terminal cleavage peptide as a model for identification of novel neuropeptides predicted by recombinant DNA analysis. *Journal of Biological Chemistry*, **257**, 2129–2136.

Amit, T., Barkey, R., Gavish, M. & Youdin, M. (1986). Anti-idiotypic antibodies raised against anti-protein (PRL) antibodies recognise the PRL receptor. *Endocrinology*, **118**, 835–843.

Bates, P., Aston, R. & Holder, A. (1992). Growth hormone control of tissue protein metabolism in dwarf mice: enhanced by a mab. *Journal of Endocrinology*, **132**, 369–375.

Benoit, R., Ling, N., Alford, B. & Guillemin, R. (1982). Seven peptides derived from pro-somatostatin in rat brain. *Biochemical and Biophysical Research Communications*, **107**, 944–950.

Blunt, S., Wood, C. A., Joplin, G. F. & Burrin, J. M. (1988). The note of a highly sensitive amplified enzyme immunoassay for thyrotropin in the evaluation of thyrotroph function in hypopituitary patients. *Clinical Endrocrinology* (Oxford), **29**, 387–393.

Branch, D. R., Shah, A. & Guilbert, L. J. (1991). A specific and reliable bioassay for the detection of femtomolar levels of human and murine tumor necrosis factors. *Journal of Immunological Methods*, **143**, 251–261.

Burlet, A., Leon-Henri, B., Robert, F., Arahmani, A., Fernette, B. & Burlet, C. (1987). Monoclonal antibodies penetrate into VP neurons, *in vivo*. *Experimental Brain Research*, **65**, 629–638.

Cayanis, E., Rajagopalan, R., Cleveland, W., Edelman, I. & Erlanger, B. (1986). Generation of an auto-anti-idiotypic antibody that binds to the glucocorticoid receptor. *Journal of Biological Chemistry*, **261**, 5094–5104.

Chen, H. & Kabat, E. (1985). Immunochemical studies on blood groups. *Journal of Biological Chemistry*, **260**, 13208–13217.

Chretien, I., Van Kimmenada, A., Pearce, M. K., Bancherewau, J. & Abrams, J. S. (1989). Development of polyclonal and monoclonal antibodies for immunoassay and neutralization of human interleukin-4. *Journal of Immunological Methods*, **117**, 67–81.

Cox, L. J., Clarke, P. M. S., Alpha, B., Crowther, N. & Hales, C. N. (1991). Sensitive enzyme-amplified immunometric assays for human insulin and intact proinsulin. In *Proceedings of the ABC National Meeting*, Glasgow, U. K. 13–17 May 1991. Published by the Association of Clinical Biochemists.

Czarnocka, B., Ruf, J., Ferrand, M., Carayon, P. & Lissitzky, S. (1985). Purification of the human thyroid peroxidase and its identification as the microsomal antigen involved in autoimmune thyroid disease. *FEBS Letters*, **190**, 147–152.

D'Andrea, A. D., Lodish, H. F. & Wong, G. G. (1989). Expression cloning of the murine erythropoietin receptor. *Cell*, **57**, 277–285.

Dechaud, H., Bador, R., Clamstrat, F. & Desuzinges, C. (1986). Laser-excited immunofluorometric assay of prolactin, with use of antibodies coupled to lanthanide-labelled diethylenetriaminepenta-acetic acid. *Clinical Chemistry*, **32**, 1323–1327.

Dhahir, F., Cook, D. & Self, C. (1992). An amplified enzyme-linked immunoassay for proinsulin. *Clinical Chemistry*, **38**, 227–232.

Ekins, R. & Dakabu, S. (1985). The development of high sensitivity, pulsed light, time-resolved fluoroimmunoassays. *Pure and Applied Chemistry*, **57**, 473–480.

Elbashir, M., Brodin, T., Akerstrom, B. & Donmer, J. (1990). Monoclonal antibodies to the pituitary growth-hormone receptor by the anti-idiotypic approach. *Journal of Biochemistry*, **266**, 467–474.

Erlich, P. & Moyle, W. (1983). Co-operative immunoassay: ultrasensitive assays with mixed monoclonal antibodies. *Science*, **221**, 279–281.

Finke, R., Seto, P. & Rapoport, B. (1990). Evidence for the highly conformational nature of the epitope(s) on human thyroid peroxidase that are recognized by sera from patients with Hashimoto's thyroiditis. *Journal of Clinical Endocrinology and Metabolism*, **71**, 53–59.

Finke, R., Seto, P., Ruf, J., Carayon, P. & Rapoport, B. (1991). Determination at the molecular level of a β-cell epitope on thyroid peroxidase likely to be associated with autoimmune thyroid disease. *Journal of Clinical Endocrinology and Metabolism*, **73**, 919–921.

Forsayeth, J., Caro, J., Sinha, M., Maddux, B. & Goldfine, I. (1987). Monoclonal antibodies to the human insulin receptor that activate glucose transport but not insulin receptor kinase activity. *Proceedings of the National Academy of Sciences U.S.A.*, **84**, 3448–3451.

Fukuda, Y., Hashimo, J., Haruyama, M., Tsuruoka, N., Nakazato, H. & Nakanishi, T. (1991). A sandwich enzyme-linked immunosorbent assay for human interleukin-5. *Journal of Immunological Methods*, **143**, 89–94.

Gill, G., Kawamoto, T., Cochet, C., Le, A., Sato, J., Masui, H., McLeod, C. & Mendelsohn, J. (1984). Monoclonal anti-epidermal growth factor receptor antibodies which are inhibitors of epidermal growth factor binding and antagonists of epidermal growth factor-stimulated tyrosine protein kinase activity. *Journal of Biological Chemistry*, **259**, 7755–7760.

Grassi, J., Frobert, Y., Pradelles, P., Chercuitte, F., Gruaz, D., Dayer, J-M. & Poubelle, P. E. (1989). Production of monoclonal antibodies against interleukin-1 alpha and -1beta. Development of two enzyme immunometric assays (EIA) using acetylcholinesterase and their application to biological media. *Journal of Immunological Methods*, **123**, 193–210.

Gray, I., Siddle, K., Docherty, K., Frank, B. & Hales, C. (1984). Proinsulin in human serum: problems in measurement and interpretation. *Clinical Endocrinology*, **21**, 43–47.

Gregoriou, M. & Rees, A. (1984). Properties of a mab to epidermal growth factor receptor with implications for the mechanism of action of EGF. *EMBO Journal*, **3**, 929–937.

Groome, N. (1991). Ultrasensitive two-site assays for inhibin-A and activin-A using monoclonal antibodies raised to synthetic peptides. *Journal of Immunological Methods*, **145**, 503–550.

Guan, X. & Dluzen, D. (1991). Castration reduces potassium-stimulated norepinephrine release from superfused olfactory bulbs of male rats. *Brain Research*, **568**, 147–151.

Helle, M., Boeije, L., de Groot, E., de Vos, A. & Aarden, L. (1991). Sensitive ELISA for interleukin-6: detection of IL-6 in biological fluids: synovial fluids and sera. *Journal of Immunological Methods*, **138**, 47–56.

Hill, B. & Erlanger, B. (1988). Monoclonal antibodies to the thyrotropin receptor raised by an autoanti-idiotypic protocol and their relationship to monoclonal antibodies from Graves' patients. *Endocrinology*, **122**, 2840–2850.

Hillyard, C., Myers, C., Abeyasekera, G., Stevenson, J., Craig, R. & MacIntyre, I. (1983). Katacalcin: a new plasma calcium-lowering hormone. *Lancet*, **1**, 846–848.

Holder, A., Aston, R., Rest, J., Hill, D., Patel, M. & Ivanyi, J. (1987). Monoclonal antibodies can enhance the action of thyrotropin. *Endocrinology*, **120**, 567–573.

Isaksson, O., Eden, S. & Jansson, J. (1985). Mode of action of pituitary growth hormone on target cells. *Annual Reviews in Physiology*, **47**, 483–499.

Ivanji, J. (1982). Study of antigenic structure and inhibition of activity of human growth hormone and chorionic somatomammotrophin by monoclonal antibodies. *Molecular Immunology*, **19**, 1611–1618.

Jacobs, S. & Cuatrecasas, P. (1986). Phosphorylation of receptors for insulin and insulin-like growth factor 1. *Journal of Biological Chemistry*, **261**, 934–939.

Kabat, E., Wu, T., Reid-Miller, M., Perry, H. & Gottesman, K. (1987). *Sequences of Proteins of Immunological Interest*, 4th edn. United States Department of Health and Human Services, National Institutes of Health, Bethesda, Maryland.

Kawano, M., Hirano, T., Matsuda, T., Taga, T., Horii, Y., Iwato, K., Asaoku, H., Tang, B., Tanabe, O., Tanaka, H., Kuramoto, A. & Kishimoto, T. (1988). Autocrine generation and requirement of BSF-2/IL-6. *Nature*, **332**, 83–85.

Konishi, J., Iida, J., Endo, K., Misaki, T., Nohara, Y., Matsuura, N., Mori, T. & Torizuka, K. (1983). Inhibition of thyrotropin-induced adenosine 3,5-monophosphate increase by immunoglobulins from patients with primary myxoedema. *Journal of Clinical Endocrinology and Metabolism*, **57**, 544–549.

Lerner, R. A. (1982). Tapping the immunological repertoire to produce antibodies of predetermined specificity. *Nature*, **299**, 592–596.

Lerner, R. (1984). Antibodies of predetermined specificity in biology and medicine. *Advances in Immunology*, **36**, 1–44.

Libert, F., Lcvort, A., Gerard, C., Parmentier, M., Perret, J., Ludgate, M., Dumont, J. & Vassart, G. (1989). Cloning, sequencing and expression of the human thyrotropin (TSH) receptor: evidence for binding of autoantibodies. *Biochemical and Biophysical Research Communications*, **165**, 1250–1255.

Linthicum, D., Bolger, M., Kussie, P., Albright, G., Linton, T., Combs, S. & Marcett, D. (1988). Analysis of idiotypic and anti-idiotypic antibodies as models of receptor and ligand. *Clinical Chemistry*, **34**, 1676–1680.

Logue, F. C., Perry, B., Chapman, R., Milne, I., James, K. & Beastall, G. (1991a). A two-site immunometric assay for PTH (1–84) using N and C-terminal specific monoclonal antibodies. *Annals of Clinical Biochemistry*, **28**, 160–166.

Logue, F. C., Perry, B., Biggart, E. M., Chapman, R. S. & Beastall, G. H. (1991b). Production and characterisation of monoclonal antibodies to parathyroid hormone (1–34). *Journal of Immunological Methods*, **137**, 159–166.

MacIntyre, I., Hillyard, C., Murphy, P., Reynolds, J., Gaines Das, R. & Craig, R. (1982). A second plasma calcium-lowering peptide from the human calcitonin precursor. *Nature*, **300**, 460–462.

McGregor, A. (1990). Autoantibodies to the TSH receptor in patients with autoimmune thyroid disease. *Clinical Endocrinology*, **33**, 683–685.

McKenzie, J. (1964). Neonatal Graves' disease. *Journal of Clinical Endocrinology and Metabolism*, **24**, 660–668.

Magnusson, R., Chazenbalk, G., Gestautas, J., Seto, P., Filetti, S. & Rapoport, B. (1987). Isolation and characterization of a cDNA clone for porcine thyroid peroxidase. *Molecular Endocrinology*, **1**, 856–861.

Mako, M., Starr, J. & Rubenstein, A. (1977). Circulating proinsulin in patients with maturity onset diabetes. *American Journal of Medicine*, **63**, 865–869.

Menzaghi, F., Burlet, A., Van Oers, J., Tilders, F., Nicolas, J. & Burlet, C. (1991). Long-term inhibition of stress-induced adrenocorticotropin release by intracerebral administration of a mab to rat corticotropin-releasing factor together with ricin A chain and monensin. *Journal of Neuroendocrinology*, **3**, 469–476.

Milton, N., Hillhouse, E. & Milton, A. (1990*b*). The involvement of CRF-41 and prostaglandins in the febrile response. *Journal of Endocrinology* **127**(suppl.), 96.

Milton, N., Hillhouse, E., Nicholson, S., Self, C. & McGregor, A. (1990*a*). Production and utilization of monoclonal antibodies to human/rat corticotrophin-releasing factor-41. *Journal of Molecular Endocrinology*, **5**, 159–166.

Morgan, D. & Roth, R. (1986). Mapping surface structures of the human insulin receptor with monoclonal antibodies: localization of main immunogenic regions to the receptor kinase domain. *Biochemistry*, **25**, 1364–1371.

Morrell, D., Dadi, H., More, J., Taylor, A., Dabestani, A., Buchanan, C., Holder, A. & Preece, M. (1989). A monoclonal antibody to human insulin-like growth factor-1: characterization use in radioimmunoassay and effect on the biological activities of the growth factor. *Journal of Molecular Endocrinology*, **2**, 201–206.

Nagayama, Y., Kaufman, K., Seto, P. & Rapoport, B. (1989). Molecular cloning, sequence and functional expression of the cDNA for the human thyrotropin receptor. *Biochemical and Biophysical Research Communications*, **165**, 1184–1190.

Nussbaum, S. R., Rosenblatt, M., Mudgett-Hunter, M. & Potts, Jr., J. T. (1981). Monoclonal antibodies directed against the biologically active regions of parathyroid hormone. In *Monoclonal Antibodies in Endocrine Research*, ed. R. Fellow & G. Eisenearth, New York, Raven Press, p. 181.

Ohbo, K., Takeshita, T., Asao, H., Kurahayashi, Y., Tada, K., Mori, H., Hatakeyama, M., Taniguchi, T. & Sugamura, K. (1991). Monoclonal antibodies defining distinct epitopes of the human IL-2 receptor beta chain and their differential effects on IL-2 responses. *Journal of Immunological Methods*, **142**, 61–72.

Paterson, N., Biggart, E., Chapman, R. & Veastall, G. (1985). Evaluation of a time-resolved immunofluorometric assay for serum thyroid stimulating hormone. *Annals of Clinical Biochemistry*, **22**, 606–611.

Pettersson, K. & Soderholm, J. (1990). Ultrasensitive two-site immunometric assay of human lutropin by time-resolved fluorimetry. *Clinical Chemistry*, **36**, 1928–1934.

Pettersson, K. & Soderholm, J. (1991). Individual differences in lutropin immuno-reactivity revealed by monoclonal antibodies. *Clinical Chemistry*, **37**, 333–340.

Phillips, A., Hahn, D., McGuire, J., Wang, M., Heap, R., Rider, V. & Yaussig, M. (1988). Inhibition of pregnancy before and after implantation in rats with mab against progesterone. *Contraception*, **38**, 109–116.

Polak, J. & Bloom, S. (1986). Somatostatin localization in tissues. *Scandinavian Journal of Gastroenterology*, **119**, 11–21.

Portmann, L., Fitch, F., Havran, W., Hamada, N., Franklin, W. & De Grott, L. (1988). Characterization of the thyroid microsomal antigen and its relationship to thyroid peroxidase, using monoclonal antibodies. *Journal of Clinical Investigation*, **81**, 1217–1224.

Raff, H. & Findling, J. (1989). A new immunoradiometric assay for corticotropin evaluated in normal subjects and patients with Cushing's syndrome. *Clinical Chemistry*, **35**, 596–600.

Ratcliffe, W. A., Hughes, S., Gilligan, M. G., Heath, D. A. & Ratcliffe, J. G. (1990). Production and characterisation of monoclonal antibodies to parathyroid hormone-related protein. *Journal of Immunological Methods*, **127**, 109–116.

Robertson, N., Kusmik, W., Grove, B., Miller-Diemer, A., Webb, M. & Litwack, G.

(1987). Characterization of a mab that probes the functional domains of the glucocorticoid receptor. *Journal of Biochemistry*, **246**, 55–65.

Roddis, M. J., Burrin, J. M., Johannssen, A., Ellis, D. H., & Self, C. H. (1985). Serum thyrotropin: a first-line discriminatory test of thyroid function. *Lancet*, **1**, 277–278.

Rohlik, Q. T., Adams, P., Kull, F. & Jacobs, S. (1987). An antibody to the receptor for insulin-like growth factor 1 inhibits the growth of MCF-7 cells in tissue culture. *Biochemical and Biophysical Research Communications*, **149**, 276–281.

Rolink, A. G., Melchers, F. & Palcios, R. (1989). Monoclonal antibodies reactive with the mouse interleukin 5 receptor. *Journal of Experimental Medicine*, **169**, 1693–1701.

Rudd, B. (1991). Growth, growth hormone and the somatomedin: an historical perspective and current concepts. *Annals of Clinical Biochemistry*, **28**, 542–555.

Russel, W., van Wyk, J. & Pledger, W. (1984). Inhibition of the mitogenic effects of plasma by a mab to somatomedin C. *Proceedings of the National Academy of Sciences U.S.A.*, **81**, 2389–2395.

Ryan, D. H., Fallon, M. A. & Horan, P. K. (1988). Flow cytometry in the clinical laboratory. *Clinica Chimica Acta*, **171**, 125–173.

Satoh, J., Prabhakar, B., Haspel, M. V., Ginsberg–Fellner, F. & Notkins, A. L. (1983). Human monoclonal autoantibodies that react with multiple endocrine organs. *New England Journal of Medicine*, **309**, 217–220.

Scammell, J., Wear, L. & von Haven, R. (1990). A monoclonal antibody which inhibits the biological activity of rat prolactin, but not prolactin from other species. *Molecular and Cellular Endocrinology*, **71**, 125–131.

Scechter, Y., Maron, R., Elias, D. & Cotter, I. (1982). Autoantibodies to insulin receptor spontaneously develop as anti-idiotypes in mice immunized with insulin. *Science*, **216**, 542–545.

Schreiber, A., Couraud, P., Andre, C., Vray, B. & Strosberg, A. (1980). Anti-alprenolol anti-idiotypic antibodies bind to β-adrenergic receptors and modulate catecholamine-sensitive adenylate cyclase. *Proceedings of the National Academy of Sciences U.S.A.*, **77**, 7385–7389.

Schreiber, A., Libermann, T., Lax, I., Yarden, Y. & Schlessinger, J. (1983). Biological role of epidermal growth factor-receptor clustering. *Journal of Biological Chemistry*, **258**, 846–853.

Schreurs, A., Sugawara, M., Arai, K.-I., Ohta, Y. & Miyajima, A. (1989). A monoclonal antibody IL-3-like activity blocks IL-3 binding and stimulates tyrosine phosphorylation. *Journal of Immunology*, **142**, 819–825.

Schumacher, J. H., O'Garra, A., Shrader, B., van Kimmmenade, A., Bond, M. W., Mosmann, T. R. & Coffman, R. L. (1988). The characterization of four monoclonal antibodies specific for mouse IL-5 and development of mouse and human IL-5 enzyme linked immunosorbent assays. *Journal of Immunology*, **141**, 1576–1581.

Sege, K. & Peterson, P. (1978). Use of anti-idiotypic antibodies as cell surface receptor probes. *Proceedings of the National Academy of Sciences U.S.A.*, **75**, 2443–2447.

Seth, J., Kellet, J., Caldwell, G., Swetting, V., Beckett, G., Gow, S. & Toft, A. (1984). A sensitive immunoradiometric assay for serum thyroid stimulating hormone: a replacement for the thyroid releasing hormone test. *British Medical Journal*, **289**, 1334–1346.

Sinton, E., Riemann, D. & Ashton, M. (1991). Antisperm antibody detection using concurrent cytofluometry and indirect immunofluorescence microscopy. *American Journal of Clinical Pathology*, **95**, 242–246.

Smith, C. & Norman, M. (1990). Prolactin and growth hormone: molecular heterogeneity and measurement in serum. *Annals of Clinical Biochemistry*, **27**, 542–550.

Sobey, W., Beer, S., Carington, C., Clark, P., Franks, B., Gray, P., Luzio, S., Owens, D., Schneider, A., Siddle, K., Temple, R. & Hales, C. (1989). Sensitive and specific two site immunoradiometric assays for human insulin, proinsulin, 65–66 split and 32–33 split proinsulins. *Biochemical Journal*, **260**, 535–541.

Spitz, M., Spitz, L., Thorpe, R. & Eugui, E. (1984). Intrasplenic primary immunization for the production of monoclonal antibodies. *Journal of Immmunological Methods*, **70**, 39–43.

Stanley, C., Johannsson, A. & Self, C. (1985). Enzyme amplification can enhance both the speed and sensitivity of immunoassays. *Journal of Immunological Methods*, **83**, 89–95.

Strasburger, C., Kostyo, J., Vogel, T., Brennard, G. & Kohen, F. (1989). The antigenic epitopes of human growth hormones as mapped by monoclonal antibodies. *Endocrinology*, **124**, 1548–1557.

Sunahara, N., Kawata, S., Kaibe, K., Furuta, R., Yamayoshi, M., Yamada, M. & Kurooka, S. (1989). Differential determination of recombinant human interleukin-1 alpha and its deamidated derivative by two sandwich enzyme immunoassays using monoclonal antibodies. Comparison with a polyclonal antibody-based competitive enzyme immunoassay. *Journal of Immunological Methods*, **119**, 75–82.

Taga, T., Hibi, M., Hirata, Y., Yamasaki, K., Yasukawa, K., Matsuda, T., Hirano, T. & Kishimoto, T. (1989). Interleukin-6 triggers the association of its receptor with a possible signal transducer, gp130. *Cell*, **58**, 573–581.

Takeshita, T., Asao, H., Suzuki, J. & Sugamura, K. (1990). An associated molecule, p64 with high-affinity for interleukin-2 receptor. *International Immunology*, **2**, 477–480.

Thompson, R. & Jackson, C. A. (1984). Cyclic complexes and high avidity antibodies. *TIBS*, **9**, 1–3.

Trischitta, V., Wong, K., Brumetti, A, Scalisi, R., Vigneri, R. & Goldfine, I. (1989). Endocytosis, recycling, and degradation of the insulin receptor. *Journal of Biological Chemistry*, **264**, 5041–5046.

Van Ness, J., Laemmli, U. K. & Pettijohn, D. E. (1984). Immunization *in vitro* and production of monoclonal antibodies specific to insoluble and weakly immunogenic proteins. *Proceedings of the National Academy of Sciences U.S.A.*, **81**, 7897–7901.

Vince, G., Starkey, P., Jackson, M., Sargent, I. & Redman, C. (1990). Flow cytometric characterization of cell populations in human pregnancy decidua and isolation of decidual macrophages. *Journal of Immunological Methods*, **132**, 181–189.

Vuhai-Luuthi, M., Jolivet, A., Jallal, B., Salesse, R., Bidart, J., Houllier, A., Guiochon-Mantel, A., Garnier, J. & Milgrom, E. (1990). Monoclonal antibodies against luteinizing hormone receptor. Immunochemical characterization of the receptor. *Endocrinology*, **127**, 2090–2098.

Wakefield, L. M., Smith, D. M., Flanders, K. C. & Sporn, M. B. (1988). Latent transforming growth factor-β from human platelets. *Journal of Biological Chemistry*, **263**, 7646–7654.

Wang, M., Whyte, A., Heap, R. & Taussig, M. (1990). Pregnancy-blocking progesterone antibody targets specifically the uterus through its progesterone-binding sites. *Journal of Molecular Endocrinology*, **4**, 283–291.

Wang, M., Whyte, A., King, I., Taussig, M. & Heap, R. (1989). Immunofluorescent localization, by use of anti-idiotypic antibody, of monoclonal anti-progesterone antibody in the mouse uterus before implantation. *Journal of Reproductive Fertility*, **86**, 211–218.

Weeks, I., Beheshti, I., McCapra, F., Campbell, A. & Woodhead, J. (1983). Acridinium esters as high specificity labels in immunoassay. *Clinical Chemistry*, **29**, 1474–1479.

Weeks, I., Sturgess, M., Siddle, K., Jones, M. K. & Woodhead, J. S. (1984). A high sensitivity immunochemiluminometric assay for human thyrotrophin. *Clinical Endocrinology*, **20**, 489–495.

White, A., Dobson, S., Gray, C. & Ratcliffe, J. (1986). Production and characterization of monoclonal antibodies to adrenocorticotrophin (ACTH) for an immunoradiometric assay. In *Monoclonal Antibodies: Basic Principles, Experimental and Clinical Applications in Endocrinology*, Serona Symposia Publications, Raven Press, vol. 30, **3**, 59–76.

White, A., Smith, H., Hoadley, M., Dobson, S. & Ratcliffe, J. (1987). Clinical evaluation of a two-site immunoradiometric assay for adrenocorticotrophin in unextracted human plasma using monoclonal antibodies. *Clinical Endocrinology*, **26**, 41–52.

Winter, G. & Milstein, C. (1991). Man-made antibodies. *Nature*, **349**, 293–299.

Wright, L., Feinstein, A., Heap, R., Saunders, J., Bennett, P. & Wang, M. (1982). Progesterone mab blocks pregnancy in mice. *Nature*, **295**, 415–417.

Wu, T. & Kabat, E. (1970). An analysis of the sequences of the variable regions of Bence–Jones proteins and myeloma light chains and their implications for antibody complementarity. *Journal of Experimental Medicine*, **132**, 211–250.

15

Monoclonal antibodies in rheumatology

J. D. ISAACS

15.1 Introduction

During the coming decade monoclonal antibodies (mab) may modify our approach to the management of autoimmunity. Evidence from animal models of human disease suggests that mab can provide a more targeted therapeutic option than conventional treatments, being aimed specifically at the cells that are involved in the immunopathological process. This will reduce and, in some cases eliminate, the need for other immunosuppressive agents such as steroids and cytotoxic agents with their associated side-effects. The ability to use mab in this way has arisen from a clearer understanding of immune physiology and the cellular interactions that make up an immune response.

In this chapter the rheumatological diseases are used to exemplify the potential of mab therapy. The fundamental immunology will be reviewed followed by a summary of the data from animal models of SLE and rheumatoid arthritis. This will set the stage for a discussion of the current data in human autoimmune and inflammatory diseases. Although mab have thus far been reserved for severe, refractory cases the results are exciting and may herald a major change in the future management of such conditions.

15.2 Normal immune response

15.2.1 Central role of the T cell

The use of mab to control unwanted immunological responses requires an understanding of the cellular interactions that are involved in their initiation. It is now generally accepted that most immune responses are initiated by the activation of a helper (usually $CD4^+$) T cell as a result of interaction with antigen. T cells cannot respond to antigen directly but require it to be 'presented' to them by an antigen-presenting cell (APC, Figure 1). The APC processes antigen into a number of small peptides which then appear on its surface in association with major histocompatibility complex (MHC) molecules (Germaine & Margulies, 1993). Crystallographic studies of MHC class I molecules demonstrate a surface structure comprising two alpha helices sup-

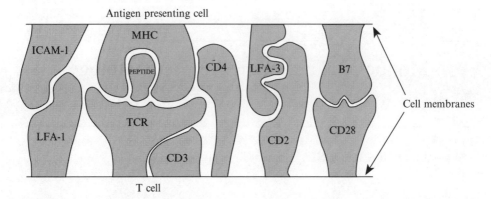

Figure 15.1. Some of the surface interactions between a T cell and an antigen-presenting cell.

ported on a beta sheet with the peptide resting in a cleft between the helices. It is stabilized there by interactions between peptide side chains and complementary pockets in the floor and sides of the cleft (Bjorkman *et al.*, 1987; Garrett *et al.*, 1989, Saper *et al.*, 1991). The primary sequence of MHC class II molecules suggests a similar structure (Brown *et al.*, 1988). Polymorphisms within MHC molecules are concentrated within the amino acids lining the cleft such that allelic variants bind their own unique set of peptides (Rammensee *et al.*, 1993). The helix–peptide–helix structure is recognized by the T cell receptor (TCR). The recognition part of this molecule comprises two polypeptide chains which resemble immunoglobulin light chains in structure. CD3 is the signalling portion and consists of five non-covalently linked peptide chains. A number of other intercellular interactions takes place during antigen recognition. CD4 on the T cell binds to an invariant portion of an MHC class II molecule on the APC. The cytoplasmic tail of CD4 is coupled to a tyrosine protein kinase, p56[lck] and this association is necessary for antigen-specific signal transduction (Glaichenhaus *et al.*, 1991). Other interactions include those between leucocyte function associated molecule 1 (LFA-1) and intercellular adhesion molecule-1 (ICAM-1), CD2 and LFA3, and CD28 and B7 (Figure 15.1).

The exact requirements for T cell activation are unknown although antigen recognition *per se* is insufficient. If T cells are presented with antigen by chemically 'fixed' APCs they actually become refractory to subsequent, otherwise adequate, stimuli (Mueller *et al.*, 1989). These observations are consistent with a two-step model in which, in addition to antigen recognition, the T cell requires certain 'second signals' to become activated (Bretscher & Cohn, 1970). The more recent experiments imply that lack of second signals (as seen with 'fixed' APCs) may result in a state of unresponsiveness and this is important for understanding the theory behind the use of mab in auto-immunity. The nature of the second signal (or signals) has proven elusive although CD28 may play a role (Linsley & Ledbetter, 1993).

Once activated, T cells secrete a variety of lymphokines which act on cells of lymphoid and non-lymphoid lineage resulting in destruction of virally-infected cells, tumours and transplanted tissue, as well as the induction of specific antibody responses. T cell activation is therefore central to the generation of a range of immune responses and the genetic linkage of many autoimmune diseases to specific MHC haplotypes supports a central role for T cells in their development also. Presumably the responsible autoaggressive T cells escaped thymic deletion (Pullen *et al.*, 1988) or peripheral inactivation (Miller & Morahan, 1992) during development of the immune system, but if it were possible to regulate their activity then control of the disease may follow.

15.2.2 Adhesion molecules

Before causing damage, lymphocytes and inflammatory cells must enter the target organ (Haynes *et al.*, 1989; Pattarayo *et al.*, 1990). The potential interactions between leucocytes and endothelium are complex, involving selectins, integrins, members of the immunoglobulin gene superfamily and other 'homing' receptors such as CD44 but the physiology is rapidly becoming clear. Initial interactions seem to occur between glycoproteins on leucocytes and selectins on endothelial cells (Lawrence & Springer, 1991; Springer & Lasky, 1991). For lymphocytes, an interaction between VLA-4 on the cell and VCAM-1 on endothelium is important for adhesion whereas LFA-1 is essential

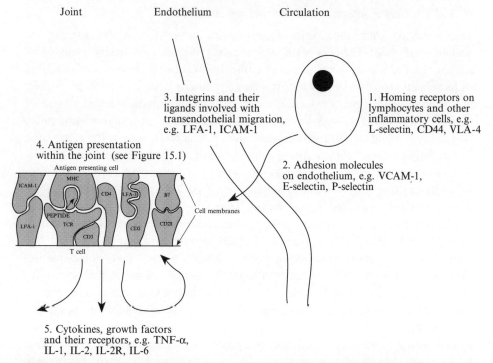

Figure 15.2. Potential therapeutic targets for monoclonal antibodies in inflammatory joint disease.

for transendothelial migration (Kavanaugh *et al.*, 1991). Already this information is being used to design new anti-inflammatory mab and other reagents. Figure 15.2 summarizes the potential targets for immunotherapy with mab.

15.3   Monoclonal antibodies to control immune responsiveness

15.3.1   *Immunosuppression with monoclonal antibodies*

Given the central role of the T cell, it is not surprising that immune responsiveness can be dampened by blocking some of the interactions depicted in Figure 15.1. Chapter 12 of this book describes the immunosuppressive properties of mab directed at some of the surface molecules present on T cells and their use in organ transplantation. A number of studies have also demonstrated that T cell mab can suppress autoimmune diseases in animals. Thus class II MHC mab were able to suppress experimental autoimmune encephalomyelitis (EAE, a model for multiple sclerosis; Steinman *et al.*, 1981), experimental myasthenia gravis (Waldor *et al.*, 1983) and the systemic lupus erythematosus (SLE)-like illness of NZB/NZW mice (Adelman *et al.*, 1983; 15.4.1). CD4 mab have also proved useful in collagen-induced arthritis (Ranges *et al.*, 1985; 15.4.2) and diabetes (Shizuru *et al.*, 1988).

15.3.2   *Tolerance induction with monoclonal antibodies*

More exciting than their immunosuppressive properties is the tolerogenic potential of mab. Patients with autoimmune diseases or organ transplants usually require life-long treatment to control unwanted immune reactivity. If it were possible to reverse this autoreactivity permanently, then perhaps disease progression or transplant rejection could be controlled with a single course of therapy. It is relatively easy to induce tolerance to foreign proteins using mab. Benjamin & Waldmann (1986) treated mice with a CD4 mab at the same time as challenging them with a foreign protein (human gamma globulin, HGG). Not only did the mice fail to make an immune response to HGG (immunosuppression) but they were also unresponsive on subsequent challenge, long after the CD4 mab had been cleared from the circulation (immunological tolerance). In a subsequent study (Benjamin *et al.*, 1988), tolerance was shown to reside at the level of the T cell and could also be obtained using an LFA-1 mab. Two important observations were made, firstly, that non-depleting F(ab')$_2$ preparations of CD4 mab could also induce tolerance and secondly, that tolerance was 'reinforceable': the tolerant state had a limited life-span of about 120 days but a further challenge with HGG during this time prolonged it for a further 120 days. Similar findings were subsequently reported using other protein antigens but an indication of the power of such therapy came when Qin *et al.* (1989) obtained tolerance to allogeneic tissues using mab. Mice were infused with allogeneic bone marrow following ablation of their own lymphocytes by CD4 and CD8 mab. The mice subsequently demonstrated haemo-poietic chimerism (their circulation contained cells of both donor and self origin) and permanently accepted skin grafts from mice of the same strain as the marrow donor. In this situation tolerance was lifelong. Again, similar effects could be achieved with non-depleting mab (Qin *et al.*, 1990).

Cobbold *et al.* (1990) recently reported findings of great significance to the therapy of autoimmune disease. Mice that were actively rejecting a foreign skin graft were treated with an intensive regimen of non-depleting CD4 and CD8 mab. Although most skin grafts were lost (treatment was started too late to salvage these), further grafts of MHC-identical skin were accepted. This was an extremely important observation because it demonstrated that mab could change the phenotype of a T cell from activated and rejecting to quiescent and tolerant. Not only were non-depleting mab used but the authors were able to demonstrate *in vitro* that potentially reactive T cells were still present in recipient mice, even though these could no longer reject *in vivo*. They termed this phenomenon 'reprogramming' of the immune system (Cobbold *et al.*, 1992). Equivalent mab effects in humans could provide long-term control of autoimmunity from short-term treatments. One option might be to temporarily ablate the cognate immune system, perhaps accompanied by a means of re-educating subsequently developing thymocytes (Qin *et al.*, 1989) but a means of changing the phenotype of autoreactive T cells without destroying them would be preferable.

15.3.3 *How is tolerance achieved with monoclonal antibodies?*

To extrapolate these impressive findings to the human situation (where there is a much larger immune system to control) it is important to understand the mechanisms behind mab-induced tolerance. Waldmann *et al.* (1988) proposed a hypothesis that could account for all of the experimental findings. It bears some relation to the Bretscher & Cohn (1970) two-signal model and suggests that when a naive T cell encounters antigen for the first time, two outcomes are possible: it can turn on (become activated) or turn off (become tolerant). The process of antigen recognition is assumed to be the same for either event, the final outcome resting on the presence or absence of 'second signals'. In this model these are provided by collaborative interactions with other T cells and their lymphokine products, insufficient interactions resulting in tolerance. Following a course of depleting mab T cells redevelop gradually and leave the thymus in small numbers. If T cells then encounter specific antigen they do so in insufficient numbers to form collaborative units and therefore default to a tolerant state. When non-depleting mab are used the blockade of accessory or adhesion molecules on the T cell surface prevents antigen recognition. As mab levels fall gradually, individual T cells can recognize antigen once more but again only in small numbers and a tolerant state ensues.

Such hypotheses based on animal experimentation are important for guiding new strategies for tolerance induction with mab. Recent data suggest that potent regulatory mechanisms exist that maintain the tolerant state once it has been established (Qin *et al.*, 1993; Waldmann & Cobbold, 1993). The recognition that such regulatory mechanisms may be activated following mab therapy reinforces the notion that short-term therapy could lead to long-term antigen-specific immunosuppression (tolerance) and control of autoimmunity.

15.4   Animal models of rheumatological disorders

Discussion will be focused on models of SLE and rheumatoid arthritis (RA), these being the most extensively studied conditions.

15.4.1   *Systemic lupus erythematosus*

NZB/NZW F_1 mice develop a syndrome which bears many similarities to human SLE (Steinberg *et al.*, 1984). The illness predominantly affects females which develop a variety of autoantibodies, including anti-double-stranded DNA. Affected animals also develop immune complex-mediated glomerulone-phritis with proteinuria and, ultimately, death from renal failure. Mab have been used both to prevent and treat this disorder. Wofsy & Seaman (1985) administered a depleting CD4 mab to mice aged between 2 months and 12 months. Compared with controls, treated mice developed significantly lower autoantibody titres, had a reduced incidence of glomerlonephritis and lived longer. Thus, 90 treated mice were alive at 12 months compared with 27 mice that received saline and 0 mice that received a control mab. The increased mortality in the latter group reflected an increased incidence of immune complex disease, secondary to sensitization to the administered mab (15.6.2). While demonstrating the importance of $CD4^+T$ cells in the initiation of SLE in this model, these data had little bearing on the treatment of established disease. In a subsequent study, 7-month-old female NZB/NZW F_1 mice with established disease were treated with weekly injections of CD4 mab (Wofsy & Seaman, 1987). Treated mice again showed a reduction in autoantibody titres and a reversal of established nephritis. They survived for more than 12 months from the initiation of therapy compared with less than 2 months for a saline control group.

Non-depleting $F(ab')_2$ fragments of this same antibody were also able to prevent disease with a reduction in associated immunosuppression (Carteron *et al.*, 1989). Other models of SLE, such as BXSB mice and MRL-lpr/lpr mice have also been modulated with CD4 mab (Wofsy, 1986; Santoro *et al.*, 1988), and anti-IA (murine class II MHC) reagents were also effective in NZB/NZW F_1 mice (Adelman *et al.*, 1983). The story is not entirely straightforward, however. While Thy-1 mab prevented disease in MRL-lpr/lpr mice, they were of no benefit to NZB/NZW F_1 mice and resulted in fatal anaphylaxis in BXSB mice (Wofsy *et al.*, 1985).

Tolerance was not demonstrated in any of the above experiments: in each case long-term administration of antibody was required to achieve therapeutic effects.

15.4.2 Rheumatoid arthritis

Whereas SLE is probably an immune complex disorder, the pathogenesis of RA is less clear. Certainly there is genetic linkage to the MHC both in human and in animal models and histologically the synovium contains CD4$^+$T cells in close association with monocytes and macrophages (Janossy *et al.*, 1981). Furthermore, T cells transfer disease in animal models such as collagen-induced and adjuvant arthritis (Holmdahl *et al.*, 1985) and human RA can be suppressed by treatment directed at T cells such as thoracic duct drainage and total lymphoid irradiation (Paulus *et al.*, 1977; Gaston *et al.*, 1988). When synovium is examined in greater detail, however, it becomes apparent that many T cells appear to be resting whereas the monocytes are activated as judged by surface phenotype and lymphokine secretion (Firestein & Zvaifler, 1990; Feldmann *et al.*, 1990). This has led some authors to suggest that although T cells are important in the initiation of RA, it is monocytes and fibroblasts that direct the irreversible damage in later stages (Firestein & Zvaifler, 1990).

Despite these reservations, T cell mab have shown benefit in animal models of RA. This was first documented by Ranges *et al.* (1985) who administered CD4 mab to mice prior to immunization with type II collagen and reduced both the incidence and the severity of subsequent arthritis. Similar effects were achieved with an IA mab (Wooley *et al.*, 1985), and an IL-2R mab (Bannerjee *et al.*, 1988). Yoshino *et al.* (1991) prevented streptococcal cell wall-induced arthritis in rats with an antibody against the $\alpha\beta$ TCR whereas Billingham *et al.* (1990) inhibited the development of adjuvant arthritis in rats by CD4, class II and pan-T cell mab but could not demonstrate an equivalent effect with an antibody against the IL-2R.

As in SLE, these experiments support a role for CD4$^+$T cells in the initiation of arthritis. A few studies have concentrated on established disease. Hom *et al.* (1988) could not retard established collagen-induced arthritis in mice with depleting CD4, CD8 or Thy-1 mab alone or with a combination of CD4 and CD8 mab. Somewhat unexpectedly, a combination of Thy-1 and CD4 mab did slow disease progression. Proposed explanations were that this combination acted on an additional population of cells than either agent alone (either Thy-1$^+$CD4$^-$ or CD4$^+$Thy-1$^-$) or, more simply, that improved depletion of the Thy-1$^+$CD4$^+$ population achieved with the combination was responsible. Yoshino *et al.* (1990) suppressed established adjuvant arthritis in rats with a mab directed at the $\alpha\beta$ TCR but disease relapsed following cessation of therapy. Billingham *et al.* (1990) studied animals with passively transferred adjuvant arthritis (in which T cells from arthritic animals transfer disease to syngeneic, naive recipients). Passive disease could be prevented with CD4 mab; established disease could be suppressed with a CD4 mab alone or in combination with a pan T cell mab but, as in the study by Yoshino *et al.* (1990), symptoms returned after cessation of therapy. A CD8 mab had no effect.

An important observation from Billingham *et al.* (1990) was the induction of non-responsiveness to arthritis induction using CD4 mab. Rats treated with CD4 mab at the time of immunization with adjuvant not only failed to develop arthritis (see above) but were refractory to a subsequent adjuvant challenge following antibody clearance. Similar observations were made in the streptococcal cell wall arthritis model (van den Broek *et al.*, 1992). As with SLE models, tolerance has yet to be achieved in established disease.

T cell mab can therefore be used both to prevent and treat SLE- and RA-like illnesses in experimental animals. The results of such experiments have been sufficiently encouraging to prompt a number of small, open studies in humans and these are summarized in the next section.

15.5   Monoclonal antibodies in human rheumatic diseases

15.5.1   *Rheumatoid arthritis*

Rheumatoid arthritis is a common condition which carries a high morbidity yet often proves refractory to a spectrum of standard treatments. Evidence for an autoimmune pathogenesis and results from animal models have made it a popular disease for studies of mab therapy in human autoimmunity. No published trials are double-blinded and placebo-controlled and, therefore, while providing useful toxicity data, cannot provide robust evidence of efficacy. Furthermore, inconsistencies in study design do not allow inter-study comparisons to be made. Nonetheless, they have contributed important suggestions and guidelines for future work in this area.

15.5.1.1 *Monoclonal antibodies against CD4*

Many early studies used CD4 mab (Table 15.1). All were of mouse origin apart from one chimeric mab (a fusion protein comprising mouse v-region and human c-region; see 15.6). Toxicity was low although many patients suffered a 'first dose reaction' on initial treatment. This comprised fever, chills and nausea, sometimes accompanied by hypotension, myalgias and rashes. It was probably due to cytokines released from $CD4^+$ lymphocytes themselves or from monocytes and macrophages and a number of studies documented a rise in circulating IL-6 levels preceding symptoms.

Notwithstanding the uncontrolled nature of these studies efficacy was impressive. Most patients had long-standing disease refractory to a number of second-line drugs yet the majority showed some response to a brief (5–10 day)

Table 15.1. *CD4 Monoclonal antibodies tested in rheumatoid arthritis*

Species	Isotype	Designation	Authors
Mouse	IgG2a	VIT4	Herzog *et al*. (1989)
Mouse	IgG2a	M-T151	Herzog *et al*. (1989)
			Reiter *et al*. (1991)
Mouse	IgG2a	BL4	Goldberg *et al*. (1991)
Mouse	IgG1	MAX.16H5	Horneff *et al*. (1991)
Mouse	IgG1	B-F5	Wendling *et al*. (1991)
Chimeric mouse/human	Human IgG1	cM-T412	Choy *et al*. (1992*b*)
			Moreland *et al*. (1993*d*)
			Van der Lubbe *et al*. (1993)

course of therapy. Average symptomatic relief was around 3 months, although occasional patients responded for longer and a few went into remission. Clinical improvement was usually seen within days of therapy. Some patients in dose-ranging studies received ineffective doses and were useful controls for confounding variables such as admission to hospital.

It is not known how CD4 mab achieve their beneficial effect in autoimmunity. Possibilities include cytotoxicity, steric hindrance of T cell/APC interaction, modulation of CD4, signalling through CD4 or even the induction of programmed cell death (Newell *et al.*, 1990; Choy *et al.*, 1992*a*). Until the requisite properties are identified development of new agents must be empiric. A major problem is the lack of a suitable animal model for preclinical assessment. While primates possess homologous cell surface antigens (Jonker, 1990) it is ethically questionable as well as expensive to routinely test all new mab in such animals. Smaller mammals cannot be used because their antigens are insufficiently homologous in structure for crossreactivity of mab. In selecting the mouse mab M-T412 for chimerization parameters such as epitope specificity, affinity, modulating index and immunosuppressive capacity were examined, although exact requirements were unknown (Riethmuller *et al.*, 1992). Furthermore, with the number of potential variables (others include pharmacokinetics and cytotoxicity), it is unlikely that controlled clinical studies will reveal optimal characteristics. Biological parameters such as antigenic modulation (Horneff *et al.*, 1993*a*), half-life, depletion of CD4$^+$ lymphocytes and suppression of *in-vitro* responsiveness to antigen and mitogen were measured in a number of the published studies but none correlated with therapeutic efficacy. In one study (Horneff *et al.*, 1991) T cell reactivity actually increased in some responding patients! It is not even simple to predict biological characteristics of different mab. For example among the mouse mab listed in Table 15.1, isotype does not correlate with modulation (most profound with BL4 [IgG2a] and MAX.16H5 [IgG1]) whereas lasting depletion occurred with MAX.16H5 but not B-F5 (both IgG1). CD4 is also expressed on monocytes and macrophages and actions on these cells may explain some of the immunomodulatory effects (Horneff *et al.*, 1993*b*).

It is possible that the actual mab used is less important than the way in which it is used. Thus single or weekly doses of cM-T412 did not relieve symptoms in RA (Choy *et al.*, 1992*b*, Moreland *et al.*, 1993*a*) and a 5-day course was more effective than 5 weekly doses (Choy *et al.*, 1993*a*). Furthermore, the amount of mab entering the joint may be an important therapeutic determinant (Choy *et al.*, 1993*b*).

15.5.1.2 *Monoclonal antibodies against T cell activation antigens*

The most specific anti-T cell therapy for autoimmunity would target just those cells causing disease but no studies in RA have convincingly demonstrated an oligoclonal T cell response. Even if the inciting autoantigen(s) were isolated, thus facilitating identification of pathogenic clones, these would probably differ between patients with different MHC haplotypes. Thus, while collagen-induced arthritis in inbred mice is modulated by mab directed against T cell receptors carrying the $V\beta8$ chain (Moder *et al.*, 1993), equivalent therapies are not possible in RA. A number of markers become expressed on activated T cells, however, and targeting these provides a more specific therapeutic approach. A murine anti-human CD7 mab improved symptoms in 2 of 6 patients with active disease (Kirkham *et al.*, 1991, Table 15.2). A chimeric version of the same mab improved joint scores in 8 of 10 patients after two doses 1 week apart but reported follow-up was limited to 3 weeks and the study was uncontrolled (Kirkham *et al.*, 1992). Both mabs reduced circulating T cell numbers but only the chimeric provoked a 'first-dose' reaction. Two of three patients treated with an IL-2 receptor (IL-2R) mab improved symptomatically for 3 months (Kyle *et al.*, 1989). Recently other biological response modifiers have been used to target IL-2R positive cells in RA. $DAB_{486}IL-2$ is a fusion protein in which the toxic moiety of diphtheria toxin has been fused to human IL-2. This binds to and kills cells expressing the high affinity IL-2 receptor and has been used in an open dose-ranging study in RA (Sewell *et al.*, 1993). Nine of 19 patients receiving medium or high doses made a therapeutic response compared with none at a lower dose. Of note, responses appeared more durable with successive courses of treatment. First dose reactions were similar to those seen with mab, although one patient developed a specific hypersensitivity reaction requiring corticosteroid therapy. Mildly elevated liver enzyme levels developed in 55% of patients.

15.5.1.3 *Monoclonal antibodies against pan-T cell antigens*

Less specific rather than more specific mab may be required to treat human autoimmunity. Animal models suggest that when there is a low frequency of antigen-reactive cells, perhaps early in the course of an autoimmune disease,

Table 15.2. *Other mab tested in rheumatoid arthritis*

Antigen	Species	Isotype	Designation	Authors
Anti-T-cell				
CD7	Mouse	IgG2a	RFT2	Kirkham *et al.* (1991)
CD7	Chimeric mouse/human	Human IgG1	SDZ-CHH-380	Kirkham *et al.* (1992)
IL-2R	Rat	IgG2b	Campath-6	Kyle *et al.* (1989)
CD52	Humanized rat	Human IgG1	Campath-1H	Isaacs *et al.* (1992*a*)
CD5	Mouse	IgG1	CD5-plus (ricin A chain conjugate)	Strand *et al.* (1993)
Anti-cytokine				
IL-6	Mouse	IgG1	B-E8	Wendling *et al.* (1993)
TNF-alpha	Chimeric mouse/human	Human IgG1	cA2	Elliott *et al.* (1993)
Anti-adhesion molecule				
ICAM-1	Mouse	?	BIRR1	Kavanaugh *et al.* (1993)

blocking CD4 mab alone may be able to switch off the disease. As the autoreactive T cell load increases, as in established disease, $CD8^+$ cells must also be targeted and, under these conditions, lymphocyte depletion may be necessary (Cobbold *et al.*, 1992). The Campath antigen (CD52) is a small glycoprotein of unknown function expressed on all lymphocytes and monocytes (Hale *et al.*, 1990). Mab binding this antigen are potently lytic for B cells and T cells both *in vitro* and *in vivo*, with relative sparing of NK cells and monocytes. A humanized Campath mab, Campath-IH (Riechmann *et al.*, 1988, 15.6.2), was administered to patients with refractory RA in an open phase I study (Isaacs *et al.*, 1992*a*). Peripheral blood lymphocytes were undetectable after the first dose, during which all patients experienced a moderate 'first-dose' reaction. Arthritic symptoms improved dramatically within 48 hours, relief lasting from 3 weeks to 7 months after a 10-day (60 mg) course. Subsequent dose-ranging studies investigated single i.v. infusions (Weinblatt *et al.*, 1992), subcutaneous dosing (Johnston *et al.*, 1992), and i.v. dosing over 5 or 10 days (Isaacs *et al.*, 1993). The latter appeared most efficacious with 13 of 39 patients maintaining a Paulus response at 3 months.

CD5 is expressed on all T cells and a subset of B cells linked with autoimmune pathogenesis (Andrew *et al.*, 1991). CD5-plus is a fusion protein comprising a mouse CD5 mab linked to ricin A chain, the toxic component of the potent plant toxin ricin. When administered to patients with RA there was a transient fall in T cell numbers (rising to 70% of baseline at 1 month) and function (Strand *et al.*, 1993). There was symptomatic benefit, although uncontrolled, lasting for 6 months in 25% of patients. Four weeks after treatment benefit was most marked in patients with recent-onset disease (less than 3 years) but this advantage disappeared with longer follow-up. There was also a trend toward greater improvement at 6 months in patients concomitantly receiving methotrexate or azathioprine. Adverse effects were more pronounced than those associated with other mab and included fluid retention (75% at higher dosing levels) and pulmonary oedema. These adverse effects are likely to be related to the ricin A chain component but the unconjugated mab has not been tested in clinical studies.

15.5.1.4 Antibodies against cytokines

While T cells may initiate inflammatory joint disease, overwhelming evidence implicates cytokines such as TNF-α, IL-1 and IL-6 as inflammatory mediators and a number of anti-cytokine reagents have been assessed in animal models and in human disease. IL-6 mab was administered to five patients with long-standing RA resulting in a short-term symptomatic improvement (Wendling *et al.*, 1993). There were no adverse effects associated with therapy which unexpectedly resulted in a rise in serum IL-6 levels, presumably via a reduction in clearance. IL-1 activity was suppressed using a recombinant pharmacological receptor antagonist and a soluble form of the type I IL-1 receptor rather than with mab (Lebsack *et al.*, 1993; Drevlow *et al.*, 1993). In pilot studies both compounds demonstrated a therapeutic effect. A murine TNF-alpha mab was used to treat collagen-induced arthritis in mice (Williams *et al.*, 1992) and a chimeric TNF-alpha mab has been used in RA (Elliott *et al.*, 1993). Therapy was well tolerated and resulted in a dramatic fall in the acute phase response associated with symptomatic relief of median duration 14 weeks. A mab against transforming growth factor-beta (TGF-beta) was tested in an animal arthritis model leading to a reduction in not only acute inflammation but also chronic joint destruction (Wahl *et al.*, 1993). TGF-beta is usually considered immunosuppressive and anti-inflammatory but these results highlight the complexity of acute inflammation and cytokine action. They advocate caution in the empiric application of anti-cytokine therapy in conditions such as RA. Recently, for example, a gamma-interferon mab was shown to worsen collagen-induced arthritis in mice (Williams *et al.*, 1993).

These preliminary studies suggest that cytokine mab can modulate disease activity in RA with fewer adverse effects and, perhaps, less immunosuppression than T cell mab. Their mode of action, however, is primarily anti-inflammatory and they are unlikely to produce long-term benefit when used alone. An exciting prospect for the future is the combination of T cell and cytokine-directed mab (15.7).

15.5.1.5 Antibodies against adhesion molecules

Adhesion molecules are expressed on leucocytes and endothelium and mediate extravasation of cells into inflammatory sites (Pattarayo *et al.*, 1990). It follows that mab directed at these markers should suppress inflammation although, like cytokine mab, they may not have disease-modifying effects. A CD54 (ICAM-1) mab has been assessed in a phase I study in refractory RA with evidence of efficacy, lasting to day 90 in three of 21 patients (Kavanaugh *et al.*, 1993). T cell numbers increased transiently after therapy but proliferative and recall responses were suppressed for approximately 1 month (Davis *et al.*, 1993). Mab directed against endothelial markers such as E-selectin may provide a more specific anti-inflammatory effect without accompanying immunosuppression. Soluble receptors again provide an alternative to mab (Watson *et al.*, 1991).

15.5.2 Other diseases

15.5.2.1 Systemic lupus erythematosus

Ten patients with SLE have been treated with CD5-plus. In the first report (Wacholtz & Lipsky, 1992) two of four patients with refractory lupus nephritis responded for 5 months and one other for at least 14 months. The latter had a sustained fall in peripheral blood T cell count. In a separate cohort (Stafford *et al.*, 1993) six patients were treated. Two with thrombocytopenia did not respond but two of four with glomerulonephritis responded for 4 months and more than 6 months. Average peripheral blood T cell count was 66% of baseline at 6 months.

Five patients with lupus nephritis refractory to corticosteroids and cyclophosphamide received CD4 mab MAX.16H5 (Hiepe *et al.*, 1991, 1993). Four responded transiently (3–4 weeks) but then entered complete remission following a methylprednisolone bolus. This report raises further questions regarding the mechanism of action and optimal use of CD4 and other mab. Modulation of disease activity may occur in the absence of a sustained clinical response, perhaps by addressing an imbalance in $CD4^+$ subsets or cytokine profiles. In such a situation responsiveness to more conventional therapies may be restored.

15.5.2.2 Systemic vasculitis

Perhaps the most impressive results of mab therapy to date have been seen in patients with systemic vasculitis (Mathieson *et al.*, 1990; Lockwood *et al.*, 1993). The first patient to be treated had a 25-year history of episodic fever, rash, pleurisy, pericarditis, arthritis, myalgias and episcleritis. Histology of skin and muscle demonstrated vasculitis with prominent lymphocytic infiltrate.

Symptoms had been partially controlled by a number of treatments including prednisolone, azathioprine, dapsone, cyclophosphamide and plasma exchanges. Many were discontinued as a result of side-effects. In 1988 the patient developed high fevers, anorexia, weight loss, rash and arthralgias. These symptoms proved refractory to standard immunosuppressive therapy and a trial of Campath-IH was initiated. This resulted in a short-lived remission and two further courses gave similar effects. On the fourth treatment Campath-IH was followed by a course of CD4 mab. This combination heralded a long-lasting remission (42 months), punctuated only by short-lived skin lesions. A second patient presented at 18 years with rash, arthritis, pleurisy, pericarditis and acalculous cholecystitis. Biopsy again showed a lymphocytic vasculitis but symptoms did not respond to standard treatments. Campath-IH alone provided transient relief but when followed by a CD4 mab remission lasted 1 year. A further patient with a variant of Sjogren's syndrome associated with pancreatitis, pneumonitis, optic neuritis and nephritis responded to high-dose Campath-IH alone after a low dose had provided temporary relief of symptoms. This patient remains well 24 months later. Apart from adrenal replacement corticosteroids none of these patients required immunosuppressive therapy once remission had been obtained.

These cases bring to the fore what is perhaps the most important question surrounding mab therapy. These agents are potently immunosuppressive but can they achieve long-term effects on disease processes in humans? As discussed earlier in this chapter, mab can modulate ongoing immune responses in animals leading to antigen-specific tolerance (Cobbold et al., 1992). Equivalent effects in humans would lead to the long-term control of autoimmune processes with short courses of therapy. Although at first sight this prospect may appear unlikely, the only obvious major difference between the immune systems of mice and humans is in size. Perseverance with animal models has led to the design of tolerogenic regimens for a variety of circumstances. In general, the stronger the antigenic stimulus and activated T cell 'load', the more aggressive therapy needs to be. In the most difficult situations, such as transplantation tolerance across MHC barriers, combinations of mab are required. The first deplete or 'debulk' a high proportion of the cells and the second blockade those that are left. Such experiments provided the rationale behind combination therapy in vasculitis patients. The long remissions obtained suggested that the underlying disease had been modified in some way and emphasize the importance of a logical progression from controlled animal data to human disease.

15.5.2.3 Miscellaneous conditions

Uncontrolled pilot studies have documented improvement following CD4 mab therapy in psoriasis (Nicolas et al., 1991; Prinz et al., 1991), inflammatory bowel disease (Emmrich et al., 1991; Riethmuller et al., 1992), chronic autoimmune hepatitis (Riethmuller *et al.*, 1992) and relapsing polychondritis (van der Lubbe *et al.*, 1991; Choy *et al.*, 1991).

15.6 Adverse effects of monoclonal antibodies

15.6.1 *Significance of lymphocyte depletion*

The chimeric mab cM-T412 was produced initially because it was likely to be less immunogenic than murine mab (15.6.2) but also because its human IgG1 c-region would interact more effectively with human complement and Fc receptors. A likely consequence of the latter is the effective and long-lasting depletion of CD4$^+$ peripheral blood lymphocytes in recipients of this mab. After 30 months, 22 patients receiving total doses of 300–700 mg had CD4$^+$ peripheral blood lymphocyte counts approximately one-third of pre-treatment values. Furthermore, these had remained static for the preceding 12 months with no compensatory increase in other lymphocyte subsets (Moreland *et al.*, 1993*b*). One patient died 18 months after therapy with *Pneumocystis carinii* pneumonia while receiving treatment with methotrexate and prednisolone (Moreland *et al.*, 1993*c*). One other patient developed *E. coli* pyelonephritis during the first 6 months of follow-up, considered to be unrelated to mab therapy (Moreland *et al.*, 1993*d*). All patients in this study also received methotrexate which may have delayed CD4$^+$ peripheral blood lymphocyte repopulation. In another study in which similar doses of mab were used without methotrexate, CD4$^+$ counts were 60% of baseline at 12 months (van der Lubbe *et al.*, 1993).

Campath-IH also results in prolonged lymphopenia which affects predominantly CD4$^+$ but also the CD8$^+$ subset (Isaacs *et al.*, 1992*a*). An increased incidence of minor infections occurs within 6–8 weeks of therapy when peripheral blood lymphocytes are at their lowest. No infections occurred during 8 months of follow-up in 13 patients receiving single i.v. infusions despite a mean CD4$^+$ count of $119 \times 10^9/l$ at 8 months (Weinblatt *et al.*, 1993). A fatal infection occurred, however, in a patient who received 100 mg Campath-IH over 5 days. Due to a poor therapeutic response this patient received methotrexate and additional prednisolone 6 days after mab therapy but died 2 weeks later despite appropriate antifungal treatment, from disseminated coccidioidomycosis.

While tolerance can be achieved in animals with non-depleting mab, depletion is still required to control large numbers of activated lymphocytes (Cobbold *et al.*, 1992). This is likely to be the situation in established human autoimmunity and therefore lymphocyte depletion may be essential for long-term control of disease. It is not clear, however, why peripheral blood lymphopenia persists for so long after clearance of cM-T412 and Campath-IH. Blood counts do not necessarily reflect total body lymphocyte numbers and the mab may, for example, interfere with recirculation dynamics. Thus, minor infections occur early after Campath-IH but are uncommon later, despite persisting blood lymphopenia. Furthermore, both fatalities (one each with cM-T412 and Campath-IH) occurred in patients receiving additional immuno-suppression which, itself, is associated with fatal opportunistic infection. Over-all there is no clear correlation between CD4$^+$ lymphocyte counts and infection rates in these patients.

Subtyping of CD4$^+$ peripheral blood lymphocytes shows a predominant loss of naive cells following Campath-IH (Ganten *et al.*, 1993) and similar findings have been reported following therapy with CD4 mab in mice (Field *et al.*, 1993). Memory responses may therefore be relatively preserved and, with an apparently intact monocyte/macrophage system and normal NK cell numbers, innate responses should remain strong. Notwithstanding this, it is clear that patients must be assessed carefully after mab therapy particularly when further treatment is indicated and, where possible, additional immunosuppression avoided for 6–8 weeks. The therapeutic ratio of depleting versus non-depleting mab urgently requires further attention.

Patients treated with OKT3 for transplant rejection have an increased incidence of malignancy, particularly non-Hodgkin's lymphomas. Available evidence suggests that the overall degree of immunosuppression rather than OKT3 *per se* provides the increased risk (Penn, 1990) but patients with persisting lymphopenia must also be monitored regularly for these complications.

15.6.2 *Antiglobulin response*

Because of their foreign protein structure, xenogeneic mab invariably provoke an 'antiglobulin response' in the recipient (Isaacs, 1990). Thus, most patients treated with murine CD4 mab became sensitized. Although antiglobulins only rarely result in adverse reactions (Reiter *et al.*, 1991) they may prevent binding of mab to target antigen and reduce the effectiveness of a second course of treatment. Chimeric mab possess a human c-region and should therefore be less immunogenic than rodent counterparts. Indeed, only two of 25 RA patients raised antiglobulins to chimeric cM-T412 and these were of low titre (Moreland *et al.*, 1993*d*). Humanization is a more sophisticated process than chimerization, in which any rodent sequences not involved in antigen recog-nition are mutated to equivalent human sequences (Riechmann *et al.*, 1988; Chapter 7). Fully humanized mab should be even less immunogenic than chimeric mab although there remains the potential for anti-idiotype and anti-allotype responses (Gorman & Clark, 1990). Campath-IH, the first humanized therapeutic mab, did not provoke antiglobulins following a single course of treatment in eight patients with RA. This compared favourably with 11 of 14 patients treated for transplant rejection with the rat parent mab Campath-IG. Furthermore, these latter patients were receiving concomitant immunosuppression which lowers the incidence of sensitization (Friend *et al.*,

1991). Three of four patients became sensitized on retreatment with Campath-IH, however, as did a patient treated for vasculitis (Lockwood *et al.*, 1993). In each instance the response was against the residual rat idiotype. Thus, while reducing immunogenicity, humanization does not prevent an antiglobulin response following multiple treatments.

15.6.3 First dose response

Many patients receiving T cell mab develop a syndrome on the first day of treatment which includes fever, chills and nausea (15.5.1.1). This is generally self-limiting although a case of possible haemolytic-uraemic syndrome may have evolved from such a reaction (Isaacs *et al.*, 1993). As the cytokines responsible for these symptoms are identified it should become possible to offer specific prophylaxis. Furthermore, genetic engineering of mab promises agents potentially free of such adverse effects (15.7.2).

15.7   The future

15.7.1 Better ways of using existing agents

As suggested throughout this chapter the future success of mab therapy probably depends less on the production of novel agents and much more on the sensible use of those that already exist, as exemplified by combination therapy in vasculitis. The heightened inflammatory environment within an arthritic joint may *per se* be a barrier to tolerance induction (Cobbold *et al.*, 1992) and the sequential use of a cytokine mab to rapidly dampen inflammation and a T cell mab to reprogram autoreactive cells may be another promising combination in future studies. Table 15.3 lists variables that require further study in controlled investigations to optimize mab therapy. It is imperative that high quality animal studies continue to provide testable hypotheses and improved protocols.

15.7.2 Genetic engineering

Genetic engineering is constantly refining the mab armamentarium. Already it has been used to produce reagents of reduced immunogenicity (15.6.2). Studies *in vitro* with matched sets of chimeric mab (which share one v-region but differ in the c-region) improved understanding of the relationship between isotype and effector function (Bruggemann *et al.*, 1987). Following from this, the identification of mab 'motifs' mediating interaction with complement and Fc receptors provided the impetus for 'designer' mab. These can be made to specification, for example with respect to their ability to kill target cells or provoke cytokine release reactions (Isaacs *et al.*, 1992*b*; Bolt *et al.*, 1993).

Table 15.3. *Factors requiring further investigation in T cell mab studies*

Monoclonal antibody
Therapeutic importance of:
  antigen recognized (narrow versus broad specificity, e.g. CD4 versus Campath)
  epitope recognized
  isotype
  affinity for target antigen
  modulating capacity for target antigen
  immunosuppressive properties *in vitro*
  lytic capacity (activation of complement, affinity for Fc receptors)
  pharmacokinetics (half-life, etc.)
  concentration in blood and synovial fluid
  coating and saturation of target cells *in vivo*
  other targets recognized, e.g. monocytes and macrophages

Patient
Stage of disease (early versus late)
Young versus old
Optimal monitoring for immunosuppression/significance of prolonged lymphopenia

Dosing regimen
Dose
Route of administration (i.v., s.c., intra-articular)
Frequency (daily, weekly, monthly)
Duration of therapy
Need for maintenance therapy

Combination therapy
Other biological response modifiers (other mab, soluble receptors)
Other anti-rheumatic drugs (prednisolone, methotrexate, etc.)

Evidence for disease modification in the absence of symptomatic relief
Enhanced sensitivity to other therapies (e.g. corticosteroids, DMARDs)
Cytokine profiles in peripheral blood or synovial fluid?
Cytokine profiles of blood or synovial lymphocytes?

DMARDs, disease-modifying anti-rheumatic drugs.

15.8   Summary

During the 1990s we may witness a revolution in the management of auto-immunity as a result of mab therapy. Not only are mab potently immuno-suppressive and anti-inflammatory but, used in the correct way, they also possess tolerogenic properties. These have been well documented in animals and in theory could provide a cure for diseases such as RA and SLE in humans. So far clinical studies are at a preliminary stage but significant remissions have been achieved in otherwise refractory cases of RA and vasculitis. Animal models have proved indispensable as a means of understanding how to use mab to their optimal advantage and future progress may depend on further logical extrapolation from animal studies to the clinic. At the same time advances in genetic engineering are providing improved mab tailor-made to the requirement of individual diseases.

15.9 Acknowledgements

The author is a Medical Research Council Clinician Scientist and a Fellow of Downing College, Cambridge. Campath is a registered trademark of Burroughs Wellcome and The Wellcome Foundation.

15.10 References

Adelman, N. E., Watling, D. L. & McDevitt, H. O. (1983). Treatment of NZB/NZW F_1 disease with anti-IA monoclonal antibodies. *Journal of Experimental Medicine*, **158**, 1350–1355.

Andrew, E. M., Plater-Zyberk, C., Brown, C. M. S., Williams, D. G. & Maini, R. N. (1991). The potential role of B-cells in the pathogenesis of rheumatoid arthritis. *British Journal of Rheumatology*, **30** (Suppl. 1), 47–52.

Bannerjee, S., Wei, B.-Y., Hillman, K., Luthra, H. S. & David, C. S. (1988). Immunosuppression of collagen-induced arthritis in mice with an anti-IL-2 receptor antibody. *Journal of Immunology*, **141**, 1150–1154.

Benjamin, R. J., Qin, S., Wise, M. P., Cobbold, S. P. & Waldmann, H. (1988). Mechanisms of monoclonal antibody-facilitated tolerance: a possible role for the CD4(L3T4) and CD11a (LFA-1) molecules in self-non-self discrimination. *European Journal of Immunology*, **18**, 1079–1088.

Benjamin, R. J. & Waldmann, H. (1986). Induction of tolerance by monoclonal antibody therapy. *Nature*, **320**, 449–451.

Billingham, M. E. J., Hicks, C. & Carney, S. (1990). Monoclonal antibodies and arthritis. *Agents and Actions*, **29**, 77–87.

Bjorkman, P. J., Saper, M. A., Samraoui, B., Bennett, W. S., Strominger, J. L. & Wiley, D. C. (1987). The foreign antigen binding site and T cell recognition regions of class I histocompatibility antigens. *Nature*, **329**, 512–518.

Bolt, S., Routledge, E., Lloyd, I., Chatenoud, L., Pope, H., Gorman, S. D., Clark, M. & Waldmann, H. (1993). The generation of a humanized, non-mitogenic CD3 monoclonal antibody which retains *in vitro* immunosuppressive properties. *European Journal of Immunology*, **23**, 403–411.

Bretscher, P. & Cohn, M. (1970). A theory of self-non-self discrimination. *Science*, **169**, 1042–1049.

Brown, J. H., Jardetzky, T., Saper, M. A., Samaroui, B., Bjorkman, P. J. & Wiley, D. C. (1988). A hypothetical model of the foreign antigen binding site of class II histocompatibility molecules. *Nature*, **332**, 845–850.

Bruggemann, M., Williams, G. T., Bindon, C. I., Clark, M. R., Walker, M. R., Jefferis, R., Waldmann, H. & Neuberger, M. S. (1987). Comparison of the effector functions of human immunoglobulins using a matched set of chimaeric antibodies. *Journal of Experimental Medicine*, **166**, 1351.

Carteron, N. L., Schimenti, C. L. & Wofsy, D. (1989). Treatment of murine lupus with F(ab′)2 fragments of monoclonal antibody to L3T4. Suppression of autoimmunity does not depend on T helper cell depletion. *Journal of Immunology*, **142**, 1470.

Choy, E. H. S., Adijaye, J., Kingsley, G. & Panayi, G. (1992a). Chimaeric anti-CD4 antibody acts by causing apoptosis (programmed cell death) of human lymphocytes. *Arthritis and Rheumatism*, **35**, S–44.

Choy, E. H. S., Chikanza, I. C., Kingsley, G. H., Corrigall, V. & Panayi, G. S. (1992b). Treatment of rheumatoid arthritis with single dose or weekly pulses of chimaeric anti-CD4 monoclonal antibody. *Scandinavian Journal of Immunology*, **36**, 291–298.

Choy, E. H. S., Chikanza, I. C., Kingsley, G. H. & Panayi, G. S. (1991). Chimaeric anti-CD4 monoclonal antibody for relapsing polychondritis. *Lancet*, **338**, 450.

Choy, E. H. S., Pitzalis, C., Bill, J. A., Kingsley, G. H. & Panayi, G. S. (1993a). The importance of dose and dosing regimen of anti-CD4 monoclonal antibody (mAb) in the treatment of rheumatoid arthritis (RA). *Arthritis and Rheumatism*, **36**, S129.

Choy, E. H. S., Pitzalis, C., Bill, J. A., Kingsley, G. H. & Panayi, G. S. (1993b). The amount of anti-CD4 monoclonal antibody (mAb) entering the rheumatoid arthritis (RA) joint may determine clinical efficacy. *Arthritis and Rheumatism*, **36**, S39.

Cobbold, S. P., Martin, G. & Waldmann, H. (1990). The induction of skin graft tolerance in major histocompatibility complex-mismatched or primed recipients: primed T cells can be tolerized in the periphery with anti-CD4 and anti-CD8 antibodies. *European Journal of Immunology*, **20**, 2747–2755.

Cobbold, S. P., Qin, S., Leong, L. Y. W., Martin, G. & Waldmann, H. (1992). Reprogramming the immune system for peripheral tolerance with CD4 and CD8 monoclonal antibodies. *Immunology Reviews*, **129**, 165–201.

Davis, L. S., Kavanaugh, A. F., Nichols, L. A. & Lipsky, P. E. (1993). Immunoregulatory changes induced by treatment of rheumatoid arthritis patients with a monoclonal antibody to intercellular adhesion molecule-1 (ICAM-1) *Arthritis and Rheumatism*, **36**, S129.

Drevlow, B., Capezio, J., Lovis, R., Jacobs, C., Landay, A. & Pope, R. M. (1993). Phase I study of recombinant human interleukin-1 receptor (RHU IL-1R) administered intra-articularly in active rheumatoid arthritis. *Arthritis and Rheumatism*, **36**, S39.

Elliott, M. J., Maini, R. N., Feldmann, M., Long-Fox, A., Charles, P., Katsikis, P., Brennan, F. M., Walker, J., Bijl, H., Ghrayeb, J. & Woody, J. N. (1993). Treatment of rheumatoid arthritis with chimeric monoclonal antibodies to TNFα. *Arthritis and Rheumatism*, **36**, 1681–1690.

Emmrich, J., Seyfarth, M., Fleig, W. E. & Emmrich, F. (1991). Treatment of inflammatory bowel disease with anti-CD4 monoclonal antibody. *Lancet*, **338**, 570–571.

Feldmann, M., Brennan, F. M., Chantry, D., Haworth, C., Turner, M., Abney, E., Buchan, G., Barrett, K., Barkley, D., Chu, A., Field, M. & Maini, R. N. (1990). Cytokine production in the rheumatoid joint: implications for treatment. *Annals of Rheumatological Disease*, **49**, 480–486.

Field, E. H., Chace, J. H. & Cowdery, J. S. (1993). Anti-CD4 preferentially eliminates naive CD4 cells and spares pre-activated CD4 cells. *Arthritis and Rheumatism*, **36**, S47.

Firestein, G. S. & Zvaifler, N. J. (1990). How important are T cells in chronic rheumatoid arthritis? *Arthritis and Rheumatism*, **33**, 768–773.

Friend, P. J., Waldmann, H., Hale, G., Cobbold, S., Rebello, P., Thiru, S., Jamieson, N. V., Johnston, P. S. & Calne, R. Y. (1991). Reversal of allograft rejection using the monoclonal antibody Campath-IG. *Transplantation Proceedings*, **23**, 2253–2254.

Ganten, T.-M., Jendro, M. C., Fulbright, J. W., Matteson, E. L., Weyand, C. M. & Goronzy, J. J. (1993). Restricted diversity of the T cell receptor repertoire after therapeutic T cell depletion with the monoclonal antibody Campath-IH. *Arthritis and Rheumatism*, **36**, S40.

Garrett, T. P., Saper, M. A., Bjorkman, P. J., Strominger, J. L. & Wiley, D. C. (1989). Specificity pockets for the side chains of peptide antigens in HLA-Aw68. *Nature*, **342**, 692–696.

Gaston, J. S. H., Strober, S., Solovera, J. J., Gandour, D., Lane, N., Schurman, D., Hoppe, R. T., Chin, R. C., Eugui, E. M., Vaughan, J. H. & Allison, A. C. (1988). Dissection of the mechanisms of immune injury in rheumatoid arthritis using total lymphoid irradiation. *Arthritis and Rheumatism*, **31**, 21–29.

Germaine, R. N. & Margulies, D. H. (1993). The biochemistry and cell biology of antigen processing and presentation. *Annual Reviews in Immunology*, **11**, 403–450.

Glaichenhaus, N., Shastri, N., Littman, D. R. & Turner, J. M. (1991). Requirement for association of p56lck with CD4 in antigen-specific signal transduction in T cells. *Cell*, **64**, 511–521.

Goldberg, D., Morel, P., Chatenoud, L., Boitard, C., Menkes, C.-J., Bertoye, P. H., Revillard, J.-P. & Bach, J.-F. (1991). Immunological effects of high dose administration of anti-CD4 antibody in rheumatoid arthritis patients. *Journal of Autoimmunity*, **4**, 617–630.

Gorman, S. D. & Clark, M. R. (1990). Humanisation of monoclonal antibodies for therapy. *Seminars in Immunology*, **2**, 457–466.

Hale, G., Xia, M.-Q., Tighe, H. P., Dyer, M. J. S. & Waldmann, H. (1990). The Campath-I antigen (CDw52). *Tissue Antigens*, **35**, 118–127.

Haynes, B. F., Hale, L. P., Denning, S. M., Le, P. T. & Singer, K. H. (1989). The role of leucocyte adhesion molecules in cellular interactions: implications for the pathogenesis of inflammatory synovitis. *Springer Seminars in Immunopathology*, **11**, 163–185.

Herzog, C., Walker, C., Muller, W., Rieber, P., Reiter, C., Riethmuller, G., Wassmer, P., Stockinger, H., Madic, O. & Pichler, W. J. (1989). Anti-CD4 antibody treatment of patients with rheumatoid arthritis: I. Effect on clinical course and circulating T cells. *Journal of Autoimmunity*, **2**, 627–642.

Hiepe, F., Thiele, B., Brink, I., Volk, H. D. & Emmrich, F. (1993). Investigations on the treatment of systemic lupus (SLE) with the monoclonal anti-CD4 antibody MAX.16H5. *Arthritis and Rheumatism*, **36**, S227.

Hiepe, F., Volk, H.-D., Apostoloff, E., Baehr, R. V. & Emmrich, F. (1991). Treatment of severe systemic lupus erythematosus with anti-CD4 monoclonal antibody. *Lancet*, **338**, 1529–1530.

Holmdahl, R., Klareskog, L., Rubin, K., Larsson, E. & Wigzell, H. (1985). T-lymphocytes in collagen II-specific T-cell lines and clones. Characterisation of arthritogenic collagen II-specific T-cell lines and clones. *Scandinavian Journal of Immunology*, **22**, 295–306.

Hom, J. T., Butler, L. D., Riedl, P. E. & Bendele, A. M. (1988). The progression of the inflammation in established collagen-induced arthritis can be altered by treatments with immunological or pharmacological agents which inhibit T cell activities. *European Journal of Immunology*, **18**, 881–888.

Horneff, G., Burmester, G. R., Emmrich, F. & Kalden, J. R. (1991). Treatment of rheumatoid arthritis with an anti-CD4 monoclonal antibody. *Arthritis and Rheumatism*, **34**, 129–140.

Horneff, G., Guse, A., Schulze-Koops, H., Kalden, J. R., Burmester, G. R. & Emmrich, F. (1993*a*). Human CD4 modulation *in vivo* induced by antibody treatment. *Clinical Immunology and Immunopathology*, **66**, 80–90.

Horneff, G., Sack, U., Kalden, J. R., Emmrich, F. & Burmester, G. R. (1993*b*). Reduction of monocyte-macrophage activation markers upon anti-CD4 treatment.

Decreased levels of IL-1, IL-6, neopterin and soluble CD14 in patients with rheumatoid arthritis. *Clinical and Experimental Immunology*, **91**, 207–213.

Isaacs, J. D. (1990). The antiglobulin response to therapeutic antibodies. *Seminars in Immunology*, **2**, 449–456.

Isaacs, J. D., Clark, M. R., Greenwood, J. & Waldmann, H. (1992*b*). Therapy with monoclonal antibodies. An *in vivo* model for the assessment of therapeutic potential. *Journal of Immunology*, **148**, 3062–3072.

Isaacs, J. D., Manna, B. L., Hazleman, B. L., Schnitzer, T. J., St. Clair, E. W., Matteson, E. L., Bulpitt, K. J. & Johnston, J. M. (1993). Campath-IH in RA – a study of multiple iv dosing. *Arthritis and Rheumatism*, **36**, S40.

Isaacs, J. D., Watts, R. A., Hazleman, B. L., Hale, G., Keogan, M. T., Cobbold, S. P. & Waldmann, H. (1992*a*). Humanised monoclonal antibody therapy for rheumatoid arthritis. *Lancet*, **340**, 748–752.

Janossy, G., Panayi, G., Duke, O., Bofill, M., Poulter, L. W. & Goldstein, G. (1981). Rheumatoid arthritis: a disease of T-lymphocyte/macrophage immuno-regulation. *Lancet*, **2**, 839–842.

Johnston, J. M., Hays, A. E., Heitman, C. K., St. Clair, E. W., Jacobs, M. R., Yocum, D. E., Thakor, M. S., Achkar, A. A. & Matteson, E. L. (1992). Treatment of rheumatoid arthritis patients by subcutaneous injection of Campath-IH. *Arthritis and Rheumatism*, **35**, S105.

Jonker, M. (1990). The importance of non-human primates for preclinical testing of immunosuppressive antibodies. *Seminars in Immunology*, **2**, 427–436.

Kavanaugh, A. F., Lightfoot, E., Lipsky, P. E. & Oppenheimer-Marks, N. (1991). Role of CD11/CD18 in adhesion and transendothelial migration of T cells. Analysis utilizing CD18-deficient T cell clones. *Journal of Immunology*, **146**, 4149–4156.

Kavanaugh, A., Nichols, L., Davis, L., Rothlein, R. & Lipsky, P., (1993). Anti-CD54 (intercellular adhesion molecule-1; ICAM-1) monoclonal antibody therapy in refractory rheumatoid arthritis. *Arthritis and Rheumatism*, **36**, S40.

Kirkham, B. W., Pitzalis, C., Kingsley, G. H., Grahame, R., Gibson, T. & Panayi, G. S. (1991). Monoclonal antibody therapy in rheumatoid arthritis: the clinical and immunological effects of a CD7 monoclonal antibody. *British Journal of Rheumatology*, **30**, 459–463.

Kirkham, B. W., Thien, F., Pelton, B. K., Pitzalis, C., Amlot, P., Denman, A. M. & Panayi, G. S. (1992). Chimeric CD7 monoclonal antibody therapy in rheumatoid arthritis. *Journal of Rheumatology*, **19**, 1348–1352.

Kyle, V., Coughlan, R. J., Tighe, H., Waldmann, H. & Hazleman, B. L. (1989). Beneficial effect of monoclonal antibody to interleukin 2 receptor on activated T cells in rheumatoid arthritis. *Annals of Rheumatic Diseases*, **48**, 428–429.

Lawrence, M. B. & Springer, T. A. (1991). Leukocytes roll on a selectin at physiologic flow rates: distinction from and prerequisite for adhesion through integrins. *Cell*, **65**, 859–873.

Lebsack, M. E., Paul, C. C., Martindale, J. J. & Catalano, M. A. (1993). A dose- and regimen-ranging study of IL-1 receptor antagonist in patients with rheumatoid arthritis. *Arthritis and Rheumatism*, **36**, S39.

Linsley, P. S. & Ledbetter, J. A. (1993). The role of the CD28 receptor during T cell responses to antigen. *Annual Reviews of Immunology*, **11**, 191–212.

Lockwood, C. M., Thiru, S., Isaacs, J. D., Hale, G. & Waldmann, H. (1993). Long-term remission of intractable systemic vasculitis with monoclonal antibody therapy. *Lancet*, **341**, 1620–1622.

Mathieson, P. W., Cobbold, S. P., Hale, G., Clark, M. R., Oliveira, D. B. G., Lockwood, C. M. & Waldmann, H., (1990). Monoclonal antibody therapy in systemic vasculitis. *New England Journal of Medicine*, **323**, 250–254.

Miller, J. F. A. P. & Morahan, G. (1992). Peripheral T cell tolerance. *Annual Reviews of Immunology*, **10**, 51–70.

Moder, K. G., Luthra, H. S., Griffiths, M. & David, C. S. (1993). Prevention of collagen-induced arthritis in mice by deletion of T cell receptor Vβ8 bearing T cells with monoclonal antibodies. *British Journal of Rheumatology*, **32**, 26–30.

Moreland, L. W., Bucy, R. P., Jackson, B., Feldman, J. & Koopman, W. J. (1993*b*). Long-term follow-up (30 months) of rheumatoid arthritis patients treated with a chimeric anti-CD4 monoclonal antibody (cMab). *Arthritis and Rheumatism*, **36**, S129.

Moreland, L. W., Bucy, R. P., Tilden, A., Pratt, P. W., Lobuglio, A. F., Khazaeli, M., Everson, M. P., Daddona, P., Ghrayeb, J., Kilgarriff, C., Sanders, M. E. & Koopman, W. J. (1993*d*). Use of a chimeric monoclonal anti-CD4 antibody in patients with refractory rheumatoid arthritis. *Arthritis and Rheumatism*, **36**, 307–318.

Moreland, L. W., Pratt, P., Mayes, M., Postlethwaite, A., Weisman, M., Schnitzer, T., Lightfoot, R., Calabrese, L. & Koopman, W. (1993*a*). Minimal efficacy of a depleting chimeric anti-CD4 (cM-T412) in treatment of patients with refractory rheumatoid arthritis (RA) receiving concomitant methotrexate (MTX). *Arthritis and Rheumatism*, **36**, S39.

Moreland, L. W., Pratt, P. W., Sanders, M. E. & Koopman, W. J. (1993*c*). Experience with a chimeric monoclonal anti-CD4 antibody in the treatment of refractory rheumatoid arthritis. *Clinical and Experimental Rheumatology*, **11** (Suppl. 8), S153–S159.

Mueller, D. L., Jenkins, M. K. & Schwartz, R. H. (1989). Clonal expansion vs functional clonal inactivation. *Annal Reviews of Immunology*, **7**, 445–480.

Newell, M. K., Haughn, L. I., Maroun, C. R. & Julius, M. H. (1990). Death of mature T cells by separate ligation of CD4 and the T cell receptor for antigen. *Nature*, **347**, 286–289.

Nicolas, J. F., Chamchick, N., Thivolet, J., Wijdenes, J., Morel, P. & Revillard, J. P. (1991). CD4 antibody treatment of severe psoriasis. *Lancet*, **338**, 321.

Pattarayo, M., Prieto, J., Rincon, J., Timonen, T., Lundberg, C., Lindbom, L., Asio, B. & Gahmberg, C. (1990). Leukocyte-cell adhesion: a molecular process fundamental in leukocyte physiology. *Immunological Reviews*, **114**, 67–108.

Paulus, H. E., Machleder, H. I., Levine, S., Yu, D. T. Y. & MacDonald, N. S. (1977). Lymphocyte involvement in rheumatoid arthritis: studies during thoracic duct drainage. *Arthritis and Rheumatism*, **20**, 1249–1262.

Penn, I. (1990). Cancers complicating organ transplantation. *New England Journal of Medicine*, **323**, 1767–1768.

Prinz, J., Braun-Falco, O., Meurer, M., Daddona, P., Reiter, C., Rieber, P. & Riethmuller, G. (1991). Chimaeric CD4 monoclonal antibody in treatment of generalised pustular psoriasis. *Lancet*, **338**, 320–321.

Pullen, A. M., Marrack, P. & Kappler, J. W. (1988). The T cell repertoire is heavily influenced by tolerance to polymorphic self-antigens. *Nature*, **335**, 796.

Qin, S., Cobbold, S., Benjamin, R. & Waldmann, H. (1989). Induction of classical transplantation tolerance in the adult. *Journal of Experimental Medicine*, **169**, 779–794.

Qin, S., Cobbold, S. P., Pope, H., Elliott, J., Kioussis, D., Davies, J. & Waldmann, H. (1993). 'Infectious' transplantation tolerance. *Science*, **259**, 974–977.

Qin, S., Wise, M., Cobbold, S. P., Leong, L., Kong Yi-Chi, M., Parnes, J. & Waldmann, H. (1990). Induction of tolerance in peripheral T cells with monoclonal antibodies. *European Journal of Immunology*, **20**, 2737–2745.

Rammensee, H.-G., Falk, K. & Rotzschke, O. (1993). Peptides naturally presented by

MHC class I molecules. *Annual Reviews of Immunology*, **11**, 213–244.

Ranges, G. E., Sriram, S. & Cooper, S. M., (1985). Prevention of type II collagen-induced arthritis by *in-vivo* treatment with anti-L3T4. *Journal of Experimental Medicine*, **162**, 1105–1110.

Reiter, C., Kakarand, B., Rieber, E. P., Schattenkirchner, M., Riethmuller, G. & Kruger, K. (1991). Treatment of rheumatoid arthritis with monoclonal anti-CD4 antibody M-T151. Clinical results and immunopharmacologic effects in an open study, including repeated administration. *Arthritis and Rheumatism*, **34**, 525–536.

Riechmann, L., Clark, M., Waldmann, H. & Winter, G., (1988). Reshaping human antibodies for therapy. *Nature*, **332**, 323–327.

Riethmuller, G., Rieber, E. P., Kiefersauer, S., Prinz, J., van der Lubbe, P., Meiser, B., Breedveld, F., Eisenburg, J., Kruger, K., Deusch, K., Sander, M. & Reiter, C. (1992). From antilymphocyte serum to therapeutic monoclonal antibodies: first experience with a chimeric CD4 antibody in the treatment of autoimmune disease. *Immunological Reviews*, **129**, 81–104.

Santoro, T. J., Portanova, J. P. & Kotzin, B. L. (1988). The contribution of L3T4$^+$ cells to lymphoproliferation and autoantibody production in MRL-lpr/lpr mice. *Journal of Experimental Medicine*, **167**, 1713–1718.

Saper, M. A., Bjorkman, P. J. & Wiley, D. C. (1991). Refined structure of the human histocompatibility antigen HLA-A2 at 2.6 A resolution. *Journal of Molecular Biology*, **219**, 277–319.

Sewell, K. L., Parker, K. C., Woodworth, T. G., Reuben, J., Swartz, W. & Trentham, D. E. (1993). DAB486IL-2 fusion toxin in refractory rheumatoid arthritis. *Arthritis and Rheumatism*, **36**, 1223–1233.

Shizuru, J. A., Taylor-Edwards, C., Banks, B. A., Gregory, A. K. & Fathmann, G. C. (1988). Immunotherapy of the non-obese diabetic mouse: treatment with an antibody to helper T-cells. *Science*, **240**, 659–662.

Springer, T. A. & Lasky, L. A. (1991). Sticky sugars for selectins. *Nature*, **349**, 196–197.

Stafford, F. J., Fleischer, T. A., Brown, M., Lee, G., Austin, H., Balow, J. E. & Klippel, J. H. (1993). Clinical and biological effects of anti-CD5 ricin A chain immunoconjugate in systemic lupus erythematosus (SLE). *Arthritis and Rheumatism*, **36**, S227.

Steinberg, A. D., Raveche, E. S., Laskin, C. A., Smith, H. R., Santoro, T., Miller, M. L. & Poltz, P. H. (1984). Systemic lupus erythematosus: insights from animal models. *Annals of Internal Medicine*, **100**, 714–727.

Steinman, L., Rosenbaum, J. T., Sriram, S. & McDevitt, H. O. (1981). *In vivo* protective effects of antibodies to immune response gene products: prevention of experimental allergic encephalitis. *Proceedings of the National Academy of Sciences of the U.S.A.*, **78**, 7111–7114.

Strand, V., Lipsky, P. E., Cannon, G. W., Calabrese, L. H., Wiesenhutter, C., Cohen, S. B., Olsen, N. J., Lee, M. L., Lorenz, T. J., Nelson, B. & the CD5 Plus Rheumatoid Arthritis Investigators Group. (1993). Effects of administration of an anti-CD5 plus immunoconjugate in rheumatoid arthritis. Results of two phase II studies. *Arthritis and Rheumatism*, **36**, 620–630.

Van den Broek, M. F., van de Langerijt, L. G. M., van Bruggen, M. C. J., Billingham, M. E. J. & van den Berg, W. B. (1992). Treatment of rats with monoclonal anti-CD4 induces long-term resistance to streptococcal cell wall-induced arthritis. *European Journal of Immunology*, **22**, 57–61.

Van der Lubbe, P. A., Miltenburg, A. M. & Breedveld, F. C. (1991). Anti-CD4 monoclonal antibody for relapsing polychondritis. *Lancet*, **337**, 1349.

Van der Lubbe, P. A., Reiter, C., Breedveld, F. C., Kruger, K., Schattenkirchner, M.,

Sanders, M. E. & Riethmuller, G. (1993). Chimeric CD4 monoclonal antibody cM-T412 as a therapeutic approach to rheumatoid arthritis. *Arthritis and Rheumatism*, **36**, 1375–1379.

Wacholtz, M. C. & Lipsky, P. E. (1992). Treatment of lupus nephritis with CD5 Plus, an immunoconjugate of an anti-CD5 monoclonal antibody and ricin A chain. *Arthritis and Rheumatism*, **35**, 837–838.

Wahl, S. M., Allen, J. B., Costa, G. L., Wong, H. L. & Dasch, J. R. (1993). Reversal of acute and chronic synovial inflammation by anti-transforming growth factor beta. *Journal of Experimental Medicine*, **177**, 225–230.

Waldmann, H. & Cobbold, S. (1993). The use of monoclonal antibodies to achieve immunological tolerance. *Immunology Today*, **14**, 247–251.

Waldmann, H., Cobbold, S., Benjamin, R. & Qin, S. (1988). A theoretical framework for self-tolerance and its relevance to therapy of autoimmune disease. *Journal of Autoimmunity*, **1**, 623–629.

Waldor, M., Sriram, S., McDevitt, H. O. & Steinman, H. L. (1983). *In vivo* therapy with monoclonal anti-IA antibody suppresses immune responses to acetylcholine receptor. *Proceedings of the National Academy of Sciences of the U.S.A.*, **80**, 2713–2717.

Watson, S. R., Fennie, C. & Lasky, L. A. (1991). Neutrophil influx into an inflammatory site inhibited by a soluble homing receptor-IgG chimaera. *Nature*, **349**, 164–167.

Weinblatt, M. E., Coblyn, J., Maier, A., Anderson, R., Helfgott, S., Thurmond, L., Spreen, W. & Johnston, J. M. (1993). Sustained lymphocyte suppression after single dose Campath-IH infusion: an 8-month follow-up. *Arthritis and Rheumatism*, **36**, S40.

Weinblatt, M. E., Johnston, J. M., Hazleman, B. L., Manna, V. K. & the Campath-IH Rheumatoid Arthritis Investigators. (1992). Treatment of rheumatoid arthritis with single dose infusion of Campath-IH. *Arthritis and Rheumatism*, **35**, S105.

Wendling, D., Racadot, E. & Wijdenes, J. (1993). Treatment of severe rheumatoid arthritis by anti-interleukin-6 monoclonal antibody. *Journal of Rheumatology*, **20**, 259–262.

Wendling, D., Wijdenes, J., Racadot, E. & Morel-Fourrier, B. (1991). Therapeutic use of monoclonal anti-CD4 antibody in rheumatoid arthritis. *Journal of Rheumatology*, **18**, 325–327.

Williams, R. O., Feldmann, M. & Maini, R. N. (1992). Anti-tumor necrosis factor ameliorates joint disease in murine collagen-induced arthritis. *Proceedings of the National Academy of Sciences of the U.S.A.*, **89**, 9784–9788.

Williams, R. O., Williams, D. G. & Feldmann, M. (1993). Increased limb involvement in murine collagen-induced arthritis following treatment with anti-interferon-gamma. *Clinical and Experimental Immunology*, **92**, 323–327.

Wofsy, D. (1986). Administration of monoclonal anti-T cell antibodies retards murine lupus in BXSB mice. *Journal of Immunology*, **136**, 4554–4560.

Wofsy, D., Ledbetter, J. A., Hendler, L. & Seaman, W. E. (1985). Treatment of murine lupus with monoclonal anti-T cell antibody. *Journal of Immunology*, **134**, 852–857.

Wofsy, D. & Seaman, W. E. (1985). Successful treatment of autoimmunity in NZB/NZW mice with monoclonal antibody to L3T4. *Journal of Experimental Medicine*, **161**, 378.

Wofsy, D. & Seaman, W. E. (1987). Reversal of advanced murine lupus in NZB/NZW mice by treatment with monoclonal antibody to L3T4. *Journal of Immunology*, **138**, 3247–3253.

Wooley, P. H., Luthra, H. S., Lafuse, W. P., Huse, A., Stuart, J. M. & David, C. S.

(1985). Type II collagen-induced arthritis in mice. III. Suppression of arthritis by using monoclonal and polyclonal anti-Ia antisera. *Journal of Immunology*, **134**, 2366–2374.

Yoshino, S., Cleland, L. G., Mayrhofer, G., Brown, R. R. & Schwab, J. H. (1991). Prevention of chronic erosive streptococcal cell wall-induced arthritis in rats by treatment with a monoclonal antibody against the T cell antigen receptor $\alpha\beta$. *Journal of Immunology*, **146**, 4187–4189.

Yoshino, S., Schlipkoter, E., Kinne, R., Hunig, T. & Emmrich, F. (1990). Suppression and prevention of adjuvant arthritis in rats by a monoclonal antibody to the $\alpha\beta$ T cell receptor. *European Journal of Immunology*, **20**, 2805–2808.

16

Technical appendix: Monoclonal antibody production methods

H. M. LADYMAN and M. A. RITTER

16.1   Immunization

To produce IgG monoclonal antibodies (mab) you should give at least three immunizations at intervals of 3 weeks, for IgM antibodies only one or two immunizations are necessary, the fusion should then be performed 3–4 days after the last immunization.

For soluble antigens an adjuvant will enhance the immune response. Whole cells require no adjuvant and tissue homogenates can be used with or without adjuvant.

The amount of antigen per immunization is dependent on the species of animal to be immunized and the type of antigen (Table 16.1). The volume of immunogen is dependent on the animal to be immunized and the route of immunization. For intraperitoneal immunization (i.p.) in mice up to 200 μl and in rats up to 500 μl can be administered. Subcutaneous (s.c.) injections should not exceed 100 μl per site, usually in four sites per animal in the neck region.

Equal amounts of antigen and Freund's adjuvant (shaken to resuspend the mycobacteria) should be mixed and emulsified, usually using two glass syringes connected with a double luer fitting needle with a 1 mm bore. This mixture should be pushed rapidly from one syringe to the other until a thick emulsion is formed. Because it is impossible to retrieve all the immunogen from this apparatus it is necessary to prepare approximately twice the required volume. The emulsion can be tested by applying a drop onto the surface of some water: it should float as a discrete droplet.

16.2   Media and general cell culture

The essence of cell culture is a good sterile technique. Firstly, you need a class II laminar flow cabinet in which to work. Remember that the flow of sterile air is directed downwards and the main source of contamination is from your hands; if you pass them across the top of open bottles or plates you will contaminate the air as it flows down and so contaminate your work. No matter how carefully you wash your hands they are never sterile. Arrange the

Table 16.1. *Amount of antigen per immunization is dependent on the species to be immunized and type of antigen*

Species to be immunized	Type of antigen	Dose of antigen
Mouse	Soluble	$1–50\ \mu g$
Mouse	Cellular (or tissue homogenate)	$10^6–10^7$ cells
Rat	Soluble	$10–200\ \mu g$
Rat	Cellular (or tissue homogenate)	$10^7–5 \times 10^7$ cells

equipment that you require inside the cabinet in such a way that you can reach each item without over-reaching one item for another and only have essential items in the cabinet.

Before you start work, switch on the cabinet and allow it to run for 20 minutes to ensure replacement of the air inside with the sterile air passing through the filter. To sterilize the work surface swab it liberally with 70% ethanol. Work well inside the cabinet, where the air flow is less disturbed, and not close to the front edge where the movement of your hands will unavoidably disturb the air flow rendering this area less 'safe'. Wipe up any spillage immediately and swab down with 70% ethanol. When removing a pipette from the can hold it only by the end which you will insert into your pipette aide, taking care not to touch the tip of it against anything. When pipetting medium from a bottle into a flask, insert the pipette straight into the medium without touching the sides or neck of the bottle, suck up the medium, remove the pipette from the bottle and transfer to the flask. Insert the pipette just inside the neck of the flask without touching it and expel the medium. Replace the caps of both bottle and flask immediately.

Dissection instruments can be sterilized by immersing in 70% ethanol. The alcohol should be allowed to evaporate before use so that you do not 'fix' the tissue.

16.3   Contamination in tissue culture

However careful you are, occasionally some contamination will occur; the most common types and how to treat them are described below.

16.3.1   *Bacteria*

These are seen at the light microscope level as rods or cocci and they can be treated with antibiotics. If penicillin and streptomycin are already added to your medium add gentamycin at $50\ \mu g/ml$. Alternatively, you can clone the cells again in antibiotics in an effort to clone out the bacteria. Provided, however, that you have more cells either in culture or frozen down in liquid nitrogen, the best solution is to discard the contents of the well and sterilize it with 70% alcohol.

16.3.2 Fungi

These are easy to see under the microscope as thin strands of hyphae. You can sometimes remove the hyphae and/or treat with fungizone. Most cells are sensitive to fungizone so, unless the cells are really valuable, it is safer to discard them and sterilize the well. Remove all the medium and fungi from the well, add chloros (sodium hypochlorite), leave for 2–3 min, remove the chloros, rinse with sterile water then remove this, leaving the well empty. It is also advizable to change the lid of the plate to minimize the possibility of further contamination.

16.3.3 Yeast

These are easily recognizable as they appear as budding microorganisms. Treat with fungizone or discard that well. Sterilize the well with 70% alcohol or chloros, as above.

16.3.4 Mycoplasma

This contamination is difficult as the organisms cannot be seen at light microscopy level but typically they slow down cell growth. Poor fusion rates result from mycoplasma contamination of myeloma cells. Kits are available commercially for testing for the presence of mycoplasma (e.g. Gen-Probe mycoplasma T C Rapid detection system; Gen-Probe Inc. USA). If you do detect mycoplasma in you cultures it is possible to rescue the cells either by special antibiotics (e.g. MRA, ICN Flow, U.K. or BM-Cycline, Boeringer Mannheim, Germany) or by passaging the cells through a mouse. To do this, inject between 5×10^6 and 1×10^7 cells i.p. into a syngeneic mouse and let them grow for a week or so, until a tumour is formed. Kill the mouse and either take out the tumour and tease it to release the cells or just aspirate the cells from the peritoneal cavity. This may have to be done twice to be sure that the cells are completely mycoplasma-free.

16.4 Cryopreservation of cells

The earliest time you can freeze hybridoma cells, with consistent success, is after the first cloning. Subsequently, aliquots of cells should be frozen at regular intervals and stored in liquid nitrogen. Sometimes hybridoma cells stop secreting antibody for no apparent reason (usually chromosomal instability) and it is important to go back occasionally to a vial that was frozen down soon after cloning.

The freezing mixture consists of fetal calf serum (FCS) 90% and dimethyl-sulphoxide (DMSO) 10%. This mixture will give good cell preservation for most hybridomas but occasionally you may have a more sensitive clone that requires less DMSO, in which case use 7% or 5%. Always prepare the DMSO in FCS (although it is expensive) because it will give good protection to the cells so that when you thaw them out you will get a higher yield of viable cells. Always choose a well or flask of very healthy cells for freezing down, as these will survive the procedure more readily.

Prepare the mixture and store at 4 °C, DMSO is toxic to cells at temperatures above 4 °C.

16.4.1 Freezing down cells

1. Harvest the cells, count them and then centrifuge at 150 *g* for 5 minutes, discard the supernatant and resuspend the cell pellet.
2. Label your cryotubes and put on ice.
3. Add cold freezing mixture to the cells so that there are between 10^5 and 5×10^6 cells/ml.
4. Transfer 1 ml aliquots into the cryotubes and start the freezing procedure.
5. If you have a freezing machine it will freeze as follows: 0 °C to −30 °C at 1°/min and −30 °C to −60 °C at 2°/min. The cells can then be safely transferred into liquid nitrogen for storage.
6. If you do not have a freezing machine you can still freeze your cells successfully as follows: leave the samples on ice for 2 h. Wrap them in insulated bubble film and pack in a polystyrene box padded with cotton wool and place in a −70 °C freezer overnight, then transfer into liquid nitrogen.

16.4.2 Thawing cells

1. When required thaw out the cells rapidly in a waterbath or incubator at 37 °C.
2. Quickly dilute into 10 ml of complete medium with 10% FCS (room temperature), it is important to dilute out the DMSO quickly as it is toxic to the cells at temperatures above 4 °C.
3. Centrifuge (150 *g* for 5 min) to pellet the cells and discard the supernatant. Resuspend the cells in fresh medium and plate them out into a flask or dish, depending on the number of cells in the vial, and transfer into the incubator.

16.4.3 *Myeloma cells*

The myeloma cells should be thawed out 10–14 days before the fusion and grown up in complete medium with 10% FCS. The cells will probably need subculturing every 3–4 days and they should be split the day before the fusion so that they will be in the exponential growth phase.

16.5 The fusion

Materials
Immunized mouse
Non-immunized mouse of same strain for macrophage preparation
2×10^7 myeloma cells
50% polyethylene glycol (PEG) (1 g of PEG autoclaved, 1 ml serum-free medium added while PEG is molten)
Serum-free medium (RPMI-1640 Hepes buffered)
20 ml RPMI medium, bicarbonate buffered, with 15% FCS
Complete medium with 10% FCS (RPMI-1640 bicarbonate buffered, plus antibiotics and 10% FCS)
70% alcohol
Dissection instruments (forceps, scissors, mounted needles)
5 ml syringe
21 and 25 G needles
Centrifuge tubes (10 and 50 ml)
1% acetic acid in phosphate buffered saline (PBS)
0.2% Trypan blue in PBS
Improved Neubauer counting chamber
50 mm petri dishes
Tissue culture plates (24-well)
HAT (hypoxanthine, aminopterin and thymidine) and HT (hypoxanthine and thymidine) concentrates.

Method
1. The last immunization should have been administered 3–4 days before the fusion and the myeloma cells should be in the exponential growth phase.
2. Place the PEG, 15% FCS, RPMI and a beaker of water into the incubator to warm to 37 °C.
3. Kill the immunized mouse by cervical dislocation or in a CO_2 chamber. Place the animal on its right side so its spleen is uppermost and swab the body with 70% ethanol. Using a pair of fine forceps and scissors (both sterilized in 70% ethanol) cut open the mouse to expose the spleen. The incision should not puncture the gut or the surrounding

splenic arteries and veins. Remove the spleen, place in a sterile Petri dish containing 5 ml of sterile Hepes (N-2-hydroxyethpiperazine-N'-2-ethanesulphonic acid) buffered RPMI medium (serum-free medium). Hepes buffer is used as it buffers better in air than sodium bicarbonate whereas the latter is better for use in the incubator with CO_2. Transfer the Petri dish and spleen to the sterile hood. Remove any adherent fat from the spleen and transfer the spleen into a fresh dish containing 5 ml of serum-free medium. Holding the spleen in the sterile forceps use a 21 G needle mounted on a 1 ml syringe to tease the spleen to release the cells. As the cells are released the medium will become cloudy with cells, pipette them into a 10 ml centrifuge tube. Add more medium to the dish and keep teasing until all the cells are released.

4. Leave the tube in a rack and allow the tissue clumps to settle out. Pipette the supernatant, single cell suspension into a fresh 10 ml tube. Make this up to 10 ml with extra serum-free medium, centrifuge at 250 *g* for 10 min, discard the supernatant and resuspend the cells in 10 ml of fresh Hepes buffered medium. Count the cells. Take 50 μl of the cells, 450 μl of 1% acetic acid in PBS and then add 500 μl of 0.2% Trypan blue in PBS. Mix well, then pipette some of the mixture into a Neubauer counting chamber.

5. The counting chamber is divided up into nine large squares. The centre square is subdivided into 25 while the surrounding eight squares are subdivided into 16. Select one of the corner squares and count all the cells in this large square (16 small squares). Count only the viable cells, i.e. not the blue ones. The red blood cells will have been lysed by the acetic acid. This number of cells (X) is then multiplied by 10^4 and then by your dilution factor, 50 μl in 1000 μl (i.e. 20). If you then multiply by the volume in ml (10), you will obtain the total number of cells (total number of leucocytes = $X \times 10^4 \times 20 \times 10$).

6. Wash the cells twice in serum-free medium. Centrifuge at 250 *g* for 10 min between washes.

7. Harvest the myeloma cells, wash them twice in serum-free medium, resuspend them in 10 ml, take a 50 μl sample and count using an equal volume of 0.2% Trypan blue, calculate the number of cells (the dilution factor this time is 2) (total number of myeloma cells = $X \times 10^4 \times 2 \times 10$).

8. Mix the spleen cells and myeloma cells in a 50 ml tube at a ratio of 10 viable spleen cells to 1 viable myeloma cell and centrifuge the cells to form a cell pellet (using all the spleen leucocytes).

9. Remove the supernatant and gently resuspend the cell pellet by tapping the tube.

10. Put the tube into the beaker of water at 37 °C. Add 1 ml of warm PEG slowly to the cells over a period of 1 min, continually stirring the mixture with the pipette tip. The cells must not be in contact with the

concentrated PEG solution for more than 2 min as it will eventually totally disrupt the cell membranes.

11. Immediately add 1 ml of serum-free medium as in step 10 and then add a further 4 ml of serum-free medium over 3–4 min, without stirring, running it slowly down the inside of the tube.

12. Add a further 20 ml of serum-free medium followed by 20 ml of medium with 15% FCS, again by running it slowly down the inside of the tube. This medium should be buffered with sodium bicarbonate. Invert the tube once and leave at 37 °C for 1–2 h to allow the cell membranes to stabilize.

13. Macrophage feeder cells can be prepared while the cells are incubating; alternatively, they can be prepared and plated out 1–2 days before the fusion. This lowers the risk of contamination as they can be checked microscopically before the fusion cells are plated out.

14. Kill a normal unimmunized mouse of the same strain as the immunized animal by cervical dislocation or in a CO_2 chamber.

15. Swab the abdomen with 70% ethanol. Lift up a small flap of skin in the middle of the abdomen and snip it off. Extend the cut forwards and backwards. Great care must be taken to ensure that the peritoneum is not punctured as this will contaminate the macrophage preparation. It is often easier to pull the skin apart as it tears away quite easily.

16. Using a 5 ml syringe with 25 G needle inject 5 ml of cold complete medium into the peritoneal cavity taking care not to puncture the gut. The cold medium causes the gut to contract and so reduces the risk of contamination.

17. Palpate the abdomen gently and withdraw the medium using a 5 ml syringe with 21 G needle. Again be careful not to puncture the gut or abdominal organs, e.g. liver, spleen, etc.

18. Usually 3–4 ml of cell suspension can be retrieved. For each 24-well plate you require 0.5 ml of macrophage suspension; therefore, one mouse should yield sufficient macrophages for 6–8 plates.

19. 1–2 h after the fusion centrifuge the hybrids (250 g for 10 min) and resuspend to between 10^5/ml and 2.5×10^5/ml (using your myeloma cell count as this will be your limiting factor) in complete medium with 10% FCS.

20. Add 0.5 ml of macrophages per 50 ml of hybridoma cell suspension.

21. Add sufficient HAT concentrate for the volume of cell suspension.

22. Plate the hybrids out in 24-well plates at 2 ml/well.

23. Put the plates into a plastic box and place in the incubator at 37 °C with 5% CO_2.

24. After 1 week, remove 1 ml of medium from each well and add 1 ml of fresh 10% FCS, bicarbonate buffered, RPMI medium with HAT.

25. After 1 further week, remove 1 ml of medium and replace with 1 ml of fresh 10% FCS, bicarbonate buffered, RPMI medium with HT.

26. Every week after this, 1 ml of medium is changed using fresh 10% FCS, bicarbonate buffered, RPMI medium, without either HAT or HT.

16.6   Cloning techniques

16.6.1   *Cloning by limiting dilution*

There are two methods that can be used for limiting dilution: either the cells can be diluted to a set concentration and plated out in a microtitre plate to give theoretically 0.3 cells/well or you can start with a higher concentration of cells and titrate them out across a microtitre plate so that only the last column will be at less than 1 cell/well. This latter method is easier to perform and also eliminates the risk of losing a clone as a result of the slow growth that sometimes occurs when the cells are plated out at a very low density. It has of course to be realized that not all the wells will contain single clones even when they are titrated to such low concentrations and the only way to be absolutely certain that you have a pure clone is to inspect the wells regularly as they start to grow up and mark the wells where you are sure that there is only one clone growing. This is very time-consuming but it does eliminate the necessity of repeating the cloning yet again.

It is important to clone as early as possible to avoid your clone of interest being overgrown by a non-producer. Therefore, as soon as you get a positive result in your screening assay you should clone that well.

16.6.1.1 *Limiting dilution by titration*

Materials
Cells to be cloned
Tissue culture plate (96-well)
Complete medium with 10% FCS
Centrifuge tubes (10 and 50 ml)
Improved Neubauer counting chamber
Macrophages from mouse peritoneal lavage, as described for fusion

Method
1. Harvest all the cells from your positive well, always check that you have not left cells behind as they do tend to adhere to the plastic.
2. Count the cells and adjust to 160 cells/ml.
3. In the 96-well microtitre plate add 100 μl of medium to each well in columns 3–12.
4. Add 100 μl of your cell suspension to each well in columns 1–4. Then double dilute from column 3 and column 4 into alternate columns. Discard 100 μl from columns 11 and 12 (Figure 16.1).

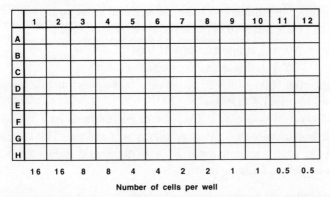

	1	2	3	4	5	6	7	8	9	10	11	12
A												
B												
C												
D												
E												
F												
G												
H												

16 16 8 8 4 4 2 2 1 1 0.5 0.5

Number of cells per well

Figure 16.1. Plate layout for cloning by titration. Cells are double-diluted across the plate into wells of alternate columns.

5. Add 100 μl of macrophage suspension (from peritoneal lavage) to each well. For each 96-well plate add 0.2 ml of macrophage suspension to 10 ml of medium.

It should take between 10 and 14 days for these clones to grow up, then they should be re-screened. Any positive clones can be grown up in bulk. Do not forget to freeze down vials of cells as soon as possible. If you are certain that there is only one clone growing in the well then you need not reclone. If you are in any doubt, then you should reclone starting your titration with 8 cells per well.

16.6.1.2 *Limiting dilution by set concentration*

With this technique you should perform at least three cloning steps. The first cloning should be plated out at 6 cells/well and the second and third cloning should be at theoretically 0.3 cell/well. This gives the best possible chance of obtaining a single clone but still you can only be certain that you have a pure clone by checking your plates for wells with single clones growing in them.

Materials
Cells to be cloned
Tissue culture plate (96-well)
Complete medium with 10% FCS
Centrifuge tubes (10 and 50 ml)
Improved Neubauer counting chamber
Macrophages from mouse peritoneal lavage, as described for fusion

Method
1. For 6 cells/well adjust to 30 cells/ml, for 0.3 cells/well adjust to 1.5 cells/ml. This should be done by serial dilution.

Example: assuming you have 10^5 cells/ml from your positive well. Make two serial 1:10 dilutions to give 1000 cells/ml.

10^5/ml, diluted 1:10 = 10^4/ml
10^4/ml, diluted 1:10 = 1000/ml

Then take 600 μl into 20 ml to give 30 cells/ml or take 30 μl into 20 ml to give 1.5 cells/ml.

Obviously you could fill a lot of plates from one fusion plate well but usually two to three plates will suffice. The excess cells can be plated into a fresh 24-well plate and grown on for 1–2 weeks before freezing down.

2. Prepare peritoneal macrophages as before.
3. Add the macrophages to the cell suspension (0.2 ml of macrophage suspension is sufficient for each 96-well plate) and then add 200 μl of the cell/macrophage mix to each well of the plate.
4. This will now take about 2 weeks to grow up and as the wells start to turn yellow or when clones of cells can be seen they should be tested. Not all the wells will be positive because of non-secreting clones or undetectable antibody concentration. You should, therefore, retest each negative well twice.
5. When you are certain that you have fully cloned your hybrids transfer them into 24-well plates, then into flasks to grow up your mab in bulk. Freeze down portions of healthy cells as soon as possible.

16.6.2 *Cloning in soft agar*

This is a modification of the method originally described by Metcalf *et al.* (1975, *J. Exp. Med.*, **142**, 1534–1549).

Medium

1. Dulbecco's modified Eagles medium (powder) (Gibco) with 4500 mg/l glucose, L-glutamine, without sodium bicarbonate. Dissolve the contents of 1 (1 l) packet in 200 ml of distilled water and make up to 250 ml. Filter sterilize through 0.2 μm filter and store at 4 °C. (This is 4 times concentrated.)
2. To make double strength medium for cloning:
Take 50 ml of the concentrated medium and add:

> 5 ml of NaHCO$_3$ (7.5% w/v)
> 1 ml of glutamine (200 mM)
> 1 ml of penicillin/streptomycin ($\times$ 100 stock)
> 1 ml of pyruvate (100 mM)

Make up to 100 ml with sterile distilled water then add 25 ml FCS.
3. Agar (Noble agar, Difco): prepare a 2 $\times$ concentration of agar (0.6%)

in distilled water. Boil until dissolved. Using a pre-warmed pipette, transfer 10 ml amounts into glass universals then autoclave (15 lb/sq in for 20 min), then keep at 37 °C.

4. Agar medium: add 10 ml of concentrated medium to each bottle of molten agar (keep at 37 °C.)

Method

1. Place three 30 mm Petri dishes inside each 100 mm dish, add 5 ml sterile water to one 30 mm dish to humidify the chamber.

2. Harvest the cells from the fusion plate count and adjust to 10^5/ml in single strength medium with 20% FCS.

3. Quickly transfer 1.5 ml of agar/medium to each cloning dish, add 100 μl of cells, mix well and allow to stand at room temperature for 30 min.

4. Transfer to the incubator at 37 °C and disturb as little as possible. After 7–10 days the clones should be detectable by inverted light microscopy.

5. When the clones of cells are visible, using an inverted light microscope (40 × objective lens) and a drawn-out pipette or microcapillary tube, pipette up each clone of cells individually and transfer to a 96-well plate containing 200 μl/well of RPMI with 20% FCS.

6. Incubate at 37 °C in 5% CO_2 in air.

7. After 3–5 days when rapid growth is apparent the supernatant can be screened and cells from positive wells subcultured and frozen down as necessary.

16.6.3 Single cell manipulation

There are two ways in which you can be sure that you plate only one cell/well in the 96-well plate. Firstly, you can do it manually, using a micropipette and inverted microscope (method 1) or secondly, you can use a fluorescence activated cell sorter (FACS) to do it automatically (method 2).

Method 1

1. Add 0.2 ml macrophages from a peritoneal lavage to 20 ml complete medium with 10% FCS and plate out into a 96-well plate at 200 μl per well.

2. Dilute the cells from a positive well into a Petri dish so that they are very diluted.

3. Using an inverted light microscope (40× objective lens) and a drawn-out pipette or microcapillary tube, pipette up a single cell and transfer it into the well of a 96-well plate.

4. Repeat step 3 for all the wells of the plate.

5. Incubate the plate at 37 °C in 5% CO_2 in air for 10–14 days, by which time the clones of cells should be visible.
6. Screen the supernatant and subculture and freeze down the cells as necessary.

Method 2

To use the FACS you have to set up the specially adapted equipment to the machine, ensure that the system is running using sterile tubing and with sterile PBS; this may have to be done by a trained technician. Once the machine is set up the procedure is simple.

1. Prepare your 96-well plates with macrophages, 0.2 ml of peritoneal lavage in 20 ml of complete medium, plated at 200 μl per well.
2. Adjust your hybridoma cells to approximately 10^6/ml in the same medium.
3. Apply the tube of cells to the machine at the inlet port.
   While the cell suspension runs through the machine, it is vibrated at a high velocity to break the cell stream up into droplets. These droplets then pass by a detector that is able to identify droplets containing a single cell, which are given a positive charge so that when they pass by a second detector they are deflected into the well of the 96-well plate. A motorized stage moves the plate so that each well systematically receives a single cell.
4. Incubate the plate at 37 °C in 5% CO_2 in air for 10–14 days, by which time the clones of cells should be visible.
5. Screen the supernatant and subculture and freeze down the cells as necessary.

Although these methods guarantee hybridoma clonality, the first is very time-consuming and the second relies on the availability of a FACS machine; therefore, they are not really recommended as routine cloning methods. They are very useful techniques if you want to be absolutely certain that you have a pure clone.

16.7   Bulk production of monoclonal antibodies

16.7.1   Tissue culture

There are many ways of growing up bulk amounts of antibody, the simplest is to grow them in large tissue culture flasks and collect the supernatant. This will yield only about 10 μg/ml of supernatant and if you want to purify the mab you will have to produce several litres of supernatant. Alternatively, you can grow the mab as ascitic fluid in a mouse or rat depending on the species in which the mab was raised; this will yield about 10 mg/ml of ascitic fluid. Another method is to use commercially available systems such as the hollow fibre bioreactors that are capable of producing from 100 mg to 75 g of mab per month, depending on the system chosen.

16.7.2 Production of ascites

Method
1. Inject each animal with 0.5 ml of Pristane i.p. (Pristane is 2,6,10,14-tetramethylpentadecane).
2. Grow up the hybridomas in culture.
3. Seven days after the first Pristane injection, harvest the cultured hybridoma cells and centrifuge them at 150 g for 5 min, discard the supernatant and resuspend the cell pellet, in sterile PBS, to a concentration of between 2×10^6 and 2×10^7 cells/ml.
4. Inject 0.5 ml of cell suspension i.p. into each animal using a 21 G needle.
5. Inspect the animals daily for swelling of the abdomen (indicating ascitic fluid production).
6. As soon as there is considerable swelling of the abdomen or if the animal is in distress, kill it and remove all the ascitic fluid using a syringe with a 19 G needle and transfer it into a 10 ml tube.
7. Remove any cells by centrifuging for 10 min at 250 *g*. Store the fluid frozen in small aliquots. The cells can be used to inoculate another animal or frozen down in liquid nitrogen for a future inoculation.

16.8 Screening techniques

16.8.1 Enzyme linked immunosorbent assay (ELISA)

Materials
96-well ELISA plate
Antigen (e.g. human serum albumin (HSA) at 25 μg/ml)
ELISA coating buffer pH 9.6
Primary antibody (e.g. mouse mab against HSA)
HRP (horse radish peroxidase) conjugated secondary antibody (e.g. anti-mouse Ig HRP)
Substrate, e.g. Ortho-phenyl diamine (OPD)
Substrate buffer
Hydrogen peroxide
PBS/Tween
3 M sulphuric acid
ELISA plate reader
Cling film
Foil

			Standard			Sample A			Sample B			
	1	2	3	4	5	6	7	8	9	10	11	12
A	B	-VE	1/2	1/2	1/2	1/2	1/2	1/2	1/2	1/2	1/2	XXX
B	L	C	1/4	1/4	1/4	1/4	1/4	1/4	1/4	1/4	1/4	XXX
C	A	O	1/8	1/8	1/8	1/8	1/8	1/8	1/8	1/8	1/8	XXX
D	N	N	1/16	1/16	1/16	XXX	XXX	XXX	XXX	XXX	XXX	XXX
E	K	T	1/32	1/32	1/32	XXX	XXX	XXX	XXX	XXX	XXX	XXX
F		R	1/64	1/64	1/64	XXX	XXX	XXX	XXX	XXX	XXX	XXX
G		O	1/128	1/128	1/128	XXX	XXX	XXX	XXX	XXX	XXX	XXX
H		L	1/256	1/256	1/256	XXX	XXX	XXX	XXX	XXX	XXX	XXX

Figure 16.2. Plate layout for ELISA example.

Method

1. Add 50 μl of antigen (HSA) in ELISA coating buffer to each well of the ELISA plate (Figure 16.2).
2. Cover with cling film and incubate for 1 h at 37 °C.
3. Wash 4 times in PBS/Tween.
4. Add 50 μl PBS/Tween to each well.
5. Add 50 μl of primary antibody, e.g. mouse anti-HSA standard to wells A3, A4 and A5; 50 μl of sample A to wells A6, A7 and A8; 50 μl of sample B to wells A9, A10 and A11. Then double dilute them down the plate by mixing and transferring 50 μl into the well below (Figure 16.2). Add PBS/Tween to all other wells.
6. Cover with cling film and incubate for 30 min at 37 °C.
7. Wash 4 times in PBS/Tween.
8. Add 50 μl of conjugated secondary antibody, e.g. HRP-anti-mouse Ig to each well except the blank (e.g. column 1).
9. Cover with cling film and incubate for 30 min at 37 °C.
10. Make up substrate solution.

N.B. WEAR GLOVES WHEN HANDLING OPD

Add 2 mg (1 tablet) of OPD to 5 ml of fresh OPD buffer. When dissolved add 15 μl of 3% hydrogen peroxide.

11. Wash the plate 4 times in PBS/Tween.
12. Add 50 μl of substrate solution to each well.
13. Incubate in the dark for approximately 10 min (wrap in foil).
14. Stop the reaction by adding 30 μl of 3 M sulphuric acid to each well.

TAKE CARE! THIS IS A STRONG ACID SOLUTION

---

15. Read plate in an ELISA plate reader (450λ)

The plate reader tells you the absolute absorbance reading for each well.

You will then have to calculate your specific absorbance by subtracting the negative control value (background) from all your other readings.

When you set up your ELISA you need to decide on a point of positivity. This is found by grouping all the negatives and all the positives into two groups. You must then decide on a point at which you will consider anything less as negative and anything greater as positive. Alternatively, if you have a supply of positive antisera from a polyclonal source you could express each value as a percentage of this known positive. After finding the percentage value of the negative controls you may consider for instance that anything greater than 25% as positive.

16.8.1.2 Recipes

ELISA coating buffer
Na_2CO_3 1.59 g/l
$NaHCO_3$ 2.93 g/l
NaN_3 0.2 g/l
Adjust to pH 9.6 if necessary

PBS/Tween
PBS + 0.05% Tween

OPD substrate buffer
0.1 M citric acid   12.2 ml
0.2 M Na_2HPO_4 12.8 ml
Distilled water   25 ml

Make this fresh each time, immediately before use add 2 mg OPD and 15 μl of 3% hydrogen peroxide to 5 ml of buffer.

> **WARNING: OPD IS A SUSPECTED CARCINOGEN, WEAR GLOVES**

16.8.2 Immunohistochemistry

16.8.2.1 Tissue preparation

Fresh tissue should be cut into small pieces using a scalpel, placed into a small soft plastic, straight sided ampoule with a push fit cap and enough saline added to just cover the tissue. This should then be put into liquid nitrogen until it is frozen. It can then be stored at $-70\,°C$ without deterioration. The saline will give protection against tissue damage caused by the formation of ice crystals in the peripheral tissue when it is transferred from $-70\,°C$ to $-30\,°C$ in the cryostat for sectioning.

Cryostat sections should be cut at about 5–6 μm and transferred to microscope slides. The most convenient slides are polytetrafluoroethylene (PTFE)-coated ones with wells left in which to place the sections. The sections should be allowed to air dry at room temperature for 2–24 h.

16.8.2.2 Cytospins

Any cell suspension can be used to prepare cytospin slides. Blood or bone marrow cell suspensions should first be layered over Ficoll or dextran. The cells should then be made up to 10^6/ml in normal saline or any other isotonic medium, preferably containing some protein (e.g. FCS or BSA (bovine serum albumin)) as this will help the cells to adhere to the slide. Two or three drops of this suspension from a Pasteur pipette can then be added to the cytospin bucket. Set the cytospin machine to 550 r.p.m. for 4 min. The cytospins should be allowed to air dry at room temperature for at least 30 min prior to fixation or storage.

16.8.2.3 Smears

Immunocytochemistry can be carried out on cell smears (e.g. blood smears) that have been prepared routinely in a hospital laboratory.

16.8.2.4 Fixation

The type of fixative used is dependent on several factors:

1. Type of antigen: the most important factor is not to degrade your antigen in the fixation step or the antibody will have no chance of binding to it. Most antigens will tolerate acetone fixation; however, if the antigen has a lipid component this will be degraded by acetone and a different fixative should be used (e.g. methanol).
2. Type of cell preparation: good tissue morphology is achieved with acetone fixation; however, red blood cells tend to be removed from the slides by acetone. This can be overcome by using a mixture of acetone and methanol (Table 16.2).
3. The antibodies to be used: some antibodies will not recognize their antigen after acetone fixation and you may need to experiment with different fixatives to achieve good staining results. Adding 10% formaldehyde can sometimes help.

It should be remembered that if an aqueous fixative is used (e.g. methanol) then the slides should not be allowed to dry out after fixation but must be transferred directly to TBS (Tris buffered saline). If they do dry out then the morphology and the staining reaction will be greatly impaired. With acetone fixation the slides should be allowed to dry until the acetone has evaporated.

Table 16.2. *Fixation conditions suitable for most antigens and antibodies*

	Fixative	Time (min)	Post-fixation
Tissue section	100% acetone	10	Air dry
Cytospin	50% acetone/50% methanol	1	Transfer to Tris buffered saline
Blood smear	45% acetone/45% methanol/10% formalin	1	Transfer to Tris buffered saline

16.8.2.5 Storage

All slides can be stored at −20 °C without deterioration for many months but they do need some attention first.

> Tissue section: Prefix in acetone for 10 min, allow to dry (if your antibody–antigen interaction is impaired by acetone, store unfixed).
> Cytospins: Do not prefix.
> Smears: Do not prefix.

The slides should then be tightly wrapped in aluminium foil, either individually or in pairs (back to back), to exclude air (this will prevent condensation forming on them while thawing). They can then be stored at −20 °C.

On removal from the freezer prior to staining they should be allowed to warm to room temperature before the aluminium foil is removed or condensation will form on them.

16.8.2.6 Immunoperoxidase staining

> *Materials*
> TBS, pH 7.6
> Fixative
> Tissue sections, cytospins or cell smears
> Haematoxylin
> Staining trough (Coplin jar)
> Wet box
> Normal human serum (if material to be stained is of human origin)
> Primary antibodies
> Secondary antibody-peroxidase conjugated
> 3,3′-diaminobenzidine tetra hydrochloride (DAB)
> Hydrogen peroxide (H_2O_2), 100 vol, 30% (v/v)
> Coverslips
> Water-based mountant

> **WARNING: DAB IS A SUSPECTED CARCINOGEN, WEAR GLOVES**

Method

1. Fix tissue section or cell preparation as previously described.
2. Label slides.
3. Place slides in wet box and apply 50 μl of mab carefully to the appropriate tissue preparation.
   This is the primary mab layer, e.g.
      (i) mouse anti-human B cell
     (ii) mouse anti-human T cell
    (iii) negative control (irrelevant antibody or buffer)
   Incubate at room temperature for 30 min.
4. Carefully tip excess antibody off the slide onto a paper tissue, then immerse in TBS for 2–5 min, agitating occasionally.
5. Carefully dry around each section or cytospin being sure not to wipe off the cells. Do not allow them to dry out or the morphology will be impaired.
6. Apply 50 μl of the second layer antibody, e.g. peroxidase-conjugated rabbit anti-mouse Ig to each section including the controls.
   Incubate at room temperature for 30 min.
7. Wash as in step 4.
8. Prepare substrate:
   To 6 mg of DAB, add 10 ml of TBS and 5 μl of 30% H_2O_2. Once prepared the substrate must be used immediately and cannot be stored.
9. Lay slides out in wet box and flood with the substrate. Incubate for 10 min at room temperature.
10. Wash in TBS.
11. Counterstain in haematoxylin, rinse in running tap water until blue (4–5 min).
12. Mount in water based mountant.
13. View under light microscopy.

16.8.2.7 *Alkaline phosphatase staining (APAAP Method)*

Materials
TBS, pH 7.6
Fixative
Tissue sections, cell smears or cytospins
Haematoxylin
Staining trough
Wet box

Normal human serum (if material to be stained is of human origin)
Primary antibodies
Bridging antibody: rabbit anti-mouse Ig
Alkaline phosphatase anti-alkaline phosphatase complex (APAAP)
Naphthol-AS-MX-phosphate
1 M levamisole
0.1 M Tris buffer, pH 8.2
Fast red TR salt
Dimethyl formamide (DMF)
Filter paper
Coverslips
Water-based mountant

Method
1. Fix tissue sections or cell preparations as previously described.
2. Label slides.
3. Place slides in wet box and apply 50 μl of appropriate mab to each section. This is the primary mab layer.
   Incubate at room temperature for 30 min.
4. Carefully tip off excess antibody from the slide onto a paper tissue then immerse in TBS for 2–5 min, agitating occasionally.
5. Carefully dry around each section or cytospin being sure not to wipe off the cells. Do not allow them to dry out or the morphology will be impaired.
6. Apply 50 μl of the second layer bridging antibody, rabbit anti-mouse Ig, to each section. (To enhance the staining intensity this antibody can be AP conjugated.)
   Incubate at room temperature for 30 min.
7. Wash as in step 4.
8. Dry around sections as in step 5, then apply third layer antibody-enzyme complex, 50 μl APAAP to each section. (This is a mouse mab specific for AP, complexed with AP which will be captured by the anti-mouse Ig bridging antibody).
   Incubate at room temperature for 30 min.
9. Wash as in step 4.
10. Prepare substrate:

**FAST RED IS A SUSPECTED CARCINOGEN,
WEAR GLOVES**

Dissolve 2 mg of naphthol-AS-MX-phosphate in 200 μl of DMF (in a fume cupboard).
Add 10 ml of 0.1 M Tris buffer, pH 8.2
   20 μl of 1 M levamisole

      10 mg of fast red

      Filter before use. Once prepared the substrate must be used immediately and cannot be stored.

11. Lay slides out in wet box and apply substrate to sections. Incubate for 20 min at room temperature.
12. Wash as in step 4.
13. Counterstain in haematoxylin, rinse in running tap water until blue (4–5 min).
14. Mount in water-based mountant.
15. View under light microscopy.

   Fast blue BB salt can be used instead of fast red; this will give a blue coloured product. It is useful when double staining, in combination with immunoperoxidase as the blue contrasts with the brown. It is not compatible with the haematoxylin counterstain which is also blue.

16.8.2.8 Immunofluorescence staining

Materials
TBS, pH 7.6
Fixative
Tissue sections, cell smears or cytospins
Staining trough
Wet box
Normal human serum (if material to be stained is of human origin)
Primary mab
Secondary antibody fluorochrome conjugated, e.g. rabbit anti-mouse FITC
Coverslips
Fluorescently inert aqueous mountant (Citifluor AF1; Citifluor, U.K.)

Method
1. Fix tissue sections or cell preparation as previously described.
2. Label slides.
3. Place slides in wet box and apply 50 μl of appropriate mab to each section. This is a primary antibody layer.
   Incubate for 30 min at room temperature.
4. Carefully tip off excess antibody from the slide onto a tissue then immerse in TBS for 2–5 min, agitating occasionally.
5. Carefully dry around each section or cytospin being sure not to wipe off the cells. Do not allow them to dry out.
6. Apply 50 μl of the second layer antibody, e.g. rabbit anti-mouse Ig FITC to each section.
   Incubate for 30 min at room temperature.

7. Wash as in step 4.
8. Mount in Citifluor mountant.
9. View under U.V. fluorescence microscopy.

16.8.2.9 Recipes

All secondary antibodies should be diluted in TBS with 10% normal serum, from the same species as the tissue, to inhibit cross-reactivity with Ig in the tissue, unless species specific secondary antibodies are used. It is also important to titrate secondary antibodies so as to use them at optimal concentration. Most companies give a recommended concentration range; therefore, you should titrate within that range to find the optimum concentration for your assay.

TBS
50 mM Tris
150 mM NaCl
Adjust to pH 7.6

Haematoxylin
5 g haematoxylin
50 ml absolute alcohol (ethanol)
100 g ammonium or potassium alum
1 l distilled water
2.5 g mercuric oxide
40 ml glacial acetic acid

1. Dissolve haematoxylin in the alcohol.
2. Dissolve alum in hot water.
3. Add (1) to (2).
4. Bring to boil.
5. Carefully add mercuric oxide, in the fume cupboard.
6. Allow to cool.
7. Filter.
8. Add glacial acetic acid.

16.9 Monoclonal antibody characterization and purification

16.9.1 Isotyping on hybridoma cytospins

Materials
Hybridoma cells
Cytospin machine
Cytospin filter papers

Glass microscope slides and coverslips
RPMI medium with 10% BSA
Water-repellent marker
Acetone/methanol (1:1 solution)
TBS, pH 7.6
Staining trough
Isotype specific antibodies (FITC or HRP-conjugated)
Water-based mountant
Improved Neubauer counting chamber
Microscope

Method

1. Harvest the hybridoma cells, wash once and resuspend to 10^6/ml. Use medium with 10% BSA as this will help the cells stick to the slides.
2. Prepare 6 cytospins for each clone, using 100 μl of the cells per slide.
3. Using a water-repellent marker inscribe a circle around each cytospin.
4. Fix the slides for 1 min in acetone/methanol and then transfer to TBS.
5. Prepare 1:20 dilutions (or dilution recommended by the manufacturer) of the conjugated (FITC or HRP) anti-isotype antisera (anti-IgG1, IgG2a, IgG2b, IgG3 and IgM) in TBS.
6. Add 50 μl of each anti-isotype to the first 5 slides adding 50 μl of TBS to the sixth as a negative control and incubate for 30–45 min in a wet box.
7. For HRP-antibodies wash briefly in TBS, then incubate for 10 min in DAB substrate. For FITC-antibodies omit this step.
8. Wash briefly in fresh TBS and mount in a water-based mountant.
9. Positive cytoplasmic and membrane staining should be seen on one slide only, indicating the mab isotype.

16.9.2 *Salt fractionation*

Salt fractionation is most suitable for IgG antibodies, IgM mab will precipitate, but some are susceptible to degradation in this method.

Materials

Antibody solution (ascites, serum or supernatant)
Sodium sulphate, anhydrous
Distilled water
Dialysis tubing or G25 column
PBS, pH 8

Method

1. Allow your antibody solution to reach room temperature, add sodium sulphate to make an 18% (w/v) solution, slowly while stirring. If added

too quickly 'hot spots' will form which will denature the antibody. Stir for a further 20–30 min at room temperature to allow full precipitation.

2. Transfer into a centrifuge tube and centrifuge at 3000 *g* for 30 min at room temperature.
3. Discard the supernatant and redissolve the precipitate in distilled water, using the minimum volume required to completely dissolve the pellet.
4. Either transfer into dialysis tubing and dialyse against 2 l of PBS, pH 8 for 48 h, changing the PBS four times, or run through a G25 column (pass through a 0.4 μm filter first), equilibrated in PBS, pH 8, to remove the sodium sulphate from the protein solution.

16.9.3 *Purification of monoclonal antibody by protein A affinity chromatography*

Materials
Mab solution (filtered through 0.2 μm filter to remove aggregates)
1–2 ml protein A Sepharose column
1 M Tris, pH 9
0.1 M phosphate buffer, pH 8
0.1 M citrate buffer, pH 4
G25 column

Method
1. Adjust the pH of the mab to pH 8.0–8.5 with 1 M Tris.
2. Equilibrate the protein A column with 0.1 M phosphate buffer, pH 8.0. Check the pH of the eluent, when it is pH 8.0 then the column is equilibrated.
3. Allow the meniscus to run down until it just touches the surface of the gel.
4. Add about 5 ml of the immunoglobulin preparation to the column, take care not to disturb the column surface.
5. You will be able to see the solution move down the column. Start collecting the eluent just before it reaches the bottom.
6. When the meniscus reaches the surface of the column add 5 ml of phosphate buffer, pH 8.0. Collect the eluent.
7. Repeat step 6.
8. When the meniscus reaches the surface add 5 ml of 0.1 M citrate buffer, pH 4.
9. You will be able to see the solution move down the column. Start to collect the eluent just before the solution reaches the bottom of the column. Collect the eluent into a tube containing 1 M Tris, pH 9, this is to neutralize the pH quickly because low pH can degrade the mab irreversibly. Use 100 μl Tris buffer to 1 ml eluent.

10. Repeat step 8.
11. Repeat from step 2, until all mab has been purified.
12. To regenerate the protein A column run through alternate 5 ml cycles of 0.1 M sodium acetate, pH 4.5, containing 500 mM NaCl and 0.1 M Tris, pH 8.5 containing 500 mM NaCl. Then re-equilibrate with 0.1 M phosphate buffer, pH 8. Always store column in buffer with 0.02% sodium azide.

16.9.3.1 Recipes

0.1 M phosphate buffer
0.1 M Na_2HPO_4
0.1 M NaH_2PO_4

Mix to give desired pH (8.0).

Citrate buffer
0.1 M trisodium citrate
0.1 M citric acid

Mix to give desired pH (4.0).

16.9.4 *Protein G affinity chromatography*

Materials
3 ml protein G Sepharose column
0.02 M sodium phosphate, pH 7
0.1 M glycine-HCl, pH 2.7 (or pH 9–10)
1 M Tris, pH 9

Method
1. Adjust the pH of the mab to pH 7 by diluting 1:1 with binding buffer (0.02 M sodium phosphate, pH 7).
2. Equilibrate the protein G column with 0.02 M sodium phosphate buffer, pH 7. Check the pH of the eluent, when it is pH 7 then the column has equilibrated.
3. Allow the meniscus to run down until it just touches the surface of the gel.
4. Add up to 5 ml of prepared ascites or concentrated immunoglobulin or a maximum of 25 ml of cell culture supernatant to the column, take care not to disturb the column surface.
5. Allow the antibody solution to run through the column until the meniscus reaches the surface of the column. Then add 30 ml of sodium

phosphate buffer, pH 7 and allow this to run through the column to wash away the unbound proteins.

6. When the meniscus reaches the surface add 15 ml of 0.1 M glycine buffer, pH 2.7, to elute the antibody from the column. Collect the eluent as 1 ml fractions into tubes containing 100 μl of 1 M Tris, pH 9, to neutralize the pH. Low pH can degrade the mab irreversibly.

7. To regenerate the protein G column, run through 30 ml of 0.01 M sodium phosphate, pH 7, then if more mab is to be purified continue from step 4. If the column is to be stored, add 30 ml of 20% ethanol solution and allow 15 ml to run through the column, then seal the column and store at 4 °C.

   If your mab is susceptible to low pH degradation elution can be performed using 0.1 M glycine-NaOH, pH 9–10.

16.9.5 *Fractionation of IgG into subclasses*

There are four main subclasses of mouse IgG (IgG1, IgG2a, IgG2b and IgG3) which differ in the structure of their heavy chain constant region and in their affinity of binding to protein A. These differences can be used to purify the subclasses by affinity chromatography. IgG1, 2a and 2b are first purified as above (IgG3 does not bind protein A and so is lost with the non-IgG components in the sample). The bound subclasses are then eluted separately by buffers of differing pH. IgG1 is eluted at pH 6.0, IgG2a at pH 4.5 and IgG2b at pH 3.5.

16.9.6 *Preparation of F(ab')₂ fragments*

To overcome the problem of Fc receptor binding of mab, the F(ab')$_2$ fraction can be prepared. This takes advantage of the fact that the Fc portion of the immunoglobulin molecule is susceptible to digestion by the enzyme pepsin. This cleaves the molecule in such a way that the antibody-binding sites are left intact and still held together by disulphide bonds as a dimer, which is known as the F(ab')$_2$ fragment (Figure 16.3).

Unfortunately, the sensitivity to pepsin is slightly different for each mab, so that various parameters must be carefully tested each time to find the optimum conditions for each mab. The variable factors for F(ab')$_2$ fragmentation are listed in Table 16.3, together with values that have been found previously to be suitable for several mab. These values can be used as a starting point and varied to achieve better results.

Materials
Purified mab
Sodium acetate buffer, pH 4.0

Table 16.3. *Parameters that need to be titrated when preparing F(ab')₂ fragments*

Variable parameter	Suggested values
pH	3.5–4.0
Monoclonal antibody concentration	10 mg/ml
Pepsin concentration	2–3% by total weight of IgG
Digestion time	6–18 h

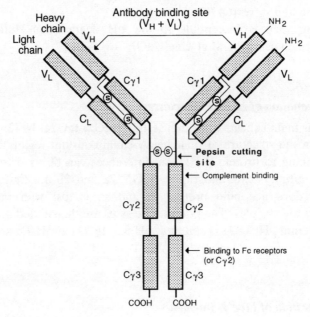

Figure 16.3. Basic structure of an antibody molecule showing the pepsin cutting site for making F(ab')₂ antibody fragments.

Pepsin
1 M Tris, pH 9

Method
This is a basic method to determine the optimum conditions for the pepsin digestion of a mab to produce a F(ab')₂ fragment.

1. Equilibrate the antibody in sodium acetate buffer, pH 4, either by dialysis or size exclusion chromatography (G25) and adjust the concentration to 10 mg/ml.
2. Add pepsin to give a concentration of 2% (w/v).
3. Incubate on a rotary mixer for a total 20 h at 37 °C, taking a 50 μl

sample every hour. To quench the pepsin reaction adjust to pH 8 by adding 1 M Tris, pH 9, and store at 4 °C.

4. Analyse the samples by SDS-PAGE (7.5%) under non-reducing conditions to determine the optimum digest conditions. This is the point where very little intact mab (MW 150 kDa) remains and the $F(ab')_2$ is not digested further into monomeric Fab' fragments. If the optimum time is greater that 8–10 h it can be decreased by adding more pepsin (i.e. 3% w/v).

5. When you have determined the optimum conditions for your mab you can then prepare a larger sample.

6. Run the digested sample through a S200 or G200 size exclusion chromatography column to separate out the $F(ab')_2$ portion.

16.9.7 Size exclusion chromatography

16.9.7.1 Preparation and use of an S200 column

1. S200 comes in methanol for storage and must be washed before use. For a 100 cm × 2.5 cm column you will need 300 ml of settled gel. Wash this three times in 1 l of elution buffer (e.g. 50 mM NaCl, 10 mM Tris, pH 6.8). Allow the gel to settle each time before decanting the buffer.

2. Set up the column in a cold room and make sure it is perfectly vertical using a plumbline. Insert the lower adaptor, tighten and clamp off the tube.

3. The gel slurry should be 75% settled gel. Degas the gel in a vacuum flask with the side arm attached to a vacuum line. Bubbles in the gel will cause flow deformities.

4. Attach an extension reservoir to the column and half fill the column with buffer (all buffers should be degassed). Open the lower adaptor and allow the buffer to run down to about 10% of the total column volume. This removes any air that has been trapped in the lower adaptor.

5. With the bottom adaptor open pour the gel down the side of the column so that it does not splash and trap any air. Fill the reservoir to the top with the gel.

6. Allow the gel to settle but make sure it does not dry out.

7. When it has all settled and a flat gel surface is obtained, insert the top adaptor. To do this fill the column to the top with buffer so that there is a positive meniscus. Insert the adaptor at an angle so that no air is trapped. Gently push it in until it just touches the gel surface. Carefully tighten up the adaptor.

8. Attach the peristaltic pump to the lower adaptor and pump buffer up through the column at 12 ml/h. The pump rate can be measured by

Table 16.4. *Reagents suitable for column calibration*

Substance	Molecular weight
Cytochrome C	12 K
Myoglobin	17 K
Ovalbumin	45 K
Bovine serum albumin	68 K
Aldolase	149 K
Catalyse	
Horse liver	221 K
Bovine liver	247 K

timing the flow into a measuring cylinder. Ensure that no air is pumped into the column. Pump it this way overnight.

9. The next day connect the pump to the top adaptor to reverse the flow and overnight pump down through the column.

10. Readjust the top adaptor so that it just touches the top of the gel bed. The column is now ready for testing and calibration.

11. Introduce 1 ml of Blue Dextran 2000 (2 mg/ml) into the column via the pump (be certain not to introduce any air bubbles into the system).

12. As soon as it enters the column put the tube from the bottom adaptor into a measuring cylinder.

13. Because of its high molecular weight the Blue Dextran is excluded from the gel. If it moves through the column in a neat well-defined band then the gel is uniform. If it does not form a neat band then the gel must be repoured.

14. When the band reaches the lower adaptor note the volume of the buffer eluted. This is the Void Volume of the column (the volume of the space in the column around the beads) and is the amount of eluent that can be discarded prior to sample collection.

15. Having established a good column, now calibrate it with a mixture of molecules of known molecular weight.

16. Choose 3 or 4 proteins from Table 16.4 that are reasonably spaced and make up a solution so that they are each at 5 mg/ml in a total volume of 2 ml. Apply to the column and set up the in-line spectrophotometer and recording system to record the protein bands as they elute from the column. Determine the elution volume for each molecular weight marker.

17. You should obtain a separate peak for each protein, thus the column is calibrated and ready to use.

18. Samples are applied in the same way in volumes not exceeding 5 ml.

16.9.7.2 Care of the column

1. Do not knock the column as this can fracture the gel.
2. Do not allow the column to run dry.
3. Ensure all buffers are sterile or contain azide (0.01%).
4. Do not allow the column temperature to fluctuate as this can create air bubbles which will interfere with the uniformity of the gel.
5. All samples should be centrifuged and filtered through a 0.2 μm filter before application to remove any impurities or aggregates that may silt up on the top of the gel bed.
6. When not in use, keep the pump running and recirculate the buffer upwards through the column (this avoids excessive packing of the column).

16.9.8 Coupling of antibody to CNBr-activated Sepharose 4B

Cyanogen bromide (CNBr) can be bound to Sepharose to form a stable cross-linked structure that has the ability to bind covalently to proteins or nucleic acids via their primary amino groups or nucleophilic groups. CNBr-activated Sepharose can be purchased ready for coupling to any protein or DNA. The coupling reaction takes place at high pH (pH 8–10) when the amino groups of the protein will be unprotonated. The choice of pH depends on the protein ligand and its subsequent activity. At higher pH more amino groups will bind to the Sepharose and this may cause immobility of the ligand or stearic hindrance. For IgG the usual pH chosen is 8.5–9.0. Due to the electrolytic nature of proteins there is a tendency for protein–protein adsorption. This is inhibited by salt ions added to the coupling reaction buffer (0.5 M NaCl). The amount of ligand that will bind to the gel is also dependent on the concentration of the ligand in the reaction. With too high a ligand to gel ratio the efficacy of the immunoadsorbant formed will be impaired due to stearic hindrance, avidity of binding or increase in non-specific binding. Therefore, in general 1–10 μmoles ligand per ml of gel is recommended and 2 μmoles ligand per ml of gel is often most successful. For protein ligands, such as immuno-globulin, 5–10 mg protein per ml gel is recommended, keeping in mind the possibility of stearic hindrance. Using a concentration towards the lower end of this scale may result in a more effective immunoadsorbant. After the reaction time the excess active groups must be blocked by hydrolysis. This is achieved by either incubating for 2 h in Tris-HCl pH 8 buffer or overnight in a milder alkaline solution. Alternatively, an excess of small primary amines can be added to block the excess sites (ethanolamine or glycine); although these will add a number of charged groups to the gel their effect can be negated by using buffers with high salt content (0.5 M NaCl) during the affinity chromatography. Excess uncoupled ligand should be removed by washing the gel with 4–5 cycles of alternate high and low pH buffers. This procedure will remove any protein that is ionically bound to the gel but not that which is covalently bound. Such ligand–Sepharose coupled gels can be stored at 4 °C in the presence of a metabolic inhibitor such as sodium azide or merthiolate.

Materials

1 g freeze-dried CNBr-activated Sepharose (this gives 3.5 ml gel volume)

Antibody sample (17.5–35 mg)

1 mM HCl

0.1 M NaHCO$_3$, 0.5 M NaCl, pH 8.5 (coupling buffer)

1 M ethanolamine or 0.2 M glycine, pH 8

0.1 M acetate, 0.5 M NaCl, pH 4

0.1 M Tris, 0.5 M NaCl, pH 8.5

0.1 M sodium acetate, 0.5 N NaCl, pH 4.5

Method

1. Take 1 g of CNBr-activated Sepharose 4B, wash and reswell the gel on a scintered glass funnel (porosity G3) over a side arm flask with vacuum suction, using 200 ml of 1 mM HCl. Use about 200 ml/g of gel.

2. Dissolve or dialyse the antibody in coupling buffer (0.1 M NaHCO$_3$, 0.5 M NaCl, pH 8.5) and adjust to 2.5–5 mg/ml.

3. Wash the gel with 5 ml of coupling buffer and immediately transfer into 7 ml of the antibody solution (do this quickly as at this pH the reactive groups on the gel will hydrolyse). Seal the tube and mix on a rotator for 2 h at room temperature or overnight at 4 °C (do not use a magnetic stirrer as this will damage the gel beads). This gives a volume ratio of 1:2, gel to antibody, and between 5–10 mg/ml of gel.

4. Allow the gel to settle, remove the supernatant buffer and add 20 ml of blocking buffer (1 M ethanolamine or 0.2 M glycine, pH 8). Incubate for 2 h at room temperature or overnight at 4 °C.

5. Transfer the gel to a scintered glass funnel and wash with 4–5 cycles of high then low pH buffer (0.1 M acetate, 0.5 M NaCl, pH 4, and coupling buffer, pH 8.5) to remove the excess non-absorbed protein and blocking buffer. Use about 100 ml of each buffer in total.

7. The antibody–Sepharose conjugate is now ready for use. Store at 4 °C with 0.1 M sodium azide.

   Use the antibody-coupled Sepharose in the same way as protein A Sepharose except that the ligand binding should be performed in PBS, pH 7.4, and the elution with 0.5 M propionic acid, pH 3 (this has the advantage of interfering with the hydrophobic interactions in addition to the low pH effect).

   Regenerate the column with alternate cycles of 0.1 M Tris, 0.5 M NaCl, pH 8.5, and 0.1 M sodium acetate, 0.5 M NaCl, pH 4.5. Then re-equilibrate in starting buffer (PBS, pH 7.4). Always store gel in buffer with sodium azide.

Table 16.5. *Volume of each stock solution required to obtain the specified percentage acrylamide gel for a running gel*

	Acrylamide (%)				
	5	7.5	10	12.5	15
Acrylamide	2.5	3.75	5.0	6.25	7.5
Tris pH 8.8	5.6	5.6	5.6	5.6	5.6
Water	6.85	5.6	4.35	3.1	1.85
10% SDS	0.15	0.15	0.15	0.15	0.15
10% APS	0.05	0.05	0.05	0.05	0.05
TEMED	0.01	0.01	0.01	0.01	0.01

Volumes in ml; APS, ammonium persulphate; SDS, sodium dodecyl sulphate.

16.10 Polyacrylamide gel electrophoresis in the presence of sodium dodecyl sulphate (SDS-PAGE) and Western blotting

16.10.1 SDS-PAGE

16.10.1.1 Minigel method

1. Prepare the running and stacking gel mixtures except for adding the tetramethylethylenediamine (TEMED) and ammonium persulphate as in Table 16.5 to give the desired percentage gel.
2. Assemble the gel plates ready to add the gel, this depends on the type of apparatus you have. Basically they consist of two specially cut plates separated by plastic spacers (0.5, 0.75 or 1.0 mm) and stand on a glass plate on a level surface. To seal the lower edge of the gel former, prepare the sealing gel as in Table 16.7. This mixture will set very quickly, so using a Pasteur pipette immediately apply the gel to the lower edge allowing the gel to run in to the bottom of the gel former by capillary action, it will seal against the glass plate. Use some of this mixture also to seal between the spacers and the plates by running some mixture down the sides, it will fill any gaps by capillary action. Leave to stand for about 5 min to be sure that the sealing gel is completely set.

   Your system may seal the bottom of the gel plates by pressing against a rubber or silicon seal, in which case you will not need to use the sealing gel.
3. Select the comb that you will use to form the sample wells and use this to measure and mark on the gel plate the level to which to fill the running gel, about 5 mm lower than the comb.

Table 16.6. *Volume of each stock solution required to make the stacking gel*

	Volume (ml)
Acrylamide	1.0
Tris, pH 6.8	0.75
Water	3.76
10% SDS	0.06
10% APS	0.03
TEMED	0.006

APS, ammonium persulphate; SDS, sodium dodecyl sulphate; TEMED, tetramethylethylene-diamine;

Table 16.7. *Volume of each stock solution required to make the sealing gel*

	Volume (ml)
Running gel mix	1.5
10% APS	0.025
TEMED	0.005

APS, ammonium persulphate; TEMED, tetramethylethylenedia-mine.

4. Add the ammonium persulphate and TEMED to the running gel mixture, mix gently and fill the gel former to the mark.
5. Very carefully apply overlay onto the gel, this is less dense than the gel so it will form a layer above the gel. This is important as the gel will polymerize more quickly and evenly when air is excluded.
6. Allow the gel to polymerize. This usually takes 30–40 min but is temperature dependent.
7. When the running gel has set, pour off the overlay and rinse the top of the gel with distilled water. Drain off the water using a tissue to absorb the last drop.
8. Insert the comb part-way into the gel former. Add the ammonium persulphate and TEMED to the stacking gel mixture, mix gently using

a Pasteur pipette. Push the comb down into place at a slight angle so that no air bubbles form in the gel; if necessary add more gel to completely fill the gel former.

9. Leave for 15–30 min to allow the stacking gel to set.

10. Prepare the samples and molecular weight markers, mix with an equal volume of sample buffer, place the tubes into a rack in a boiling water bath for 3 min.

11. When the stacking gel has set, carefully remove the comb so that none of the partitions are broken. Rinse the top of the gel with electrophoresis buffer. Transfer the gel into the apparatus and add electrophoresis buffer to the top reservoir so that it floods into the top of the gel (Figure 16.4).

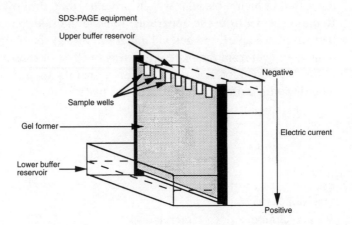

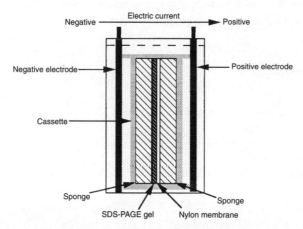

Figure 16.4. SDS-PAGE and Western blotting.

12. Using a Hamilton syringe apply the molecular weight markers and samples into the wells of the gel. As the sample buffer contains glycerol it is more dense than the electrophoresis buffer and will sink to the bottom of the well. The amount of sample added depends on the size of well. Usually 10 μl of molecular weight markers will be sufficient but if you are not sure how much of your sample to add, then use sufficient to fill the well without overflowing.
13. Fill bottom reservoir with electrophoresis buffer.
14. Assemble the apparatus and connect to the power pack, set the controls to constant voltage and to 50 volts.
15. When the dye front reaches the end of the stacking gel, increase the voltage to 100 volts.
16. Allow the gel to run until the dye front is about 0.5 cm from the bottom of the gel (approximately 1.5 h) or longer if you are only interested in high molecular weight proteins, then turn off the current. Remove the gel from the apparatus, remove the side spacers and lever the two plates apart, the gel will adhere to one of the plates. Carefully remove the gel from the plate into a tray of PBS, or transfer buffer if it is for Western blotting, using either a spatula to peel it off or by pipetting with buffer to wash it from the plate.

16.10.1.2 Recipes

Acrylamide stock
30 g acrylamide + 0.8 g bisacrylamide

Make up to 100 ml and filter. Store in a dark bottle at 4 °C. Acrylamide is a very powerful neurotoxin so DO NOT inhale the powder and always wear gloves. The acrylamide should be weighed out in a fume cupboard. Acrylamide is now available in solution or as preweighed powder which avoids handling the hazardous power.

Electrophoresis buffer

	g/500 ml	g/l
0.025 M Tris	1.5	3.0
0.192 M glycine	7.21	14.42
0.1% SDS	0.5	1.0

Adjust to pH 8.3 if necessary.

SDS stock
10% SDS in distilled water

Heat to 37 °C to dissolve, store at room temperature.

TEMED
Tetramethylethylenediamine available commercially. Store in a dark bottle at room temperature.

Ammonium persulphate stock
10% Ammonium persulphate in distilled water

Prepare fresh daily.

Bromophenol blue
0.1% Bromophenol blue in distilled water. Stir until all dye is dissolved then filter and store at 4 °C.

Sample buffer
1 ml 10% SDS
1 ml glycerol
0.8 ml 1 M Tris, pH 6.8
0.1 ml of 0.1% bromophenol blue
Make up to 10 ml with distilled water

This is a non-reducing buffer. For reducing conditions add 2-mercaptoethanol to make a 5% final concentration or add 15.4 mg dithiothreitol per ml of sample buffer.

Overlay
Distilled water or
10% ethanol in distilled water

Destain
5 parts H_2O + 4 parts ethanol + 1 part glacial acetic acid

Stain
0.1% Coomassie Blue in destain

16.10.2 Western blotting

16.10.2.1 Transfer of proteins from SDS-PAGE onto nitrocellulose membrane

Method
1. Remove the gel cassette from the tank and remove the two formers that remain at the sides. Lever off one of the glass plates and transfer the gel into a tray of transfer buffer.

2. Cut a piece of nitrocellulose or nylon membrane to approximately the same size as the gel (usually 10×8 cm) and pre-wet it according to the manufacturer's instructions. Slide the membrane underneath the gel in the tray of buffer.

3. Cut 2 pieces of filter paper to fit the size of the transfer cassette, pre-wet them in transfer buffer. Then slide one piece underneath the membrane and place the other on top of the gel being careful not to trap any air bubbles, thus forming a 'sandwich'.

4. Soak the sponges from the transfer cassette in transfer buffer and assemble the gel/membrane 'sandwich' between the sponges in the cassette and load into the tank (Figure 16.4) (gel towards the negative and membrane towards the positive electrodes).

5. Fill the tank with transfer buffer. Then connect to the power pack.

6. Set on constant current and 300 mA the run for 1 h 15 min.

7. Switch off the current and remove the cassette from the tank. Remove the membrane into PBS. At this stage then membrane can be stored at 4 °C in PBS with 0.02% sodium azide.

8. If you want to stain a strip of the membrane with Amido Black then cut a small strip from the membrane and put into the Amido Black stain. Put the rest of the blot in blocking buffer (2.5% milk power in PBS) which will block any unbound protein-binding sites on the paper. Leave this for up to 24 h at 4 °C or 2 h at room temperature.

9. Meanwhile the strip of membrane can be destained in Amido Black destain solution. The gel itself can also be stained in Coomassie Blue to check that all the protein has been transferred but this is not usually necessary, particularly if you have used pre-stained molecular weight markers as these will be visible on the membrane.

10. Rinse the blot in washing buffer (0.5% milk powder in PBS) and then wash for at least 1 h on a rocking table.

16.10.2.2 Recipes

Transfer buffer
25 mM Tris-HCl   (3.03 g/l)
192 mM glycine   (14.42 g/l)
20% (v/v) methanol
Adjust to pH 8.3 if necessary

Blocking buffer
2.5% milk powder in PBS

Washing buffer
0.5% milk powder in PBS

Amido Black destain
90% methanol
3% acetic acid
8% distilled water

16.10.2.2 *Immunostaining of Western blot*

Materials and equipment
Membrane with transferred proteins (pre-blocked in blocking buffer, as above)
Primary antibodies (e.g. mouse mab)
Peroxidase-conjugated antibody specific for the primary antibody (e.g. rabbit anti-mouse Ig)
Diaminobenzidine substrate DAB
Washing buffer (0.5% milk powder in PBS)
Rocker or shaker

Method
1. Rinse the paper briefly in some washing buffer.
2. Remove paper from the buffer, place on a clean glass plate or plastic tray and cut into strips about 7 mm wide. Using pencil label each strip and mark the top, then transfer each strip into a separate tube, staining trough or seal in plastic film to make a bag.
3. Add your primary antibodies to each tube, trough or bag, seal and incubate on a rotator or rocking platform for 1–2 h.
4. Transfer the strips into tubes or troughs containing washing buffer and wash for 30 min on rotator or rocking platform, change the buffer after 10 min.
5. Transfer the strips into tubes or troughs containing secondary antibody (peroxidase conjugated), incubate for 1 h on the rotator or rocking platform.
6. Wash strips again as in step 4.
7. Put into clean tubes and add freshly prepared diaminobenzidine substrate.
   Incubate until bands appear but no more than 10 min.
8. Wash in tap water for 5 min.
9. Remove paper and allow to air dry.

N.B. THE COLOUR SOMETIMES FADES WITH TIME

16.10.2.3 Recipes

   DAB substrate
To 30 mg of DAB, add 50 ml PBS and 15 μl of 30% H_2O_2

Index